The Essential Handbook for GP Training and Education

Edited by

DR. RAMESH MEHAY

Creator of <u>www.bradfordvts.co.uk</u>
GP Trainer (Ashcroft Surgery, Bradford, UK)
Former Training Programme Director (Bradford GP Training Scheme)

<u>www.essentialgptrainingbook.com</u>

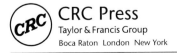

CRC Press
Taylor & Francis Group
Boca Raton London New York

CRC Press is an imprint of the
Taylor & Francis Group, an **informa** business

First published 2012 by Radcliffe Publishing

Published 2021 by CRC Press
Taylor & Francis Group
6000 Broken Sound Parkway NW, Suite 300
Boca Raton, FL 33487-2742

© 2012 by Dr Ramesh Mehay
CRC Press is an imprint of Taylor & Francis Group, an Informa business

No claim to original U.S. Government works

ISBN 13: 978-1-84619-593-8 (pbk)
ISBN 13: 978-1-138-44715-8 (hbk)
ISBN 13: 978-1-84619-791-8 (ebk)

DOI: 10.1201/9781846197918

Visit the Taylor & Francis Web site at
http://www.taylorandfrancis.com

and the CRC Press Web site at
http//www.crcpress.com

Ramesh Mehay has asserted his right under the Copyright, Designs and Patents Act 1988 to be identified as the author of this work.

Every effort has been made to ensure that the information in this book is accurate. This does not diminish the requirement to exercise clinical judgement, and neither the publisher nor the author can accept any responsibility for its use in practice.

British Library Cataloguing in Publication Data

A catalogue record for this book is available from the British Library.

By carbon balancing the material used to produce this publication we have saved
3535 kg of CO_2 and preserved 297 m^2 of land.

Cover image © 2007 Matthew Martin. This cartoon, entitled 'The Teacher', was published in *The Times* on 5th January 2007. We are grateful to both Matthew Martin and *The Times* for their kind permission to reproduce this image.

Typeset by Darkriver Design, Auckland, New Zealand

*For all our competencies, we are nothing
without compassion . . . and it's not always easy
to remember that compassion is a verb.*

AMAR RUGHANI
GP (Sheffield)

Contents

Preface

Over the last ten years I have seen how the world of GP training has changed. There are more GP educators than ever before, training is more structured and very comprehensive. You can't become a GP Trainer by simply being a GP for x number of years, or by showing a tad of interest alone. You have to *know* some educational 'stuff' and have some educational *skills* (and quite right too!). So here is a book to help you with that. But of course – I would say that. So how might I convince you? I could make one thousand and one promises – but I am not going to. The book speaks for itself and I'm sure our thoughts and personal examples will stimulate and inspire you. In the meantime, here are ten interesting facts about this book:

1. Over 80 hands-on educators have been involved in this book (some are doctors, some are not). The idea behind this balanced mix of contributors is to add new textures and flavours difficult to find in other books.
2. Our educators were chosen on strict selection criteria. For instance, those who had *developed* a project or *enacted* learning theory scored more 'brownie' points than those who had merely written about it. Too many educational books these days are written by academics alone but ours is different; we've got the do-ers too!
3. Each chapter has a lead author supported by a set of 'buddy' authors. This ensures the content of each chapter is balanced, equilibrated and not skewed by any strong views.
4. Lead and buddy authors were allocated to topics they were passionate about - beyond a simple interest in or familiarity with. We believe that writing something you're passionate about helps capture pearls of practical wisdom difficult to find elsewhere.
5. Guidance was given to all authors, detailing a minimum syllabus required of their text. Thus, each chapter covers the basics and beyond.
6. All authors were asked to write in a relaxed style, with a sprinkling of humour; a move away from the pompous language used in many traditional medical texts. We wanted to give you a text that was light-hearted and easy to grasp on the first read. Perhaps even light-hearted enough for you to take into the garden on a nice warm summer's day, to read over a glass of wine or a cup of tea!
7. Our chapters are dotted with tables, flowcharts, interesting anecdotes and colourful diagrams. We are positive that this varied format will help the content come alive and consolidate your learning.
8. Each chapter combines theory and practice. There's a wealth of practical material, suggestions and templates that you can use straight away.
9. Every chapter is linked to additional web material for those of you who want to delve deeper. Our website has over 300 academic and practical resources.
10. And finally, the authors have not been paid anything for contributing; they have given their time and expertise freely and willingly. That's how committed to GP education they are. Now, isn't that a sign of true dedication? And I hope a reflection of what you're likely to get from this book.

Is there any other book about GP education that offers you the same?
(Answers on a postcard . . .)

Ramesh Mehay
November 2016

Why developing teaching skills is important

You will see from our dedication list that there have been many legendary educators that have gone before us who have shaped and influenced our thinking. In fact, there are so many teachers in all parts of our lives. Those that have played significant roles have helped carve out our life's journey. We know who they are, and we cherish them forever.

As an educator, you too will have a significant impact on your learners for the rest of their lives. Your actions will shape their life journeys. Your learners will inherit or emulate some of these. Therefore, adopting positive attitudes and behaviours is incredibly important and we hope this book will show you the right path. This poem by Gervase Phinn reminds us never to underestimate the power of our actions on others.

Remember Me?
"Do you remember me?" asked the young man.
The old man at the bus stop,
Shabby, standing in the sun, alone,
Looked round.
He stared for a moment screwing up his eyes,
Then shook his head.
"No, I don't remember you".
"You used to teach me," said the young man.
"I've taught so many," said the old man, sighing.
"I forget."
"I was the boy you said was useless
Good for nothing, a waste of space.
Who always left your classroom crying,
And dreaded every lesson that you taught."
The old man shook his head and turned away.
"No, I don't remember you," he murmured.
"Well, I remember you," the young man said.

(Many thanks to Gervase Phinn for allowing us to use his poem. www.gervase-phinn.com)

How to use this book

It is up to you how you use this book. Yes, this book lends itself well to being read from cover to cover. It's light-hearted, it's alive and it's engaging. However, you can also dip in and out of sections too – perhaps reading something when the time is right.

Don't forget to check out our website: www.essentialgptrainingbook.com. There's practical material for those who are puzzled over implementation and academic material for those who are simply hungry for more.

There's only one thing we ask of you in return – feedback! After you have read a chapter, give us feedback so we can improve it for the next edition. Be part of our next edition by helping to steer the content and format.

To give feedback…

- Go to www.essentialgptrainingbook.com
- Click the chapter you've just read
- Click the button which says 'give feedback'
- Detail a few words – it needn't be lengthy if you don't want it to be.

About the editor

Dr Ramesh Mehay qualified from Leeds University in 1993. A little lost after his house officer year, he tried out various hospital specialties in Northern Ireland and Greater Manchester. After five years of roaming, he decided to give General Practice a shot and fell in love with it through a training post in Sherburn-In-Elmet offered by the York GP scheme. His second GP placement in Acomb (also York) ignited his passion for teaching, inspired by an extremely enthusiastic GP Trainer, Peter Harrison.

Once qualified, Ramesh's first taste of teaching came from the local Yorkshire MRCGP course, run by Neal Maskrey. There he met Nick Price, who coaxed him into joining him and Maggie Eisner as Course Organisers (the old term for Training Programme Directors) for what was then known as the Bradford Vocational Training Scheme (now Bradford GP Training Scheme). He applied and was appointed in 2001 by Jamie Bahrami - the founder of the Association of Course Organisers - who said it was time to take a risk before his retirement!

Since then, Ramesh has come to be well-known for two main things. The first is his popular GP training website: www.bradfordvts.co.uk. This holds an extraordinarily diverse number of online resources for both GP trainers and trainees, and he received the Paul Freeling Award in 2008 for it (awarded for innovative or meritorious work in the field of vocational training for general practice).

The second thing he is well-known for is the immense guidance he has developed for trainers and trainees around the MRCGP, Educational Supervision and ARCPs - especially at a time when support was generally and nationally deficient. His resources are popular because of his ability to simplify the complex – turning dull lengthy documents into bite-sized visually engaging chunks of information. It is because of this that the UK Association of Programme Directors (UKAPD) approached him to lead and develop this book back in 2009. The book was completed by 2012. In 2013, Ramesh received the Paul Freeling Award for a second time – this time for the contribution this book has made to GP training. It is hoped that this book will be the third thing that he becomes well-known for.

Ramesh continues to be a GP trainer and partner at Ashcroft Surgery in Bradford and is still committed to developing more and more online resources. And for those of you who know him and get emails at 3 am – yes, he sleeps an average of 5 hours per day and has done so since reckless student days. Some things never change!

Dedication

This book is dedicated to the legendary educator colleagues and trainees who have gone before us. These unsung heroes have shaped us during our time with them, and thereon after. All of us stand on the shoulders of giants, and ideas thought of as new and original are often built upon the principles and foundations laid down by others. This book serves to honour our lost friends.

We'd also like to dedicate this book to Jamie Bahrami (former Yorkshire Deanery) and Patrick McEvoy (Northern Ireland). Jamie's determination and energy helped get GP training off the ground and he became the founding father of the Association of Course Organisers back in 1984 (which became UKAPD in 2008). Patrick (or 'Paddy') wrote the first recognised 'manual' for Course Organisers called *Educating the Future GP* in 1993. It is his inspirational work that led to the natural evolution of this book. We hope the educational philosophy of his book continues to live on through ours.

And finally, we would also like to dedicate this book to our partners in life, our partners at work and our families – who have given us space, time and support in our writing.

All contributing authors
The Essential Handbook, 2012

Acknowledgements from the Editor

I would like to start by thanking Roger Burns (Pembrokeshire), Mike Tomson (Sheffield) and the prevailing UKAPD executive committee of 2009 for the opportunity to lead on this book when the project was being conceived.

Having never written a book before, I would like to extend my thanks to the following established authors for their words of wisdom: Sheena McMain, Adrian Dunbar, Jonathan Lloyd, Liz Moulton, Emma Storr, Roger Higson and Elaine Powley. I am also deeply grateful to Maggie Eisner (Bradford), Ruth Nisbet (Kelso, Scotland) and Anna Romito (London). I'm not the greatest guru on grammar and punctuation and these 'Grammar Girls' helped keep me on track.

I am deeply grateful to several trainers up and down the country who kindly offered to read and comment on initial chapter versions. A special thanks to Amar Rughani and Prit Chahal for keeping my spirits in good form, especially during the maelstrom. And of course, to all the other authors for showing faith in me.

To be honest - I have lots of things to be thankful for and I could just go on and on. I don't come from the most privileged of beginnings and I don't believe I would be leading the privileged life that I am living today if I wasn't so divinely nurtured by my late parents, Dharam Pal Mehay and Gurmit Kaur Seniaray.

My final gratitude goes to my other half, Robert Hartley, who is my ultimate soul mate in life, and who has been and always will be my rock.

PART ONE

GP Training in the UK

The Structure of GP Training in the UK

RAMESH MEHAY – TPD (Bradford) & lead author   MIKE TOMSON – APD (Yorkshire & the Humber)
IAIN LAMB – Associate Advisor (SE Scotland)   JAMES MEADE – TPD (Northern Ireland)
MALCOLM LEWIS – Director of General Practice (Wales Deanery)

It has been my experience that being relatively young is no barrier to getting involved in medical educa-tion. If you are interested, get in touch with people who are (or have been) involved in your training. Talk to them about what it is like to be involved in medical education. You could gain first-hand experi-ence by doing some training. You could run a session at the local training scheme, or apply to the local undergraduate medical school to become involved in some teaching. . . . Do not be scared to apply – it is a rewarding job.

Sanjiv Ahluwalia, Deputy Head of GP School, London Deanery[1]

This chapter is intentionally small because . . .

1 We don't want to bore you to death.
2 We don't think it is too taxing to understand the structure of GP training in the UK.
3 Things might change soon (e.g. with the GP consortia) so there is no point talking about the structure in too much depth.
4 There is more detailed guidance on our website (which we will periodically update). Your dean-ery will give you specific advice for your region too.

Who cares about the structure of training in the UK?

Many GP Trainers (and some Training Programme Directors) go about their business without knowing much about the structure – and, yes, they do get by. However, knowing about the structure would help them understand the roles and responsibilities different people play, as well as understanding who is accountable to whom.

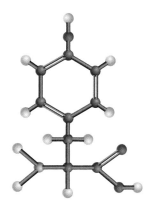

This information is particularly helpful in situations where advice from others would be most valued. A typical scenario would be where they're struggling with a trainee in difficulty or a GP trainee making an unusual request for leave.

 Red Alert: The structure in Scotland is different to the rest of the UK. NHS Education Scotland is a special health board responsible for supporting NHS services delivered to the people of Scotland by developing and delivering education and training for those who work in NHS Scotland.

Isn't the structure just overly bureaucratic?

We don't think so. Trainees deliver much of the NHS service. The quality of the patient care they provide depends on the quality of training they receive. *And*, none of that matters if there aren't enough people to do the job in the first place! Therefore, to provide quality patient care, you need a structured organisation to do the following.

1 Ensure recruitment selects enough people to do the job.
2 Ensure recruitment selects the right people for the job.
3 Make sure that we train them up properly (quality training).
4 Double check we have trained them properly (quality assurance).

That's a heck of a job.

The current GP training system, in a nutshell

- There is a common set of guidelines and regulations covering all medical training (including GP). This is commonly called the Gold Guide (or even GG) though formally titled *A Reference Guide for Postgraduate Speciality Training in the UK*. There's more about this later, and you can find a link to it from our website.
- All GP trainees must complete three years of an approved training programme of which 18 months has to be in GP land (this may in time become five years). The 3 years are often referred to as ST1, ST2 and ST3 (ST = specialty training year). When a trainee joins a programme, they are given a National Training Number (NTN) which stays with them until they complete their training.
- During the three years, the trainee receives Clinical and Educational Supervision. Clinical Supervision is about helping them to acquire clinical knowledge, skills and attitudes (and thus gain competence) as they rotate through the posts. Educational Supervision focuses on their educational development (through learning gaps) and helps keep them on track for their training programme overall.
- Throughout the training programme, the trainee is assessed using Workplace-Based Assessments (WPBA) – things like case-based discussions (CBDs), multi-source feedback (MSF) from colleagues, direct observation of procedural (clinical) skills (DOPS) and so on. The trainee needs to demonstrate competency progression throughout their training period through these WPBA assessments and a log of their learning/clinical experiences. All of this is kept in an electronic folder called the ePortfolio.
- Towards the end of every ST year, an independent panel called the Annual Review of Competency Progression (ARCP) panel assesses each trainee's ePortfolio. If progress is good, the panel will give an 'Outcome 1' and allow them to proceed to the next year. If the panel has some concerns, but progress is still good enough for the trainee to carry onto the next job, an 'Outcome 2' is likely to be given. On the other hand, if there are concerns about the trainee's progress such that the panel feels repeating a training period would be beneficial, an 'Outcome 3' is given.
- By the end of training, the trainee is required to have taken and successfully passed two examinations. One is a multiple-choice paper testing knowledge (called the Applied Knowledge Test or AKT), and the other is a special OSCE type exam where they are tested on a variety of clinical and communication skills using simulated patients (called Clinical Skills Assessment or CSA).

- When the ST3 trainee has successfully completed everything and is deemed competent, they receive a certificate to signpost that they've reached the level required for independent safe general practice (called the Certificate of Completion of Training – CCT; also known as ARCP 'Outcome 4').

 Top Tip: Don't worry about all the acronyms and outcomes, especially if you're new to GP training. They will come to you naturally after a few months.

Who decides what is what?

The General Medical Council (GMC)

The GMC is ultimately 'top dog': it is the independent regulator for doctors in the UK. Its statutory purpose is '*to protect, promote and maintain the health and safety of the public*', and its powers are set out in the Medical Act 1983.[2] In brief, this is what it does:

> ### The Medical Act 1983
> - It determines the principles and values that underpin good medical practice.
> - It has a general function to promote high standards and coordinate all stages of medical education.
> - It is responsible for (and actually sets) the standards of postgraduate medical education and training.
> - It quality assures that these standards are being met by approved training programmes and institutions (e.g. through its visiting programme).
> - It certifies doctors who apply for their CCT and makes that doctor eligible for inclusion on the GMC's Specialist or GP Register.

The Medical Royal Colleges

The Medical Royal Colleges/Faculties are 'deputy dogs'. They develop entry criteria, curricula and exit criteria for their particular specialty in accordance with the guidance set by the GMC. The GMC reviews these criteria. Once approved, the colleges (via college tutors/regional advisors) work with deaneries to help them deliver the curricula at a local level (and help to quality assure and manage them).

The deaneries

The deaneries are independent organisations whose aim is to ensure a training programme is delivered to specialty doctors in training according to GMC standards. At the head of the deanery sits the Postgraduate Dean and his or her team, but more about them later. The deaneries cover all medical specialties, not just general practice (although general practice comprises a large part of their work). The deaneries work closely with the Royal Colleges and local education providers, and employ Training Programme Directors (TPDs) in order to deliver the programmes. (Yes! The medical specialties have TPDs too – not just general practice.)

Training Programme Directors

The TPDs are the people who make things happen at a shop floor level – developing a training programme across local educational provider units (hospital departments and GP posts).

Higher specialist training is managed by more than one organisation

We hope you have not come to the conclusion that one organisation simply dumps their training objective over to the organisation beneath them. What actually happens is that a number of representatives from each of the organisations above meet and work with one another through deanery specialty training committees. A useful analogy is to think about the construction of a house. The GMC and RCGP are a bit like the local council who, through their policies and permissions, say what you can and cannot do. The deanery and TPDs are the architects who have to design something that fits in with these policies and permissions. Finally, the TPDs, Clinical and Educational Supervisors are the builders who start making the plans come to life. Once it is built the trainees, of course, become the new tenants.

The Gold Guide[3]

This is a reference guide for postgraduate training in the UK for all medical specialties including general practice. Written by the UK Scrutiny Group (led by the four UK Chief Medical Officers – England, Scotland, Northern Ireland and Wales), the first edition appeared in August 2007 and has

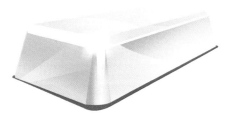

been updated periodically ever since through an iterative process of feedback from various stakeholders. The standards and requirements set by the GMC are extensively quoted in the Gold Guide to ensure that its recommendations are underpinned by them and the GMC's other publication, *Good Medical Practice*.[4]

It primarily deals with the operational side of things – providing recommendations such as approving training programmes, flexible training, Educational Supervision, ARCP panels, remedial training and so on. In short, if you're uncertain about anything in relation to training, look it up in the Gold Guide first (although it is primarily aimed at Royal Colleges, deaneries, local education providers and TPDs). The Gold Guide is available online on the Modernising Medical Careers (MMC) website: www.mmc.nhs.uk

> *A note on the CMOs: England, Scotland, Wales and Northern Ireland each have a Chief Medical Officer. The CMO provides independent professional advice and guidance on healthcare matters to the First Minister or Ministers for Health (Scotland, Wales and Northern Ireland) or Secretary of State (England). Things like medical regulation, education and training, standards and performance.*

How does the money stuff work?

It's complicated, there are some variations (especially in Scotland), and the amounts are large, but we'll keep it simple. Basically, the deanery covers:

- 50% of the basic salaries of most doctors in hospital training posts (the hospital trust is responsible for the rest)
- 100% of the salary in the case of Foundation Year doctors, public health doctors, GP Specialty Trainees, supernumerary flexible trainees and those on extensions to their programmes
- all study leave
- the funding for the postgraduate centres (including the library) and its staff.

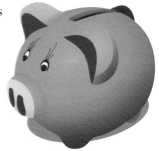

Question: In terms of spending, who are deaneries accountable to?
Answer: The NHS Executive (and they do double-check to see if it is spent as intended).

Is it mandatory to provide flexible training?

Well, it depends on the circumstances. The answer is yes if the doctor has difficulty pursuing full-time training through illness or disability. Flexible training may also be provided for trainees with domestic commitments, unique opportunities in personal or professional development and for those with a religious commitment. Each case will be judged on its merits. Flexible training can be arranged by reducing sessions in an established post, job sharing, or creating a supernumerary placement, and demand is rising. Each flexible trainee requires an annual review of progress to make sure they're on track *as well as* a review every time they cross from one speciality training year to another.

A bit more about the deanery

You can now appreciate the onerous set of tasks the deanery has to coordinate, deliver and quality assure. The Postgraduate Dean is assisted by a GP Director, a number of Deputy Deans, Associate

CAUTION 1: *The configuration in some deaneries might be at variance with our map. For example, Scotland does not have APDs – instead, they have Associate Advisors who cover a variety of roles. The presence of Deputy Directors depends on the size of the deanery. Some deaneries will have a team of Associate Postgraduate Deans, who cover all specialties including GP. It would be impractical to present a spectrum of different deanery configurations. Our aim here is to give you a rough idea about how things might look in your deanery – which is better than nothing.*

CAUTION 2: *Some of the terms may be different in different deaneries. For example, some areas use the term Course Organisers for TPDs – both having the same role and responsibilities.*

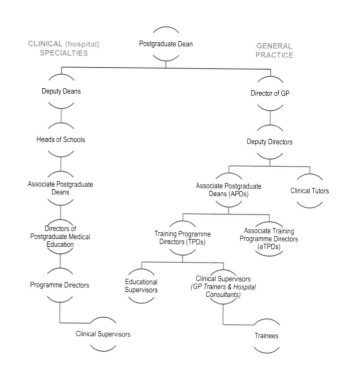

Postgraduate Deans and other administrative staff (including a business manager). The size of the deanery depends on the patch it covers (and hence the number of trainees). Most medical staff employed by the deanery will be employed on a part-time basis and will continue to hold other clinical jobs. The important thing to remember is that all of them do the job because they are committed to improving medical training and ultimately improving the quality of patient care.

The hierarchical map on the previous page shows you who is who in the deanery (and who is accountable to whom). For more detailed information on each person's role, please go to our website. There's another document there detailing organisations and educational institutions that you might also want to check out – many of whom will support you in your current educational role.

What happens after training?
The First Five Initiative
This initiative aims to provide educational and peer support for newly qualified GPs (up to five years). They usually run conferences, meetings and social events to help new GPs network and find their bearings. Contact your local RCGP office to find out more: www.rcgp.org.uk/new_professionals/first5.aspx

After that?
The education available to all well-established and new GPs is variable and depends on what the locality trust provides. For example, nearly all trusts provide educational afternoons where medical cover is provided for the practice. One is also expected to engage regularly in practice-based learning – where the practice comes together to learn from and solve local problems and issues in a collaborative way. Then there are evening courses – some sponsored, others not. Local RCGP offices have educational leads who aim to help us with our professional development. Most faculties put on an educational programme of events – check out what yours provides (go to www.rcgp.org. uk and scroll to the bottom right where it says 'Find the local RCGP'). However, what you decide ultimately to learn about depends on what you've identified in the annual GP appraisal.

Closing statement

We started this chapter with a quote from Sanjiv Ahluwalia, and we'd like to finish with another quote from him. It shows that there are many doors open to you in the field of GP training and education. Which ones you choose to open and explore is entirely up to you. If you've got commitment and passion, you'll be supported along the way.

> I qualified as a GP in 2000. Having nearly made the decision to give up medicine several times during my short career, it was only when I became a GP trainee that I finally found the support, guidance, and inspiration to be good at being a GP. It was my GP Trainer, the Training Programme Directors, and fellow trainees who provided this inspiration. I very quickly realised that being an educator is both rewarding and inspiring. In 2002, I applied to become a GP Training Programme Director, and in 2003 a GP Trainer. After gaining experience in both these roles I applied to become an Associate Director in 2007. I felt it was time to take a management responsibility over an area larger than my scheme.
>
> Sanjiv Ahluwalia, Deputy Head of GP School, London Deanery[1]

A sample of resources on our website
- An updated version of this chapter.
- Who is who in the deanery.
- Organisations worth exploring.

Please give us some feedback on this chapter to help shape it for the next edition.
Go to www.essentialgptrainingbook.com and simply click on the title of this chapter.

References

1 www.londonDeanery.ac.uk/general-practice/continuing-professional-development-for-gps/developing-your-career/non-clinical-roles/testimonials/associate-director
2 Medical Act 1983, available at: www.gmc-uk.org/about/legislation/medical_act.asp
3 The Gold Guide, available at: www.mmc.nhs.uk/
4 GMC's *Good Medical Practice*, available at: www.gmc-uk.org/guidance/good_medical_practice.asp

The GP Trainer and Practice Manager

GLYNIS BUCKLE – Head of GP School (Oxford Deanery) & lead author; formerly a Practice Manager
RAMESH MEHAY – TPD & Trainer (Bradford) **JOHN HART** – TPD & Trainer (Kettering)

This chapter has been written for intending/new GP Trainers, their Practice Managers, new Training Programme Directors (TPD) and any other colleagues in the practice who are interested.

Throughout, we make several references to your deanery's website. This is because although there are many similarities in the way in which different deaneries work towards the same ultimate goals, there are also some differences. Sometimes it is important to check out exactly what your deanery requires of you and your practice.

So, you're thinking of becoming a GP training practice?

Before you even start thinking about filling in that application form, do the following.

● Make contact with the local Training Programme Director (TPD) and arrange an informal meeting – if you don't know who they are, contact your deanery. Try to think of what you'd like to get out of this meeting and what you'd like to be clearer about. Jot these down to remind you.

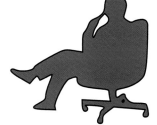

● Then spend some time with others from your practice (including your Practice Manager (PM)) defining your reasons why you want to get involved in GP training. Do something like a SWOT analysis – divide an A4 page into four quadrants, and work out the strengths, weaknesses, opportunities and threats that are associated with getting involved in GP training.

● Define the practice ethos towards GP training. Double-check that everyone agrees to GP training being a practice activity – not one which is shoved back to the GP Trainer when things go wrong. In other words, everyone agrees to play a part in GP training, and that it's 'the collective' that is responsible for it. Make sure the PM is part of this discussion, and you have his or her buy-in.

● Work out precisely what the steps are to becoming (1) a GP Trainer and (2) a training practice. (3) Define what the expectations of GP training are. (4) Make sure the PM is clear about this too.

The pros and cons of GP training

Why should I become a trainer? You'd be right to ask that question, especially as it is not very well paid. To help you make that decision, we've created a specific document looking at this question in more detail. It's on our website, and it's called *A Comprehensive Look at the Pros and Cons of GP Training.*

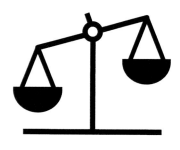

Positives include the contact with young doctors, which is stimulating and keeps everyone more in touch with developments in general practice. It helps develop your educational skills and helps keep you and the practice up to date clinically. Being a training practice is very valuable for GP recruitment. The pleasure of seeing young people develop and their overt appreciation for your help is immeasurable. Being part of the training scheme puts you in touch with others (e.g. Trainers) beyond the limits of your practice boundary and opens up the opportunity to work creatively with them.

Negatives include the occasional perception of a lack of commitment of the younger generation, and that they simply don't have the same work ethic as the older generations, though they might argue they have a better work-life balance! The disruption to continuity of patient care (trainee changes every 6–12 months) often means that the Trainer picks up what's left behind. If you get a poorly performing trainee, that in itself can be demotivating (it still happens even though the recruitment process is much more robust and geared towards selecting high-quality trainees). Finally, GP training isn't a particularly high earner – this sometimes means it can lose priority within the practice.

Remember, you have to make the right decision for your practice *and* you. If either one of you is not 'hooked' into *doing* the training, you're more likely to have a miserable and stressful time. Training is a practice activity – not like the old days where it was just the Trainer who took complete responsibility; it's really important to secure the support of the practice. In addition, if you get the rest of the practice on board you can share the workload and when you do that, training becomes an enjoyable activity, and everyone's a winner.

What's the Practice Manager got to do with it?

As with most other areas of practice activity, the Practice Manager (PM) plays a crucial role in the establishment and performance of a successful GP training practice. The PM is the key to making things happen; they're your right arm! Therefore, make sure the PM is part of all discussions and shares the same attitude towards taking on GP training as you.

 Top Tip: Having a Practice Manager who is fully engaged with the practice's ethos for wanting to become a training practice enables you as the Trainer to focus on education. The support of your Practice Manager is as important as the support of the other doctors.

The Practice Manager from a practice down the road from us rang for advice on two things. They usually give their trainees three hours' worth of teaching/educational activity a week. However, their present trainee, although hard-working, diligent and committed, wasn't [as] up to the mark as the others and, therefore, needed more input and that meant extra educational time. She wanted to know how we would get the trainee to give the time back. The trainee also wanted to go on a three-day communication skills course but the practice thought that as the Half-Day Release ate up most of the study leave, he wasn't actually entitled to any. Did we agree?

We were a bit shocked that the practice was so rigid in their thinking. In our practice, if a trainee needs more input, they need more input – end of the story! Why all the unnecessary fuss about paying back time? As for the 3 hours per week of educational time – well that's just a minimum, not the expected.

With respect to Study Leave – yes, Half-Day Release does eat it all up but if this trainee is hard-working and diligent and would benefit from going, what's an extra three days of Study Leave? As long as they're not taking the Mickey! We felt this practice needed to get a grip and revisit their reasons for engaging in GP training in the first place. Was it for an extra pair of hands or was it because they truly wanted to help new young trainees flourish? We wonder . . .

So:
- even if you're an established training practice but have just appointed a new PM – go back to basics and go through the practice ethos towards training with them
- and if you're an existing training practice with an established PM make sure that, annually, you're reviewing and developing his or her role in GP training.

The role of the Practice Manager in GP training

GP training requires skilled organisation in order for it to become an integrated (rather than an added on) part of practice activity, and organisational skills are one of the reasons you employed your PM. Just as there is no definitive model General Practice, there is no definitive job description or person specification for a PM. Therefore, in the context of this chapter, the title of Practice Manager refers to the person in your practice who can influence both strategic planning and monitor what actually happens at the operational level.

So why are you becoming a Trainer/training practice?

- If we did not believe it was a worthwhile thing to do, we would not be writing this chapter.
- If you did not think it was a worthwhile thing to do you would not be reading this chapter, let alone this book.

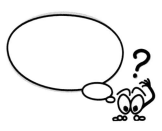

So, let's start with these two questions:
1 Why are you thinking of becoming a Trainer?
2 Why now?

If your answer is:
- *'The existing Trainer is giving up and someone needs to take over'*
  You need to think again and give it some serious thought because GP training involves commitment and hard work. The previous Trainer may have made it look so easy, but that's probably because they were so experienced, committed and had the right attitude.
- *'I've always wanted to be a Trainer and now seems to be the right time'* or *'The practice wants to train so I thought I'd volunteer'*.
- Good – at least your heart (attitude) seems to be in the right place. But you still need to think more deeply; GP training is not a pushover! Be prepared for a steep learning curve with initial rough waters that will settle quite quickly if you're truly committed. For most of us, it's worth it.

The types of responses we like to hear are:

- *'I had a fab Trainer/training practice and I want to give something back.'*
- *'I want to help new young seedlings flower.'*
- *'I want to be part of a educational/training community – who continuously want to learn and improve.'*
- *'I love teaching and feel I have lots to offer but I'd really like to develop my educational skills.'*

The key ingredients of successful GP training

It's simple really. Many of you might think that the key to being successful at GP training is familiarity with protocol and assessments. All of that helps, but it all breaks down if the following key ingredients are missing.

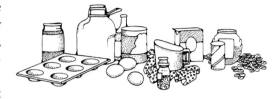

1 Your desire to becoming a GP Trainer must marry with the practice's desire to train (or continue to train).

2 Your colleagues (not just the doctors) must see GP training as a practice activity (*not* a sole Trainer activity of which they want no part).

3 The entire practice (or most of them) are supportive of GP training.

If any of these three things are not quite right, go back to the drawing board and work on them *before* going down the training route. Becoming a Trainer is hard but rewarding work and perhaps not something to do because you feel under pressure from your partners – especially if you would rather be developing your talents as a GP with Special Interest (GPwSI) in dermatology or as chair of your Local Medical Committee (LMC). Equally, going it alone because you desperately want to be a Trainer and hoping that the practice will eventually catch up with the idea is usually a recipe for disaster and resentment.

Is now the right time for me to become a Trainer?

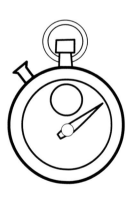

Some doctors know as soon as they start their own training (or even before) that they want to be a Trainer fairly early on in their career, while others grow into the idea. It doesn't matter which camp you fall into. However, how quickly you can become a Trainer after qualifying as a GP varies slightly from deanery to deanery. It is usually around three years (but check your deanery's website or with your local TPD).

Other than being able to meet the deanery's criteria, there is no right or wrong time to become a Trainer. The important thing is that it is something you want to do, that it feels like the right time, and that you have the support of your practice. If you're the type with many fingers in different pies, something has to go if you want to take up GP training.

The effect of GP training on your practice

There will be considerable organisational issues by way of rearranging timetables and schedules (and not just yours) to accommodate your new role in the practice. Your PM and your colleagues need to understand the impact that getting involved in GP training will have on the practice; in particular the following.

- Your time away from patient contact to allow you protected time for training.
- Time away from patient contact for other doctors who will also be helping to deliver GP training (e.g. through tutorials, etc.).
- Your time attending Trainers' meetings and workshops.
- Making protected time for debriefing sessions and tutorials.
- Interrupted surgeries to assist the GP trainee.
- Time for Educational Supervision (most Trainers are *Clinical* Supervisors for their *own* trainees but also *Educational* Supervisors for *other* trainees in their area).
- Room allocation changes to integrate the GP trainee.

Sometimes, other colleagues may see you as 'not pulling your weight' because of your intermittent absences (without realising that most of your absences are because of a training requirement, and overlooking the fact that your attendance shows your diligence and commitment). This is why we keep saying it is always much better to get these sort of things agreed in principle before you start training – it helps prevent resentment afterwards from others.

 Top Tip: If you're a new training practice, it may be difficult to define exactly how much time you will need for training, so it is useful to talk to other Trainers (a buddy perhaps?) and to look at your deanery's guidelines. Your PM could benefit too from finding a PM buddy or mentor from another local training practice. Even if you're in an existing training practice, the very fact that you're a new Trainer means you are likely to need more time than an established Trainer who is more experienced.

What needs to be organised?

This is the bit where your PM is instrumental.

The types of things that need organising

The new trainee's induction

Please read our *Web Chapter: Induction*. Induction should cover everything from how the computer system works to 'How do I get a cup of coffee'! Don't forget about the opportunity for the trainee to sit in not only with the doctors but also the nursing and administrative team – to see 'how things are done around here'. Remember that the trainee may only have had experience of working in the hierarchical system of hospitals, which is almost absent in 21st-century general practice.

GP timetable and workload

Service delivery versus education can often be a tricky balance to achieve. GP trainees must get protected time for sufficient education, and must not be abused in terms of workload. However, seeing patients is equally important so that they can get a real feel for the job and be able to develop skills to cope with all its demands.

Sometimes your partners may question how much they are getting in return for having a GP trainee in the practice (to which we would say, re-examine the practice ethos towards training).

Some deaneries go on about GP trainees being regarded as supernumerary – probably because they want to protect trainees from abuse. We believe that trainees should not be regarded as supernumerary because this devalues the work they do and the contribution they make to patient care. As part of their training the GP trainee needs to gain an understanding of what it is like to be part of a practice team and what that means in terms of negotiating annual leave and giving adequate notice of planned educational activity which will take them out of the practice. So, while we feel they should not be regarded as supernumerary, the practice must not depend on them to ensure that it meets its patient demands in terms of access.

The guidelines:
● GP trainees should work 10 sessions each week
● 7 sessions should be direct patient contact and 3 should be on educational activity (though of course seeing patients is one of the best ways of learning to be a GP)
● One of these educational activity days may be Half or Full-Day Release – organised by the Programme Directors; find out if this is the case and which day this is on.

Clinical supervision
Remember that a doctor in training must always be supervised by either their Trainer or another GP who works permanently in the practice. They cannot be supervised by a locum GP.

Timetabling debriefs
● It is essential that you build in time at the end of each of the trainee's surgeries for them to be debriefed by a qualified GP.
● This does not have to be the Trainer and often works well on a rota basis so that all the doctors in the practice feel involved with the trainee.
● The primary aim of debriefs is to make sure that what the trainee has done is clinically safe (i.e. for patient safety). The secondary aim is to identify and fill in some of their learning gaps.
● Be wary of the learner who says they do not want to be debriefed. Remember that they don't always know what they don't know (cf. Johari's Window[1]).
● At the start, you should glance over every patient seen. With time, as you get a good 'feel' for the trainee's competence, you'll know whether you need to cast an eye over every patient or not (and whether surveying random ones will do).
● Outcomes should be identified in terms of Patient's Unmet Needs (PUNs) and Doctor's Educational Needs (DENs).[2]

Trainer's timetable
You and your PM should talk – to see what changes need to be made to your timetable to enable you to provide the GP training. Borrow a neighbouring training practice's Trainer timetable if you feel you're totally in the dark.
● Tutorial time should happen *during* your working week – *not* on your half-day off!
● The tutorial time needn't be delivered in one 3-hour lump (and actually is better split because one's attention span cannot extend this far). Many Trainers do 1½ hours twice a week.
● You should not have to 'repay' the practice the time for going on Trainers' Workshops and so on.
● Your PM will have an overview of workload and patient demand for access and should be able to help to present some timetable options that work well with the practice.

- Consider building some 'blank' time in your own surgery so that you can field initial GP trainee queries during their own surgery. Remember, training is a shared responsibility: the other doctors need to 'take turns' in this clinical supervision process.

Who covers you when you're away

While training is the responsibility of the practice as a whole, you are the named Trainer and the person ultimately responsible for the GP trainee. When you are on annual leave, it is important that someone else in the practice is nominated to take on this role so that everyone knows who to turn to in the unlikely event of there being a problem.

If you are a single-handed practitioner, you will have to ensure that you have proper formal arrangements to cover your annual leave, e.g. getting your GP trainee to work in another training practice (this will need to be approved by your Programme Director). By the way, you don't have to be a full-timer to be a Trainer. There are loads of part-time Trainers out there. You just need to make sure there is structured nominated cover for the trainee on those days that you're not scheduled to be in the surgery.

Surely the trainee doesn't need to attend the practice meetings?

It is an expectation that your trainee *will* attend all practice meetings – how else are they going to learn about the planning, decision-making process and the business systems within 21st-century general practice? Sometimes your partners may be uncomfortable with this idea, but unless the subject for discussion is deeply private and confidential, e.g. the health or personal relationship of another doctor in the practice, there is really no reason for the trainee not to attend. Some practices can be a little sensitive about money issues, but the trainee has to learn about general practice as a business – warts and all! Obviously, they're bound by the rules of confidentiality, so what is there really to worry about?

Practice business meetings	Primary Health Care Team meetings	Significant event meetings
Referral - Prescribing - ProActive Care meetings	Practice Based Commissioning or Locality meetings	Local Medical Council and PCT meetings

Modern general practice has a multitude of meetings and GP trainees should attend as many as possible. (ProActive Care meetings are designed to keep vulnerable people out of hospital.)

What else can the Practice Manager help with?

Your PM is an expert at managing staff and dealing with all those tricky HR issues. Your GP trainee is an employee and from time to time there may be employment and contractual issues to be sorted out, e.g. annual leave, study leave, maternity/paternity leave, even the occasional salary or expenses query. Your manager is more likely than you to understand the 'language' of these queries and will therefore find it easier to take up the queries with the appropriate organisation.

Your manager is also likely to be a good listener and probably noted for his or her people skills as well as business acumen. The pastoral role played by the PM towards the GP trainee should never be underestimated. The GP trainee may sometimes find it easier to confide in the PM about personal issues such as child care, sick parents, relationship issues or the stress of travelling.

Your manager may not be trained as an educator, but they do have a wealth of knowledge on the subject of management to pass on to the trainee. We're going to leave it at that for now but hope you are convinced (if you needed any convincing) that your PM is an essential part of the practice training set-up.

 Top Tip: Most deaneries will hold faculty development days for Trainers. These will often include an invitation to PMs. Some schemes even run training events for PMs – a good place for your PM to start networking with others.

So what about the preparation to become a Trainer? I hear it's hard work

Every deanery has its own version of what new Trainers need to do. We've tried to cover the full range of what different deaneries do here, but not all of these will be required. Your best bet is to go onto your local deanery's website and check.

1 Some will want you to do a Trainer's course, others, **an educational diploma or certificate** and some even both! Being a learner and meeting deadlines while working and dealing with all the normal and usual pressures of life will certainly help you to empathise with your learners. The diagram on the right shows some of the types of things educational courses will cover.

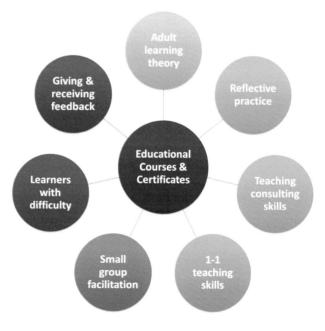

2 Some deaneries expect you to have **'borrowed' a GP trainee** and practised some of the things you will be expected to do as a fully fledged GP Trainer – like COTs and CBDs (if you don't know what these are, read Chapter 25 on MRCGP).

3 To make sure you're educating the 'borrowed' trainee in the right way, some deaneries will expect you to engage in a series of **Educational Supervision meetings** with a nominated experienced Trainer (where you look constructively at videos of your educational sessions).

4 During this time, the TPD will periodically contact you, inviting you to **help at the local Half/Full-Day Release programme and attend Trainers' Workshops/meetings**. Attendance to some degree is expected by most deaneries – because it should enrich your educational skills further.

5 Both the Educational Supervisor and local TPD may be expected to write a report on you – they will have got to know you by now.

6 Then it's the final hurdle – the formal interview process (though some deaneries may do this as part of the approval visit). Be open and honest during this interview. Don't fudge things, and make sure all the organisational bits like the timetable are perfect. Ask your local TPD for a bit more about the interview process.

However much support you get from your practice, there will always be some degree of anxiety.
- If you are a new Trainer in a new practice, you will be concerned that you are doing the right thing, and that you are good enough to be a Trainer.
- If you are a new Trainer in an existing training practice, you will be concerned that you are as good as the previous or more experienced Trainer.
- And, of course, there is the anxiety from wanting to try to do things differently without appearing to criticise what has gone before.

 Top Tip: If your deanery does not require you to engage with an Educational Supervisor or Mentor, join your Trainers' Group as soon as you can and buddy up with one of the experienced people (not someone from your own practice). Try to take every opportunity you can to get involved with the other educational activities run by your local GP training scheme.

Help is always at hand

Once you've been approved, there will undoubtedly be some anxiety as you take responsibility for your first GP trainee – especially if they do not appear to be making the progress you expect. However, don't forget that help is always on hand (see diagram right).

It's always better to ask for help *early* rather than late – even if you think the concern is minor, or if you feel you might be overreacting. Things are easier to fix early on than at the end when it's just one big chaotic mess. **Seeking reassurance can show insight not weakness.**

Your Training Programme Director

A fellow trainer in your practice	A trainer from another practice

The Trainers' Group	Your Educational Mentor	A fellow practice colleague/PM

Your PM may well be the person to help you to sound out the opinions of other members of your practice team. Again, their skills will enable them to do so in a detached non-judgemental way and filter out a fact from opinion. Sometimes, as a Trainer, you can end up being a little too protective of your learner to maintain an objective view.

Meeting the deanery criteria to become a training practice

If you want a GP trainee in your practice, there are two things that need to be satisfied first:

1 **You** need to do all the deanery-prescribed things necessary to become an **approved Trainer** (discussed above).
2 **The practice** needs to meet all the deanery criteria to become an **approved training practice**.

We're now going to concentrate on meeting the 'practice' criteria. Again, your PM will be invaluable in getting you through this challenge. Get hold of your deanery's training practice criteria (from their website) and work through it bit by bit (with your PM). Don't forget the basic principles of planning:

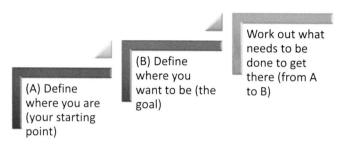

If there is still a long way to go, get your colleagues to help out – it's a great way of getting real practice ownership for training. Even if you are nearly there, keep everyone appraised of the progress you are making (it makes them feel part of it). Keep in touch with the local TPD; they'll make sure you're on track (besides, they have to write a 'practice report' towards the end anyway).

What's this I hear about a practice visit?

The final stage usually takes the form of a visit to you and your practice. The visit will last somewhere between three hours and a whole day – best to cancel your own surgeries for that day. The visiting team are there simply to:

- check that you and the practice fully understand what it means to have responsibility for a GP trainee
- check that the practice environment is one which is conducive to learning
- check that you're already providing a good level of patient care
- and to make sure everything is generally in order.

The visiting team is usually a combination of:

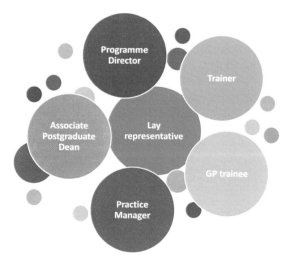

What, they're going to be judging us on patient quality! How?

Relax, they're not looking for you to be wonderfully brilliant – just good enough. They're not out to trip you up either. What they'll look at varies from deanery to deanery. Ask your local TPD. Once again, your PM is instrumental in making sure all of this looks and *is* good. The types of things they *might* look at are as follows.

● Your Quality and Outcomes Framework (QOF) report – no surprise there!

● Clinical note summaries – to ensure that someone new seeing the patient can easily access all the necessary information that they need in order to continue the appropriate care.

● Patient demographics – to make sure the trainee is going to be exposed to a variety of cases and, therefore, experience. If your practice population is skewed towards young families, the trainee may not get sufficient exposure to the care of the elderly and chronic disease. This will not preclude you from training, but you would have to address the imbalance. We are not suggesting that you take on a whole load of different patients, but an organised swap with another practice can work very well.

● The practice weekly timetable – to see how organised the practice is, how busy the practice is and whether there is 'time space' for the GP trainee to be able to ask for help when they need it.

● A review of systems and protocols – to ensure patient safety. Examples include your protocol for yielding and following up positive cervical smear results, updating the child protection register, procedure for requesting an urgent home visit – you get the idea.

● You may also be asked to show the visiting team a video of your teaching. This enables them to assess how much you have learnt so far particularly around learner-centred adult education.

At the end, the team will give you feedback on the areas in which you are doing well and can be proud of. Of course, they will also talk about those areas that need a bit more work – and discuss ideas with you. Some of these may not be 'big enough' to preclude you from training, but others like the following will.

● The Trainer is not in practice enough to give the GP trainee the support they need.

● The timetable does not have adequate protected time for training.

In cases where they do decide to let you carry on with training, it's likely they'll also ask for an interim report (either from you or a Programme Director visit) to ensure the suggested improvements have been implemented.

The visiting team will then write a report detailing their observations and recommendations to the GP Dean/Director for consideration and approval by the appropriate deanery committee.

The Practice Manager as an educator

Some PMs have undertaken Certificates in Medical Education – in other words, they are Primary Care Educators in their own right; but they are few and far between. Most PMs can undoubtedly help with the meaty bit of the trainee's education too – particularly with regard to practice management and organisation – we're not just talking about finances here.

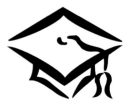

The Practice Manager's curriculum – things they can teach on

Change management and strategic planning
- Use a real example, e.g. becoming a training practice.
- Why did you do it, how did you do it, who was involved?
- What were the challenges and issues, what were the benefits?
- Integrate with the theories of change management and strategic planning.

Time management and personal organisation
- This is often a big issue for several people in the practice (not just GP trainees).
- Exploring where this is an issue within the practice.
- The impact that this can have on other team members and patients.
- Unpicking why it might be an issue and suggesting some solutions.

Meetings
- Why do we have meetings?
- How often should we have them? Who should be there? Group dynamics.
- How should they be organised? Methods of chairing them, taking minutes/notes.
- Maybe giving the trainee the opportunity to chair a meeting and then reflect on what it felt like – experiential learning.

Being an employer
- What does it mean to be an employer?
- How much employment law do you need to know?
- Equal opportunities, recruitment, interviewing, appraisal. (Next time you do recruitment and interviewing, get the GP trainee involved – experiential learning.)
- Where do you get help if things go wrong?

Complaints
Never a pleasant experience and always to be taken seriously, no matter how apparently trivial or unfounded.
- Effect on the individual and the support measures in the practice.
- How does the practice *view* them – significant event; are they seen as a learning opportunity?
- How does the practice *deal* with them – protocol, who gets involved, etc?

Finance
- Where does the money come from? Where does the money go?
- How can you protect it? How can you maximise on it?
- Money-making decision pathways. Who controls the purse strings?
- The practice accountant – is one really necessary?

Top Tip: How can you expect people to teach who haven't been trained to teach? So, how about providing some personal training on the basic principles of adult education to those who will be involved (PM, other docs, nurses)? Could you dedicate a couple of the practice's weekly protected learning time events to do this? Read Chapter 6: Teaching from Scratch for some ideas or see a PowerPoint on our website called *A Beginner's Guide to Teaching*. Some deaneries run short teacher courses for doctors who are not Trainers – and many extend their invitation to PMs and nurses too.

Closing statement

We'd just like to close with this personal statement from a Trainer:

Getting involved in GP training is one of the best things we did recently. Why? Personally, I felt my working life was becoming a bit humdrum. In fact, I felt the whole practice was a bit like this – you know, where everyone goes about their job okay but something is missing. The new trainee brought that spark back into our working lives.

In our practice, the whole practice has signed up to help with GP training and education – as a GP Trainer, I am merely the lead. I'm not the only one that does tutorials – others are involved too and they like it. They also like clinically supervising the trainee and sitting in with them. They even like being quizzed by the trainee (perhaps it makes them feel valued). And let's not forget all the other things the GP trainee does for us – providing extra appointment slots, taking home visits and so on.

I've heard some GPs from intending training practices being concerned about their QOF values going down or their prescribing/referral budgets going through the roof. This is a perception more than it is real. Yes, they do go up a bit at first but they soon come back down.

Anyway, I love doing GP training, and our practice loves having a trainee (and I don't just mean the doctors and nurses). If the daily work at the practice could be likened to a broth or stew, then the GP trainee would be the herbs and spices. It's the trainee who brings the flavour back home. If I wanted to write a whole chapter on the benefits the GP trainee brings with them, I could.

A sample of resources on our website

- A comprehensive look at the pros and cons of GP training.
- Some FAQs from intending Trainers and their PMs.
- Framework on competencies and attributes for GP educators.

Other chapters you may like to read

- Chapter 1: The Structure of GP Training in the UK
- Web chapter: Induction – how trainers can help trainees settle into their practices.

Please give us some feedback on this chapter to help shape it for the next edition.
Go to www.essentialgptrainingbook.com and simply click on the title of this chapter.

References

1 Luft J, Ingham H. *The Johari Window: a graphic model of interpersonal awareness. Proceedings of the Western Training Laboratory in group development.* Los Angeles: UCLA; 1955.

2 Eve R. Learning with PUNs and DENs: a method for determining educational needs and the evaluation of its use in primary care. *Educ Gen Pract.* 2000: **11**: 73–9.

3 The Training Programme Director*

ROGER BURNS – ex-TPD (Haverfordwest) & lead author   RAMESH MEHAY – TPD (Bradford) & lead author
MIKE TOMSON – APD (Yorkshire & the Humber Deanery)   BRAD CHEEK – ex-TPD (East Cumbria)

*Training Programme Directors were formerly called Course Organisers. The term Programme Directors (PD) is often used interchangeably with Training Programme Directors (TPDs). Many schemes also employ **Associate** Programme Directors (aPDs – not to be confused with APDs which stands for Associate Postgraduate Deans), who are generally people new to programme directing and who work alongside the Programme Directors helping with a couple of specific areas like Half-Day Release, developing modular programmes and so on.

What TPDs actually do

A TPD is a facilitator of GP education after the foundation years. He or she is usually skilled in working in small groups: their job description comes from their deanery. Each deanery may have a slightly different job description, based on a national template. The mind map on the following page summarises all the roles and responsibilities of the TPD.

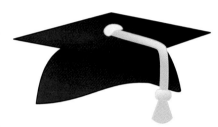

Although you may be blown over by the number of things a TPD does, what the mind map fails to convey is the satisfaction that can be obtained when things go well and the freedom that exists for innovative work together. But, above all, it doesn't convey the sense of shared achievement that is realised when GP trainees are seen to develop the knowledge, skills and attitudes necessary for general practice.

A conversational piece

There is a document on our website which is a conversational piece between an established PD and

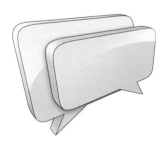

someone contemplating the role. If you're a new PD or thinking of applying, please go and download it now. It will help you make your decision or induct you into your role.

The document is called: *What do Programme Directors Do? A conversational piece.*

What do Programme Directors do?

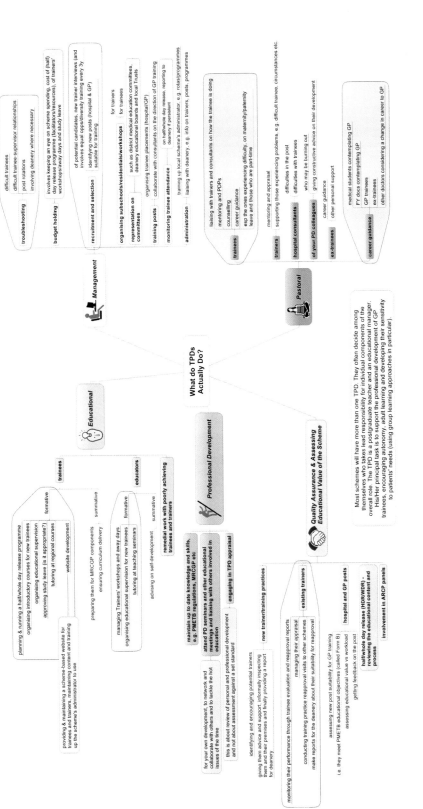

What do TPDs Actually Do?

Management

troubleshooting
- difficult trainees
- difficult trainee-supervisor relationships
- involving deanery where necessary

budget holding
- involves keeping an eye on scheme spending, cost of (half) day release programme (facilitators/resources), of trainers' workshops/away days and study leave

recruitment and selection
- of potential candidates, new trainer interviews (and involves equal opps/diversity training every 3y
- identifying new posts (hospital & GP)
- post rotations suitable for training

organising subschools/residentials/workshops
- for trainers
- for trainees

representation on committees
- such as district medical education committees, deanery educational boards and local Trusts

training posts
- organising trainee placements (hospital/GP)
- collaborate with consultants on the direction of GP training

monitoring trainee attendance
- on half/whole day release, reporting to deanery if persistent

administration
- training up local scheme's administrator. e.g. rotas/programmes
- liaising with deanery. e.g. info on trainers, posts, programmes

Pastoral

- liaising with trainers and consultants on how the trainee is doing
- mentoring and PDPs
- career guidance
- counselling
- esp the ones experiencing difficulty, on maternity/paternity leave and those who are part-time

trainers
- mentoring and appraisal
- supporting those experiencing problems, e.g. difficult trainee, circumstances etc.

hospital consultants
- difficulties in the post
- difficulties with trainees

of your PD colleagues
- who may be burning out
- giving constructive advice on their development

ex-trainees
- career guidance
- other personal support

career guidance
- medical students contemplating GP
- FY docs contemplating GP
- GP trainees
- ex-trainees
- other doctors considering a change in career to GP

Most schemes will have more than one TPD. They often decide among themselves who takes lead responsibility for individual components of the overall role. The TPD is a postgraduate teacher and an educational manager. His/Her principal task is to support the professional development of GP trainees, encouraging autonomy, adult learning and developing their sensitivity to patients' needs (using group learning approaches in particular).

Educational

trainees
- planning & running a half/whole day release programme
- organising introductory courses for new trainees
- organising educational supervision
- approving study leave (is it appropriate?)
- tutoring at regional courses
  - formative
  - website development
- providing & maintaining a scheme-based website for trainees and trainers, maintaining content and training up the scheme's administrator to use
- preparing them for MRCGP components
  - summative
  - ensuring curriculum delivery

educators
- managing Trainers' workshops and away days
- organising educational supervision for new trainees
  - formative
- tutoring at teaching seminars
  - summative
- advising on self-development

remedial work with poorly achieving trainees and trainers

Professional Development

maintain up to date knowledge and skills, e.g. PMETB regulations, MRCGP etc

attend PD seminars and other educational meetings and liaising with others involved in education

engaging in TPD appraisal

- for your own development, to network and collaborate with others and to tackle the hot issues of the time
- this is about review of personal and professional development and not about assessment against a set standard

Quality Assurance & Assessing Educational Value of the Scheme

new trainer/training practices
- identifying and encouraging potential trainers
- giving them advice and support, informally inspecting them and their premises and finally providing a report for deanery

existing trainers
- monitoring their performance through trainee evaluation and reapproval reports
- managing their appraisal
- conducting training practice reapproval visits to other schemes
- make reports for the deanery about their suitability for reapproval

hospital and GP posts
- assessing new post suitability for GP training
- i.e. they meet PMETB educational objectives (called Form B)
- assessing educational value vs workload
- getting feedback on the post

involvement in ARCP panels

half/whole day release (HDR/WDR) - reviewing the educational content and process

But I don't think I've got the right skills to be a TPD . . .

Don't worry! TPDs acquire these during the job. Actually, it's not just skills either – it's all of knowledge, skills and attitudes. The most important thing at this stage is to aspire to the right attitudes which we have listed below. Not everything in this list is *essential* in the beginning; some are just *desirable*.

The knowledge, skills and attitudes a TPD needs to have or develop

Knowledge
- An understanding of the structure of GP training and the role of educational organisations like RCGP, COGPED, UKCEA, APCE (formerly UKAPD and NAPCE).
- Being familiar with the training pathways for GP trainees and prospective GP Trainers.
- Having an understanding of the various assessment instruments used in GP training: especially, the MRCGP components and the ePortfolio.
- A knowledge of some educational theory (but don't let this put you off as most of us develop this on the job). For example: the principles of adult education, types of learning, modalities of learning, learning styles, understanding the influence of the environment on learning, formative vs summative assessment, professional development (would you believe – all covered in this book).
- Knowing the difference between facilitator, mentor and advocate.
- Understanding the role of the educator as a researcher and educational manager.
- Having a sound base of medical knowledge. Don't be put off by this. You don't have to be brilliant, just good enough. Actually, your medical knowledge improves as you help other trainees learn. *And* in some schemes, there are non-doctor TPDs who work alongside doctor TPDs – and it works just fine.

Skills
- Administrative skills: report writing, being able to locate or develop learning resources, being able to organise conferences/seminars/residentials (e.g. induction), good marketing skills.
- Communication skills and the skilful art of giving constructive feedback.
- Clinical skills: maintaining a high standard of clinical competence; being able to teach clinical and practical skills. (Again, not necessary if you are a non-doctor TPD, as long as you have fellow TPDs on your scheme who are.)
- Leadership skills: prioritising, decision-making, diplomacy, chairperson skills.
- Management skills: negotiating, delegating, team working, time management and being flexible.
- IT skills: being able to store, retrieve and share documents, email, ePortfolio use (in enough detail to be able to answer enquires from coalface educators), employing new educational technologies.
- Educational skills: being able to assess educational needs and curriculum planning, facilitating skills (1-1 and small-group work), presentation skills, creative thinking, problem-solving, using evidence-based education as a basis for teaching, motivational techniques, etc.
- Assessment skills: written, oral and clinical.
- Development skills: appraisal, revalidation, mentoring, Educational and Clinical Supervision.
- Counselling skills: on educational, career and personal matters (one of the most important skills).
- Money skills: being able to plan financially and hold a budget.

Attitudes
- Showing interest in people and different societies; cultural competence; being impartial, objective and non-discriminatory; demonstrating empathy and interest in learners; being sensitive and

responsive to others' educational needs; avoiding Educational Iatrogenesis (The doctor is the disease – Illich); encouraging a multi-professional approach to learning.

- Demonstrating probity and upholding the law and relevant regulations. Holding the improvement of the patient's health as a main priority; taking appropriate action if patient safety is threatened.
- Being highly self-motivated, committed and having a positive demeanour (approaching work with enthusiasm); willingness to go the extra mile; paying attention to detail.
- Self-awareness: being aware of own strengths, weaknesses and limitations; accepting and responding positively to feedback/evaluation.
- Being flexible and being able to cope with change; mindfulness skills: patience, diplomacy, pragmatism.
- Being committed to undertaking further training and development, demonstrating intellectual curiosity; auditing and evaluating own teaching.
- Having a mutually appreciative and respectful relationship with colleagues.
- Being able to balance clinical work, teaching and home life (even we haven't got this right yet!).

Now consider this imaginary advertisement

Newposts Deanery would like to take this opportunity to invite people with an interest in medical education to apply to become a Programme Director. Currently, we have two posts in Cityrise and one post in Remoteshire. If you are interested, please contact me@here.com

Desirable criteria:
Applicants for either of the posts will possess full GMC registration, MRCGP or equivalent, and be either currently in practice or eligible to be appointed. They will have evidence of experience in teaching, good IT skills, and effective communication, team working and organisational skills. Applicants for Training Programme Director level appointments would possess or plan to acquire a qualification in medical education. Being an active Trainer is desirable although not an essential requirement.

Perhaps you have seen the advert above and are interested in one of the posts. Here are some things to mull over:

		Popular City	Semi-Rural	Some Things to Think Over
Where		City Hospital Postgraduate Centre.	Rural District General Hospital Postgraduate Centre.	
Resources		Full-time administrator dedicated to GP training.	Part-time administrator or you may get a full-time administrator who is shared with other specialties.	Less admin support usually means the TPD has to do a lot more him/herself (although TPDs in central areas say they have lots of admin work too).
PD sessions		Most large schemes have around 3–4 TPDs each doing around 2–3 sessions each.	Usually, 1–2 TPDs doing 2–3 sessions.	There is currently some inequality between schemes in the number of TPD sessions allocated. This is being addressed in most deaneries.

	Popular City	Semi-Rural	Some Things to Think Over
Trainers	Around 40+ Trainers – many of whom wear other educational 'hats' such as training FY doctors, medical students and nurse practitioners. There will usually be a steady stream of GPs applying to do training, but also regular retirements.	Usually around 10–20 Trainers. Some of the Trainers will probably have been doing it for years, and the turnover rate might be slow too.	Recruitment of new Trainers in central areas can sometimes be difficult as there are too many other things they can earn more money doing. In rural practices, there too can be a problem recruiting new Trainers as other training practices that have experienced difficulty can put them off.
Trainees	Anywhere from 50 to 100 trainees at any one time.	Usually around 20–30 trainees	Large schemes = lots of trainees = • Finding more people to do things like Ed. Supervision. • Keeping track of individual trainees is more difficult. • The need for different TPDs to take on specialised roles and responsibilities. With smaller schemes, things are a lot more personal and easier.
Colleagues	There are usually 3–4 TPDs on moderately large schemes. Some really big schemes can have up to 8–10 TPDs. However, you can also get further support from TPDs in neighbouring schemes.	You might be the only TPD for your scheme. Alternatively, you might have another TPD (both of you doing 1.5 sessions each, for instance) – not much time for supporting each other (unless you both just agree to extra commitment. Neighbouring schemes won't be that close to you either.	Having more colleagues means you can share the workload, be creative and provide support to each other. In rural areas, there is only so much you can physically do, which leaves less space for anything else. Most schemes have an Associate Postgraduate Dean linked to them, although the availability and involvement varies.
IT skills	You need to be good with email and office software like Microsoft Word and PowerPoint. You also need to have a good paper management system (many schemes employ some sort of electronic filing system). You need to have an understanding of databases to the level that you can access this information with the help of a scheme administrator.	Again, need to be good with email and office software like Microsoft Word and PowerPoint. Again, a good paper management system is important. However, because you have fewer trainees to worry about, it doesn't need to be over-complicated. Complex databases are not necessary. One side of A4 will probably do.	The increasing complexity of the medical education system and the demand by GMC for robust quality assurance is likely to result in increasing complexity in data collection and retrieval in the future.
Type of Work	You'll do quite a bit of coal face teaching but will also end up doing some work on ARCP panels, committee meetings and other deanery-related work. However, as there are several of you, you can share this workload.	You might be the only one doing all the teaching, but it is more usual to get your local Trainers involved to free you up. As you're the only representative of your area, you might end up going to all the 'additional' deanery stuff.	It is important to have a voice at higher levels. However, you will need to create a balance of time used in these activities and time used in day-to-day scheme work.

Quick question–answer round

Do I have to be a Trainer for x number of years before I can become a TPD?

No. There are many PDs who are salaried GPs or locums. You don't have to be a Trainer or a doctor for that matter. Some GPs find this difficult to understand and accept, but if you think about it, it is not illogical. The PD has to have an understanding and zest for GP education. They need to know *how* that education 'works' and *how* to advise others. For instance, a football coach isn't the best performer in his team, but he's the best person to coach the others into performing well. So, as long as PDs have a good understanding of the requirements for GP training and how it is and could be delivered, then they are usually suitable.

Most GPs just out of vocational training are therefore suitable. Seriously, if you are a newly qualified GP think about applying: you might feel you don't have much to offer, but you do. While you may be working with other TPDs who are well established (and will usually mentor or buddy up with you), you're in the unique position of being the only one who understands it from the trainee's perspective. So, go and ring your deanery and find out if there are any jobs going.

Arghh! I don't have a degree in Medical Education

Don't worry! The minimum requirement is that you have MRCGP. Many but not all PDs have a higher educational qualification. Some deaneries are now asking prospective educators to do a Masters in Medical Education or an equivalent (e.g. Masters in Medical Ethics or in Primary Care) – perhaps you'd like to do that anyway? Despite this academic language, the most important qualification for anyone involved in medical education is **enthusiasm**.

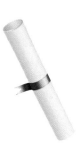

Can non-doctors apply to become Programme Directors?

You bet they can and it is not uncommon to have educationalists who are not doctors. Their contribution has been just as valuable as those of the doctors, and they add an educational dimension and experience which is lacking in those of us who have followed the traditional narrow course into our jobs as PDs.

What makes a good Half-Day Release programme?

Most GP training schemes employ a *heuristic* approach to running their Whole-Day Release (WDR) or Half-Day Release (HDR) programmes. A heuristic approach is one that enables a person to discover or learn things for themselves; a sort of 'hands on' or interactive approach to learning – very much like the way things are in modern general practice.

TPDs are enthusiastic GPs modelling good general practice within an environment that requires and models effective team working and educational principles. For example, some schemes run Balint group sessions[1] in order to model reflective practice that deals with many aspects of the new curriculum[2] which are often difficult to reach in other ways. The promotion of *reflective practice*[4] alongside the development of *positive attitudes* to the doctor–patient relationship, based on a *deeper understanding* of the doctor–patient relationship,[1] is a unique and integral experience of all GP training schemes.

'Setting an example is not the main means of influencing another, it is the only means.'

Albert Einstein

Due to the nature of small-group work, such as occurs in Balint Groups and in Problem-Based Learning (PBL),[3] many aspects of the complexity of general practice are addressed. Group work, in particular, has been shown to help address many aspects of the curriculum that are often elusive in other activities. Examples include changing attitudes and values, personal and professional development, teamwork and collaborative learning.

Should WDR/HDR be replaced by solid blocks of protected teaching time?

Recently, some schemes have switched from a *weekly* educational programme (like Half-Day Release) to teaching in solid blocks of protected time (i.e. whole weeks at different times of the year). This arrangement is not necessarily as popular with trainees as they are with TPDs, because trainees feel that they lose the peer support they gain from weekly teaching and contact. It really depends on what fits in with your local arrangement and what satisfies *most* of the stakeholders.

How do you manage to map your scheme to the delivery of the GP curriculum?[2]

The six domains (Person-centredness, Primary Care Management, Problem Solving, Comprehensive, Community-based and Holistic practice) and the three essential features (Context, Scientific Basis and Attitude) are delivered within GP schemes in an integrated fashion.

- Person-centredness, Comprehensive and Holistic approaches are incorporated within schemes through their educational approach, which values learner-centredness.
- Problem Solving, Primary Care Management and a Community Orientation form the remainder of the educational approach and can be found in every corner of a GP training post.
- Attitude, a Scientific Basis and the Context of learning provide the environmental setting and climate for an effective GP training scheme.

As a Trainer, I have a really good relationship with my GP trainees. What's the TPD–trainee relationship like?

There is a strong pastoral element to the PD–trainee relationship, but usually not as strong as that with the Trainer. However, that's not to say a TPD may not have close knowledge of most trainees on his scheme, particularly those in their final year, who are near to becoming GPs (though this can depend on the size of the scheme and the TPD's role). Besides, some trainees feel they would rather approach their TPD than the Trainer (usually for issues concerning their practice placement). How close that relationship is depends on:

1 how approachable you are
2 the personality of the trainee and
3 the size of your scheme (much easier to get to know trainees on a 1–1 level in a small scheme).

What's the point of Trainers' workshops?

Trainers' workshops run monthly, quarterly or bi-annually depending on local arrangements. The object of the Trainers' workshop is to foster best practice. Here are some things that happen in a Trainers' workshop.

- Through peer support it helps Trainers with their personal development (**incredibly important**).
- It provides some educational content, e.g. discussing new teaching methods.
- It quality assures the approaches to the assessment tools (like COTs and CBDs).
- It enables Trainers to express their views and concerns.
- It helps TPDs disseminate literature and material from the deanery to Trainers.

- It provides a forum where trainees experiencing difficulty can be discussed in order to facilitate a remedial package for them.
- It provides a platform to discuss any 'business' in relation to GP training.

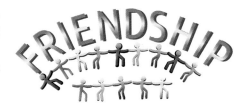

Some Trainers' workshops have trainee representatives. Some prefer the membership just to be open to Trainers – where TPDs are only invited if their expert resource is needed. If you're a Trainer and TPD and thinking of attending your local Trainers' workshop, ask yourself in which role are you attending – TPD or Trainer? Ask other Trainers what their preference is.

If I become a Programme Director, my GP partners would like to know what's in it for the practice. What do I say?

Some of the points below might appear a bit nebulous and, therefore, it's really important to say them with conviction.

- The education–organisation skills that you will pick up can be useful in all kinds of practice events: for example, designing effective in-house educational events, chairing practice meetings and the different approaches to solving practice issues.

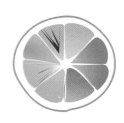

- There will be educational material generated from small-group work or visiting other practices that might be helpful with practice systems and protocols, thus avoiding duplication of work or reinventing the wheel. Examples: home visiting guidelines, chaperone policies, simplifying protocols for complex clinical areas like CKD, etc.
- You'll be 'in the know' about many things (at a strategic level) relating to the future of general practice, GP training and education. This can be advantageous for the practice too in terms of helping with future strategic planning.
- If the practice needs to appoint new doctors, you are in a very good position to head-hunt them (a bit of a perverse incentive!).
- The practice's reputation with people who are interested in education may be enhanced.
- The new challenge may refresh you and make you a more positive person around the practice.

How does GP trainee recruitment work these days?

Prospective GPs who are applying for training apply to a single deanery. Applications are received at deanery level which then arranges a fair and equitable system of assessment (often involving a written assessment, patient simulation exercises plus one or two other things). Following this assessment, the candidates are ranked, and having indicated their preferences for schemes within the deanery on their application forms, posts are allocated accordingly. APDs, PDs, aPDs and Trainers are usually involved in the recruitment process.

This system has the great advantage of being overt and fair. However, it does have disadvantages. Rural or smaller vocational training schemes, which are often remote from their deanery centres and big cities, may suffer from a lack of interest and applications. This system is also a problem for couples and families, who can be separated by large distances.

What about the set-up in Scotland, Northern Ireland and Wales? Similar to the UK?

Except for Scotland, the answer is yes. In Scotland, there are neither TPDs nor Course Organisers. Instead, they have Associate Directors who do everything TPDs do but also carry out additional regional duties (like being the local CME tutor too). Come along to one of their meetings and start networking more widely within the UK.

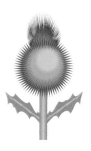

Getting support and inspiration

There will normally be some support from fellow PDs in your deanery, and most deaneries will  have some variety of time-out and induction programmes for GP Educators. The level and type of contact between PDs and the more senior educators at deanery level can be variable: in some places a happy family, in others more corporate and formal perhaps. Wherever you are you can get support and ideas from the national organisation for Programme Directors/ Course Organisers/Trainers/Associate Postgraduate Deans and other Group Facilitators: APCE. They even welcome educators outside of primary care (to encourage multi-professional learning).

Okay, enough of the name dropping; tell me more about APCE

APCE (short for Association of Primary Care Educators) is a new educational organisation whose birth is planned for 2012. They aim to represent *all* educators in Primary Care including Appraisers, Trainers, Programme Directors, GP Tutors amongst others. UKAPD (UK Association of Programme Directors) and NAPCE (National Association of Primary Care Educators) will probably come to an end but it is hoped that their members will subscribe to APCE instead.

You should join APCE for the following reasons.

- Membership is open to *all* primary care educators – Trainers, Training Programme Directors, APDs, Appraisers and so on.
- Their annual membership fee is pretty low, and some deaneries will reimburse it.
- The annual membership includes a subscription to the highly informative *Education in Primary Care* journal (often referred to as the 'Green Journal'); a separate subscription to this costs more!
- They run some educational workshops for new and established TPDs.
- Their website provides some useful online resources and a forum (where you can chat to other colleagues).
- And, finally, their exceptional annual conference is a place where you can meet new people, share exciting ways of doing things, help resolve problems, have some time out, recharge your batteries, find some personal support and have some fun! It's often held in a wonderful location in different parts of the country.

Embracing challenges and changes

APCE particularly welcomes the opportunity to build on current educational practice in GP training schemes while embracing the challenges of the future. Principles of adult education[4] are central to delivery of the new curriculum, and APCE has core educational values such as:

- creating a climate conducive to learning
- utilising the learners' prior knowledge and experience
- delivering learning that has a practical application for trainees
- creating self-directed lifelong learners (by engaging trainees in all aspects of the learning activities).

The purpose of adult education is to help them to learn, not to teach them all they know and thus stop them from carrying on learning.

Rogers[5]

Helping construct meaning and making sense of learning

APCE and its members are committed to providing educational programmes which are constructively aligned[6] with the new curriculum for GPs. There is recognition of the continuing need to provide and support a wide range of teaching and learning activities for GP trainees. By aligning these educational activities, we believe the opportunities are maximised for trainees to construct meaning and make sense of their learning on GP training schemes.

Closing statement

It is great fun being a TPD: being a Programme Director can be a very enjoyable job. Most TPDs do the job because they love it, and not for the money. It widens your circle of contacts and interest. It keeps a doctor in touch with changing educational ideas and standards, and is a motivator. For those of us who've been TPDs for many years we take great pride in watching the achievements and development of our trainees.

We believe that we are developing adult learners with those skills which allow them to enjoy a lifetime of learning. In the final analysis, and speaking as facilitators, the main irony is that a TPD knows when he is being successful by how often he feels redundant! The more redundant you feel, the more likely your trainees have become self-directed learners.

It would be useful to have more hard 'evidence' of our worth, but the reader might reflect that of all the parts of the NHS that other world governments would like to emulate, the UK Primary Care service is what they're most envious of. We remain convinced that we have been doing a public 'good' in being TPDs, and the evidence that this is true is in the young, and not so young, doctors we see in the National Health Service. General practice is one of the most challenging jobs, and the opportunity to train future general practitioners is a great privilege.

A sample of resources on our website
- What do TPDs do? – a conversational piece.
- Acronymania – a useful list of acronyms in GP training and what they mean.
- Money Matters for GP Educators – how the pay scale for GP educators works.

Websites you may like to check out
- **The GP Curriculum**
  The knowledge, skills and attitudes that a GP scheme is expected to provide:
  www.gpcurriculum.co.uk/
  www.rcgp-curriculum.org.uk/
- **The Gold Guide**
  This document tells you about the 'rules' of postgraduate training for all doctors. It's available from the MMC website. Best to type 'gold guide' into Google and then click on the www.mmc. nhs.uk weblink.
- **Bradford VTS Website**
  MRCGP; online resources for trainees and Trainers:
  www.bradfordvts.co.uk
- **GP-training.net**
  MRCGP; online resources for trainees and Trainers:
  www.gp-training.net

Please give us some feedback on this chapter to help shape it for the next edition.
Go to www.essentialgptrainingbook.com and simply click on the title of this chapter.

References
1 Balint M. *The Doctor, His Patient and the Illness*. 2nd ed. London: Pitman Medical; 1964.
2 RCGP. *2010 Curriculum*. Available at: www.rcgp-curriculum.org.uk/rcgp_-_gp_curriculum_documents/gp_curriculum_statements.aspx for general points.
3 Barrows HS, Tamblyn RM. *Problem-based Learning.* New York: Springer; 1980.
4 Brookfield SD. *Understanding and Facilitating Adult Learning.* Milton Keynes: Open University Press; 1986.
5 Rogers A. *Teaching Adults.* Milton Keynes: Open University Press; 1988.
6 Biggs J. *Teaching for Quality Learning at University.* Milton Keynes: Open University Press; 2003.

PART TWO

The Fundamentals of Teaching

4

Powerful Hooks – aims, objectives and ILOs

RAMESH MEHAY – TPD (Bradford) & lead author   JUDY MCKIMM – Dean and Prof. of Medical Education (Univ. Swansea)
MARK WATERS – GP Trainer (Hereford)   DAMIAN KENNY – GP Educationalist (Severn Deanery)
ANNA ROMITO – Researcher in Clinical Education (London Deanery)

What's the point?

Whenever you do *anything* in life, one of the first questions you might ask yourself is that of purpose. Questions like:

- *'What's the point?'*
- *'What am I trying to do/achieve?'*
- *'What do I/they get out of it?'*

The same applies to any teaching session you do: you've got to figure out what you're trying to do. Aims, objectives and learning outcomes help you with that; they're the fundamental building blocks of any teaching session. And if you don't spend time getting your foundations right (and by that we mean really trying to tease out what you're trying to do in some considerable detail), then your teaching session will crumble and fall.

Educators often get mixed up between the terms aims, objectives and intended learning outcomes. We give you a working definition below which should help you make sense of the different levels of activity and who is the focus of the learning intervention.

Defining an aim, objective and learning outcome

Aims, objectives and ILOs

- An aim is a <u>broad</u> statement of intent about the teaching activity:
  - what the teacher plans to cover/achieve in the teaching activity in broad terms
  - e.g. by the end of this chapter, you'll be clearer about aims, objectives and intended learning outcomes (ILOs) and their significance.
- An objective is a <u>specific</u> statement of intent about the teaching activity:
  - what the teacher plans to cover/achieve in the teaching activity/programme in specific terms
  - e.g. by the end of this chapter, we will have covered the definition of an ILO and have gone through the process of writing one up.
- An intended learning outcome (ILO) defines what it is you expect learners to be able to do as a result of the learning experience:
  - it's a bit like an objective except it is from the learner's perspective rather than the teacher's
  - e.g. by the end of this chapter, *you* will be able to *recite* the definition of an ILO and *write up* some examples of ILOs.

Aims and objectives describe the *hopeful* results of teaching activities. However, intended learning outcomes (ILOs) are statements that describe the important knowledge, skills and attitudes you *expect* the learners to *demonstrate* at the end of a programme/event. The ability to *demonstrate* learning is the key point with ILOs and the key word is *doing*. ILOs help us adopt an outcomes-based approach to learning – in contrast to the traditional method of teaching where it is hoped that the learners have learnt something (without checking what or the impact it has had on their personal and/or professional lives). Aims are usually pitched at an aspirational level. Objectives and ILOs are more specific and pitched at a pragmatic level: they help us to achieve our aims. Aims and objectives are teacher-centred – they're often defined by the teacher alone and are usually about where the teacher wants to go with the session. ILOs put the learner back on centre stage and get you to explore the question *'What do I want our learners to do as a result of my teaching activity?'*

> If students are to learn *desired outcomes* in a *reasonably effective manner*, then the teacher's fundamental task is to *get students to engage in learning* activities that are likely to result in their achieving those outcomes. . . . It is helpful to remember that *what the student does* is actually more important in determining what is learned than what the teacher does.
>
> (Shuell, 1986: 429)[1]

Forget about objectives and think of aims and ILOs instead

Most educators have been taught to think in terms of 'aims' and 'objectives'. Unfortunately, the way objectives are written is so variable. Some educationalists write them up in terms of the teaching intention (*'We will look at xxx in this session to help us understand more about yyy'*). Others write them in terms of the expected learning outcome (*'After this session, you will be expected to be able to do xxx whenever you come across yyy'*). For that reason, we would say ditch the objectives and use ILOs instead. See ILOs as the new objectives – they are learner-centred and get you to question what you are really expecting them to do as a result of the teaching activity.

> Aims are where you want to go.
> Objectives are how you get there.
> ILOs are where the learners will arrive.

Can we scrap the aims too and just stick with the ILOs?

Before we answer this, consider travelling from Leeds to Birmingham.

- The aim in this case would be *'to get to Birmingham from Leeds'* (**the destination**).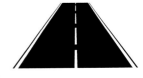
- The objectives would be the individual directions to get to the destination: *'take the M1, then the M42 and finally, the M6'* (**the steps of the journey**).
- The ILO might be map reading – working out which route to take in the first place (**the outcome**) – which in this case might not be the M1 if it happens to be clogged up with traffic that day.

If you scrap the aims, the ILOs become meaningless because you're then in the situation where you have a route, but you don't know where you're heading! Think of aims and ILOs as partners – never consider one without the other. Also note how ILOs are all about developing learners for new challenges – not just about getting from Leeds to Birmingham, but developing their skills to navigate other journeys.

Why defining ILOs *properly* is important

Before the teaching activity

- ILOs encourage teachers to focus on what they want their **learners to be able to do** as a direct result of their teaching activity rather than on what they simply wish to cover. Learners become the central focus (as they should be).
- ILOs help you work out the **content and structure** of the session. The process of defining ILOs helps you (the teacher) clarify **what is important**. For example, educators often formulate learning sessions which are over-ambitious and over-inclusive. An ILO approach reminds the teacher to keep things in the **real world**: what is realistically achievable given the time and resources?
- ILOs ensure that **all stakeholders** (learners, teachers, teaching establishment, etc.) are clear about **what is expected of learners** right from the start. If you can tweak the ILOs to really whet your audience's appetite, you can use them to '**hook**' people effortlessly into your session.
- And now that you've worked out what is expected, selecting **appropriate educational methods** to help achieve that becomes so much easier.

During the teaching activity

- ILOs help you keep the teaching session on track: either reminding you where you are at or, if a session goes off at a tangent, helping you to bring it back and refocus.

After the teaching activity

- ILOs provide a framework to help you **evaluate** your teaching session and determine whether you have achieved what you set out to achieve – simply check out your ILOs.
- ILOs help you develop appropriate **assessment** tools or methods – again, simply build up something around the original ILOs. When all the different bits (ILOs, methods and assessment) are nicely in tune with each other, we call this **constructive alignment**.

Constructive alignment:[2] the alignment of methods and assessments to the learning activities in the ILOs is called constructive alignment. It ensures that all parts of the teaching system are in accord in supporting appropriate student learning. It is based on the notion that meaning cannot be imposed or transmitted by direct instruction. Instead, meaning is personal – it depends on motives, intentions, prior knowledge and experience; it is created (constructed) by the learners individually for themselves when they *engage* in learning activities. It's covered in more detail in Chapter 6: Teaching from Scratch.

Top Tip: If you spend time on working out the aims and ILOs of your teaching session, planning the rest of it becomes a breeze.

Give me an example . . .

 Let's say you're getting repeated requests from your learners for a teaching session on telephone consultations. Having discussed their particular difficulties via email and in person, it transpires that while most don't have a problem with giving clinical advice over the phone, their *discomfort* stems from not knowing whether they've tackled the patient's agenda.

From this, your broad **aim** might be: *'How to do telephone consultations and feel happier'*. The word 'happier' is the antithesis of 'discomfort' and hopefully this will hook them in.

Your **ILOs** might be (note the verbs in italics):

After this session:
1 You will be able to *identify* the communication skills required to explore a patient's ideas, concerns and expectations.
2 You will be able to *apply* those skills in practice during telephone consultations.
3 You will be able to *formulate* a management plan (including an explanation) which incorporates those ideas, concerns and expectations.
4 You will check for the patient's understanding and agreement before finishing the telephone consultation.

These ILOs now tell you what **content** to put into your session *and* suggest how to deliver it (the **methodology**). For example, you may wish to achieve ILO 1 via group discussion after hearing a selection of audio recordings. Do you think a lecture presentation to cover ILOs 2 and 3 will suffice? No – because you need something practical, not theoretical. Perhaps a demonstration followed by practice or role play. To **evaluate** your session you will need to know whether the session made a difference for the learners: are they happier with telephone consultations now? You can do this by initiating a discussion at a follow-up session. **Can you see how clearly setting the aims and ILOs from the start makes the next steps (defining content, methodology and evaluation) so much easier?**

 Top Tip: Some facilitators have aims and objectives written out separately on a flip chart or displayed on an overhead projector throughout their session. This is an easy way of helping the facilitator *and* the learners keep track of where they're at in the session.

ILOs should tackle learning needs

A learning need can be thought of as a developmental need – something the learner needs to develop or improve on. An ILO is a direct response to satisfying a learning need. The more time you invest in identifying the learning needs in the first place, the easier it is to develop ILOs and plan the rest of the teaching session. This doesn't have to take lots of time. It can be a quick 'check-in' with the learners at the start of the session. You might also stop and check understanding during a session in order to define additional evolving learning needs. Clearly, you need to provide the right learning environment so that learners are comfortable voicing what they don't understand or what they want you to cover (even though that may be different from what you had planned). Your job as a teacher is to balance what learners need to achieve (based on a pre-defined curriculum) and meeting specific (maybe individual) demands on the day.

Domains of learning

Learning needs (and thus ILOs) usually fall into three categories (called the domains of learning): **K**nowledge, **S**kills and **A**ttitudes (KSA).

The knowledge domain (sometimes called the **cognitive domain**) explores understanding of facts, concepts and principles.

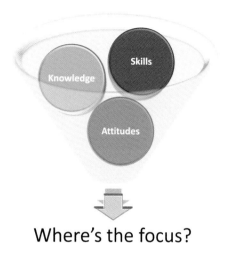

Where's the focus?

The skills domain (sometimes called the **psycho-motor domain**) is about the acquisition of specific skills like communication skills, clinical skills and problem-solving. It has three phases: (1) *the cognitive phase* (where one has to think about what one is doing); (2) *the fixative phase* (where one practises and practises to get it right); and (3) *the autonomous phase* (where the skill eventually becomes automatic). Think back to when you started to learn how to drive a car: do these three phases now make sense?

The attitudes domain (sometimes called the **affective domain**) explores *values and attitudes*. Examples of values are honesty, justice and equality. Examples of attitudes are safety, cooperation and personal care for patients.

Here is the earlier set of ILOs but this time expressed in KSO terms:

After this session:

1 You will have *explored* the value of ascertaining a patient's ideas, concerns and expectations for yourself. (attitudes)
2 You will be able to *identify* the communication skills required to explore a patient's ideas, concerns and expectations. (knowledge)
3 You will be able to *apply* those skills in practice. (skills)
4 You will be able to *formulate* a management plan (including explanation) which incorporates those ideas, concerns and expectations. (skills)

Note how the KSA method encourages a balanced approach to setting intended learning outcomes – we added an extra ILO to cover the attitudinal domain (although you don't have to cover each domain).

How do I actually work out their learning needs?

Use Johari's Window! Joseph Luft and Harry Ingham[3] created this tool in 1955 (Johari comes from **Jo**seph and **Har**ry). This model reminds us that while learners may be aware of some of their learning needs, there are some that they are not aware of, though others around them are. It encourages us to take a comprehensive approach to exploring learning needs – looking at them from all sorts of perspectives and angles. Extra learning needs are uncovered to both parties as you both explore the blind spot, façade and unknown boxes. Consequently, the arena becomes bigger (i.e. where both parties know) and the other boxes become smaller – the ultimate aim of the Johari Window.

THE LEARNER

	Things I know	Things I don't know
Others know	**ARENA** — We both are aware of something about me	**BLIND SPOT** — Others are aware of something about me that I am not
Others don't know	**FACADE** — I am aware of something about me that others are not	**UNKNOWN** — Neither of us is aware (just yet)

OTHERS

The façade box tells us that there are things the learners *themselves* know that they need to learn and develop. So, how about asking them!

- Ask your current trainee – or email the intended audience (or a subset of them) – what they want to get from the session; what difficulties they have.
- You could do an online survey (MisterPoll: www.misterpoll.com or Survey Monkey: www.surveymonkey.com).

However, the blind spot reminds us that there are things the learners might not know about themselves but others do. For instance, a trainee might be doing the same thing for all patients who come in for a repeat prescription of the contraceptive pill and may not realise there is something amiss. One of the other doctors may pick up on the lack of a BP recording and self-breast examination counselling. Another example – a trainee might feel he is plodding on with patients okay, but the receptionists might mention to the Trainer how a number of patients have unofficially expressed how rude he is. This tells us that the learners are not the only stakeholders who can determine their learning needs. People around them are invaluable too. Here, the Johari Window gives a framework for learners to learn more about themselves and their practice by others telling them or giving feedback on performance. So the arena is expanded through a combination of asking and telling.

- First, ask yourself what it is you want your learners to be able to do as a result of your teaching-learning session. You may want to refer to important checklists to help you, like NICE guidance and the RCGP's curriculum. What common learning themes have emerged from informal feedback or the educational tools (CBDs, RCAs, COTs etc.) you have used with trainees so far? Alternatively, think about the types of difficulty you had as a trainee or are still having as a jobbing GP (which is what all trainees are aspiring to be). Your opinion counts because you've been through the training process, and you may well have insights that they don't just yet.

- Ask other new young doctors in your practice – what would have been helpful when they were trainees?
- What are the experiences and opinions of your fellow Trainers and Training Programme Directors?
- And don't forget about non-medical staff: they can give you insights on non-clinical areas like communication skills, organisational abilities and attitudes.

 Top Tip: The Johari Window can be used in another way – namely, to explore relationships. Check out: www.wisc-online.com/objects/ViewObject.aspx?ID=OIC2101a

---

How to write up an ILO – five easy steps

Some educationalists are very particular about how you write ILOs. Writing ILOs is actually quite a difficult task which gets easier the more you do it (like any skill). There is a guide on our website that describes in detail the rules for writing up ILOs in true educational terms. However, what we're going to provide here is a rough and ready practical guide for those who aren't particularly interested in a PhD in formulating ILOs.

1 Work out the **learning needs** for your learning audience. This might already be specified in a curriculum or syllabus. Your learners might have identified them for you, or you might need to think about them for yourself.
2 From your learning list, formulate **your aim** – which should be a general statement of intent. Write down what you plan to achieve in your teaching session in one sentence.
3 From your aim formulate some **ILOs in KSA specific terms** (Knowledge, Skills & Attitudes). Remember, ILOs answer the question *'What is it that I want my learners to be able to do as a result of the teaching session?'*. To make things easier, grab a sheet of A4, fold it to make three columns and then consider each KSA domain systematically in turn. Refer to the list of learning needs when doing this (and you don't have to end up with something in each area).

   Miller's Pyramid[4] can help you refine each ILO you develop by reminding you to consider which level of performance (or competence) you are aiming for – is it cognition or behaviour?

The Fundamentals of Teaching

Miller's Prism of Clinical Competence (a.k.a. Miller's Pyramid)

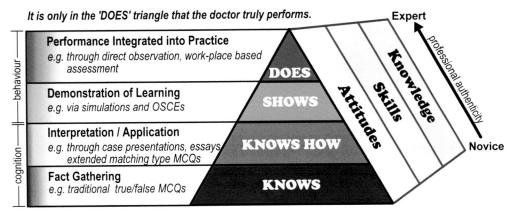

It is only in the 'DOES' triangle that the doctor truly performs.

Performance Integrated into Practice
e.g. through direct observation, work-place based assessment — **DOES**

Demonstration of Learning
e.g. via simulations and OSCEs — **SHOWS**

Interpretation / Application
e.g. through case presentations, essays, extended matching type MCQs — **KNOWS HOW**

Fact Gathering
e.g. traditional true/false MCQs — **KNOWS**

Based on work by Miller GE. The Assessment of Clinical Skills/Competence/Performance. *Acad Med.* 1990; **65**(9): 63-7.
Adapted by Drs. Ramesh Mehay and Roger Burns (January 2009).

In this pyramid, the lower levels only test cognition (or knowledge), and this is where inexperienced trainees usually sit: they either *know* or *know how* to do something. The higher levels test behaviour. That is, whether they can apply (*show* or *do*) what they know in practice. Ultimately, the best is the *'does'* level because it is at that level a doctor truly performs. However, that's not to say that the lower-level cognition zones are of low-level importance – learners usually progress through the zones, and they have to start somewhere! Perhaps your audience consists of relatively new inexperienced ST1 trainees? Note how this particular diagram also illustrates which assessment method you might use for each level. For further information on Miller's Pyramid *see* Chapter 29: Assessment and Competence.

4 Now refine each ILO to make sure it contains an **active 'doing' verb** – like explore, perform, examine, analyse and so on. There's a whole list of verbs available for each of the knowledge, skills and attitudes domains that you might want to refer to. This list is called **Bloom's taxonomy** of learning objectives and is covered in detail in Chapter 10: Five Pearls of Educational Theory. For example, if you were planning to deliver a teaching session focused on knowledge, you would use verbs from the cognitive taxonomy provided below.[5]

LOWER ORDER THINKING SKILLS (LOTS)			HIGHER ORDER THINKING SKILLS (HOTS)		
REMEMBER	**UNDERSTAND**	**APPLY**	**ANALYSE**	**EVALUATE**	**CREATE**
• describe or state • define or identify • list, state or tell • tabulate, match or select • reproduce	• compare or contrast • distinguish or differentiate • discuss or explain • group together or put in order	• apply, transfer or relate • classify or chart • demonstrate or illustrate • solve or calculate • construct, modify or develop	• analyse, infer or correlate • compare or contrast • connect, divide, separate or classify • prioritise, arrange, or order	• assess, measure, rank or grade • judge, decide, appraise, criticise, defend, justify, persuade, convince or conclude • reframe	• combine, integrate or rearrange • create, design, devise, formulate or compose • speculate or anticipate • facilitate or negotiate • generalise away from the specific

New Bloom's Taxonomy for the Cognitive Domain (after Anderson & Krathwohl, 2001)

First, you would need to decide which level of performance within this domain you are aiming for. Are you hoping that learners can simply *understand* what you say, *apply* it, or *create* new ways of using that information? Then you pick a verb from the appropriate column. Don't forget to look at the other taxonomies, which you can find in Chapter 10: Five Pearls of Educational Theory.

 Top Tip: There are some action verbs to avoid like the plague: *have awareness, appreciate, become familiar with, grasp, have critical awareness* and *understand*. They are poor because they are either too vague or difficult to demonstrate. For example, how do you demonstrate having better awareness?

5 **Final checks**
- Make sure **each ILO refers to the learner**. Each ILO needs to describe student rather than teacher behaviour. '*You will be able to examine for xxxx.*'
- Double-check that each ILO **describes a learning outcome, not a process**.
- Aim for **3–5 ILOs**. If you have loads more than this, it's likely that you're being too ambitious, and you will run out of time. Remember, ILOs focus on items that are '**essential**' (*important* for the learners to know) rather than the '**desirable**' (*nice* to know). Scrap any that do not fit this bill. If there are still too many, consider delivering your event over a number of sessions.
- Prefix your 'ILO set' with the **introductory phrase**: '*After this session:*'

And that's it. You're done.

How to add spice to ILOs and really hook people in

It's important to create ILOs that whet the appetites of individual learners within the learner audience. How can you expect them to engage otherwise? And when we refer to the 'hook', we mean really pulling them in – getting them to that state where they say, '*Yes, I want some of that, and I want it now!*' in contrast to '*Mmmm . . . that sounds interesting*'. The hook is the single most powerful element of a teaching session that can help you mesmerise, entice and even seduce your learners. The title and agenda (the aims and ILOs) provide the ideal opportunity to get your powerful hooks in so that you can attract your learners towards a change in behaviour.

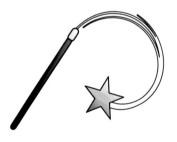

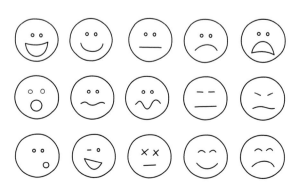

A lot of people think it is *logic* that leads to a change in behaviour, but we would argue that it is *feelings*. For example, nearly all smokers know that smoking has ill-health effects – but does that stop them smoking? No! A lot of them stop after they've had their first *scary* heart attack, or because they're getting to that age where they're *afraid* of some ill-health effect kicking in. It's feelings that matter. Each ILO is a logical statement. However, if you want to hook people in, *add* an emotive element that resonates and stirs up feelings within them. For example, which of these two tickles your taste buds that little bit more?

● *'After this session, you will be able to do a neurological examination.'*
● *'After this session, you will be able to do a neurological examination easily in 10 minutes and **feel flustered about time no more**'.*

A few more examples:
● *'After this session, you will **feel confident** in applying some basic CBT techniques to help patients.'*
● *'After this session, you will be able to apply some useful reattribution techniques to heart-sink patients and therefore **feel more positive** about them.'*

The first step to formulating the emotive element is to identify the learners' fears, concerns and frustrations. Then it's a case of signposting that your session will help resolve that feeling. Publishers of diet books are masters at hooking people through their feelings. Look at this selection of diet book titles:

● *Lose Weight without having to Exercise* (this hook works on people's **fear** of exercise).
● *Don't Lose your Mind, Lose your Weight!* (this hook works on the **concern** that losing weight might stress them out).
● *You Can Be Thin: the Ultimate Programme to End Dieting . . . Forever* (this hook works on the **frustration** from repeated diet failures).

The next time you run an educational session, see how you can refine the title and the ILOs to incorporate emotive elements in a similar way. Maybe some of these will help:

Emotive elements to hook your audience

● 'be trouble-free'
● 'working through the chaos'
● 'to re-energise you'
● 'helping you to . . .'

● 'don't be confused, be clear'
● 'the easy-peasy way'
● 'be guilt-free'
● 'effortlessly in 10 minutes'

Try and make **negative** statements sound **positive** as we have done here.

 Top Tip: If you'd like a few more 'emotive' phrases, surf an online book store and type in something like 'lose weight' or 'stop smoking' to see the variety of ways authors and publishing houses do it.

Closing statement

We'd like to end by saying that although defining aims and ILOs for any teaching session is a fundamental necessity, it's by no means an easy task. You'll become better at it with repeated practice but, even then, most of us don't get it right on the first go. Formulating good ILOs is an iterative process requiring repeated refinements on the initial attempts. Hang on in there and don't move on until you're happy with what you've developed.

A sample of resources on our website

- The Johari Window.
- Formulating ILOs and Constructive Alignment.
- Do Intended Learning Outcomes (ILOs) Stifle Creativity?

Other chapters you may like to read

- Chapter 6: Teaching from Scratch
- Chapter 8: Teaching Gems
- Chapter 10: Five Pearls of Educational Theory.

Please give us some feedback on this chapter to help shape it for the next edition.
Go to www.essentialgptrainingbook.com and simply click on the title of this chapter.

References

1 Shuell TJ. Cognitive conceptions of learning. *RER.* 1986; **56**: 411–36.
2 Biggs JB. *Teaching for Quality Learning at University.* 2nd ed. Buckingham: Open University Press; 2003.
3 Luft J, Ingham H. *The Johari Window: a graphic model of interpersonal awareness.* Los Angeles: UCLA; 1955.
4 Miller GE. The assessment of clinical skills/competence/performance. *Acad Med.* 1990; **65**(9): 63–7.
5 Anderson LW, Krathwohl D, editors. *A Taxonomy for Learning, Teaching and Assessing: a revision of Bloom's taxonomy of educational objectives.* New York: Longman; 2001.

A Smorgasbord of Educational Methods

5

ELIZABETH (BITTY) MULLER – TPD (Burton on Trent) & lead author   RAMESH MEHAY – TPD (Bradford)
SHAKE SEIGEL – TPD (Burton on Trent)   IAIN LAMB – Associate Advisor (SE Scotland)

Introduction

There are a great number of educational methods and teaching techniques available. Having a set lecture every week at the Day/Half-Day Release course gets boring. We would encourage you to employ a number of educational methods when you run a session. Here are our reasons why.

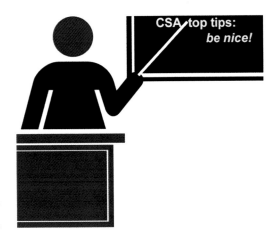

The research shows that the more *interactive* the methods you use, the more effective the learning (by effective, they mean the longer it stays in the brain).

Furthermore, if you use a variety of methods, you are more likely to stimulate a variety of *senses* in the learner (multi-modal learning). This will mean that the information will be encoded onto the brain in multiple areas and hopefully stored in long-term memory.

Our final reason is that any large group will have individuals with different learning styles and preferences (*see* Chapter 11: Learning and Personality Styles in Practice). Using a variety of methods which trigger different senses will help you to engage a greater proportion of your audience (each of whom is different).

Alignment

In this chapter, we're going to provide you with a big list of different educational methods and the pros and cons of each. This should help you to 'pick and mix' methods and match them to the type of session you are running. It is important to stop for a moment, look at your aims, objectives and intended learning outcomes and marry your educational methods to them. For example, if you want to help trainees *do* a shoulder examination, a lecture with pretty pictures is not the best way. What you want is a practical, 'hands on' session.

The lecture

Let's start with the familiar – this is an oral presentation to convey information to a group of people. The speaker (the lecturer) usually stands at the front of the room while the audience sits at the back. The lecturer talks and the audience listens.

Pros

- Lectures often receive a lot of criticism from educationalists. However, lectures are good for presenting specific information about a topic to a large group in a limited time frame.
- Some lectures are engaging – probably due to a combination of a talented speaker showing energy and dynamism who also makes sure the subject matter has 'pulling' power.
- In terms of Honey and Mumford's learning styles,[1] Theorist and Reflectors get more from lectures than do Activists and Pragmatists (*see* Chapter 11: Learning and Personality Styles in Practice).

Cons

- Lecturing is a one-way method of communication. Lectures tend to be non-participatory and the learning tends to be passive. The lecturer transmits knowledge while the audience is expected to receive it. Whether that actually happens is highly variable. Active learning does not happen.
- The lecturer will often transmit knowledge that they deem as important, which may be at variance with the audience's learning needs.
- Unless the speaker is well-prepared and lively, lectures can result in 'death by PowerPoint', and very little learning takes place.

Facilitator tips

- Ask your audience in advance of the lecture what their learning needs are. Make these the focus of your session.
- Speak for around 40 minutes and make some provision for questions.
- Consider breaking the lecture down into chunks and employ other educational methods in between the chunks (like buzz groups – see below). So, you might start off by talking about something for 10–15 minutes, then breaking by giving the audience a task to do – perhaps discussing something in pairs, then coming back to draw conclusions from those discussions before resuming the lecture again. And so the process continues.
- Finally, if you're running a course and getting others to speak, brief them on these tips. We've seen a number of awful lectures from guest or expert speakers, but you can't blame them if they've never been properly briefed.

Buzz groups (as part of a lecture)

Lectures can become boring and the purpose of buzz groups is to combat this. At some stage in a lecture, audience members are invited to turn to a neighbour and share opinion or reaction for a short time. Alternatively, the whole audience may be broken into smaller groups for discussion and feedback during a plenary session.

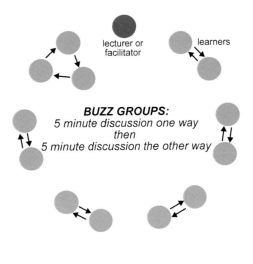

BUZZ GROUPS:
5 minute discussion one way
then
5 minute discussion the other way

Pros

- Combats boredom and inactivity.
- It helps generate questions and thoughts for the rest of the session – makes learning an active process.

Cons

- Difficult to manage if the audience is large – re: summarising the discussions.
- It can be time-consuming, i.e. breaking up, discussing and then feeding back.

The mini-lecture

In a mini-lecture, there is a short burst of fact or theory *during* a group activity. The idea is to tease out key 'take home' messages from a discussion and to summarise or place some sort of structure to them in order to 'scaffold' the learning.

Pros

- A good way of doing 'master classes'.
- It breaks a teaching and learning session – stops it from becoming dry.
- Adds structure to what could otherwise be chaotic group activity.

Cons

- If you're a verbose presenter, you will revert to talking too much!

Facilitator tips

- Be fairly rigid about timekeeping and the mini format.
- Facilitate by asking a few questions to help direct the discussion. Display your own ignorance or lack of understanding to encourage other trainees to feel safe enough to do the same (i.e. to rid their fear of looking daft to their peers).
- Get group members involved – help them develop their presentation skills. Demonstrate that PowerPoint is not the only way of getting points across. If PowerPoint is used, encourage them to use pictures as well as words.

Some learners will moan, saying, *'Why did we have to go through the discussion? Why could you not have just distilled the key messages – it would have saved half the time?'* You may need to revisit learning theory with them – how simply telling someone doesn't mean it will stay in their brains for long, *but* if they synthesise the key points themselves, it just might. *See* Kolb's learning cycle[2] in Chapter 10: Five Pearls of Educational Theory.

Debate

Derived from the old French word for 'quarrel', it has come to mean a public discussion; it allows teams of individuals to argue the merits of a proposition, without necessarily owning the opinions expressed. It can be used on a course – especially if there is currently a hot controversial issue like commissioning, management costs, consortia, prescribing and expensive treatments. By arranging a debate it allows trainees to explore the issues in greater depth, exploring both pros and cons.

Pros
- Good for dealing with controversial issues (especially if no right or wrong answer).
- It helps develop analytic, presentation and fluency skills.
- Good for trainees with medico-political aspirations.

Cons
- Point scoring rather than deep analysis of the issue can take over!
- Group members are often passive as their 'leader' takes the stand.
- Only the more flamboyant and expressive outgoing trainees may get involved; quieter, more reflective trainees may be left out of the process.

Facilitator tips
- Give enough time for each group to formulate their argument/defence.
- Using a yellow and red card system to indicate to the speaker when to close his or her speech to allow the other person their turn. Yellow card – 1 minute left; red card – stop now.
- You may wish to invite a 'subject expert' along to listen to the debate and comment afterwards on the quality and accuracy of information presented, e.g. chair or secretary of your LMC or consortium.

Seminar/workshop

A seminar is a systematic educational group session which is under the direction of a teacher or group of teachers (who usually have some expertise in the given subject).

In a seminar, the focus is on a particular topic around which everyone has some knowledge or experience (no matter how strong or mild). The purpose of the seminar is to help the participants get a better grounding of the topic, practise skills, generate practical ideas and generally help them overcome any obstacles. Part of this is achieved through engaging in dialogue with others. It is a relatively informal affair, but for it to work all members must actively participate. Seminars are often run by academic, professional and commercial organisations. The seminar may run over a few days and may consist of parts that run periodically throughout the year.

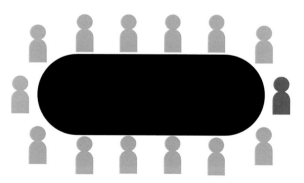

Pros
- It's interactive – participants share ideas with each other.
- Seminars usually have some flexibility about them – the group's learning needs are likely to be identified and tackled.
- It's cost-effective – allows exploration of a subject with one expert resource.

Cons
- Teaching a large group with only one 'expert' can be exhausting and sometimes difficult to manage.

Facilitator tips
- Try not to think of the bare minimum – if you've got a large group, get in some additional 'helping' facilitators. A seminar can be very poorly evaluated if there is only one expert with no flexibility to provide 1–1 support when it is needed; you will end up spreading yourself too thinly.

Cluster group teaching

Cluster grouping is an educational process where you split a large group into clusters based on a particular focus. The purpose is to be able to provide teaching and learning that is contextually relevant to that particular group. It originally came from clustering gifted school children from their peers (research showed that gifted children did not do well when placed in mixed ability groups). However, in our context, think of a focus other than intellect. For 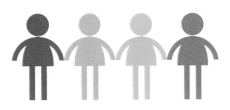 example, at Half-Day Release, you might want to run some sessions by grouping the trainees according to their ST training year.

> At our local day release programme we ran a communication skills session for all GP trainees on our scheme. When it came to evaluating the session, we noticed that most ST3s (in GP posts) loved the session, but those in hospital posts didn't. The most regular comment was that they couldn't see how to apply it back on the wards. Perhaps we would have fared better if we had two groups with two facilitators – one for communication skills in general practice and the other for the hospital setting.

Pros
- Clustering is a good way of delivering a teaching session that is contextually relevant to a large group with different groups of learning needs.
- The intellectual, social and emotional needs of each particular cluster group can be addressed.
- The pace of the teaching session can be adjusted to the cluster group.

Cons
- We all have different experiences. Splitting a group restricts the cross-fertilisation of ideas. An ST1 can learn lots from an ST3 and vice versa.
- You need a facilitator for each of the cluster groups.

Facilitator tips
- Be learner centred. Spend some time teasing out what your cluster group's particular learning needs or difficulties are.
- Remain flexible in your teaching style and value the differences within your 'classroom'.

Task groups

This is where you break down a complex problem into manageable tasks to aid its resolution. A large audience is then split into subgroups, and each is allocated one of the tasks. They work to resolve the tasks (which might take hours, days or weeks) and then the large group re-forms to share what each has found.

Pros
- Active learning, peer learning, syndicate learning (which mimics general practice).
- A good way of breaking down a large complex topic or issue.
- A collaborative way of problem-solving.
- Self-resourcing and thus economical.

Cons
- Reporting can be laborious.
- Sometimes trainees don't take others' contributions seriously.
- New trainees might find it more difficult to tackle issues and process large amounts of new knowledge in such a short time.

Peer-led learning groups

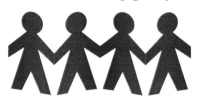

Peer-to-peer learning involves trainees sharing their knowledge and experience with one another. Peer-led learning involves getting a group of learners (or an individual learner) to teach something to another group of learners. It is based on the notion that the preparation and process of teaching is also an effective form of learning.

Our Half-Day Release (HDR) consists of four groups of trainees (of mixed ST years) who stay in their group throughout the three year programme – primarily to help build a little 'community' of learners. We always have some peer-led learning sessions on our programme, and it works like this. A learning list for the whole scheme is identified first. Then we ask each subgroup to pick a learning theme from the list, and then they are allocated their own particular half day to 'run their show'. For the rest of the half day, they go off into their small groups and start the planning process. Each group has a facilitator, just in case they go off track or need help. Before home time, each group decides when, where and how to continue the planning process until the performance day.

Pros
- It recognises that every participant can be a teacher and a learner. Learning is reinforced by the teaching process.
- It is learner and participant driven. Peers understand the goals, issues and pressures their other peers face. They speak the same language and can help each other distil critical pieces of

information. Others are also more likely to hear and internalise messages if they can relate to the messenger – often with a resultant change in attitudes and behaviours!

- Individuals learn planning, teaching and presentation skills.
- Good for teaching multifaceted aspects of the GP curriculum.

Cons

- Agreeing on a date and time for all individuals within a teaching group to meet up can be difficult to say the least.
- Newbies may not have crisp/effective teaching and presentation skills to hold the attention of fellow participants.

Facilitator tips

- Get the group to start working out their aims and objectives before they go on to methodology and delivery (i.e. teach them about lesson planning).
- Set limits on PowerPoint presentations – suggest a maximum of five slides for any given session. Encourage interactive methods, video clips, etc.
- Watch out for some people who don't engage. Even if participants can't be there on the day they can always do some sort of preparation to help the others (and ultimately 'do their bit' for their little 'community' of learners).
- At the end of the first session, make sure future *planning* sessions are set.
- If the group seems to run autonomously (i.e. without your help), let them run by themselves (even if you feel redundant). You must support the self-sustaining nature of peer networks.
- The ultimate role of the Programme Directors is to create learning spaces where peers can meet and learn from each other.

Brainstorming

This is a group creativity technique which aims to generate a great variety and quantity of ideas in relation to a problem in a short space of time. Given a problem, members are asked to suspend their critical faculty and produce *any* ideas and approaches to the question that occur to them. The group then proceeds to evaluate, elaborate, discuss and resolve.

Osborn's four ground rules for brainstorming[3]

These have been formulated to stimulate ideas and creativity and reduce inhibitions:

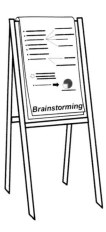
Brainstorming

1 **Focus on quantity** – the greater the number of ideas generated, the greater the chance of producing an effective (and creative) solution.
2 **Withhold criticism** – all ideas are recorded unchallenged no matter how bizarre they may seem. If you challenge people as soon as they say something, it will put them and others off. So, suspend judgement!
3 **Welcome unusual ideas** – encourages others to think laterally too. Unusual ideas often result in radical ways of doing things more effectively.
4 **Combine and improve ideas** – one idea on its own might not hold much value but when combined with another idea it might lead to something totally new, innovative and effective.

Pros

- It is fun, stimulating, participatory and enhances group cohesion.
- Quick and easy.
- Good for solving problems, making decisions and exploring judgements/values.

Cons

- Most people can't come up with creative ideas 'on the spot'. Creative ideas occur spontaneously in places like the shower.
- One person can dominate the discussion, and not allow others to express their opinions.
- Research suggests that good ideas often depend on whether there are equally good incentives for generating the ideas in the first place.[4]
- Research suggests that a volume of ideas must not be confused with productivity. Many ideas from brainstorming are of low quality and simply impractical.[5]

Facilitator tips

- Discussions can drift – you may need to keep them on track.
- Make sure quieter group members get to have their say, e.g. having a round-robin check with each group member being asked for their opinion.
- Electronic brainstorming (e.g. brainstorming anonymously on the web or via peer–peer electronic systems) works better than face-to-face brainstorming.[6] This is probably due to anonymity and fewer inhibitions or anxieties. People can think carefully before they type and there is no requirement for an immediate response. There are often greater volumes of people involved too. How about giving this a go?

Reverse brainstorming

The problem with traditional brainstorming is that coming up with a good idea on the spot is difficult! As we said, creative ideas and solutions usually occur in the shower or on the loo. So, an alternative creative and more effective way is the reverse brainstorm. The concept is simple: rather than brainstorm what you want, brainstorm the opposite of what you want – what you don't want or how to make sure something is unsuccessful. Then, *reverse* those ideas into possible positive solutions.

Reverse brainstorming – instructions

1 Identify/define problem or challenge. Write it down.
2 Either ask *'How can I **cause** the problem'* or *'How can I **make things worse?'***
3 Tell the audience: *'The more outrageous or destructive the idea the better!'*
4 Brainstorm the reverse problem and note down ideas. (Do not reject anything.)
5 Now look at the ideas and reverse them into solutions for the original problem.
6 Evaluate each solution.

I was asked to run a session on dysfunctional consultations. I was prepared and ready, but on the day could not get the blasted IT equipment to work. I asked the trainees to talk among themselves for 15 minutes, while I thought about how I might do things. Even the techies couldn't fathom the computer problems.

And, finally, it came – I'd just read about the reverse brainstorm technique, and I wanted to put it to the test – what better place than to do it here. So, without any IT stuff I simply asked the audience the question: 'If I was one of your regular heart-sink patients, how could you upset me?' Rather than brainstorming the responses, I split them into small groups to role play the scenario first (picking out some trainees beforehand to give them specific patient instructions). In the role play people were alive and dynamic; I could see some having fun. Afterwards, we brainstormed the things that really ticked the patient off. Everyone contributed, including the trainees playing the patient.

With the list generated, we grouped them into themes and then reversed them to form solutions. By the end, we'd generated so many practical ways of handling heart-sinks. The group came up with things that I hadn't even considered in my slide notes! And so many commented on how useful the session was (and probably tonnes better than my original plan).

We hope you can see how this alternative approach harnesses negative energy such as cynicism, sarcasm and hostility to spark creativity.

Pros
- It focuses on generating robust solutions rather than a volume of them.
- It imparts new perspectives to the trainee – encourages lateral thinking.
- It's a fun way of doing things – learners have a laugh while learning.

Cons
- It takes time!

Facilitator tips
- Follow the basic rules for brainstorming.
- Have faith in the process.

The Disney creativity strategy

Walt Disney was very good at turning fantasy (creative ideas) into reality. When he was creating stories, Disney used three perceptual fields. The model was refined by neurolinguistic programming (NLP) expert Robert Dilts.[7] The following three phases should be given equal time and investment.

1 **The Dreaming phase** – where ideas are explored without constraints of reality to get maximum creativity out of an idea: *the visionary*.
2 **The Realistic phase** – where the ideas created are honed down into a realistic set of goals to make things happen: *the pragmatic producer*.
3 **The Critic or evaluator phase** – where the idea and goals (i.e. what the dreamer and realist produce) are evaluated and checked for possible problems and constraints: *the eagle-eyed evaluator*.

Creativity as a total process involves the coordination of these three sub-processes: dreamer, realist and critic. A dreamer without a realist cannot turn ideas into tangible expressions. A critic and a dreamer without a realist just become stuck in a perpetual conflict. The dreamer and a realist might create things, but they might not achieve a high degree of quality without a critic. The critic helps to evaluate and refine the products of creativity.

Robert Dilts[7]

Pros
- It helps your team be creative and test out whether their ideas can be realised.
- It's a balanced approach to problem-solving – the three areas represent different pull and push forces.

Cons
- Allowing criticism during the dreaming phase may abort and stifle contribution and creativity.

Facilitation tips
- Keep each perceptual phase separate.
- Explicitly signpost which phase you are in so that everyone is clear.

Snowballing

This is a method for reaching a consensus of ideas and thoughts on a particular topic. Participants are divided into pairs to discuss a topic; they distil their thoughts and write down key issues. After 5–10 minutes, they are asked to join another pair and are asked to marry up their thoughts as a foursome. The foursome then joins another foursome and so on.

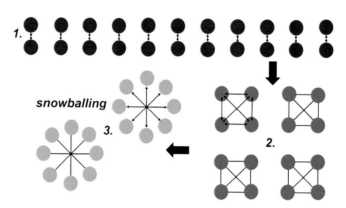

Pros
- It gets all the individuals in a group involved – comprehensive collaboration.
- It starts off with the safety of two people sharing their thoughts before gradually becoming bigger and bigger.
- A very effective way of concisely pulling together (summarising) the thoughts, ideas and issues a large group has around a particular topic.

Cons
- Participants can become bored with repeated discussion of the same points.

Facilitator tips
- Provide Post-it notes for participants to write down their ideas.
- Put flip chart paper up on the walls. Get participants to cluster their Post-it notes into themes.
- You can set increasingly sophisticated tasks as the groups get larger.

Envoying

An envoy is another word for messenger or representative. Envoying is a way of getting several small groups to share their ideas about an issue while retaining their own small-group identity. They use that additional information to help them develop their ideas further.

Let's say you have four small groups who have been set the same task. Once they've all come up with their initial solution, you ask each group to select a representative (or envoy). That envoy goes around each group (in a clockwise direction, 5 minutes per group) asking what sorts of things they came up with and notes these down. Eventually, each envoy returns to their group and 'spills the beans'. Each small group then picks out some of these ideas to help refine their own solutions (or even come up with something totally new). At the end, each group presents their final solution.

Pros

- It's collaborative, fun and dynamic.
- Envoying is a way of sharing ideas – picking out ones that aid the cause and ditching the rest.
- Although all ideas are shared, different groups will pick different ideas to help progress their initial thoughts. At the end, each small group will come up with different (and hopefully innovative) approaches.

Cons

- The exercise can take some time.
- Not particularly good for more than five small groups.
- Although envoying is a way of sharing ideas, some argue that all you get is an increasing volume of ideas – one idea is dumped onto another, which doesn't necessarily improve productivity.

Facilitator tips

- Explain the process so everyone is clear about the aim of the exercise.

Triadic teaching (working in trios)

This is a way of involving all members of a large or small group in a teaching and learning session. There are three key participants in triadic teaching, often referred to as 1st, 2nd and 3rd position (or person A, B and C).

- Person A is 1st position = presenter or explorer.
- Person B is 2nd position = listener or guide.
- Person C is 3rd position = observer.

Person A: presents or explores a problem. In an educational context, they are the learner. In a medical context, they are they patient.

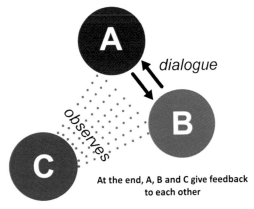

dialogue

observes

At the end, A, B and C give feedback to each other

Person B: listens to person A in order to understand and respond to their concerns. In an educational context, this is the facilitator or Trainer. In a medical context, this is the doctor or therapist.

Person C: observes (and possibly records) the interaction between Person A and Person B in terms of what they *see*, *hear* or *feel*. This will be used for feedback later. They can also act as the timekeeper for the exercise.

After the interaction between A and B, all three participants are given the opportunity to reflect on what went well, what could have gone better, key moments/phrases/interventions in the interaction, and the feelings that were generated in each position.

Pros
- It is particularly good for learning communication skills.
- It helps learners see a different perspective to a situation from that of their own – 'walking a mile in someone else's shoes'.
- It helps develop sensitivity to the emotional content of interactions.
- It helps develop feedback skills – by focusing on what was seen, heard or felt.
- It provides a safe climate within which to do all of this (a small trio).

Cons
- Not a good method for imparting factual information.

Facilitator tips
- Ground rules are needed in any exercise where feedback from fellow learners is involved (so that they don't destroy each other).
- Pendleton's rules[8] are a good starting point, although you can probably use a variety of feedback methods (*see* Chapter 7: The Skilful Art of Giving Feedback).
- Set a time limit for the exercise – 10 minutes in each chair is usually enough.

Case discussion

Case discussions are rooted in real life, and in the personal experience of the learners involved. They pose real questions for practical solutions. However, they are also flexible enough to range beyond the immediate, and they have many of the characteristics of an *ideal* problem-based learning tool.

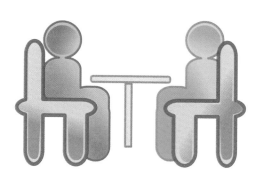

Case discussions are an indispensable educational tool. You can focus on the clinical content, process, communication, decision-making and/or consultation techniques. You can employ role play, microteaching, group work and critical incident techniques. In summary, they are reality based, versatile and economical.

Case discussions are not about having a nice friendly cosy chat with the trainee over a cup of tea and biscuits. You need to provide them with *challenge*. However, challenge is *not* destroying the trainee so that they feel small. Challenge is simply questioning what they did and why in a neutral way – pushing them to their limits (not over their limits). The trainee does not learn anything if they are not challenged.

Types of case discussions

- **Case-based discussion (CBD)** – This is covered in detail in Chapter 25: MRCGP in a Nutshell. Basically, it is a focused and structured discussion about a real patient's case. The basis for the discussion depends on what *themes* are chosen to explore. The themes are defined by the RCGP's 12 professional competency domains and include things like 'practising holistically' and 'working with colleagues'. The important thing about the case-based discussion (as part of MRCGP) is that the questioning must stick to what the trainee *actually did* and why. Refrain from hypothetical (future) questioning like *'what else could you have done'* or asking *'what if . . .'* questions. You might wish to exercise more freedom with CBDs *if* you plan to use them as a formative developmental tool at Half-Day Release.
- **Random case analysis (RCA)** – This is where cases are picked randomly from a trainee's surgery list without prejudice. The trainee presents the case while the Trainer thinks about possible themes to explore with the trainee (based on what they have said). Unlike CBDs, the Trainer is allowed to explore futuristic hypothetical issues by using *'What if . . .'* questions. For instance, *'What if she told you that her headaches were waking her up from her sleep? What would you have done then? Anything different?'* You can explore anything you like: clinical, management, ethical issues – the list is endless. This can reveal gaps in the trainee's learning which might never have been realised by looking at selected cases or only those in which the trainee had problems. A lot of random cases fail to make an impact on learning because the Trainer is often not challenging enough.
- **Problem case analysis (PCA)** – where a trainee would like you to review a particular case they had some sort of difficulty with, in order to resolve it. The problem with PCAs is that they only tackle what the trainee knows they have a problem with (the open and hidden areas of the Johari Window[9]); they fail to identify and tackle what they don't yet realise – their blind spots. Blind spots and unknown areas are, however, picked up by RCAs (hence the reason why experienced Trainers prefer to do RCAs over PCAs). The Johari Window is covered in detail in Chapter 4: Powerful Hooks – aims, objectives and ILOs.

Pros
- You can explore all sorts of things with case discussions like attitudes, ethics, decision-making, problem-solving, clinical and communication skills.
- Results in 'action learning' if used with follow-up discussion.

Cons
- If trainees self-select cases, they may be trying to hide their weaknesses.
- If you fail to challenge the trainee, little learning happens.

Facilitator tips

- Before the session starts, tell the trainee to be open and honest. Tell them that it's okay to say, *'I didn't explore that'* or *'I don't know'* – we can't know the answer to everything. Remind them that lying can paint such a black picture of them – far blacker than the lack of knowledge or a skill.
- Allow the presenter to tell their story uninterrupted (like at the start of a consultation) and *listen*. It will add context and tell you where to focus.
- The key to exploring the true depth of a trainee's ability is to listen to them carefully and then ask the right questions. If you feel you can't judge their ability because their response is too vague, superficial, or you don't quite believe they're telling the truth – stay there, dig deeper and ask more exploratory questions. Don't move on until you are clearer in your mind.
- Keep the discussion focused on the case and do not introduce other case experiences.
- Signpost the domain you are exploring: *'I'd like to now focus on practising holistically. You said . . .'*.
- Take a look at 'The One-Minute Preceptor Model' on our website.

Role play and simulated patients

There is a whole chapter devoted to working with simulated patients: Chapter 18: The Simulated Patient – your walking, talking, learning tool. We will cover the salient points here. For some reason, the word 'role play' instigates sighing and squirming among trainees. Yet role play is a powerful educational tool. Instead of that word say something like *'Let's rehearse that'*, *'Let's have a go at that'*, or *'Let's practise that'*.

Role play works best when it arises naturally in the process of one-to-one teaching or group work. Characters are allocated and given an outline of the situation, and a scenario is then enacted. Participants can find themselves in the shoes of a patient, nurse or doctor – gaining insights into other perspectives (see triadic teaching for a similar approach). If a trainee brings a problem case, get them to see both sides of the story – consider getting them to play the doctor first and then the patient on replay.

Pros

- Good for acquiring communication skills – especially difficult ones like handling the angry patient, breaking bad news, the demanding patient, etc.
- A powerful educational tool – looking at emotions and attitudes like empathy.
- Opportunity to practise and try different approaches in a safe setting.
- Good practice for the CSA examination.

Cons

- It takes a lot of time and energy (also need to 'hook' the trainees into it).
- Can be costly if using external patient simulators.

Facilitator tips

- Ground rules and feedback principles must be explicitly shared with the group to stop them being naughty or nasty.
- Don't forget to use the simulator to give feedback on performance.
- At the end, it is important to 'de-role': emotions can run high, and it is essential to neutralise them. Saying *'Priya, can you come out of role and be yourself'* should be enough.

Video or DVD teaching

Video consultations form the basis of the MRCGP's Consultation Observation Tool or COT (*see* Chapter 25: MRCGP in a Nutshell). However, videos can be used in a whole variety of formative (developmental) ways. They can be looked at on a 1–1 basis or in a group setting (if the trainee is willing). Alternatively, you can use pre-prepared trigger tapes (available from YouTube, the RCGP and other organisations) which demonstrate a particular skill or its absence. Chapter 23: Road Maps for Teaching on the Consultation goes into depth about the different ways you can use videos in teaching.

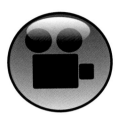

Pros

- It adds an extra visual dimension to teaching and learning sessions.
- You can stop, start and replay 'bits' (unlike observing in surgery).
- Good for communication skills analysis and group dynamic analysis. Trainees can also be encouraged to make their own topic-based videos for Half-Day Release (e.g. interviewing members of the primary care team on their roles).
- You can show motion pictures (in full or in part) to explore a particular theme (*see* Chapter 17: Using the Creative Arts).

Cons

- It takes courage to show a video of yourself.
- Simply watching a video and making comment is a bit passive.
- Full length movies are time consuming – might need to show clips instead.

Facilitator tips

- Technical glitches high – so check equipment *before* the session.
- Encourage the trainee to rewind the tape to the bit they want to show *before* the session starts (saves time and faffing about).
- Explicitly acknowledge the tape as an educational 'gift' from the trainee.
- Ensure negative feedback is controlled and does not destroy the trainee (discuss ground rules and feedback principles).
- Be prepared to use your own video to role model the use of video as a learning tool before expecting the trainee to expose their work. For instance, one Trainer said that they prepared a video of their worst consulting of the year to break the ice and explore with their new trainee how difficult general practice is to get right.

De Bono's Six Thinking Hats[10]

De Bono's hats provide a structured and comprehensive way of looking at the consequences of something. The idea is that if someone proposes a new intervention, one can *comprehensively* look at the consequences from six windows (or hats).

De Bono's Six Thinking Hats			
White hat	Information/facts	**Green hat**	Creativity
Red hat	Emotions	**Blue hat**	Thinking about thinking (the process)
Black hat	Bad points, flaws, barriers	**Yellow hat**	Good points, benefits

The aim is to gather a group of appropriate people to engage in some *parallel* thinking – discussing each hat in turn (with everybody wearing the same hat at the same time so that they don't end up trying to score points against each other). As you explore each hat, it is important to say things which are only in keeping with the value of that hat. At the end, you try to collaboratively form a general picture and consensus and decide how to move on.

> Hats may be used in some structured sequence depending on the nature of the issue. Here is an *example agenda* for a typical six hats workshop:
>
> Step 1: Present facts of the case (*White Hat*)
> Step 2: Generate ideas on how the case could be handled (*Green Hat*)
> Step 3: Evaluate the merits of the ideas – list the benefits (*Yellow Hat*)
> Step 4: List the drawbacks (*Black Hat*)
> Step 5: Get everybody's gut feelings about the alternatives (*Red Hat*)
> Step 6: Summarise and adjourn the meeting (*Blue Hat*)
>
> You don't have to stick to this sequence. Depending on the situation and the mix of people, it might be better to let people get their negative thoughts out first, or their intuitive sense, and then use yellow or green to move ahead. The blue hat comments on the thinking being used, asks for conclusions and decisions (even with regards to which hat to wear next).

For instance, a Trainer and his or her final-year GP trainee might use this method to look at the implications of future work as a locum, salaried doctor or partner in general practice.

Pros
- A comprehensive approach to examining consequences.
- No conflict between members as they are all wearing the same hat at the same time – means the group doesn't get stuck.
- Discussion is often very robust – helps people reach decisions rather than fudging them.

Cons
- If white hat information is not available, it can lead to inconclusive use of the other hats. (But this is a problem with most meetings anyway.)

The Fundamentals of Teaching

Facilitator tips

- The blue hat is the hardest one to understand. It deals with controlling the thinking process. The blue hat is often 'given' to one person, who controls what hat will be 'worn', hence controlling the type of thinking being used.
- There is a more detailed facilitator's guide on our website.

The fishbowl technique

The fishbowl technique is a fabulous way of getting all members in a group (large or small) into activity. Some individuals will hopefully volunteer to engage in an interaction (like role play) and they will then take centre stage. The rest of the large group sits around them and observes the interactions. After the interaction, the 'central performers' are asked for feedback first before the external observers give a comment.

Pros

- It can be used *in conjunction* with a variety of other educational methods – role play, De Bono's six thinking hats, debate, etc.
- Particularly good for looking at group dynamics
  – interdisciplinary teamwork mechanisms, case conferences, practice partnership meetings.
- Feedback is derived on two levels – from central stage and the audience.

Cons

- In very large groups, central stage performers can feel very intimidated, and observers can become disengaged and bored.

Facilitator tips

- You can give the external observers separate roles, e.g. one arc to watch the patient, another the doctor, another non-verbals and so on. In this way, they can give *focused* specific descriptive feedback and perhaps even enter the role play arena to try things out for themselves.
- Control negative feedback carefully so that people are not destroyed.
- At the end, ensure the central performers are all (emotionally) okay.

Action research[11]

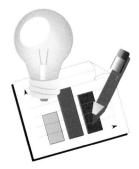

This is based on the idea that the best way of learning is by doing (action) – getting people involved in a project as a result of a problem that's raised its head. Action research is an *interactive* and *collaborative* process where members of a team resolve a problem by understanding the *underlying causes* through *data analysis or research*, *reflecting* on the findings, and making *further enquiries* before making *recommendations for change*. People learn through experimenting and researching.

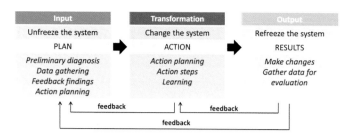

Input	Transformation	Output
Unfreeze the system	Change the system	Refreeze the system
PLAN	ACTION	RESULTS
Preliminary diagnosis	*Action planning*	*Make changes*
Data gathering	*Action steps*	*Gather data for*
Feedback findings	*Learning*	*evaluation*
Action planning		

feedback   feedback

feedback

So, each team member will work on a task that will hopefully help resolve the bigger problem. As they work through and research the task, they learn from things that work well, things that don't and any further issues they encounter along the way. They report regularly on progress.

Pros
- It encourages learners to 'experiment and play': a learning by doing strategy.
- It promotes learning in real time with collaborative reflection.
- Suits all learning styles: activists and pragmatists through doing; reflectors and theorists through researching and reflecting.
- It stretches the trainees' abilities – development of organisational, management, audit, research, problem-solving and writing skills.

Cons
- It requires preparation, supervision and time.
- Converting words and ideas into actions may not materialise.

Facilitator tips
- Keep things simple! Intervene if they end up making things unnecessarily complicated – otherwise they'll end up ripping their hair out!
- It works even better if you encourage the group to move towards the ethos of a 'community of practice'[12] (*see* Chapter 22: Interprofessional Learning).

Problem-based learning (PBL)[13]
Problem-based learning is a way of learning in fixed small groups where the trainees define a set of learning needs after analysing and working through a piece of 'trigger' text related to a clinical or management scenario. Learning is driven by a challenging, open-ended, ill-defined and ill-structured problem. The learning list is reviewed and prioritised before each group member goes away and learns about one defined area. At a subsequent meeting, they report on their learning using a variety of presentation techniques; other members are encouraged to ask questions in order to deepen everyone's understanding of the topic(s). Further material about PBL is available on our website.

Pros
- It promotes presentation, leadership, problem-solving and communication skills.
- It promotes collaborative working – learners learn to negotiate the complex nature of problems and the different ways of proceeding forwards. The truth is socially negotiated but internally constructed.[14]
- It encourages self-directed learning (learners construct their own knowledge).
- Learning is contextual and relevant – simulates real-world working.

Cons
- It requires a minimum of two sessions (i.e. at least one follow-on session).
- Reporting can be laboured and boring.
- It can lead to resentment if some do their homework and others don't.

Facilitator tips
- Select a scribe to write down the issues as they arise.
- Don't take on an expert role; you are meant to be the facilitator – there to scaffold the process. Help people make sense of their learning. Ask probing and exploratory questions like *'That's interesting. What makes you say that?'* Provide the appropriate resources and encourage the group to 'flower'.
- If discussions appear to be going off track or the group seems stuck, take over and lead discussions.

Objective Structured Clinical Examination (OSCE)
An OSCE is a set of clinical scenarios, which may or may not involve a patient simulator. Individual learners go through the clinical stations one by one and are assessed on them in a formal (summative) way. Trainees may be asked to take a history, examine, interpret results (such as ECGs) or develop a management plan. Each station has a different examiner/assessor, and each one takes around 10–20 minutes to complete. The MRCGP Clinical Skills Assessment (CSA) is a sophisticated OSCE. You can also use OSCEs in a less summative and more formative way:
- where learners assess themselves and identify their own learning needs
- where learners develop their own OSCEs for one another. In this way they learn by covering several parts of the GP curriculum, understanding what is required of them (the competencies), and then through teaching them.

Pros
- A good way of covering various bits of the GP curriculum.
- Good for testing clinical, problem-solving, communication and interpretation skills. And it tests these in an *objective* and *structured* way.
- It raises self-awareness through reflection on self-performance.
- Each station has its own examiner/assessor (reduces examiner bias).

Cons
- It takes a lot of work and planning to create OSCE scenarios.
- The logistics of running an OSCE session can be challenging.
- You need enough breakout rooms for the separate OSCE stations.
- If using simulated patients and Trainers as assessors, costs can run high.

Facilitator tips
- Use professional simulated patients if you can afford it.
- Use your admin team to help with the organisation – don't forget the stopwatch and ringing bell.
- Consider getting trainees to act (in turn) as patients, doctors and assessors (promotes understanding of different perspectives and is cheaper).

Intensive Structured Collaborative Educational Experience (ISCEE)[15]

In an OSCE, individual trainees go around various clinical stations; each station is designed to test a set of competencies. An ISCEE is similar to an OSCE except that instead of individuals, small groupettes (or a 'family of learners') go around the stations. Each member of the family takes it in turn to have a go at the different stations. The rest of the 'siblings' are there to support and help each other through the exercises (perhaps swapping places at times to demonstrate alternative ways of doing things). It's basically a way of doing OSCEs but ensuring a formative (developmental) approach.

Pros

- It provides a safe small environment in which members can be open and honest.
- It's collaborative and encourages peer-to-peer problem-solving and learning.
- It's an active and dynamic way to learn.
- Stations are based on real-life experiences (e.g. communication skills).
- Large groups can be accommodated for. A set of eight ISCEE stations can easily accommodate 40–48 trainees (whereas seven OSCE stations can only accommodate seven trainees at any one time).

Cons

- It takes a lot of work and planning to create ISCEE scenarios – just like OSCEs. You need patient simulator, facilitator and trainee instruction sheets.
- You need enough breakout rooms for each ISCEE station or alternatively a large hall with enough screens.
- Using simulated patients and Trainers as assessors means costs can run high.

Facilitator tips

- Diversify the groups – balance them in terms of gender, age, ethnicity, ST year and so on.
- Strict time keeping is essential for its success. Get someone to ring the bell!

The Balint group[16]

The Balint *group* method is a way to discuss cases or situations arising in practice, which have aroused feelings in the trainees. The small group focuses on relationships and feelings (and *not* problem-solving or clinical management). *See* Chapter 24: Doing Balint for exact details on how you do it.

Pros

- It allows for safe disclosure of uncertainty in a trusting group. It gives participants permission to be fallible and admit to feelings.
- It results in a deep sense of trust and caring within a group.
- Good method for seeing things from other perspectives.
- It liberates creative thinking, which can sometimes help doctors who may feel stuck in some way.

Cons

- Too 'touchy-feely' for some.
- Some find it frustrating not being able to talk about clinical problems.

Facilitator tips

- Aim to explore the **interpersonal dynamics**, and not the clinical questions.
- Remember that the purpose is to **deepen understanding of what's going on**; it is not an exercise in solving a problem.
- Encourage **imagination and speculation** about the case, fully acknowledging that this is not necessarily the reality of the case.
- Reinforce the rule that 'this is **not about right or wrong** practice'.
- Allow the **presenter to sit back** in a 'safe haven' and simply listen to the bulk of the discussion. During this time, they must not contribute or chip into the discussion.
- Keep the **focus on the presented case**. Avoid a new case being introduced when some part of the discussion reminds someone of a similar case they experienced.

Significant Event Analysis (SEA)

Most of you are familiar with this. It refers to the discussion and analysis of a real-life event which had a significant impact or consequences for a patient, trainee, doctor, other staff or the practice. Although most people dig up crises and errors, don't forget that you can focus on something that had an unanticipated significant positive impact too. In the case of an error or crisis, the purpose of SEAs is not only to fix the immediate problem but to identify ways of preventing it happening again in the future. It's this latter bit that people don't explore very well. It's also important to instil a 'no blame' culture so that people are comfortable with bringing these things into the open and discussing them. The emphasis should be on fixing things and making systems even better.

Pros

- It encourages analytical and systems-based thinking.
- It results in real-time learning and encourages a collaborative team approach to learning.
- It encourages a holistic approach – looking at whole practice systems.

Cons

- It requires skilful facilitation and feelings must not be overlooked – otherwise people can end up going for each other's throats or being defensive!

Facilitator tips

- Always explore people's feelings – especially those closely involved. Acknowledge, validate and settle them, otherwise you can emotionally scar them forever, and they'll never trust you again.
- If there is any hint of a 'blame culture', *stop!* Reset the climate.
- Even at the end, check everyone is (emotionally) okay. Make time for anyone who feels upset – reminding them that we all face critical moments in our medical careers where things do not go as well as we would have hoped.

Modular learning

Modules are units of education based on a particular theme (e.g. substance misuse). They are usually part of e-learning or distance learning courses, and some GP training schemes even run 1–2-day modular courses (especially for trainees doing hospital posts who find it difficult to get to HDR every week). There are a variety of e-learning modules available (BMJ, RCGP, Doctors. net) – encourage trainees to do them in advance of a HDR session on a particular topic (tops up their knowledge and allows a trainee to focus on a deeper understanding during the HDR session).

Pros
- Most e-modules enlist patient cases to help with the application of knowledge.
- There are e-modules for nearly everything! Trainees can do them in a contextual and relevant way.

Cons
- Not much room for collaborative learning with peers.
- Doing e-modules repeatedly can get boring.
- Developing modules is a resource-intensive process.

Portfolio-based learning

The ePortfolio is now a third of every GP trainee's assessment for their membership of the RCGP. Portfolio-based learning is linked to sound educational principles – gathering evidence of learning and development and collecting it over a period of time in order to demonstrate acquisition of the knowledge, skills and attitudes. It has been described by one GP educator as a wheelbarrow into which trainees gather seasonal fruits and vegetables in their journey through the orchards and veggie patches of GP training posts. This evidence is gathered in electronic format and organised into various categories.

Pros
- It encourages a trainee to reflect on experience.
- It's a good journal of where the trainee is at.
- It provides a wealth of evidence and experience which you can pick to discuss, teach and learn.

Cons
- The RCGP's ePortfolio is still a bit 'clunky and chunky'.
- The ePortfolio suits some styles (e.g. Reflectors and Theorists) better than others (Activists and Pragmatists).

Facilitator tips
- Some trainees don't use it well, and some trainees need help in learning how to reflect.

Which method for the size of the group?

We bet you're exhausted after reading all of that. We apologise if we have overwhelmed you. The table below lists the methods we've covered so far and which ones work with which size of groups. It should help you with lesson planning.

Large group	Small group	Individuals
Symposium		
Cluster group teaching		
ISCEE		
The lecture, the mini-lecture and buzz groups		
Seminar/Workshop		
Debate		
Peer-led teaching		
Brainstorming/Reverse brainstorming		
Disney creative strategy		
Task groups		
Triadic teaching		
Snowballing		
Envoying		
Fishbowling		
	OSCE	
	Balint group case discussions	
	De Bono's Six Hats	
	Role play	
	Problem-based learning (PBL) – best in small groups	
	Action learning	
	Project-based learning	
	Case-based discussion	
	Problem case analysis	
		Random case analysis
		Modular learning
		Portfolio-based learning
Video		
Critical incident analysis/Significant event analysis		

Note: you can combine some of these. For example, if you've got a large audience, you could gather a small group to sit in a small circle and consider a problem using the de Bono method. The others can then form a larger circle and sit around the smaller group and observe what's going on (the fishbowl technique). Think and be creative!

A sample of resources on our website

- Problem Based Learning – a practical guide for facilitators.
- De Bono's Six Thinking Hats – facilitator instructions.
- Random Case Analysis – facilitator instructions.
- SNAPPS, The One Minute Preceptor and lots more . . .

Other chapters you may like to read

- Chapter 10: Five Pearls of Educational Theory
- Chapter 13: Teaching and Facilitating Small Groups
- Chapter 7: The Skilful Art of Giving Feedback.

Acknowledgements

Many thanks to Mark David Jones for the section on Envoying. Mark is an ex-primary school teacher who now works as a cataloguer for Rosebery's Auctioneers in London.

Please give us some feedback on this chapter to help shape it for the next edition.
Go to www.essentialgptrainingbook.com and simply click on the title of this chapter.

References

1 Honey P, Mumford A. *The Manual of Learning Styles*. Maidenhead, UK: Peter Honey Publications; 1982.

2 Kolb D. *Experiential Learning: experience as the source of learning and development*. Englewood Cliffs, NJ: Prentice-Hall, Inc.; 1984.

3 Osborn AF. *Applied Imagination: principles and procedures of creative problem solving*. 3rd ed. New York, NY: Charles Scribner's Son; 1963.

4 Toubia O. Idea generation, creativity, and incentives. *Marketing Science*. 2006; **25**(5): 411–25.

5 Rickards T. Brainstorming revisited: a question of context. *IJMR*. 1999; **1**(1): 91–110.

6 Nunamaker J, Dennis AR, Valacich JS, *et al.* Electronic meeting systems to support group work. *Communications of the ACM*. 1991; **34**(7): 40–61.

7 Dilts Robert. *Strategies of Genius*. Capitola, California: Meta Publications; 1994.

8 Pendleton D, Schofield D, Tate P, Havelock P. *The New Consultation: developing doctor-patient communication*. Oxford: Oxford University Press; 2003. pp. 75–80.

9 Luft J, Ingham H. *The Johari Window: a graphic model of interpersonal awareness*. Los Angeles: UCLA; 1955.

10 De Bono E. *Six Thinking Hats: an essential approach to business management*. Boston, Mass: Little, Brown, & Company; 1985.

11 Lewin K. Action research and minority problems. *J Soc Issues*. 1946; **2**(4): 34–46.

12 Wenger E. *Communities of Practice: learning, meaning, and identity*. Cambridge: Cambridge University Press; 1998.

13 Barrows HS, Tamblyn RM. *Problem-based Learning*. New York: Springer; 1980.

14 Savery JR, Duffy TM. Problem based learning: an instructional model and its constructivist framework. *Educ Technol*. 1995; **35**(5): 31–7.

15 Originally coined by Nick Price– a Programme Director in Bradford.

16 Balint M. *The Doctor, his Patient and the Illness*. London: Pitman Medical; 1957 (Millennium edition, Edinburgh: Churchill Livingstone, 2000).

6

Teaching from Scratch

RAMESH MEHAY – TPD (Bradford) & lead author
ANNA ROMITO – Researcher in Clinical Education (London Deanery)

Are you looking for a few quick tips to help you teach effectively? Are you a doctor who has been asked to teach medical students, but you have had no training in how to teach? Are you a practice nurse or manager who wishes to run some educational sessions, but you feel apprehensive and ill prepared?

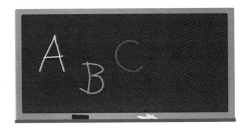

If so, don't worry – this chapter is designed for you. If you are *totally* new to education and training, then you might find it useful to first read Chapter 10: Five Pearls of Educational Theory and Chapter 4: Powerful Hooks – aims, objectives and ILOs. However, if you don't fancy that, this chapter should still get you up and running.

Four teaching tenets for newbies

Tenet 1: 'Learning' is more important than 'teaching'

When we *teach*, we are thinking about what we (as a teacher) are saying and doing. However, what we really ought to be doing is concentrating on what the learner is trying to *learn*. In this way, we focus on the learner and their outcomes rather than our own desires. Think of yourself as a *facilitator* of learning instead of a *teacher* – it helps keep the learner at the centre of attention.

Tenet 2: Try to promote adult learning (andragogy)[1]

You will see the terms andragogy and pedagogy come up time and time again in educational theory. They are fancy names for two simple things. **Pedagogy** means *child-like learning*, where children are spoon-fed knowledge by a school teacher. It is the teacher who decides what is going to be taught, not the child. The child does not usually play an active role in the learning process, other than simply absorbing knowledge. Traditional medical schools before the 1990s were like this, where the lecturer talked and the student listened and obeyed.

Andragogy means *adult learning*. Here, the learner reflects and evaluates what important things they need to know and how they are going to fill the gaps. The teacher's role in this context is to *help* them with this process.

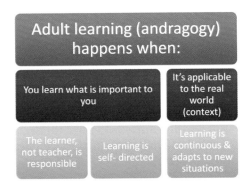

Think of andragogy and pedagogy as two ends of a spectrum. A purely pedagogic way of teaching (such as a lecture) is *not* an effective way of getting people to learn. By six months, most individuals will have forgotten about 80% of what was said. Although this figure is a lot less with an andragogic method, purely employing this approach is not ideal either. Take the example of a tutorial on the diagnosis and management of chest pain; your learners would soon become disgruntled and lose interest if you persistently failed to provide any answers, reflected all their questions back to them or signposted where they might look. Sometimes learners just want a simple straightforward answer to a question! There are some things which simply need to be 'told', usually facts and usually because of time pressure. What we are suggesting is to veer towards an andragogic approach, but not necessarily to exclude all elements of the pedagogic. In the chest pain scenario, getting learners to interact with a clinical case and trickle feeding information as they ask for it would fare better.

Tenet 3: Identify and define your aims and learning outcomes

Most things in life have a purpose. Similarly, before delivering any sort of teaching, the first step is to define your purpose (= your aims + learning outcomes). Not doing this is like getting into your car and driving off but not knowing what or where you are heading for! An effective teaching session requires a destination (= the intended learning outcome or ILO).

When I was a medical student at a very traditional school it was the norm to be interrogated at a ward round by the consultant in front of the patient, nursing staff and your peers. While the majority coped well with this others found it extremely difficult, particularly with some consultants. Retrospectively, this has been labelled as 'learning by humiliation' or perceived as 'bullying' as gaps in knowledge were exposed for all to see.

Yet a good educator in my view should be able to lead a learner to the moment of saying, 'I don't know!' Learning begins at that moment. It does not have to be a 'moment of humiliation'. It has now become something of a standing joke in our training practice that we call this 'a moment of celebration' rather than 'humiliation', on the understanding that the learner then takes responsibility for addressing the deficiency.

Prit Chahal, GP, Nottingham

Tenet 4: Constructive alignment[2]

Constructive alignment is actually a simple concept. ILOs clarify what it is the learner should be able to do as a result of the learning session. However, the ILOs won't happen just by setting them; you have to select educational methods for your lesson that will help the learners get there. In other words, these educational methods need marrying up or aligning to the ILOs. And if you really want your learners to achieve the ILOs, then make sure that you also design and align any exam or end assessment to the ILOs. After all, learners learn what they think they're ultimately going to be tested on.

The 'alignment' part of constructive alignment is thus where you align the educational methods and the end assessment to the ILOs (in order to help achieve them). The 'constructive' part refers to the three Cs of constructivism: helping learners to learn through *collaborating* with each other; in the *context* of the real world; and through *constructing* new knowledge in light of what is already known. There's more about constructive alignment on our website.

How to design *any* teaching session: the ACME way

This is a simple universal framework that Ramesh Mehay has developed for planning any teaching session, whether it is a tutorial, presentation or anything else! By the way, it has nothing to do with the fictional corporation that exists in the *Looney Tunes* universe!

Designing a teaching session – the ACME way

1 **A** is for setting Aims and Intended Learning Outcomes (ILOs)
2 **C** is for defining Content
3 **M** is for exploring Methodologies
4 **E** is for the Ending (= **S**ummarising, **E**valuation, **A**ssessment & future **L**earning)

The beauty of this model is that:
1 It is easy to remember, especially for new educators.
2 It simplifies some of the over-fussy educational theory out there.

And it works like this.
- Define the Aims and ILOs (A). This is the most crucial step. Then:
- Use the Aims & ILOs (A) to define the Content (C)
- Use the Aims & ILOs (A) to select the Methodology (M)
- Use the Aims & ILOs (A) to construct the Evaluation (E).

Aligning everything to (A) ensures that all parts of the teaching session are geared towards achieving the aims and ILOs, which is ultimately what matters. It really is that simple! Unsuccessful teaching sessions are often due to a lack of attention to one or more of the ACME areas.

Setting the Aims and ILOs

We cannot stress how important it is to spend time teasing out and setting the aims and ILOs. It is a bit like a consultation: if you don't pay sufficient attention to the beginning, the middle and the end fall apart. We are not going to spend much time talking about aims and ILOs because they have been covered comprehensively in Chapter 4: Powerful Hooks – aims, objectives and ILOs. Key points are as follows.
- Aims and ILOs are all about the purpose, *e.g. define what it is that you expect learners to be able to do as a result of the session.*
- Aims are a **broad** statement of what you are trying to achieve, *e.g. at the end of this chapter, you'll be better at designing teaching sessions that work well.*
- Intended learning outcomes are more **specific** statements about what you expect the learners to be able to do, *e.g. at the end of this chapter, you'll be able to plan a teaching session using the ACME framework.*
- Aims are teacher-focused whereas ILOs are learner-centred. What the student does is actually more important in determining what is learned than what the teacher does.[3]

- Try to define ILOs in terms of knowledge, skills and attitudes (KSA). No doubt there are things that you feel the learner should know and/or be able to do (in KSA terms). This is called the teacher's agenda. There are things the learner feels they should know and/or be able to do (again in KSA terms). This is called the learner's agenda. Incorporate items from both agendas into your ILO set.
- Review your ILOs: decide which are essential and important for them to know and which are desirable or nice for them to know. Too many ILOs will pressure you for time – you may need to ditch the 'nice to know'.
- Once you have your aims and ILOs, try to tweak them to serve as powerful hooks. You can 'spice' them up by incorporating words and phrases that:
  - acknowledge potential feelings, such as fear, concerns and frustrations
  - help move them on from those feelings (e.g. *'be troubled no more'*, *'the easy-peasy way'*, *'all in 10 minutes'* etc.).

Defining the content

You can now use the ILOs to help you define the content. An ILO such as: *'the learner will be able to apply the ACME framework to his or her next teaching session'* tells you that the session's content has to include some information about the ACME framework.

Argghhh! I have too much content but not enough time!

- Go back to your aims and ILOs and work out what is *essential* and what is *desirable*. Remove some of the desirables, or put them on hold for another session.
- Breadth vs depth. Do you want to cover a lot of material but superficially, or a few things but in detail? Depth helps your learners to get a real flavour of the subject, whereas breadth provides the overview. One shrinks the other: if you need depth, focus on fewer items; if you need breadth cut back on the depth.
- Re-evaluate your delivery, e.g. could a handout save you time?

Exploring methodologies

There are several different ways you can deliver the same session, and it is tempting to teach in the way that we ourselves learn best. However, be careful; just because some methods work for us does not mean they will work equally well for others.

- Refer to your aims and ILOs; try to select educational methods that maximise the chances of your learners achieving them. Different methods have different **levels of effectiveness**. The level of effectiveness correlates with the *nature* of knowledge necessary for competence when in an authentic situation. Learning is most effective when there is consistency between the context in which knowledge is learnt and that where it needs to be applied.[4] Therefore, the level of effectiveness that you want to achieve will determine what method you use. For example, if you want to help your learners to *manage* chest pain, you might choose a realistic case-based approach over a non-interactive lecture. If you want your learners to be able *to do* a shoulder joint injection, demonstration with practice will be more effective than discussing it.

- Try to select more than one method. This will help make the session more varied and interactive. It is also more likely to cater for different learners and their varied **learning styles**. More on learning styles later.
- Pick a method that matches the **level of competence** you are aiming for: think Miller's Pyramid.

Miller's Pyramid[5] encourages you to think about how deeply you want to get someone to learn something. The higher up the pyramid you take them, the more competent they will be.

Miller's Prism of Clinical Competence (a.k.a. Miller's Pyramid)

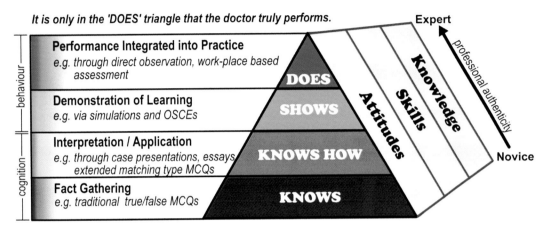

Based on work by Miller GE. The Assessment of Clinical Skills/Competence/Performance. *Acad Med.* 1990; **65**(9): 63-7. Adapted by Drs. Ramesh Mehay and Roger Burns (January 2009).

Starting with the bottom level, at the **knows** level, a learner might *know something* about (say) chest pain. That's good, but it doesn't mean they can manage a real patient with chest pain. Even better would be to **know how** to do something; for example, *knowing how* to examine a chest. But, again, that doesn't mean you can actually do a chest examination. To **show** how to do something might give you more faith in the learner. For example, a learner who *demonstrates* that they can be empathic with a patient shows they have the skill. It tells you they can do it, but it doesn't tell you whether they do it on a regular basis with a high degree of skill with their other patients. Perhaps you would have more faith if they could provide *natural* evidence for empathy on the **does** level – where they show you *several snapshots of being* empathic, say through video or direct observation.

So, when it comes to teaching, you should ask yourself which of these levels you are aiming for. It is okay to aim for 'knows something' or 'knows how' level – especially for learners who are early on in their training programme, but for those who are more experienced, aim to take them higher up. Knowing which level you are aiming for informs your methodology:

- **Knows** or **knows how**: consider lectures, independent reading, case-based discussions, problem-based learning or group discussion, brainstorming, snowballing and so on.
- **Shows**: use direct observation, video, role play, patient simulation, OSCE, task groups and so on.
- **Does**: undertake recurrent observations, use multiple work-place based assessments, compose a video portfolio and so on.

For more information on Miller, please *see* Chapter 29: Assessment and Competence.

Learning styles

Look at this picture and think about what you see. This is a classic example of how *different individuals have different ways of perceiving the same thing*: some of you see an old lady, others a young one. What this shows is that we all *receive, process* and *make sense* of information in different ways. This is also true of how we learn and that means *one* method of teaching cannot cater for us all. This picture also demonstrates the value of **collaborative learning**. Some of us who instinctively see a young woman are able to see the old woman when this is explained to us, and vice versa. Working with each other helps us to appreciate different points of view and helps reduce our blind spots.

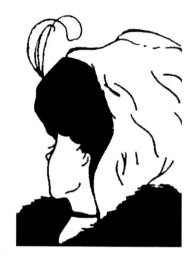

Therefore, never think of just one method for delivering a teaching session: try to use several to expand the way a trainee thinks. In groups, individuals will have different learning styles and you will *need* to use a variety of methods. Using a range of methodologies will liven up and add dynamism to your session. Learners benefit from being actively involved during the learning process and can be deeply motivated by it.[6] Methods involving a *high level of interactivity* generally work better than more passive methods. This is the reason why educationalists are often scornful about lectures, but short bursts of lectures can be very effective when punctuated with other more interactive methods.

HIGH INTERACTIVITY	Practising repeatedly	Patient simulation	Role play	Balint	Games & Quizzes	Task groups	Triadic teaching	Debate	Snowballing	Significant event analysis	Problem-based learning	Case-based discussion	Group discussion	Film, art and poetry	Buzz groups	Q&A/FAQs	Brainstorming	Field trips	Modified interactive lecture	Demonstration	The traditional lecture	Trainee reading	LOW INTERACTIVITY

Choosing your educational methods

- There are a variety of ways of delivering the same thing. Your choice will be influenced by your aims, ILOs, your learner, yourself and your environment.
- Consider using a mixture of ways even in one session, especially in group learning.
- Keep the session lively – encourage a cross-fertilisation of ideas; encourage interactivity between learners (collaborative learning).
- Try to avoid bombarding the learner with too much information.
- If it is a skill that is being taught, the session must involve learners practising.
- Periodically, summarise what you have covered so far and the key learning points.
- Build in regular breaks. Remember, the average attention span is only 20 minutes. Consider the occasional energising activity.

 Top Tip: Read Chapter 11: Learning and Personality Styles in Practice and Chapter 5: A Smorgasbord of Educational Methods.

Ending the session

Ending the session has four components: **Summarising**, **Evaluation**, **Assessment** and **Learning** (i.e. SEAL the End). For each of these components, refer back to (A) – your initial Aims and ILOs.

- Use (A) to **Summarise** key learning points and concepts. Consider using visual aids, like a flip chart, to help your learners organise learning and concepts within their own minds.
- Use (A) to **Evaluate** your session. Ask the audience how they feel; the most important question is whether your learners feel that they have achieved the ILOs. Use this as an opportunity to seek feedback – what things went well and not so well, and how could the session be improved in terms of content and methodology? Don't forget to reflect on and evaluate the session yourself.
- Use (A) to develop an **Assessment** tool. Your learning establishment might expect you to devise an end-assessment (for example, for a particular learning module). If so, make its link to the ILOs clear. As well as being a motivator for learning, learning can also take place during the assessment itself – you can set assessment tasks to help consolidate the learning.
- Use (A) to define future **Learning**. Were any of the ILOs difficult to achieve? Were any additional learning needs uncovered? Do these need revisiting in the future? What is next on the agenda now that this particular set of ILOs has been covered?

An extra little note on evaluation

No matter how experienced a teacher or facilitator you are, you should always try to get some sort of feedback on the sessions you run. We see lots of well-established trainers who no longer bother with evaluation: possibly because they have done it for so many years that they feel there is very little to be gained. However, just because you perceive a session to have gone well doesn't mean that is how it was for the punters. We hope you can see how perception is unidirectional; *perception is not necessarily the same as reality* and one needs to 'check things out'.

Sessions start becoming dry, off-target and uninteresting when people stop 'checking things out'. Ultimately, they become ineffective. We often find that newly appointed trainers deliver far more effective and dynamic sessions than some well-established trainers. Don't become complacent! Besides, evaluating yourself and being evaluated will prevent your life as a GP educator from becoming humdrum.

 Top Tip: In order to *ask evaluation questions*, you need to be in the right frame of mind for *receiving the 'answers'*. The answers may not be to your heart's content and if you're generally having a bad week, perhaps now's not the time to evaluate.

When we refer to evaluation, we don't just mean the written feedback many of you are familiar with. Learners are often bombarded with so many feedback forms that they get bored and fill them in half-heartedly, thus lessening their value. Be creative and think of other ways of evaluating your session.

- You may just want to ask for some verbal feedback.
- You could leave a dictaphone on a table near the exit door for learners to make one or two comments about the session.
- You could even ask a series of questions and get them to respond by forming a human bar chart where one side of the room is zero, and the other side is 10.

Whatever method you employ, giving an indication that the feedback received will be both embraced and considered will help motivate your learners to engage in the evaluation process.

Teaching/lesson plan templates

Teaching/lesson plan templates are invaluable for planning any teaching session. They:
- give you an overall snapshot of what you have planned
- help you see which sections are specifically tackling which ILOs
- let you see if you have got a good balance of things within your planned methods, level of interactivity, assessments and so on
- define exactly what presentation aids you will need
- help you get your timings right.

I have been a Training Programme Director for more than 10 years, and I still use teaching plans for my educational sessions. It never ceases to amaze me how incredibly easy, simple and effective this tool is. The other week I ran a session to help realign a training practice's ethos towards training. Knowing what the practice had been through, I had a rough idea of what to do. Mulling it over the following week generated more thoughts. And when I mapped things out on a teaching plan template, *more* refinements were necessary. The session went very well. On reflection, these final tweaks were instrumental in the session's success. I don't think I am ever going to stop using teaching plan templates.

Here is part of a teaching plan so you have some idea of what we are talking about. There are more detailed examples on our website, as well as a blank template for you to download and use.

Time grid for a learning session. Remember not to make the timings too tight: leave some flexibility to anticipate the unexpected!

Session Title:	Spirometry in General Practice (a workshop)				
Time	**Content** *(what information is to be given)* **& Facilitator Activity**	**Educational Method** *(e.g. brainstorming, trios, large group discussion etc.)*	**Audience Activity** *(level of interactivity)*	**Presentation Aids Needed** *(e.g. flip chart, PowerPoint, laptop etc.)*	**Objective(s) being met**
2.00	Introductions, welcome, explain today's topic Formulate session objectives	Brainstorm ideas, concerns and expectations. Negotiate agenda.	*medium*	Flip chart Working pens	[These refer to a numbered list of *intended learning outcomes* which are not supplied here]
2.20	Demonstration of how to do spirometry. Need a volunteer.	Listen and watch Allow to ask questions	*low*	Spirometer	1, 2

Session Title:	Spirometry in General Practice (a workshop)				
Time	**Content** *(what information is to be given)* **& Facilitator Activity**	**Educational Method** *(e.g. brainstorming, trios, large group discussion etc.)*	**Audience Activity** *(level of interactivity)*	**Presentation Aids Needed** *(e.g. flip chart, PowerPoint, laptop etc.)*	**Objective(s) being met**
2.35	Doctor, patient, observer, rotate twice so each has a turn. Then swap with other 3 students. Clarify and help as needed	Practise in trios	*high*	Spirometer	1, 2
3.10	Show how to read a chart. Explain the percentages using a poster prepared earlier	Listen Allow to ask questions	*low*	Poster	3, 4
3.30	Interpret some spirometry charts, discuss, make conclusions about whether obstructive etc. Clarify and help as needed	Practise	*high*	Spirometry charts	3, 4

> ## A few extra final tips
>
> - In advance of the session, consider setting your learners some homework.
> - Set some time at the beginning to acclimatise – to allow for a rapport, offload baggage or current stresses that might otherwise interfere with learning etc.
> - Incorporate the learners' knowledge and experience in your session; give the session a meaningful context by linking it to that experience.
> - Use a variety of educational tools/methods – match it to what the situation commands.
> - Maintain interest through dynamism – ask open questions, interact, vary the content, vary the method, use humour – and have fun!

Closing comments

Teaching is enjoyable and both of you, the teacher and the learner, should get something out of it. New young learners will stimulate you, and you will inspire them. They add spice to what might otherwise be quite a muted, mundane working way of life. When you start delivering powerful sessions that *have an impact*, your learners will sing your praises through their gratitude and their successes. Teaching makes you feel valued. Teaching makes you feel you have contributed something back to the world. Teaching simply makes you feel good! So, why wouldn't you want to do it? Get involved in teaching and learning – you don't know what you are missing! Life is about contribution.

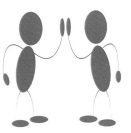

A sample of resources on our website
- The Johari Window: identifying learning needs.
- Giving Great Tutorials.
- The four stages of competence.
- Teaching plan – an example and a blank.

Other chapters you may like to read
- Chapter 10: Five Pearls of Educational Theory
- Chapter 11: Learning and Personality Styles in Practice
- Chapter 4: Powerful Hooks – aims, objectives and ILOs
- Chapter 5: A Smorgasbord of Educational Methods
- Chapter 12: How Groups Work – the dynamics
- Chapter 13: Teaching and Facilitating Small Groups
- Chapter 8: Teaching Gems
- Chapter 7: The Skilful Art of Giving Feedback.

Please give us some feedback on this chapter to help shape it for the next edition.
Go to www.essentialgptrainingbook.com and simply click on the title of this chapter.

References

1 Knowles M, Holton E, Swanson R. *The Adult Learner.* 6th ed. Burlington, MA: Elsevier Butterworth-Heinemann; 2005 (originally published 1973).

2 Biggs J. *Teaching for Quality Learning at University.* 2nd ed. Buckingham: Open University Press/Society for Research into Higher Education; 2003.

3 Shuell T. Cognitive conceptions of learning. *RER.* 1986; **56**: 411–36.

4 Seeley Brown J, Collins A, Duguid P. Situated cognition and the culture of learning. *ER.* 1989; **18**(1): 32–42.

5 Miller GE. The assessment of clinical skills/competence/performance. *Acad Med.* 1990; **65**(9): 63–7.

6 Benware C, Deci E. Quality of learning with an active versus passive motivational set. *AERJ.* 1984; **21**(4): 755–65.

The Skilful Art of Giving Feedback

FERGUS DONAGHY – TPD (Northern Ireland) & lead author   **RAMESH MEHAY** – TPD (Bradford) & lead author
SHAKE SEIGEL – TPD (Burton on Trent)   **PRIT CHAHAL** – TPD (Nottingham)

'Oh what power the gift could give us. To see ourselves as others see us'

Robert Burns (Scottish poet), 'To a Louse', 1786

Introduction

Feedback is a must for people who want to have honest relationships. It connects us and our behaviour to the world around us.[1] This chapter considers the importance of participating in feedback – to avoid it is dangerous for your emotional health! And your practice team may fall apart all around you. However, it comes with a hefty price – there are pitfalls in giving and receiving feedback from a practical aspect . . .

> I played golf for 10 years – regularly and poorly. I had a faulty grip, and I didn't care – but I practised so hard I could compensate – to a point. Folk often kindly mentioned that I needed to change the position of my right little finger – but I had invested many years' practice and my way felt so comfortable, indeed the ball usually travelled quite a long way; pity the ball was seldom straight. Then I received Ben Hogan's[2] book for Christmas. He explained the little finger must not be used as it brings other muscles into play that distort the swing. For the first time I believed, because his explanation made sense and was practical. At first, it was a little uncomfortable, but then I got used to the new grip and won my first ever golf competition with 50 points. One minor adjustment had a major transformation. But why did it take 10 years for me to change?

Why you should read this chapter

1   The most powerful single modification that *enhances achievement* is feedback. Feedback is one of those core ingredients which permeates the whole of training.

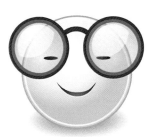

2   Feedback can either encourage or discourage behaviour and therefore it's important to get it right. *Improper* guidance/feedback is the single largest contributor to incompetence in the world of work.[3] We will be looking at what works and what doesn't in this chapter.

3   As educators we have a greater responsibility to *lead teams* and develop relationships: not just with trainees but also for any member of the primary healthcare team. Being skilful in feedback is essential for leadership, and teams can become dysfunctional if it is ignored.

4   Feedback is something that features in *all* aspects of our lives – not just our working lives! If you find that you're engaged in numerous arguments with your partner, relative or even your child, it might be because of the way you are giving feedback. Reading this chapter and learning the skill can dramatically change your relationships and thus your life.

The Jesuits often said, *'Give me the boy till he is seven and I will show you the man.'* So many of our behavioural traits are developed early in life by nature and nurture. If so much is ingrained, what chance have we of altering behaviour in grown adults who are highly intelligent and sophisticated? Yes, it is challenging, but it is possible. The benefits are enormous, the process is interesting and that's what makes it so worthwhile.

Definition and purpose

> ### Definition of feedback
> Providing information about performance or behaviour with the aim of:
> 1 affirming what you do well
> 2 helping you develop in areas you do less well.

Feedback is a form of communication that lets us know how *effective we are* and how *we affect others*. It helps us to become better the next time around; as the description of what we did is fed back to us, we come to understand more clearly what we did and did not do, and what we need to do more and less of. If we know how other people see us, we can overcome problems in how we interact with them, thus helping to close the gap between *our intent* and *the effect* we actually produced.

⚠ **Red Alert:** Feedback is not about blame, approval or disapproval. *Feedback* is more neutral – it merely describes what you did or did not accomplish given a standard or intent.

An incy-wincy bit of educational theory
A fundamental purpose of feedback is to help people *learn* through their mistakes. Therefore, before we can give feedback, we need to know *how people learn*. Kolb's learning cycle[4] describes how people learn **from their experience**.

In this cycle, immediate or *'concrete experiences'* provide a basis for *'observations and reflections'*. These are assimilated and distilled into *'abstract concepts'* producing new implications for action, which can be *'actively tested'*, in turn creating *new experiences*. However, different people have different strengths – some will be better at reflecting, others at conceptualising or experimenting. As educators we need to be aware of individual styles and preferences – this allows us to connect with them more closely. Feedback is simply facilitating people through Kolb's learning cycle and thus helping them connect with and strengthen all four bases.

1. EXPERIENCING
Concrete Experience

4. EXPERIMENTING
Testing implications of concepts in new situations

act   explore

2. REFLECTING
Observations & Reflections

decide   analyse

Formation of abstract concepts and generalisations
3. CONCEPTUALISING

Some personal reflections (Fergus Donaghy)

I was teaching medical students for 10 years and received unanimously positive feedback. I even became immune to comments like 'best attachment ever'. Then I started a Masters in Education, which added theory to my teaching experience and encouraged me to vary my instructional method and to structure the sessions, even to link them to the curriculum and to define learning objectives.

Empowered by this I eagerly awaited feedback from the six second-year students I had taken for 12 consecutive Friday afternoons for clinical skills. I had received a box of chocolates and a card signed by them all thanking me! As each session had ended, I asked for ideas how to run next week's meeting, but no suggestions were forthcoming, so I foolishly believed all was well.

On the same day, one student wrote to the university 'worst attachment ever, he has put me off medicine for life. I want to change my career'. I was hurt, cross and embarrassed. Initially, I blamed the Masters – 'Paralysis by Analysis' – was I trying to structure the sessions too much instead of 'winging it' and going with the flow where the students needed to go? It was an all-girl group so surely that must have contributed adversely to the dynamics? But, no, it was this individual where the fault lay fairly and squarely; she had every opportunity to contribute to the development of the sessions, and she chose not to. She ambushed me in the end; she waited in the long grass and reported me to the university. She disliked the sessions; perhaps she even disliked me and got her own back in the end.

I was quite experienced at teaching so I knew how to deal with this in proportion, and so I wrote my letter of resignation to the University! After all, this comment proved that all students were an ungrateful and sneaky bunch and unworthy of my talent. But then a young doctor, whom I had taught many years previously, brought me back to reality and made me consider things more objectively. She showed me learning notes she had kept from my teaching sessions eight years ago and she exemplified how I had been a role model to her and thus encouraged her to enter general practice so she could in turn teach students. I believed her and was heartened. It helped me put some negative criticism in perspective.

Recognise this?

If giving feedback is difficult, then receiving it is an even greater challenge. However, as educators and as doctors we cannot shirk this responsibility.

Strange how we feel so comfortable, some say smug, pontificating to our patients about the effects of lifestyle on their diabetes or weight. But perhaps we are not so vocal when we see our staff misbehaving, or our trainees underperforming.

If we keep our antennae out, if we are truly receptive, we get feedback every day from our personal interactions. This non-verbal leakage is so informative – if we want it to be.

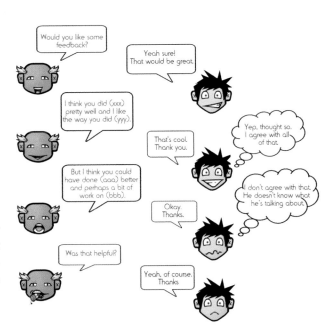

Can you remember a time when you were given feedback badly?

If you want to figure out how to give feedback effectively, a good starting point would be to know how *not* to do it. So, think back (maybe at school, college, university or even in your workplace) to a time when you were given feedback that made you feel humiliated, embarrassed or torn to shreds. Make a mental note of it. Take a couple of minutes to jot down your responses to the following.

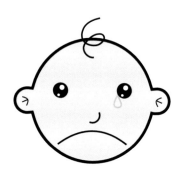

1 What was it about the *content* of that feedback that made you feel this way?
2 What was it about the *process* of that feedback that made you feel this way?
3 Was there anything about *you* that didn't help either?

You now have a list of what you shouldn't do. Can you reverse each item so that you have a list of what you should do? For instance, one of your items might be '*he made wrong judgements about me – said I was stupid*'. From that, you can conclude '*feedback should be based on observed behaviour, not judgements*'.

> When I go for golf lessons, I don't just want praise. I want to know exactly what I am being praised for. But that's not enough either. I want to improve, so I need correction; I want to know what part of my swing is faulty. And even more important I want to know how to fix it; so I can then practise a drill and work on it. However, often things get worse before they get better – and this must be accepted and tolerated.

The billion-dollar question: how do I give effective feedback?

Let's go back to our definition of feedback for a moment: '*information about performance or behaviour that leads to action to affirm or develop that performance or behaviour*'.

The key words in this definition give us a clue on how to do it.

1 **Information:** hard facts, concrete data, observable examples of performance and behaviour and *not* personal hunches *or* assumptions!
2 About **performance or behaviour:** what the person does and says and *not* about who they are.
3 That **leads to action:** in other words, a very specific intention. What's the point of giving feedback if there is no specific intention or action?
4 To **affirm or develop performance or behaviour:** the giver must be clear about the outcome they wish to see. If this is not clear to the feedback giver, what hope has the receiver got?

 Top Tip: In terms of the MRCGP, if you're trying to help learners improve their work in relation to a set standard, you've got to get rid of the secrecy about that standard. They need to know what they should be aiming for so that they can reflect on their experience and say, '*Mmm . . . What do I need to do to get there?*'

Giving feedback in the real world – a worked scenario (FD)

So now we've had a look at the background, let's see what goes on in the real world. Afterwards, we'll pick out themes from this to help formulate a more generalised framework.

Scenario

Jack is a 45-year-old trainee doctor in a rural general practice. He has worked in the practice for over 10 months; he is always very dutiful, conscientious and loyal. Clinically, he is safe and the patients respect him; perhaps even fear him a little. He is old school, prefers to keep his distance and quite private; no time for 'tittle-tattle'. He is so private that this blocks his contribution to practice debates. However, he is stressed travelling long distances to work each morning and often arrives late. His manner can be abrupt when stressed. He slams doors, bangs the keyboard and throws notes on the ground. He has a dry sense of humour, which includes sarcasm. He can be untidy at times in his appearance, and patients have commented. The staff are now at their wits' end because they find him so unpredictable. When he is in bad form he seems to let everyone know. Jack has a superior attitude when it comes to dealing with ancillary staff; it seems like they are less important.

What would you do? Take 3 minutes to either jot down or make a mental note of your approach (and, remember, the intention of feedback is for the benefit of the learner in order to make things better).

Here's what actually happened:

What happened	Conclusion(s)
I have to admit that I was cross when the staff came to me with an ultimatum about Jack's behaviour. I had previously intimated subtly to Jack about his communication skills; but obviously, I was too subtle! On other occasions, I was busy and chose not to act, thinking (and hoping) this would just blow over (or under the carpet). So now I felt I should act quickly before the moment passed. But I knew this emotive approach would be invariably counterproductive: the tone used in these circumstances is often accusatory and unbalanced. So I decided to take a breath, pick a mutually convenient time (and to allow my feelings to settle) and prepare.	Be controlled – not impulsive.
I knew that Jack could adopt a defensive attitude when confronted with feedback; he had previously protested in denial or blamed others. I needed to make sure that I triangulated the information I had – checking it with several sources and making sure it was either directly observed or corroborated so that I had confidence in it. Otherwise I knew this would end up as a debate about what happened rather than focusing on what went wrong and how to correct it.	Check that you've got the correct information.

What happened	Conclusion(s)
The staff were distressed with Jack's persistent behaviour and could tolerate it no longer. There was a danger someone would react inappropriately towards Jack, either through tears or even retaliation. I had asked them to make him aware of his actions – but they had failed at this subtle approach. So it fell to me as Trainer to do something at the earliest opportunity, otherwise the 'moment' would be lost. I informed Jack that we all undergo annual feedback and appraisal sessions; we agreed a suitable time for the following week. Jack's patient appointments were blocked for that afternoon and he was free to go home straight after the feedback.	Feedback has to be planned, protected and given in a timely way.
The following week came and Jack and I started off by discussing the purpose of feedback. My intention was to get him to realise that this was about making things better for him (and everyone else) and not retribution. Getting him to see and feel a more positive future helped with getting him on board. That made the process a whole lot smoother. We then engaged in a discussion which looked at ownership of feedback. Jack needed to know this feedback was specifically for him and not just bland guidance for any trainee in the practice; it was a direct reflection of his behaviour towards the practice team. We explored this in quite some detail, clarified facts and made space for him to air his feelings and his views.	Set the scene – feedback has to be owned and its intention clear. Clarify facts. Encourage a two-way dialogue through open questions.
Jack was untidy in his dress and appearance; patients had commented on this through our suggestion box – saying they thought he could not be bothered, looked unprofessional or was lazy. I knew Jack would react angrily and defensively to these judgemental statements (lazy, unprofessional) – who wouldn't? Therefore, to get Jack to accept and make changes, we focused on the descriptive elements – the fact that to others his shirt was not ironed, he was unshaven and his hair a bit of a mess. We then went on to have a fruitful discussion about how he would feel if he was seeing a caring professional who appeared this way.	Feedback has to be descriptive and specific – not judgemental.
It wasn't just his appearance though – he also left his room very untidy for the next user: his desk was a mess and there were even papers thrown on the floor. We explored how he would feel if he was due to work in someone else's room that was left in a similar manner. Although he knew others used his room, he did not fully realise the implications of leaving the room in that state. He agreed that this needed to change, and that he would no longer leave paper messages and notes on the table and would clear up after himself. In fact, he even asked if he could have some extra filing trays to help organise himself better.	Feedback must focus on change.

What happened	Conclusion(s)
There was no point telling Jack the staff didn't like him. He needed to know exactly why: in this case, it was his attitude and not his clinical competence that was creating problems. More specifically it was his attitude towards the non-medical staff. Even more specifically, it was his tone of voice and his sarcasm that upset others. It made them feel less valued and therefore, less appreciated. He wasn't aware of this, but he agreed that whether he meant it or not the consequence is the same, and it needed to change. He could see how improving this behaviour could earn him more respect and make him feel valued.	Feedback has to be based on observed behaviour (not personality or physical attributes).
Jack himself brought up his lateness issue and explained that it was related to the long travelling distance, road works, frequent accidents and punctures. He had quite a range of excuses. I thanked him for texting us in advance when he knew he was going to be late, giving us the chance to update the waiting patients. However, the recurring lateness caused logistical problems for patients with work commitments and staff trying to run an appointment system in a confined waiting area. We discussed ways in which the situation could be bettered and agreed on changing his duty hours to allow a later start and thus avoid peak traffic. I then finished this off by praising his commitment to work, considering the onerous journey twice daily.	Avoid being sucked into collusion (re: his excuses). Negotiate rather than being prescriptive. Give balanced feedback: positive feedback where it is due.
Having discussed things and set specific changes, both Jack and I wrote this up in his ePortfolio. Actually, I got Jack to do all the writing. I finally checked with him to make sure he was okay with what was discussed and there were no ill feelings lingering around. Despite a slightly defensive and negative start, he appeared to be more positive: explicitly stating he found the session useful and could see how it might result in a better future for him. Although he never mentioned how it would be better for everyone else too, at least I felt we 'hooked' him into change.	Agree on a plan and check you are both happy.

A practical approach to feedback

Let's see how we can *generalise away from the specific* case above to help generate a practically useable framework. We've split this bit into three sections to make it easier to understand and remember.

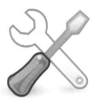

- Step 1 – Preparing to give feedback: things you need to do *before* you give any sort of feedback.
- Step 2 – Giving feedback: concentrating on *content* of your feedback.
- Step 3 – Feedback models: looking at the *process* of giving feedback.

Step 1: *Preparing* to give feedback

If you don't spend time preparing to give feedback, there is a high chance it will go belly up. The person on the receiving end may then engender ill feelings. You need to prepare – tradesmen tell us to measure twice and cut once. With feedback, there are five measurements you need to make beforehand.

1 Have I got the **facts** right?

Expect the session to run into disagreements and chaos if you've not double-checked on the facts from a variety of sources. The receiver will lose faith in you if this happens.

2 What is my **intention** behind giving this person feedback?

Will this feedback truly help the receiver or not? Is the giver just showing off? When dealing with doctors in training, we are often called to give feedback on their medical skills in relation to the various areas of competence – holistic care, professionalism or diagnostic or clinical ability. In terms of GP training, the RCGP gives excellent guidance on what is expected in each domain.[5] It clearly exemplifies what constitutes 'needs development', 'competent' and 'excellent'. It's worthwhile spending some time structuring the feedback you're planning to give in this way as it standardises judgements and is clear on how trainees can improve.

3 Is the **receiver in a fit enough state** to receive it?

How brittle are they? Put yourself in the trainee's shoes. How would it feel to receive the feedback you're planning to give? Doing this will not only help you fine-tune the way you give feedback but will also help you anticipate the various reactions from the trainee.

Furthermore, check whether something acute has happened in that person's personal life. It's almost pointless giving feedback to a trainee whose house has been burgled over the weekend – they'll be preoccupied with that. And if you do give it, they may react to it badly – making it a horrible experience for all. Explicitly ask them how life has been before giving feedback.

4 **Am I in a fit enough state** to give it?

Similarly, if you've been upset by something in your own personal life, you may end up giving feedback in a bad way and adversely handling any reactions to it. You need to be in a positive state of mind with a positive tone of voice. When life is hard, consider delaying the feedback to a calmer moment.

5 Am I giving feedback in a **timely** way?

Don't give feedback on a 'cold' topic that happened months ago. People will have difficulty recalling events. Misunderstandings start to fester and there are fewer chances of improvement. Give feedback as close to the event as possible – unless the situation is so emotionally charged that you need to give time for rough waters to settle. The right time also means making sure you give enough protected time to allow a fruitful, uninterrupted discussion.

Step 2: *Giving* feedback – concentrating on the content of your feedback

Brown and Leigh[6] devised some rules for constructive feedback. Feedback should be:

1 **Descriptive**, i.e. non-judgemental; based on behaviour not personality:

> ☹ BAD: 'Jack, you seem to have a low opinion of non-medical staff around you.'
> ☺ GOOD: 'I notice that you don't look at people when they are talking to you, particularly other staff.'

Both apply to the same situation, but the first is judgemental (and more likely to provoke a defensive reaction). The second describes what is happening and is more likely to be accepted – it's hard to argue against the evidence.

2 **Specific** or focused. In order to focus developmental feedback:

(a) avoid personal comments:

> ☹ BAD: 'Jack, you really are a scruffy looking git. Sometimes you look like a tramp!'
> ☺ GOOD: 'Jack, can we talk about your appearance? Some patients have said . . .'

(b) avoid mixed messages:

> ☹ BAD: 'Jack, you always look as if you have just got out of bed but your work is good on the whole.'
> ☺ GOOD: 'Jack, can we talk to you about your appearance in order to make a better impression?'

(c) avoid diffusion:

> ☹ BAD: 'Jack, this lateness is becoming ridiculous. Please sort it out.'
> ☺ GOOD: 'Jack, can we sit down and specifically work out how we can make this lateness better?'

3 **Directed** towards *observed* behaviour that *can be changed*:

> ☹ BAD: 'Admin staff find you intimidating; perhaps it's because you're too tall and bulky. And what's with the permanent poker face?'
> ☺ GOOD: 'Do you think staff might feel more comfortable around you if you simply smiled more?'

By observed behaviour we mean what the individual has *said* or *done*. It is not helpful to give a person feedback over which they have no choice (height, weight etc.).

4 **Timely:** given as close to the event as possible. There's no point in feedback on something that happened 3 months back.

5 **Selective:** addressing 2–3 key issues rather than 20!

And we'd like to add a sixth:

6 **Offer solutions as suggestions, not prescriptions.**

> ☹ BAD: 'From now on, I think you should do . . .'
> ☺ GOOD: 'How would you feel if I suggested . . .?'; 'Do you think it might have been helpful if . . .?'; 'Have you any thoughts on . . .?'; 'What if . . .?' What do you think?'

Step 3: Ways of giving feedback – feedback models (*process*)

I once remember asking an eminent surgeon for some feedback as a Senior House Officer; this was in the 80s before the 'West Wing' promoted the 'walk & talk' philosophy. He continued to walk down the corridor so I had to follow him clinging onto every word, not wanting to miss the moment. He opened the toilet door and proceeded to relieve himself while talking to me, then left me standing – I can't actually remember a word he said, but I will never forget the process!

There are several different models that focus on the *process* of giving feedback. All of them give you a structure for delivering your feedback. We suggest you play around with the different models: all of them can be used with either individuals or groups.

We're going to look at four different models of feedback.

1 Modified Pendleton's principles
2 SET-GO
3 Gibbs's reflective cycle
4 ALOBA.

ALOBA is described only briefly here but there is a more comprehensive guide on our website.

 Top Tip: Remember to observe Brown and Leigh's rules of feedback (the *content*) when using any model of feedback.

 Top Tip: The key to all models described below is to provide *both* challenge and support. By challenge, we mean really getting them to discuss, grow and improve. By support, we mean doing this in a way that does not dampen their self-esteem.

Modified Pendleton's[7] principles (2003 version)

Pendleton's principles focus on **providing *challenge* in a sea of *support***. It seeks to understand how and why some tasks are done well but others are not:

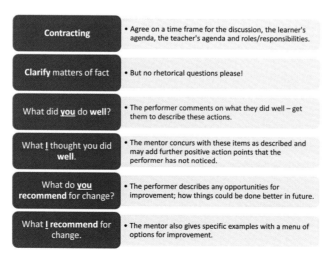

The first two stages (contracting and clarifying) were not explicitly formalised in their original version (hence now called 'Modified Pendleton's'). The focus of this model is on recommendations rather than weaknesses because the trainee is more likely to adopt these if phrased in this way (less threatening and more supportive).

Some important points about Pendleton's principles of feedback

Most of us have been brought up on Pendleton's rules, and it's a **particularly good model to use with relatively new GP trainees** (because of its supportive nature). But it has its fair share of critics, who say:

1 Once the performer (the trainee in our case) becomes familiar with the model, they end up thinking: *'Yeah, yeah, yeah . . . let's just get to the bad bits.'*
2 You're simply postponing the discovery of the learner's agenda by talking about the good bits first and that this is an inefficient use of time.

In their book, Pendleton *et al.*[7] state that these should be seen as guidelines or principles, not rules (and should not be called 'Pendleton's Rules'). That means that you don't need to follow them in the exact order illustrated in the diagram on the previous page. This gets rid of the artificiality about the feedback process. It also means that if you want to tackle the learner's agenda first, then by all means do so, but at some point, don't forget to do the positive bits to provide balanced feedback. However, following the order sequence is useful with new learners: giving the positives first makes sense because it establishes the strengths, allowing you to create a positive mindset right from the start.

One final thing to say about Pendleton's principles (and they say this too): you must *not* use them *blindly* without having explicit standards first. For example, if you're evaluating someone's consultation, use some sort of yardstick against which to assess it: something like the MRCGP COT crib sheet. Only then use Pendleton's guidelines to help communicate what you have picked up from the assessment sheet. If you don't use some sort of criteria, you'll end up bombarding the poor trainee with a load of unexpected unstructured criticism, which lacks focus and is not tailored to any agenda.

 Top Tip: When the performer is being asked to reflect on his or her own performance, it is important that they are discouraged from <u>judging</u> themselves (*'I was rubbish at exploring her concerns'*). Instead, encourage them to focus on <u>describing</u> actions (*'She mentioned rheumatoid arthritis a few times; I wonder if that was her concern? I think it was a cue that I should have explored further.'*).

The SET-GO[8] approach to feedback

Trainees usually react defensively to judgemental comments like *'I thought you were uninterested in the patient'*. Judgemental comments are subjective opinions – some people will agree with you, and others will not. The SET-GO model helps prevent this by **helping us to be more objective**. By focusing on observed behaviour – what you *see* or what you *hear* – it's difficult for a trainee to argue against it: *'I noticed that you looked at the computer screen a fair bit at the beginning while the patient was talking to you. Put yourself in the patient's shoes for a moment. What effect would it have had on you?'*

What did you **S**ee?

- Get the trainee to describe what was seen or experienced. Get them to be descriptive, specific and non-judgemental.

What **E**lse?

- Probe to discover what else was seen or experienced. What happened next in descriptive terms? If in a group what did others see? What did you see as the trainer?

What do you **T**hink, John?

- Get the trainee to reflect on the experience, and then give them an opportunity to acknowledge and problem solve by themself first.

What **G**oal would you like to achieve?

- To promote an outcomes based approach, clarify what goal the trainee would like to achieve. If in a group, what would others like to achieve?

Any **O**ffers of how we should get there?

- Explore ways of achieving the goal. Get the trainee to come up with suggestions. Invite others if in a group. **Rehearse** any suggestions. Rehearsal is a key step: new behaviour can only be acquired through actual practice.

Gibbs's Reflective Cycle[9]

Gibbs's cycle is a neat little tool because it provides you with a structure for tackling any **case discussions and consultations** learners have experienced – **especially the emotionally charged ones**. It encourages learners to reflect on what happened so that they can somehow *make sense* of the experiences. However, reflection is not enough: one has to put the new learning and understanding into practice.

ACTION PLAN
- If it arose again, what would you do differently?

DESCRIPTION
- What happened?

FEELINGS
- What were you thinking and feeling?

EVALUATION
- What was good and bad about the experience?

ANALYSIS
- Can you make sense of the experience?

CONCLUSION
- What else could you have done?

How to use it

- Use the individual stages to structure the feedback discussion.
- Encourage trainees to write learning events in their ePortfolios in this way.
- Make sure the learners are not too hard on themselves: the evaluation phase should help tease out what was *good* and bad about the experience.

ALOBA[10] – **A**genda **L**ed **O**utcomes **B**ased **A**nalysis

This model[10] was primarily developed for giving feedback on experiential learning activities (like videos of consultations, simulated patient sessions). However, it can be adapted to giving feedback on more general areas.

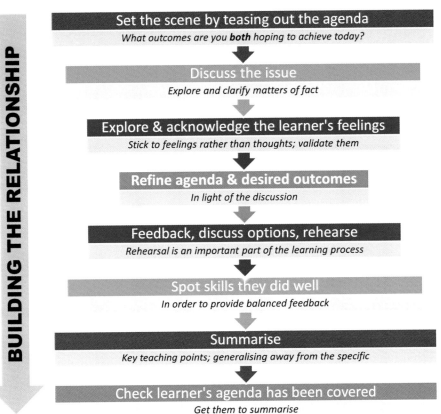

Imagine a trainee has just had an argument with one of the reception staff. You've come to hear about it. You mention it to your trainee, and he agrees it would be good to talk about it. How would you proceed? Does this modified version of ALOBA help you in any way? Follow it through and see.

The great thing about ALOBA is the fact **you can go straight to the hot issue – it is agenda led!** In other words, you don't have to do the good bits first. Why? Because both you and the learner have agreed that this is what you want to do and both of you can see the positive benefits that will emerge. In essence, you've 'hooked' the learner in: they can see what's in it for them.

We've only covered ALOBA very briefly here. A comprehensive set of ALOBA manuals is available on our website. Although there are separate versions for running a 1–1 session, a group session and a simulated patient session, the bare bones of the ALOBA model is roughly the same for all (*see* the ALOBA summary flowchart on our website).

 Top Tip: Teasing out the agenda – the most common reason educators struggle with ALOBA is because of not drilling down to a specific and detailed agenda.

Teasing out the agenda . . .

Trainer: 'So is there anything specific you wanted to get from this particular session looking at your consultation tape?'

Trainee: 'Yeah, in this consultation, I found it difficult to engage the patient' (*This is too wide an agenda – drill down to the specifics.*)

Trainer: 'What specific area of engaging the patient did you have difficulty with in this particular consultation?'

Trainee: 'I dunno really.'

Trainer: 'Was it something to do with building rapport, for instance?'

Trainee: 'No, I don't think it was rapport. In this particular case, I found it difficult to get them on board with my management plan.'

Trainer: 'Ahhh . . . so do you think it was something relating to your explanation – maybe the way you phrased and pitched it or something to do with formulating a joint management plan?'

Trainee: 'Actually, I think it was both of those. Can we look at both?'

Trainer: 'Okay, so we'll look at the tape focusing on two things: (a) your explanation and (b) formulating a joint management plan.'

What sort of material can you give feedback on?

There are loads of things in practice that you can review and give feedback on. Here are just a few: video analysis (formally or informally), random or problem cases analysis, significant events, complaints, referral and prescribing reviews, feedback from other members of the healthcare team (informal 'off the cuff' remarks or more formally via multi-source feedback) and patient feedback (again, 'off the cuff' remarks or more formally via a patient satisfaction questionnaire).

Practise giving feedback

Remember: feedback doesn't just happen in GP training; it's a feature of our daily life – at work, home and socially. *Informally*, try some of these feedback skills on your partner, a friend or even your own children. Children don't play by the rules, but they are very forgiving! Don't be surprised if suddenly you find yourself in a life that's a smooth and easy ride with fewer arguments and bickering. In addition, when you're at your Trainers' workshops (which generally provide a safe environment), have a go at giving feedback on videotaped consultations. You've nothing to lose and plenty to gain.

Don't forget to ask for feedback on yourself

By doing this, the trainee will learn the art of giving feedback and will realise that you don't have to be an educator to give feedback – it's a two-way thing. It also gives you an opportunity to stop and think how you are doing as an educator and how your practice or department is doing as a teaching and learning organisation. Besides, it reminds you of how it feels to receive feedback, thus not losing sight of how trainees can feel.

And finally . . .

We're going to finish off with a few words by Jennifer King[11] and a variation of the cartoon you saw earlier on in this chapter.

'Giving feedback is not just to provide a judgement or evaluation. It is to provide insight. Without insight into their own strengths and limitations, (the receiver) cannot progress or resolve difficulties.'

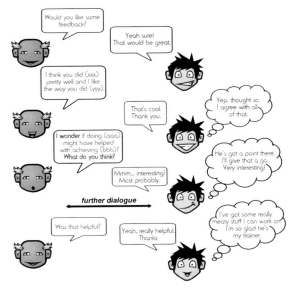

There's a lot more to it than this, but you get the idea

A sample of resources on our website
- ALOBA manuals.
- Common pitfalls in giving feedback (really worth a read).
- Handling undesirable reactions to feedback (really worth a read).
- Feedback handout for trainees.

Other chapters you may like to read
- Chapter 9: Exploring and Creating a Learning Culture
- Chapter 4: Powerful Hooks – aims, objectives and ILOs
- Chapter 13: Teaching and Facilitating Small Groups.

Please give us some feedback on this chapter to help shape it for the next edition.
Go to www.essentialgptrainingbook.com and simply click on the title of this chapter.

References

1 www.selfhelpmagazine.com/about/staff/biorich.php (accessed February 2010).
2 Hogan B. *Ben Hogan's Five Lessons: the modern fundamentals of golf.* London: Simon & Schuster Ltd; 2006.
3 Gilbert TF. *Human Competence: engineering worthy performance.* New York: McGraw-Hill; 1978.
4 Kolb D. *Experiential Learning.* New Jersey: Prentice Hall; 1984.
5 RCGP. Available at: www.rcgp-curriculum.org.uk/ (accessed February 2010).
6 Brown SP, Leigh TW. A new look at psychological climate and its relationship to job involvement, effort and performance. *J Appl Psychol.* 1996; **81**: 358–68.
7 Pendleton D, Schofield D, Tate P, Havelock P. *The New Consultation: developing doctor-patient communication.* Oxford: Oxford University Press; 2003. pp. 75–80.
8 Silverman, J Draper J, Kurtz SM. The Calgary-Cambridge approach to communication skills teaching: the SET-GO method of descriptive feedback, *Educ Gen Pract.* 1997; **8**: 16–23.
9 Gibbs G. *Learning by Doing: a guide to teaching and learning methods.* Oxford: Oxford Polytechnic; 1988.
10 Kurtz SM, Silverman J, Draper J. *Teaching and Learning Communication Skills in Medicine.* 2nd ed. Oxford: Radcliffe Publishing; 2005.
11 King J. Giving feedback. *BMJ Classifieds.* 1999; **318**: 2.

8

Teaching Gems

DAMIAN KENNY – GP Educationalist (Severn Deanery) & lead author
RAMESH MEHAY – TPD (Bradford) & lead author   **JAMES MEADE** – TPD (NIMDTA, Northern Ireland)
RODGER CHARLTON – Professor of Medical Education (Univ. Swansea)

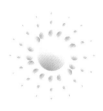

As an educator, try to encourage your learners to become really good at doing what you're trying to get them to do, rather than aiming for them being just about okay. Teaching and learning is not only about filling learners' minds with knowledge, but also about helping them to do things in practice, do them well, and aspire to do them even better! Below is a set of questions that we've been asked frequently by new educators. We think you will find them helpful.

How do I build a relationship and a 'good' educational climate that encourages the learner to interact, be honest and be open?

Ways to build the relationship
- *Your own* **language, behaviour and attitude** has a lot to do with whether learners will mirror that (why not video yourself?). If you come over as an 'expert' or an 'oracle', you may inhibit your learners from revealing how they really feel. Show a passion for teaching and they'll hopefully show some passion for wanting to learn. Show them your weaknesses (like your own learning gaps), and they'll show you theirs.
- Understand the **learner's feelings and perspective**: it's important to acknowledge and empathise with their feelings while being supportive and sensitive at the same time.

Ways to promote interaction
- Provide an **agenda which really hooks them** (*see* Chapter 4: Powerful Hooks – aims, objectives and ILOs). Make the session **interactive**: brainstorm, share thoughts, discuss issues and interact with the learner at his or her level. **Be flexible**: if a 'new' important learning issue comes up during the session, be prepared to change the initial agenda and go with the flow. And, finally, **inject humour** to make it light-hearted and fun (where appropriate).

Promoting a good educational climate
Promoting a good educational climate starts the very day your trainee arrives at your practice and continues throughout their attachment. It's a bit more difficult when you've been asked to give a tutorial to a learner or a group of learners you've never met before. Here are some tips.
- Encourage the learners to be open and honest about the way they *feel* about things and be prepared to show them *your* feelings too.
- Encourage the learners to be open and honest about their *uncertainties/knowledge gaps* and be prepared to show them *your own* uncertainties/knowledge gaps too.
- Read Chapter 9: Exploring and Creating a Learning Culture.

Explicitly signpost that it's okay to reveal their feelings, uncertainties and knowledge gaps. *'For this session to work, I need you to reveal any feelings you have like fears, concerns, uncertainties and knowledge gaps. Remember, we all have fears and uncertainties; I still do after 10 years of practising! But this session is for YOU and for that to happen, I need you to show me your inner feelings. Is that possible?'*

I'm new at all of this teaching stuff and I don't feel very confident. I'm sure it shows. Have you any tips?

Looking confident is important, even if you don't feel it. Ever been to a travel agent where the agent doesn't look as if they know what they're doing? And then you start to lose faith in them as you wonder whether you've really got a good holiday package? It's the same for learners: how can you expect them to engage in your session, have faith and be inspired by you if you're not being confident in what you're saying?

Some tips to come across as confident

- Look confident even if you don't feel it: hold your head up and speak confidently. You manage to do it with patients when they ask you about something you're not quite sure about. Do it with learners too.
- Avoid putting yourself down or starting with negative statements like:
  'Sorry, but I didn't quite have time to prepare much stuff."
  'It's not my strong subject, but I'll have a go.'
- Prepare! A lack of confidence usually occurs because of a lack of preparation either about content or methodology. If you fail to prepare, then prepare to fail!
- If you're worried about what questions the learners might ask you, don't be! Simply reflect the questions back to them (more on this below).
- In a similar fashion, if you're worried about how to approach and tackle an issue raised by a learner, reflect it back to them (more below).
- Remember, your role is to be a facilitator of learning rather than an expert. If you've created a safe learning environment where learners can openly and honestly discuss their fears, concerns and knowledge gaps, then so can you. It's good 'role-modelling' behaviour too: *'Mmm . . . that's an interesting question Naresh, and thanks for being open and honest about what you don't know. I have to admit, I don't know either. Can someone help us out? Does anyone know?'*

I get all flustered about teaching in case they ask me questions I cannot answer. I'm sure they'll lose faith in me. What can I do?

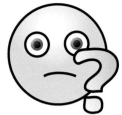

New educators often worry too much about being asked a question and being unable to answer it. Remember: a group of learners, as a whole, has far more knowledge than any one individual (including you). So rather than acting like an expert, take on the facilitative role and reflect questions back to the group at large. You'll find that there is at least one person who will respond. This also imparts a subliminal message that the responsibility for facilitating learning is shared by the group.

'That's an interesting question. Mmm . . .
  . . . have you any idea in your mind how you might go about that?'
  . . . what do you think you might do?'

'That's a good question. Mmm . . .
  . . . I wonder what other people think about that?'
  . . . Would anyone else like to reply to that?'
  . . . Does any bright spark know the answer to that?'

Apply the same principle when you're unsure about the *approach* to an issue:
  'That's interesting; I wonder how we should approach that? Does anyone have any suggestions?'

Going back to the issue about questions, should I allow learners to interrupt my teaching session with questions or should I dedicate some time space at the end?
Personally, we feel that if there is a 'hot potato', it should be tackled there and then. Besides, questions raised in this manner are based on where the session is at that particular moment (i.e. the questions are context driven). It seems illogical to cover them at the end when that 'moment' has passed. Allowing interruptions with questions can add 'dynamism' to your session too. However, if you're being *bombarded* with questions that are interrupting the natural flow of your session, you may need to manage the questions in a different way. Some of us like learners interrupting our teaching sessions while others prefer to provide time at the end.

I feel I put an awful lot of effort and planning into my teaching sessions, and I still seem to run out of time. It's exhausting and, afterwards, I don't feel particularly satisfied that 'it was worth it'.

There are two things you've mentioned here and they're both linked: over-planning and running out of time.

Over-planning: You're putting in more effort than the session needs.
- Start planning your session well before the delivery date: last-minute planning (like the day before) always leads to chaos and overload. Do the planning in bite-sized chunks. Do a bit every few days; it's more enjoyable and less overwhelming that way. It's a bit like decorating your whole house – doing it bit by bit over six months would be more fun than doing the whole lot in a couple of days!
- Be systematic in your planning approach. Chapter 6: Teaching from Scratch tells you to work out the aims first, and from that derive the contents and the methodology.

- Plotting things out on a mind map might help you. You can then cross things off as you complete them (which will also give you a sense of satisfaction that you are making progress).
- Maybe you are simply covering too much, and it's no wonder that there's a lot of work involved. If your agenda (aims and objectives) is large, the following suggestions might help.
  1 Split items into two columns – those which are essential (important to know) and those which are desirable (nice to know but not essential). Now look at the desirable list and just cross off what you think can go. Your new agenda should be lots shorter now.
  2 It may be that you're covering too much breadth **and** depth. Clearly, if you're trying to give an overview, you need to focus on the breadth and let go of some of the depth. If you're after understanding, focus on depth and narrow the breadth.
  3 Can anything be set as a homework task so you don't have to cover it – like the basics? Can some of the content go into a handout?

Running out of time during the session

- Cutting down the agenda (as in the section on over-planning above) will stop you being over-inclusive and will help with time management too.
- However, sometimes people run out of time not because there was too much stuff to cover, but because they put tight time limits in their session's plan in the first place. Set wider times in your teaching plan.
- You will almost definitely run out of time if you haven't built time in your session plan for people interjecting with their queries. It is important that you allow these queries to be voiced or discussed. A query signposts a significant ('hot') area for the individual; in a group setting, it's likely to be important for others too. If you're going to run out of time by covering a query, perhaps something else in your predefined agenda has to go. **It's completely fine not to cover everything**, providing you (a) see depth as more important than breadth and (b) you tackle what's 'hot' and not what's not.

According to feedback, the problem with my teaching sessions is that they go in all sorts of directions and therefore feel a bit unstructured. How can I add structure?
First, let's explore why structure is important.

- It provides a **framework** from which you (the facilitator) can hang things off.
- It provides a **framework** onto which the learner can construct their own knowledge.
- It shows you and the audience **where you are** and where you are going next.
- It makes the session **easy to follow**, understand and recall.
- It shows the learner how **one thing links** with another.

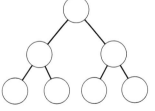

Some educationalists believe that the learners themselves should be responsible for constructing their own framework, and that imposing structure can sometimes limit creativity. Personally, we feel that if you don't provide at least a basic structure for your teaching session, all the different bits of your session will appear disjointed, and your learners may become confused.

How to add structure

1 Before your session – use a **teaching plan template** (available on our website under the resources section for Chapter 6: Teaching from Scratch).
2 At the start of your session – **set the agenda** (aims and objectives) with the learner and display it for all to see (PowerPoint, flip chart, handout, etc.)
3 Throughout your session – **signpost and summarise** frequently.
   - Signposting means telling the learner where you're going next.
     'Okay, so you said you had a problem with identifying the patient's concerns. So let's look at that next.'
   - Summarise periodically throughout your session, not just at the end.
     'Okay, before we go onto talking about explanation and management planning with the patient, shall we recap what we've covered so far?'

Sometimes my teaching session becomes a bit dull and dry. The learner seems to yawn, and it feels like hard work. How can I make it more dynamic?

- As we mentioned before, *your* **behaviour** can affect your learners. The more lively and enthusiastic you are, the more they will be too; it's infectious!
- A dull and dry session can also mean a lack of interactivity. You need to go back to the drawing board and re-examine the educational methods you used. Next time, pick a **selection of different methods** that encourage **interactivity**. For instance, if a trainee doesn't know 'the management of COPD' why not get up and go to a computer, log onto the Internet and find that out together (rather than just telling them). This also teaches them that important skill of looking for information when you don't know it.
- **Continuously monitor and 'read' your audience**. If you see a yawn or one or two people dozing off, it's time to change tack and use a different method.
- Ask the audience – **reflect back what you see**: *'It looks like some of you are flagging. How can we make the session a bit more lively and fun?'*
- Maybe your session is simply too long, and that you need to **build in a break** to recharge the learner. If you have a group of learners, introduce an energising game.
- Many group teaching sessions involve sitting in a circle discussing a particular topic or issue. While this promotes equality, sitting down for too long can promote a mindset for laziness. Occasionally getting up to write on a flip chart (or getting one of the group members to do so) might counteract this.

Trainees hate role play. As soon as I try to get them to practise a consultation skill by saying, 'Let's try that with role play', they start wincing

First of all, it's good that you understand that a skill cannot be acquired without repeat practice and you're right, one way of doing this is role play. And, yes, they do hate the words 'role play'. The answer is simple: ***don't* use the term role play**. For some reason they have negative connotations for trainees. Instead of the term 'role play', use a different phrase like one of the following.

- *'Let's practise that.'*
- *'Let's rehearse that.'*
- Or better still, don't call it anything at all – just do it! *'That's interesting. Okay, I'm going to be the patient, and let's go back to that point where she said . . . and let's try that different phrase.'*

In this way, trainees engage without realising that they're doing role play! Weird, we know, but try it and see. For example, an experienced doctor and a GP trainee may have a conversation in between patients during a joint surgery:

> *Trainer:* I have noticed that you always open the consultation by asking 'How can I help you today?' I was wondering if you had considered any other opening phrases?
>
> *Trainee:* I haven't thought about it. What do you usually say?
>
> *Trainer:* I usually try to be silent, but if the patient seems to expect me to say something, then I say: 'What would you like to talk about today?'
>
> *Trainee:* I'm not sure I'd be any good with just using gestures and stuff.
>
> *Trainer:* Well, how's about me pretending to be that patient we've just talked about and I'll walk in and you can give it your best shot? Wanna try?
>
> *Trainee:* Yeah . . . why not. If I don't get it, will you show me how you do it?
>
> *Trainer:* You got a deal.

Do you have a framework for teaching the clinical stuff in relation to patients seen?

While doing our ordinary work, there are many brief opportunities for learning and teaching, even if we only have five minutes available during a busy surgery. There are two techniques that you can use: 'SNAPPS' and 'one-minute teacher'.

SNAPPS[1] is a learner-centred model. It encourages learners to think and interact with you. One great thing about SNAPPS is that it relieves you of having to think of questions and makes the teaching session interactive, interesting and easy.

> **SNAPPS:** The learner is encouraged by the teacher to:
> S   Summarise the case
> N   Narrow the differential diagnosis
> A   Analyse the differential diagnosis
> P   Probe (ask about areas they don't fully understand)
> P   Plan management
> S   Select an issue for self-directed learning

One-minute teacher:[2] Compared to SNAPPS, this model incorporates the important step of feedback. That's not to say it is a better model: play around with both. There are documents on our website covering both in more detail.

> **One Minute Teacher:** there are five things you get the learner to focus on.
> 1   Ask the learner to outline the **diagnosis or management plan**.
> 2   Question the learner for **their reasoning** (justifying).
> 3   Teach the learner some **key take-home messages or general rules**.
> 4   Give the learner **feedback on what was done well**.
> 5   Correct errors and give the learner **feedback on what could be done better**.

What about a framework for helping me help them reflect on difficult situations?

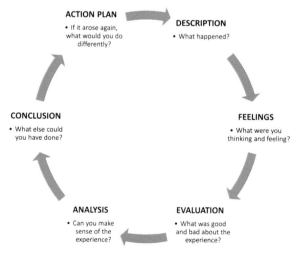

Gibbs's reflective cycle[3] can help you with this. It is particularly good when learners want to reflect on **an event which did not go as desired**: maybe identified through a significant event analysis, a difficult consultation or viewing a consultation video. Going through the cycle will help your learners figure out the key causal elements and thus what they might do differently the next time around.

It's also good for teaching sessions which involve an **exploration of the learner's feelings** (in dysfunctional consultations, for example).

I've heard about this technique called 'reflection through reframing'; can you explain a bit more about that?

Sometimes a colleague might describe a patient or a situation in a negative way, or with words that imply a **negative frame of mind**. That negativity can interfere with learning. We can help them to reflect on this in a different way by listening carefully, and then 'reframing' the comments, hoping that this may then allow them to explore the issues in a **more positive way**.

For example, if someone describes a patient as 'heart-sink', we could reframe the event and describe the patient's story as 'medically unexplained symptoms'. This is more neutral. We could even attempt positive reframing by calling them 'medically unexplored stories', which opens the possibility of discussing the perplexing symptoms as narrative medicine rather than medical symptoms. So, if a trainee begrudgingly says, *'The patient wasn't particularly interested in all the other options I offered'*, you could reframe it and alter their mindset by saying, *'It's good how you discussed the various options and gave the patient choice.'*

I've heard others talk about poems and other creative arts in teaching and encouraging reflection. Can you tell me more?

There's a whole chapter in this book dedicated to using the creative arts (Chapter 17) in teaching and learning. Reading a poem in a learning group can be an effective way of considering the Learner's emotional response to some problems, e.g. bereavement, unemployment, etc. Some learners find writing a poem helpful as a way of understanding the patient's emotional experience. We can also discuss a relevant book, podcast, play or film to explore issues, for example, about an autistic person, ethical dilemmas, or caring for someone with dementia.

> I have used poetry to help a junior doctor to focus his thoughts. The doctor was taking several minutes to make a case presentation and included every fine detail. Asking him to give the presentation in a short poem helped him to focus on the main issues and leave out less important details. (Of course, we did not bother about the rhyme or metre of the poem: it was just a tool for helping to focus thoughts).

A sample of resources on our website
- SNAPPS.
- The One Minute Preceptor.

Other chapters you may like to read
- Chapter 4: Powerful Hooks – aims, objectives and ILOs
- Chapter 6: Teaching from Scratch
- Chapter 10: Five Pearls of Educational Theory.

Please give us some feedback on this chapter to help shape it for the next edition.
Go to www.essentialgptrainingbook.com and simply click on the title of this chapter.

References

1 Wolpaw TM, Wolpaw DR, Papp KK. SNAPPS: a learner centred approach for outpatient education. *Acad Med.* 2003; **78**: 893–8.
2 Furney SL, Orsini AL, Orsetti KE. Teaching the one minute preceptor. A randomised control trial. *J Gen Intern Med.* 2001; **16**: 620–4.
3 Gibbs G. *Learning by Doing: a guide to teaching and learning methods.* Oxford: Oxford Polytechnic; 1988.

PART THREE

Educational Theory that Matters

9

Exploring and Creating a Learning Culture

DAVID PEARSON – Head of Primary Care Learning & Teaching (Univ. Leeds) & lead author
PAUL MILNE – Senior Lecturer in General Practice (Univ. Central Lancashire)
MOHAN KUMAR – Associate Director (North West Deanery)

Exploring and creating a learning what?

We all know that clinical learning doesn't occur in a vacuum. What you need is social interaction and discourse with colleagues. The *educational environment* and *learning ethos* of an educational establishment (be it a practice, hospital or training scheme) are key players in promoting social interaction and discourse. And that's where this chapter comes in – we'll be exploring the relationship between these two things.

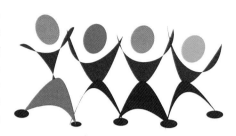

What makes someone engage and participate in their own learning?

Experience and reflection on experiences are important in clinical education (*see* Kolb and Schon in Chapter 10: Five Pearls of Educational Theory) but not enough on their own to *drive* learning. Somehow, you've got to get learners to engage before they will participate in any form of reflection.

To engage people in learning from their experience requires:

1   challenge
2   some sort of emotion and
3   an external stimulus – either from the patient, a colleague or an educator.

The theory says that transformative learning occurs where frames of reference are challenged through new experiences or perspectives and allow a construction of new meaning through critical reflection.[1] Ideas may change radically, changing the person and their world view (if you want to know more, look up Habermas[3] on critical theory and Freire[4] on emancipatory learning).

Encouraging 'communities of practice'

At the beginning of this chapter we said that learning doesn't happen in a vacuum – individual transformative learning occurs through social interaction within organisations, teams or groups.

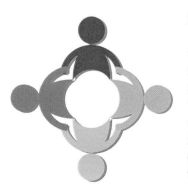

This comes from **sociocultural learning theory** but Vygotsky says it's normal for humans to interact with others anyway.[5]

But Jean Lave and Etienne Wenger[6,7] argue that learning occurs through *meaningful* involvement in activity, and specifically through negotiating the meaning of that involvement with peers, tutors or similar – which they call a 'community of practice'. A 'community of practice' is defined as 'a group of people who share a concern or a passion for something they do and learn how to do it better as they interact regularly'. A supportive and activity-rich environment is crucial for learning, but so is the role modelling that makes the trajectory from junior learner to involved player explicit. (For more detail on Wenger's communities of practice, there's an excellent resource on our website).

> The theory on 'communities of practice' helps explain why GP trainees might find hospital posts more supportive and stimulating and why having multiple trainees, other learners, or salaried doctors in a GP practice may be as valuable as having an experienced Trainer.

The learning culture, climate and ethos

These terms are very closely related but let's start with another term first – organisational culture. Understanding that will help with the others.

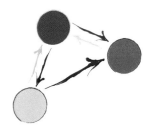

Organisational culture in its simplest form is about 'how we do things around here'. Why an organisation does things usually stems from:

1 what has gone on before (traditions, a historical perspective)
2 their core values (importance)
3 their current attitudes (commitment).

Learning culture is pretty much the same thing, but in the context of education. *Learning climate* is often used interchangeably with *learning culture*; but culture implies a historical perspective whereas the learning climate may be no more than the current perceptions on learning according to members of an organisation or team. Having a good *learning ethos* (e.g. towards GP training) equates with most individuals in an organisation having a belief in it and committing to it with their *minds, bodies and souls*.

> We've always trained since the year dot [tradition]. However, I think GP training has become so much better over the last five years. Before that, the Trainer in our practice always banged on about it being important to give him protected time to do various training activities. We used to give in – it was less of a hassle that way and it saved our eardrums!
>
> When he left the practice, one of the other partners took over. He started to do things differently. For a start, he wanted to know how we all felt about GP training, what we thought about the trainees we'd had to date and whether we wanted to become more involved. We all liked the idea of being involved. It was nice seeing young doctors develop and knowing that you had a part to play in that process [core value]. We also realised how previous trainees added dynamism to our practice (and even bonded us together at times) [attitude]. And nearly everyone felt good about 'giving something back' to the world by training up good doctors [core value].
>
> So, in our practice, the Trainer is the overall 'champion' for training, and the rest of us are like mini-Trainers. Helping trainees makes you feel good, and they add a bit of sparkle to your life too. The whole practice (not just us doctors) loves having a trainee around and each of us goes out of our way to help them [commitment].
>
> GP Trainer, Bradford

In this scenario, it's great how the second Trainer instigated the new *collaborative* approach to GP training. However, notice how it required sanctioning from the other doctors first. Hodkinson and colleagues emphasised the importance of power, hierarchy and conflict on the learning environment.[8] Some learning environments are 'expansive' with a workplace highly supportive of education, others 'restrictive' where opportunities to learn are closely linked to organisational and not learner needs, and opportunities for external support and participation limited.[9]

CREATING A LEARNING CULTURE – A CASE STUDY

One of the authors [PM] has studied Engeström's activity theory (covered in Chapter 22: Interprofessional Learning) and how it relates to GP education. The research was a four-year ethnographic study of the relationship between a training practice's culture and how it learns.

In the training practice it was found that the reception staff constructed their learning from their interactions with the computer (mediating artefact). While entering data on the computer about INR results the receptionist (subject) asks the practice nurse about their relevance to patient care (object). This learning was encouraged by the GP Trainer through engendering a learning culture that incorporated the practice's internal rules, community of practice and good organisation.

In the same practice and as part of its contract (external rules and regulations) the practice was required to produce a practice and professional development plan (PPDP: mediating artefact). The practice team (community of practice) developed the plan at a superficial level and expressed little desire to engage with it. The PPDP did not fit the practice's workload organisation and had poor face validity with patient care (object).

The research concluded that activity theory alone did not explain the learning process. The geography of the practice building, social capital, and complex adaptive system theory were needed to explain the overall learning process in the practice studied.

Social learning in a virtual world

A huge change to social learning and learning environments has come from the recent proliferation of virtual communities, social-networking sites (e.g. Facebook, MySpace) and opportunities for learning through iPods, iPads, phones and other mobile devices. What are referred to as 'communities of practice' with an implication of interaction, discussion and engagement are often simply networks.[10,11] The online learning environment offers great potential to enhance the education of GP trainees, but only with appropriate encouragement, training and support.

The educational environment

The **learning climate** within a workplace or organisation will be affected by *physical factors* making up the learning architecture. When running an educational session, don't forget about things like:

- the space and design of the room
- the temperature of the room
- lighting (especially poor lighting)
- visual distractions
- background noise
- the way chairs and tables are laid out (e.g. for a more inclusive discussion, consider moving away from the typical board room type of set-up)
- comfort of seating.

So what does all of this mean for me?

Smith and Wiener-Ogilvie[12] explored the perceptions of postgraduate GP learners in Scotland to the learning environment in their teaching practice. From that it appears that there are three characteristics which define a good training practice.

A good training practice is one in which there is:

- a happy practice environment: feeling part of the team and being able to ask questions
- good practice organisation: well-organised teaching, protected time for learning
- a Trainer who is supportive, well organised, knowledgeable and good at feedback.

To create a good learning ethos, you need to engage everyone, not just the doctors!
Respect for the staff that support clinical learning is essential for a positive learning environment. Involve them right from the start in new decisions about teaching. Quince and colleagues[13] found that some general practice staff considered it a benefit to have medical students: for themselves (in terms of variety and interest) and the practice. Involvement in teaching improved practice image and self-esteem. Conversely, some staff commented on the pressure on appointments and the increased complexity of their role, and they resented not being involved in the initial decision to teach students. What attitude do you think they'll have when the next set of medical students arrive?

CASE STUDY: PORTRAIT OF A TEACHING PRACTICE
Sunnybank Medical Centre, Bradford: a positive learning environment

One of the authors [DP] undertook a year-long study of a GP training practice. Over a series of interviews with GP trainees and Trainers the following words (among others) and phrases were frequently used to describe the practice's learning environment.

- About the practice: friendly, supportive, challenging, committed, experience, opportunity, excellence: real patients, whole practice and whole team involved.
- About the tutors: helpful, passionate, actively involved, and skilled.

GP trainees felt secure, supported, stimulated and engaged; they believed all these factors helped them develop their learning. Various elements appeared to come together to create this positive learning environment:

- a history of involvement with education
- a whole-practice commitment
- a high-quality practice
- an excellent (low) clinician: patient ratio
- a wide range of learners alongside the GP trainees
- an excellent management and administrative support system.

All these are perhaps of equal importance, but one conclusion of the research was that the wide range of learners within the practice emphasised the trajectory of learning within a professional progression. This was a significant factor in facilitating and supporting learning for undergraduate medical students, GP trainees and for established GPs and Trainers.

See Pearson D, Lucas B. What are the key elements of a primary care teaching practice? *Educ Prim Care*. 2011; **22**(3): 159–65.

What of the undergraduate learning environment?

Grant and Robling[14] conducted research with a Welsh practice taking undergraduate medical students. This was a single practice, recently formed. A picture emerged of an enhancement of team spirit and pride in the practice. The suggestion that learning activity helped to strengthen team spirit may reflect more the freshness of the team or its small size. The positive climate certainly supported learning.

Evaluating your practice learning environment

Many of you will be interested in the learning environment from a desire to enhance your own practice and better support GP trainees or other clinical learners. There are many useful tools to explore the elements of individual and social learning. None is perfect for a clinical practice setting in primary care and none fully embraces social learning theory, communities of practice or activity theory. However, most of them do focus on the physical characteristics of the learning environment and tutor attributes. They also emphasise the need for:

• Structure • Support • Safety • Stimulation • Challenge

A mini diagnostic tool for assessing your learning environment

Ask your current trainee:
- Was it clear who to speak to?
- Were they friendly and welcoming?
- Did they return your call/email?
- Did they send information you asked for or show you where to find it?

Talk to outgoing trainees (or medical students, or nurse learners):
- Did they feel welcomed, supported, part of the team and engaged with practice life?
- Were there other learners to share ideas with, or colleagues of a similar age, outlook or experience?
- Did they have time to talk and share experiences? Were they encouraged to do so?

Contact the local training scheme
- Do they allocate trainees to practices according to their learning styles? What sort of marrying up process do they use?
- Which practices are the most supportive (and chat to them to see how they do things)?
- Decide what's best for you, and why.

There are other models out there such as *The Dundee Readiness for Educational Environment Measure (DREEM)*[15] and *The Postgraduate Hospital Educational Environment Measure (PHEEM)*[16]

One of the authors (MK) reviewed the criteria for learning environments for North West Deanery and developed a self-evaluation questionnaire based on various models and pertinent to a GP training environment. The questionnaire (available on our website) helps practices to rank themselves against set standards and identify areas for development even before applying to become a training practice. Prospective Trainers in the North West Deanery use this tool during their Basic Trainer's Course. Whether new to training or an established training practice, the tool helps identify gaps *and* highlight areas of good practice and innovation. The model has enabled ownership and team participation in developing the physical, psychological and the educational milieu* for learning.

See also:
Mohan Kumar (2010) Formative assessment document for potential speciality Trainers and practices. Available from North West Deanery, Manchester www.nwpgmd.nhs.uk
  You may also value an article by Cotton et al.[2] in which an expert working party considered the learning environment in undergraduate teaching practices. The criteria they developed offer a useful framework for considering postgraduate GP training.

> * *Milieu refers to the entirety of the surrounding state and environmental conditions that influence one's growth or development. It refers to one's ambience or one's environmental surroundings. It is the atmosphere or climate one is situated in. It is the totality of your surroundings or the setting you are in.*

Bringing it all together

OK. You've had the theory, had some tasks to do, thought about how this relates to your situation and to primary care education. But you want to get on. Talk to your partners and colleagues and make the learning environment for your GP trainee as good as you possibly can. Let us offer you some top tips on how to do that.

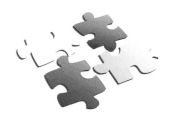

Get the practice sorted out first
● Aim for the highest possible clinical standards.
● Have systems to support personal learning, practice learning, appraisal and learning from critical events (whether positive or negative).
● Have systems that value the informal learning that takes place every day in the practice.

Get the philosophy and infrastructure right
● Get the whole team on board with the idea of being a learning and teaching practice.
● Learning is for everyone – the most junior and the most experienced should learn together.
● Aim for a range of learners, a range of levels, a range of professionals.
● Get the management and administrative support for learning in place.
● Prioritise education, protect time, encourage attendance and involvement.
● Pull together the tools and resources used daily in the practice that influence learning.
● Think about how the geography of the practice building and how its social spaces might influence informal learning.

When your learners arrive
● Make time to support learners, make time to support colleagues.
● Create time for learners to meet together and share ideas, encourage networking.
● Make learning as *real* as you are able: *real* patients, *real* cases, *real* responsibilities.
● Don't be afraid to challenge your learners; challenge stimulates learning.
● Be proud of your learners and of being a learning and teaching practice.
● Share your successes with other practices; it will help them and you.

Conclusion

We hope that you can see how the social and learning environment provides the foundation for the development of any learner. Without this foundation, the remaining architectural design for learning and education isn't particularly robust.

By now, you should have some ideas on what you might improve in your own learning organisation. If not, use one of the questionnaires to seek this information out. If we've managed to stimulate or stir up something inside you, we strongly urge you to read some of the resources in our Essential Reading list below. We've been very selective about this list – it includes resources which have had an instrumental impact on our lives, and we hope they will do so in yours too.

A sample of resources on our website

- Social learning models.
- Communities of practice (Wenger).
- North West Deanery self-evaluation of learning organisations.

Essential reading list

- Senge P. *The Fifth Discipline: the art and practice of the learning organisation.* New York: Currency and Doubleday; 1990.
- Argyris C, Schon DA. *Organizational Learning II: theory, method, and practice.* Reading: Addison-Wesley; 1996. This book has some really good stuff on single and double loop learning in organisations.
- Dowd JF. Learning organizations: an introduction. *Managed Care Quarterly.* 1999; **7**(2): 43–50. Talks about organisational leadership.
- Stinson L, Pearson D, Lucas B. Developing a learning culture: twelve tips for individuals, teams and organizations. *Med Teacher.* 2006; **28**(4): 309–12. Summarises all of these ideas.
- Milne P. Contesting the freedom to learn: the role of the Practice and Professional Development Plan in a British general practice. *Work Based Learning.* 2009. Available at http://wblearning-ejournal.com/archive/11-08-10/fullpaperpeerreview6.pdfe-journal (accessed November 2011).

Please give us some feedback on this chapter to help shape it for the next edition.
Go to www.essentialgptrainingbook.com and simply click on the title of this chapter.

References

1 Mezirow JD. *Transformative Dimensions of Adult Learning.* San Francisco: Jossey-Bass; 1991.
2 Cotton P, Sharp D, Howe A, *et al.* Developing a set of quality criteria for community-based medical education in the UK. *Educ Prim Care.* 2009; **20**: 143–51.
3 Habermas J. *Erkenntnis und Interesse. English Knowledge and Human Interests.* Boston, Mass: Beacon Press; 1970.
4 Freire P. *Pedagogy of the Oppressed.* New York: Herder and Herder; 1970.
5 Vygotsky LS. *Mind in Society: the development of higher psychological processes.* Cambridge, Mass: Harvard University Press; 1978.
6 Lave J, Wenger E. *Situated Learning: legitimate peripheral participation.* Cambridge: Cambridge University Press; 1991.
7 Wenger E. *Communities of Practice: learning, meaning, and identity.* Cambridge: Cambridge University Press; 1998.
8 Hodkinson P, Biesta G, James D. Understanding learning culturally: overcoming the dualism between social and individual views of learning. *Vocations and Learning.* 2008; **1**: 27–47.

9 Fuller A, Unwin L. Learning as apprentices in the contemporary UK workplace: creating and managing expansive and restrictive participation. *J Educ Work.* 2003; **16**(4): 407–26.

10 Sandars J. The use of new technology to facilitate learning through personal networks. *Work Based Learning Prim Care.* 2007; **5**(1): 5–11.

11 Sandars J. Online communities of practice for healthcare professionals: when hype meets reality. 2008. Available from: www.leeds.ac.uk/medicine/meu/lifelong08/papers.html (accessed 19 February 2010).

12 Smith VC, Wiener-Ogilvie S. Describing the learning climate of general practice training: the learner's perspective. *Educ Prim Care.* 2009; **20**: 435–40.

13 Quince T, Benson J, Hibble A, Emery J. The impact of expanded general practice-based student teaching: the practices' story. *Educ Prim Care.* 2007; **18**: 593–601.

14 Grant A, Robling M. Introducing medical student teaching into general practice: an action research study. *Med Teach.* 2006; **28**(7): 192–7.

15 Roff S, McAleer S, Harden RM, *et al.* Development and validation of the Dundee Ready Education Environment Measure (DREEM). *Med Teach.* 1997; **19**(4): 295–9.

16 Roff S MS, Skinner A. The Postgraduate Hospital Educational Environment Measure [PHEEM]. *Med Teach.* 2005; **27**: 326–31.

10

Five Pearls of Educational Theory

RAMESH MEHAY – TPD (Bradford) & lead author
ANNA ROMITO – Lecturer in Clinical Education (London Deanery)
MARK WATERS – GP Trainer (Hereford) & Course Organiser (Scaling the Heights)
KIRSTY BALDWIN – Postgraduate Programme Director (MSc Primary Care, Univ. Leeds)
HASNA BEGUM – TPD (Bradford)

It is the supreme art of the teacher to awaken joy in creative expression and knowledge.

Albert Einstein

Here is a selection of educational theories which we feel have made a big difference to us since we took up our roles as educators in general practice. They are not presented in any particular order of importance because they are all important.

Educational theory is fun!

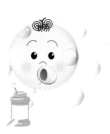

- It is the academic scaffold that structures the evidence for what we do.
- It encourages you to think about how learning happens.
- It gives you a tool to challenge assumptions.
- It can help you provide a learning framework for your learner.

We will cover the following *five* pearls of educational theories:

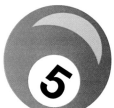

1 Adult Learning Strategies (also called andragogy)
2 Constructivism
3 Reflective Learning Cycles like Gibbs and Kolb
4 Motivational theories: Maslow's, The 6 Cs of Motivation and the ARCS Model
5 Bloom's Taxonomy for Learning Objectives: the cognitive, affective and psychomotor domains.

These are the things that make a real difference at ground level and that you really need to know as an educator. There are other educational theories that have also had a significant impact on us (such as Grow's SSDL model and Johari's Window), which are available on our website for you when you are ready.

The purpose of adult education is to help them to learn, not to teach them all they know and thus stop them from carrying on learning.

Rodgers[1]

Educational pearl number 1: adult learning

Also known as andragogy, pronounced *an-druh-goh-jee*.

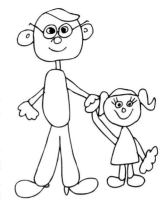

To help us get an understanding of andragogy let us first take a peek at pedagogy (or 'child learning'). Pedagogy embodies teacher-focused education: learning is based on the teacher's agenda, rather than the learner's. The teacher has full responsibility for making decisions about what will be learned, how it will be learnt and when it will be learnt. Learners assume a submissive, child-like role and are dependent upon being 'spoon fed' knowledge by their teacher.

Andragogy is the complete opposite. In andragogy the teacher and learner are on a level playing field – what is taught depends on what the two negotiate and agree on. It is defined as: 'Any intentional and professionally guided activity that aims at a change in adult persons,'[2] where change means a shift in knowledge, skills, attitudes and thus behaviour. In andragogy, the educator does not control or feed the learner. Instead, the educator helps (or facilitates) the learner with their learning.

Pedagogy is often referred to as the art and science of teaching children, whereas andragogy often refers to adults. However, this distinction isn't quite right because children can learn effectively from andragogical techniques, and some pedagogical techniques are good for adults too. Andragogy and pedagogy are best seen *not* as separate entities but as two ends of a spectrum; what methods you wish to employ depend on your target audience and the educational objectives set. For example, if your intention is to give your learners factual knowledge in a relatively short space of time, the pedagogical lecture method is absolutely fine.

 Top Tip: For an excellent critique of andragogy vs pedagogy visit: www-distance.syr.edu/andragogy.html

---

We will now go on to explore some of the key players in andragogy and their principles. The four players we will concentrate on are Knowles, Brookfield, Vella and Billington. There's quite a significant overlap in their principles (and that's not surprising because they're all talking about the same thing – adult learning!). However, some of them unfortunately use a lot of educational jargon. Don't stress too much over this – if something is not well explained in one set of principles, it probably will be in another. Nevertheless, reading all of the next section, even if you don't understand bits here and there, should give you a gist of what adult learning (andragogy) is all about.

Knowles' assumptions about adult learning[3]		
1	**Adults need to know**	• Adult learners need to know why they need to learn something before undertaking to learn it. • Therefore, survey your learners and identify their learning needs. • Make sure your teaching session is orientated to their goals.
2	**Adults have self-concept**	• Adults need to be responsible for their own decisions and to be treated as capable of self-direction. • They are independent learners who need to be free to direct themselves and not be imprisoned by rules. • Therefore, treat your learners as equals and show them respect. Encourage them to be independent, self-directed and creative.
3	**Adults have experience**	• Adult learners have a variety of experiences of life which represent the richest resource for learning. These experiences are, however, imbued with bias and presupposition. • Reflective learning becomes *transformative* whenever assumptions are found to be distorting, inauthentic or otherwise invalid. • Therefore, try to weave their experience into new learning and connect new knowledge to their experience; provide insight into their biases.
4	**Adults have readiness to learn**	• Adults are ready to learn those things they need to know in order to cope effectively with life situations. • Therefore, tailor your learning programme to their current roles and the challenges therein.
5	**Orientation to learning**	• Adults are motivated to learn the things that they perceive will help them perform tasks they confront in their life situations. • Therefore, make sure your teaching session includes learning that is relevant and can be immediately applied.
6	**Motivation to learn**	• As a person matures, the motivation to learn becomes internal. • Therefore, empower your learners by building their self-esteem and imparting a sense of achievement.

Brookfield's Principles of Adult Learning[4]

Brookfield places greater emphasis on collaboration, experiential learning and critical reflection.

1 Adults should be **voluntary participants** in the learning situation (and they should be able to withdraw voluntarily).
2 Adult learning should be characterised by **mutual respect** among participants.
3 Adult education can and should be viewed as a **collaborative** activity.
4 **Praxis** needs to happen. Praxis is a continual process of activity, followed by reflection, refinement and then implementation.[5]

Praxis = Experience + Reflection → Refinement → Implementation

5 Learning should involve a **critical reflection** of the basis of one's beliefs.
6 Adult education should strive towards developing **self-directed** and **empowered** learners.

Vella's 12 Principles for Effective Adult Learning[6]

Vella amalgamates both Knowles' and Brookfield's work with a few extras on top.

1 **Needs assessment**: Learners need to participate in what is to be learned, such that expectations and needs are established both accurately and early.
2 **Safety:** You need to provide a safe educational environment where the learner can feel comfortable revealing their true inner feelings.

3 **A sound relationship:** Between learners, and between the learners and the educator.

4 **Sequence and reinforcement:** Carefully order that which you are trying to teach in a logical way and reinforce key elements as you progress (to help learners remember).

5 **Action with reflection (praxis):** Encourage a continual process of activity, followed by reflection, refinement and then implementation (*see* Kolb's learning cycle below).

6 **Learners as subjects of their own learning:** Respect learners as decision-makers by supporting their autonomy and freedom to be creative.

7 **Learning with ideas, feelings, actions:** Explore your learners' knowledge, skills, behaviour, emotions and attitudes.

8 **Immediacy:** For learning to hold meaning, it needs to be both useful and transferable to authentic situations *in the near future.*

9 **Clear roles:** Both teacher and learners must know of their own and each other's role in the learning process. For example, does the teacher give the impression of being an 'expert' who is not to be questioned or are learners free to debate and disagree?

10 **Teamwork:** Encourage collaboration among the learners, e.g. small-group work.

11 **Engagement:** Of learners in what they are learning and their learning process.

12 **Accountability:** Evaluating or monitoring your learners' progress will help both of you to check that they are learning what was intended.

How to design an effective adult teaching programme – Billington's 7 Characteristics[7,8]

1 An environment in which learners feel **safe and supported**, where personal needs and individuality are honoured.

2 An environment that promotes **intellectual freedom**, experimentation and creativity.

3 An environment where the educational department treats adult learners as peers – who are to be accepted and **respected as intelligent, experienced adults** whose opinions are considered and appreciated. Such regard can help faculty members enjoy reciprocity of the learning experience.

4 **Self-directed learning**, where learners take responsibility for their own growth. This can take the form of designing their own learning programmes in order to address what each learner needs and wants to develop in order to function optimally.

5 **Pacing or intellectual challenge**. Optimal pacing is achieved by **challenging people marginally beyond their present level of ability**. Excess challenge can encourage people to give up. Too little challenge can precipitate boredom and limit learning. Adults who report high levels of intellectual stimulation appear to develop more.

6 **Active involvement in learning**, in contrast to passively listening or simple attendance. Interaction, experimentation and dialogue help cement learnt facts and theory.

7 **Regular feedback**, where learners are able to inform their educational faculty of their learning needs and experiences, and where mechanisms are in place to permit responsive change to occur.

Top Tip: If we subscribe to the core principles of adult learning, we get a three-fold benefit: our learners learn best; learning is stimulating for them; and both we and they have fun in the process.

Educational pearl number 2: the 3 Cs of constructivism

Constructivism is the theory that people construct their own understanding and knowledge of the world, through experiencing things and reflecting on those experiences. When learners encounter something new, they reconcile it with previous knowledge and experience. They may change what they believe, or they may discard the new information as irrelevant. To be active creators of their knowledge, however, they must be able to ask questions, explore and assess what they know. In the classroom, the constructivist view of learning means encouraging students to use active techniques such as experiments and real-world problem-solving using authentic data if possible, and to create knowledge and reflect on their understanding.

Faculty of Education, University of Alberta[9]

Constructivism proposes that people learn best by actively constructing their own concepts, ideas and understanding. This activity usually involves applying new information together with what they already know. Its emphasis is on the learner rather than the educator, where the learner's own individual construct of meaning is what is important. There are three elements to constructivism (the three Cs) as illustrated in the diagram on the right.

Construction

• *knowledge builds on **what is already known.***

Context

• *prior understanding must be used in concert **with current experiences** to construct, elaborate or restructure knowledge.*

Collaboration

• ***working with others** helps explore different perspectives because knowledge varies in different contexts and cultures.*

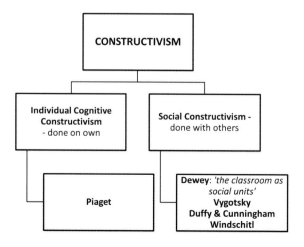

Constructivism is attributed to a number of originators: Vico[10] (1700s), Dewey[11] (1938), Piaget[12] (1950) and Vygotsky[13] (1978). Vico is well known for his *verum esse ipsum factum* (1710) in which he says that the 'truth' (or knowledge) has to be **made, constructed, created or invented**. It cannot be verified through observation alone.[10] Dewey takes this further by talking about the spark-generating dynamic that has to occur between the individual and those around him for this to happen.

Only by wrestling with the conditions of the problem at hand, seeking and finding his own solution (not in isolation but in correspondence with the teacher and other pupils) does one learn.

Dewey[14]

This emphasis on interaction makes it clear that one of the most fundamental principles of constructivism is that **there are no universal truths, and meaning is socially negotiated**.[15,16] This is a concept educators often have difficulty adopting. In constructivism, knowledge is seen as a socially negotiated human construct, i.e. it is built as a result of social interaction. Therefore, constructivism proposes new definitions for knowledge and truth – ones based on inter-subjectivity instead of the classical objectivity. For example, if you give a group of adults a novel to read, and then ask them individually to describe it, each will have their own interpretation with some commonalities. However, if you engage them in a group discussion, you will find that some of them change their viewpoints and understanding as they acquire new insights from others. This illustrates how knowledge is entirely a context-dependent, socially negotiated construct, where new knowledge is created as a result of a dynamic social interaction and application within the learner's environment. **Constructivism, therefore, emphasises the social nature of learning**, and its focus is the rich learning a group environment provides us with.

Caine and Caine's 12 Principles of Constructivism[17]

1 **The brain is a parallel processor:** Our amazing brains can handle a whole host of information of differing nature at the same time, such as thoughts, feelings, facts, sounds and so on. Therefore, effective teaching must employ a variety of teaching methods and textures to mirror this.

2 **Learning engages the entire physiology:** Meaningful teaching has to encompass the whole that includes knowledge, skills, attitudes, culture and experience.

3 **The search for meaning is innate:** Every learner brings with them their own unique experiences, which give unique meaning to whatever is taught. The effective teacher needs to recognise and incorporate prior and current experiences into the educational session.

4 **The search for meaning occurs through 'patterning':** To teach effectively, one has to connect isolated ideas to global concepts and themes. In order to help learners make sense of new concepts, the educator needs to help establish a learning framework from which they can hang things.

5 **Emotions are critical to patterning:** The educator needs to acknowledge and incorporate emotions, feelings and attitudes into any learning taking place.

6 **The brain processes parts and wholes simultaneously:** The educator needs to use both and not explore one at the expense of the other. Aim to situate the isolated ideas and knowledge within global concepts and themes at the right time.

7 **Learning involves both focused attention and peripheral perception:** We have seen that learning is influenced not only by the subject matter but also by the environment. Consider the impact of culture and situation, and aim to create a climate conducive to learning.

8 **Learning always involves conscious and unconscious processes:** Lapses of time can be used to promote learner reflection. Revisiting an educational session after a time interval can allow learners to 'mull' the learning over and give them a chance to try out new ideas.

9 **We have at least two different types of memory: a spatial memory system and a set of systems for rote learning:** Again, the educator needs to balance both and not explore one at the expense of the other. Too much rote learning and inadequate room for experiential (or spatial) learning can seriously limit true understanding.

10 **We understand and remember best when facts and skills are embedded in natural, spatial memory:** In other words, when combined with experiential learning in an authentic environment.

11 **Learning is enhanced by challenge and inhibited by threat:** Echoing Billington's[7,8] characteristic of pacing and intellectual challenge, learners need to be stretched without feeling destroyed.

12 **Each brain is unique:** Thus, each learner has an individual way of learning. Therefore, teaching should be offered in a variety of formats to enable learners to 'cherry pick' what would work best for them.

How to design a classroom based on constructivism

A pedagogical classroom teacher would say:	A constructivist classroom teacher would say:
• Curriculum begins with dividing the whole into parts and examining those parts, i.e. examine the micro-skills first. • Stick to a rigid, fixed and defined curriculum. • Learning is based on repetition. • Learners work mainly alone. • Educators impart information; learners are there to soak it all up. • Educator is directive and authoritarian. • Knowledge is seen as inert. • Refer to books/workbooks where necessary. • Assessment is via knowledge tests, e.g. true/false questions, recall of facts.	• Examine the whole first and then derive the component parts, i.e. introduce concepts first. • Go down the path where the learners take you: focus on their questions, interests and areas of unmet needs. • Learning is interactive and based on building upon what learners already know. • Learners work mainly in groups. • Educators interact with their learners and help them 'construct' their own knowledge. • Educator is on a level playing field, engages in dialogue with the learner(s) and negotiates the agenda. • Knowledge is seen as dynamic; forever evolving with our experiences. • Refer to a variety of creative teaching material. • Assessment is through a workplace-based assessment, i.e. what they do in real life as a result of learning.

Practical points

When you are running an educational session, it is important to identify your learners' prior understanding from real experiences first (context). Then use methods that enable learners to build on this and form their own constructs (construction). Start off with familiar ideas before introducing new ones. Learners should be encouraged to explore possibilities, try them out and rethink problems. Encourage self-initiative, creative autonomy *and* collaboration with others – including you! Hopefully, there will be some new learning concepts that emerge.

- Remember that every learner is an individual, who will approach learning their own way; aim to construct meaning that is unique to them. *(construction)*
- Aid understanding by organising the concepts into frameworks, such as mind maps. *(construction)*
- Teach by getting learners to question and explore for themselves; use *'why'* (analysing), *'how could . . .'* (creating) and *'what do you think'* (evaluating) questions. *(context)*
- Use case studies to help test newly formed concepts and encourage application. *(context)*
- Get them to explain their understanding to each other. *(collaboration)*.

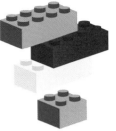

⚠ **Red Alert:** Not everyone finds the idea of constructivism works for them. There was a recent aggressive critique of the use of constructivism in qualitative research published in the BMJ (*BMJ.* 2011; **342**: d424). Have a read, see what you think . . . Read the online responses too. We still think constructivism makes a lot of sense – what about you?

Educational pearl number 3: reflective learning cycles

The GMC states that the most influential factor in postgraduate learning is *through experience*.[18] They recommended a change in clinical education that incorporates 'curiosity-driven self-directed learning', with intent to enable learners to gain full meaning from their experiences.[18] This drive to capitalise on experiences has generated a renewed enthusiasm for reflection as a concept for learning. Reflection is an integral part of experience; you cannot learn from experience without it. Reflecting on experience helps us to determine what new things we will do the next time around. This **cyclical learning strategy** can be repeated numerous times, with knowledge developing and expanding with each cycle.[19]

Gibbs's Reflective Cycle[20]

Gibbs's Reflective Cycle is a neat tool to help learners reflect on and consider their experiences. Use the headings to structure a reflective discussion around any experiential event. It is particularly good for looking at emotionally charged cases. You can even encourage trainees to write up log entries in their ePortfolios in this *reflective* way.

 Top Tip: Gibbs's Cycle: Make sure the learners are not too hard on themselves when talking about their bad bits in the evaluation phase.

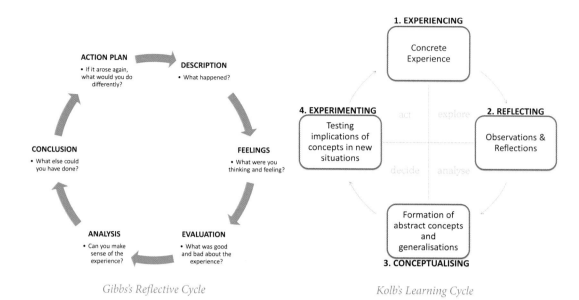

Gibbs's Reflective Cycle   Kolb's Learning Cycle

Kolb's Experiential Learning Cycle[21]

Kolb's learning cycle presents a similar theory for how we learn but takes it one step further. Reflection in itself is not enough; we need to put new understanding into *active* practice to fully crystallise that which has been learnt. This process means that the learner can explore, analyse, decide and influence their behaviour as part of learning. The cycle consists of four stages of learning from experience. You can come into the cycle at any point, but then you must follow the other stages in sequence in order to ensure learning happens. As with Gibbs's cycle, you can use Kolb's framework to structure group or individual discussion on any experiential event.

Educational pearl number 4: motivational theories

Never underestimate the power of motivation: it encourages learners to become active and curious. This makes learning more powerful, which in turn has a positive effect on performance. Motivating our learners requires two things.

1 A **valuing** judgement: the learner has to feel some value towards what is to be learnt.
2 An **expectancy** judgement: they must feel able to achieve the desired outcome.

Maslow's Hierarchy of Needs[22]

Maslow's hierarchy is a useful model in understanding the 'valuing' arm of motivation. His hierarchy is usually presented as a pyramid; this basically demonstrates that each of us is motivated by needs, and that fundamental basal level needs must be satisfied in order for higher level needs to be met. The basal levels can be divided into *physiological* needs and *psychological* needs. If these lower levels are made unstable (e.g. through health and disease), then maintaining the higher levels becomes less important to us.

At the top of the pyramid is Self-actualisation. This is all about fulfilling one's own unique potential through morality, creativity, problem-solving and expressing one's own ideas or points of view. At this level, people *become themselves*. It is where learners truly engage in their own learning and can place value on what is taught to them. However, this cannot happen if the levels below Self-actualisation are not met. The levels below Self-actualisation are often referred to as 'Deficiency Needs' (or 'D-needs'). If these D-needs (like being loved or having a sense of belonging)

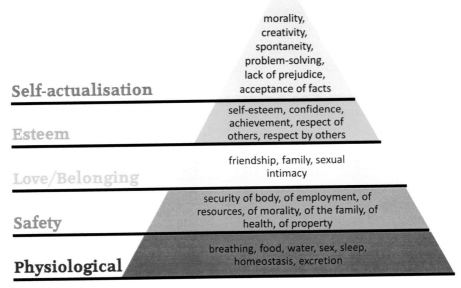

Maslow's Hierarchy of Needs

are not met, a learner can become preoccupied and stuck here. This will prevent them from truly engaging in learning: they are unlikely to have a strong motivation for anything else until matters pertaining to their D-needs are resolved.

- Humans need to feel a sense of belonging and acceptance (from families, friends etc.)
- Humans need to love and be loved (sexually and non-sexually).
- Humans need to have food, water and shelter and to feel safe.

 An Extra Note: Maslow later added another level called Transcendence Needs – that of helping others to achieve Self-actualisation.

For those of us who live in the 'First World', one must be *extra careful* about overlooking physiological or safety needs and assuming they are automatically satisfied. Consider the trainee who is in severe debt or with five young children to feed, who has not had enough sleep because he's doing night shifts (moonlighting) to make some extra money, as well as trying to get an education. How motivated do you think he will be the next day at your teaching session with eyes half open? Or, perhaps something closer to home: think back to a lecture where you were desperate for the loo or sat in a hot stuffy room – were you still concerned with learning?

This model is only a concept to help guide you! **It is not a fully responsive model to life.** Humans are complex beings who will move up and down this hierarchy throughout their lives. This changeability means you need to be flexible in the way you use it too. For instance, someone who is going through marital difficulties (Love/Belonging) does not necessarily mean they will not respect others (Esteem). And life is not as neatly delineated as Maslow's model would suggest: helping others, e.g. at the homeless centre in the evenings (Transcendence level, i.e. beyond Self-actualisation), might actually improve your perception of self-worth (the lower 'Esteem' level).

Practical points

Harkin *et al*[23] have redrawn Maslow's hierarchy as applied to the classroom (see diagram on the right). Don't automatically label a trainee who (for example) is not preparing his CBDs in advance as lazy. Instead, consider whether there are any D-needs that are making it difficult for him to prepare – things like marital, financial or housing difficulties. If this is the case, perhaps you can create a positive educational climate that temporarily separates the learner from their difficulties. For instance, making the leaner feel valued and respected might help place them at the higher levels of Belonging and Esteem, thus

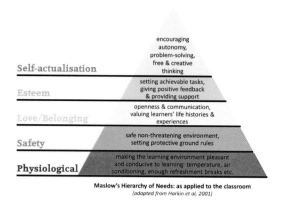

Maslow's Hierarchy of Needs: as applied to the classroom
(adapted from Harkin et al, 2001)

helping them to engage with learning more readily. Programme Directors can use this model in a similar way with Trainers who are all of a sudden struggling or behaving atypically.

The 6 Cs of Motivation[24]

	The 6 Cs of Motivation
1	*Choice* When people choose something to do, they generally do it. So give learners choices. For example, if you are planning a peer-led training session, identify an array of learning needs from the group and then allow smaller groups to choose which topic they would like to do and how.
2	*Challenge* Push them just beyond their skill level; try to get them to yearn for more knowledge or exploration. Tread carefully; we have seen how very hard tasks can create anxiety and demotivate, while easy tasks can result in boredom.
3	*Control* The more control learners have the more responsible, independent and self-directed they will be. Give them control over decision making, organisation and methodology. A facilitator just needs to guide with a light touch where possible. Again, be careful: too much handover with inadequate support can lead to anxiety.
4	*Collaboration* Do you need to build up team spirit? Working in groups promotes sharing of different perspectives, which can lead to inspiration and, therefore, deeper engagement. It also encourages learners to negotiate learning strategies and tasks among themselves. By working in collaboration and 'belonging' to a group, individuals will feel they cannot let the group down; often, they end up motivating each other.
5	*Construct meaning* Be clear about the aims and objectives of the educational session. One of the biggest reasons why learners appear disinterested is because the session does not provide a powerful enough 'hook'. So, spell out what they will get from the session and how it will enrich their lives. Make it sound juicy!

The 6 Cs of Motivation

6	Consequences
	You may need to try to link a reward to the intended outcome (to highlight achievement). Examples of this include poster displays of work, publishing or distributing written works to a bigger audience or even creating a bit of competition with others. Something as simple as a small box of chocolates as the winning prize can do wonders!

These principles are based on the notion that people are more likely to get deeply involved in things that **involve their own choices and goals**. In which case the role of the educator is to facilitate the learner to: make appropriate choices and weave in a sense of personal meaning through the task. If you have a group of learners who seem to lack that spark of dynamism of wanting to learn, think of these 6 Cs and see whether any of these will help relight their fire!

The ARCS Model for Motivation[25]

The ARCS model: a pragmatic framework for motivational teaching

- **Attention** – 'Hook' the learners and stimulate an attitude of inquiry.
  Focus your session around their fears, concerns and frustrations.
- **Relevance** – making the educational session relevant to the learners' needs.
  Survey group experience and determine what they need help with to do their job.
- **Confidence** – create a positive educational ethos which promotes success.
  Give them confidence that 'they can do it'. Your own positivity will infiltrate others!
- **Satisfaction** – ensure they continue to enjoy the learning experience.
  Periodically check how they are feeling. Get them back into a positive frame of mind.

Educational pearl number 5: Bloom's Taxonomy of Learning Objectives[26]

Bloom's Taxonomy of Learning Objectives

According to Bloom, when somebody learns something, what is learnt usually falls into one or more of the following three categories.
- Cognitive Domain, where knowledge is gained.
- Psychomotor Domain, where skills are acquired.
- Affective Domain, where attitudes are changed.

These are referred to as the three domains of learning. However, there are varying learning depths to each of these learning domains. For example, for the knowledge domain: being able to use a mathematical formula and *apply* it to a real situation is far more impressive than just being able to *recite* it. The spectrum of learning depths, subdivisions and layers is called Bloom's Taxonomy (taxonomy is another word for classification). Each taxonomy is hierarchical – by which we mean that higher levels cannot be reached if lower ones are not attained. For instance, if you look at the knowledge domain (see below), one must be able to 'remember', 'understand' and 'apply' before being able to 'analyse'.

Educators often refer to Bloom's Taxonomy to help them formulate learning outcomes. Formulating learning outcomes is an essential skill in planning any educational event. Identifying the learning outcomes then helps you to examine and decide which methods will help you to achieve them. And to take it one step further, you can then use your learning outcomes to formulate an assessment or evaluation tool to check whether learning outcomes have been achieved. This process of aligning everything back to the initial learning outcomes is called constructive alignment. It's covered in more detail in Chapter 4: Powerful Hooks – aims, objectives and ILOs and Chapter 6: Teaching from Scratch. Let's look at each learning domain in a bit more detail.

Cognitive (knowledge) domain[27]

This cognitive domain addresses *knowledge structures*. Simply *knowing the facts* is at the bottom rung of this educational ladder. We have provided a list of action words linked to this hierarchy that can be usefully employed when trying to write learning objectives or outcomes.

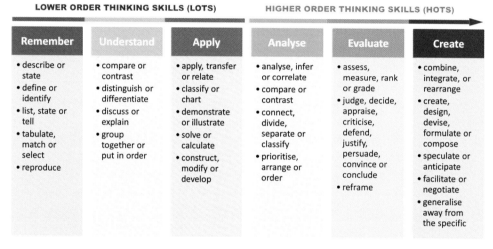

LOWER ORDER THINKING SKILLS (LOTS)			**HIGHER ORDER THINKING SKILLS (HOTS)** →		
Remember	**Understand**	**Apply**	**Analyse**	**Evaluate**	**Create**
• describe or state • define or identify • list, state or tell • tabulate, match or select • reproduce	• compare or contrast • distinguish or differentiate • discuss or explain • group together or put in order	• apply, transfer or relate • classify or chart • demonstrate or illustrate • solve or calculate • construct, modify or develop	• analyse, infer or correlate • compare or contrast • connect, divide, separate or classify • prioritise, arrange or order	• assess, measure, rank or grade • judge, decide, appraise, criticise, defend, justify, persuade, convince or conclude • reframe	• combine, integrate, or rearrange • create, design, devise, formulate or compose • speculate or anticipate • facilitate or negotiate • generalise away from the specific

New Bloom's Taxonomy for the Cognitive Domain (after Anderson & Krathwohl, 2001)

Remember = recall of knowledge
Understand = interpret knowledge
Apply = applying ideas to old and new situations
Analyse = teasing out important ideas
Evaluate = deciding for oneself whether ideas are flawed or appropriate
Create = weaving new ideas with old to create something new

- Before we can **understand** a concept, we have to **remember** it.
- Before we can **apply** the concept, we must **understand and remember** it.
- Before we **analyse** it, we must be able to **apply, understand and remember** it.
- Before we can **evaluate** its impact, we must have **analysed, applied, understood and remembered** it.
- Before we can **create**, we must have **evaluated, analysed, applied, understood and remembered** it.

Affective (attitude) domain[27]

Many of you will remember learning lots of knowledge (e.g. anatomy) and skills (e.g. examination of various systems) from your medical school days. Attitudes were primarily ignored. The attitudinal domain is often overlooked because it is the most nebulous and hardest to evaluate of the three domains. Even so, **attitudes are important** and should form an equal – if not greater – part of the overall curriculum of learning; things pertaining to this domain cannot be readily picked up by books or the Internet. And it is our attitudes that hold everything else

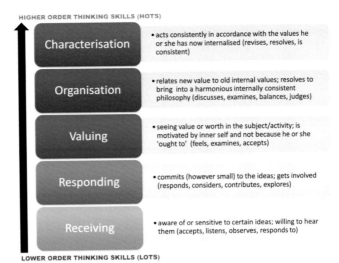

HIGHER ORDER THINKING SKILLS (HOTS)

Characterisation • acts consistently in accordance with the values he or she has now internalised (revises, resolves, is consistent)

Organisation • relates new value to old internal values; resolves to bring into a harmonious internally consistent philosophy (discusses, examines, balances, judges)

Valuing • seeing value or worth in the subject/activity; is motivated by inner self and not because he or she 'ought to' (feels, examines, accepts)

Responding • commits (however small) to the ideas; gets involved (responds, considers, contributes, explores)

Receiving • aware of or sensitive to certain ideas; willing to hear them (accepts, listens, observes, responds to)

LOWER ORDER THINKING SKILLS (LOTS)

New Bloom's Taxonomy for the Affective Domain (after Anderson & Krathwohl, 2001)

together! The affective learning domain addresses a *'feeling* tone' which incorporates attitudes, opinions, appreciations, values and emotional sets. In this diagram, characterisation refers to the process whereby an individual's affect towards something passes from a general awareness level to an internalised level. Once internalised, it becomes a core value which strongly guides future behaviour in a long-term and consistent way.

Psychomotor (skills) domain[28,29]

Bloom never completed his work on the psychomotor domain, which was instead achieved by one of his students, Dave.[28] Dave's model was further refined by Simpson,[29] which is that presented below.

Level	Category	Notes
1	Perception	**AWARENESS** – the point where a learner **recognises** that they need to start building a particular skill. *Example: a child who sees another child riding a bicycle and thinks, 'I wouldn't mind having a go at that.'*
2	Set	**READINESS** – where a learner **gets ready** or **prepares** for the challenge (new skill). *Example: the child decides it's time to pluck up the courage and ask his dad for a bike (and keeps pestering him until he gives in).*
3	Guided Response	**ATTEMPT** – the learner starts training or learning sessions. They **follow instruction**, **imitate** or **practise** the skill which is very rusty at this stage. *Example: the child rides the bike under guided instruction from his dad. Falls off quite a bit but sometimes manages to ride it!*

Level	Category	Notes
4	Mechanism	**BASIC PROFICIENCY** – the leaner is getting the hang of it and can **make**, **perform** or **complete** basic manoeuvres. However, he still has to think about them and they are not performed with smoothness. *Example: the child can now ride the bike. He hardly ever falls off but he can only ride up and down and can't turn around yet. He is still wobbly, and you can clearly see him think hard about what he is doing.*
5	Complex Overt Response	**EXPERT PROFICIENCY** – the learner is becoming good, **coordinated** and can **demonstrate** manoeuvres with ease. Motions are smooth and automatic, without prior thinking either! *Example: the child is now riding well. He can turn corners and performs biking manoeuvres that are smooth and without stopping to think.*
6.	Adaptation	**ADAPTABLE PROFICIENCY** – the learner is not only good but can perform manoeuvres tailored to a variety of different stimuli. The learner can **adjust** or **flex** performance according to context. *Example: the child can ride extremely well. He does not mind if others are on the street as he can easily manoeuvre around them.*
7	Origination	**CREATIVE PROFICIENCY** – the learner not only performs manoeuvres effortlessly but can also think independently to **formulate** and **execute** new integrated activities. The learner can **modify**, **redesign** and **troubleshoot**. *Example: the child is really exceptional on the bike. He has found out that he can do wheelies and all sorts of tricks just by experimenting.*

We prefer using the terms in capitals; they are easier to interpret. We have used the example of a child learning to ride a bike. Can you apply the model to a trainee learning about consultation skills? Try it now; it will only take you five minutes!

Closing comment

So far, we have talked about five educational pearls which we hope will serve you for life. If we have managed to ignite some interest, then we are happy! There are more educational pearls on our website. Why not go over there sometime and take a peek?

A sample of resources on our website

- Five more pearls of educational theory.
- A deeper look at constructivism.
- Emotional intelligence.
- Complexity and chaos in teaching.
- Cognitive dissonance in a nutshell.

Educational theory and pearls elsewhere . . .

Further resources on educational theory (as applied to medicine)
- Bradford VTS: www.bradfordvts.co.uk (click online resources then section 03.7)
- GPtraining.net: www.gp-training.net

Acknowledgements
We would like to thank Dorothy Billington's permission for reproducing her work. Available at: www.newhorizons.org/lifelong/workplace/billington.htm

Please give us some feedback on this chapter to help shape it for the next edition.
Go to www.essentialgptrainingbook.com and simply click on the title of this chapter.

References

1 Rogers A. *Teaching Adults*. Milton Keynes: Open University Press; 1988.

2 Knowles M, Holton E, Swanson R. *The Adult Learner*. 6th ed. Burlington, Mass: Elsevier Butterworth-Heinemann; 2005 (originally published 1973).

3 Knowles M *et al. Andragogy in Action: applying modern principles of adult education*. San Francisco: Jossey Bass; 1984.

4 Brookfield S. *Understanding and Facilitating Adult Learning*. San Francisco: Jossey-Bass; 1990.

5 Dewey J. *Experience and Education*. New York: Kappa Delta, then Collier; 1938.

6 Vella J. *Learning to Listen, Learning to Teach*. San Francisco: Jossey-Bass; 1994.

7 Billington D. *Ego Development and Adult Education*. Doctoral Dissertation, The Fielding Institute. Dissertation Abstracts International. 1988; **49**(7). (University Microfilms No. 88-16, 275).

8 Billington D. Available at: www.newhorizons.org/lifelong/workplace/billington.htm (accessed 17 February 2009).

9 Faculty of Education. Available at: www.quasar.ualberta.ca/techcur/THEORY/constructivism.htm (accessed 17 May 2011).

10 Croce B. *The Philosophy of Giambattista Vico*. (Trans. RG Collingwood) London: Howard Latimer; 1913.

11 Dewey J. *How We Think*. Boston: DC Heath & Company; 1910.

12 Piaget J. *The Psychology of Intelligence*. New York: Routledge; 1950.

13 Vygotsky L. *Mind in Society: the development of higher psychological processes*. Cambridge, Mass: Harvard University Press; 1978.

14 Dewey J. *Experience and Education*. New York: Macmillan; 1938.

15 Duffy T, Cunningham D. Constructivism: implications for the design and delivery of instruction. In: Jonnasen D, editor. *Handbook of Research for Educational Communications and Technology*. Mahwah, New Jersey: Lawrence Erlbaum Associates; 1996.

16 Windschitl M. Framing constructivism in practice as the negotiation of dilemmas: an analysis of the conceptual, pedagogical, cultural, and political challenges facing teachers. *Rev Educ Res*. 2002; **72**(2): 131–75.

17 Caine R, Caine G. *Making Connections: teaching and the human brain*. Alexandria, VA: Association for Supervision and Curriculum Development; 1991.

18 Cited in Maudsley G, Strivens J. Promoting professional knowledge, 'experiential learning' and 'critical thinking' for medical students. *Med Educ*. 2000; **34**(7): 535–44.

19 Sandars J. The use of reflection in medical education: AMEE Guide No. 44. *Med Teach*. 2009; **31**: 685–95.

20 Gibbs G. *Learning by Doing: a guide to teaching and learning methods*. Oxford: Further Education Unit, Oxford Polytechnic; 1988.

21 Kolb D. *Experiential Learning*. New Jersey: Prentice Hall; 1984.

22 Maslow A. *Motivation and Personality*. New York: Harper; 1954.

23 Harkin J, Turner G, Dawn T. *Teaching Young Adults: a handbook for teachers*. London: Routledge; 2001.

24 Turner J, Paris S. How literacy tasks influence children's motivation for literacy. *The Reading Teacher*. 1995; **48**(8): 662–73.

25 Keller J. Available at: www.arcsmodel.com/Mot%20dsgn.htm (accessed 17 February 2009).

26 Bloom B, editor. *Taxonomy of Educational Objectives: the classification of educational goals*. Susan Fauer Company, Inc; 1956.

27 Anderson L, Krathwohl D, editors. *A Taxonomy for Learning, Teaching and Assessing: a revision of Bloom's taxonomy of educational objectives*. New York: Longman; 2001.

28 Dave R. Psychomotor levels. In: Armstrong R, editor. *Developing and Writing Educational Objectives*. Tucson, Arizona: Educational Innovators Press; 1970. pp. 33–4.

29 Simpson E. *The Classification of Educational Objectives in the Psychomotor Domain*. 1st ed. Washington: Gryphon House; 1972.

Learning and Personality Styles in Practice

11

MARK WATERS – GP Trainer (Hereford) & lead author
IAIN LAMB – Associate Advisor (SE Scotland)
RAMESH MEHAY – TPD (Bradford)

(We) live in a rich learning environment, constantly involved in and surrounded by professional interaction and conversation, educational events, information and feedback. The search for the one best or 'right' way of learning is a counsel of despair . . .

Grant, Chambers and Jackson 'The Good CPD Guide' 1999[1]

Introduction

This chapter will focus on our **unique nature as individual human beings**, and how this impacts on teaching and learning. Conversations with educationists (and books like this one) tend to

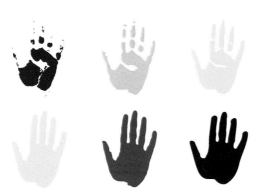

involve a lot of generic references to 'learners', and it's a reasonable term. However, we need to be watchful we don't lose sight of our own humanity. **Before we are learners, or teachers, we are individual people.**

We'll review some of the ways that **learning can be affected by personality, learning styles, values and beliefs**. Then we'll explore how an awareness of these factors can be put to practical use. There will also be some theoretical discussion to provide a sound basis for all this lovely woolly personal stuff. There will be some examples and some anecdotes from our own experience. You'll be encouraged to think about what this means to you as well. But first, a memory:

> I play the guitar. I'm not fantastic, but I know my way around. I learnt as a teenager, and have played fairly regularly since then. So when one of my teenage sons was interested to learn, it seemed natural that I should give him a few lessons. 'What a lovely thing to do together,' I thought to myself. Even so, things didn't work out as well as I had hoped. The things I thought were pretty obvious he seemed to struggle with. Progress was slow, and we both got upset. I gave up, thinking he would maybe just not be able to play . . .
>
> Then a few months later he started playing the guitar for himself, and he downloaded chord charts and tablature for his favourite songs from the Internet. Now he plays the guitar really well, as well as mandola and a range of homemade instruments. So what went wrong – was it my teaching, was he just not ready, or was it something else? Maybe the problem was in the assumptions I made about the way he would learn?

Learning doesn't just 'happen'. There are a number of theoretical models, which attempt to describe the process. But that's just it – it's a process. Whichever model makes most sense to you, what all of them share is the idea that learning requires dynamic and active engagement.

When teaching, ask yourself these questions.
- Who is this learner?
- What do I know about him or her?
- What motivates him or her?
- How does he or she like to learn?
- What does he or she find difficult about learning?

It seems obvious to say that learners are an integral part of the activity of teaching and learning, but it is surprisingly easy in practice to forget this. And, quite simply, because **learners are involved in their own learning**, they will find some approaches more successful than others. This chapter will focus on understanding what it is that makes some approaches more successful.

OK, so we're all different. Can you be more specific?

Yes indeed. However, let's just do a bit of eavesdropping first. We can learn a lot from listening to other people's conversation. Here's a conversation between a GP Trainer and his trainee. The Trainer is Martin, and the trainee Gabriel, although those aren't their real names.

Gabriel: You've mentioned the 'process of learning' a couple of times – what exactly do you mean?

Martin: Well . . . what do you think happens when you learn something?

Gabriel: Well . . . I suppose maybe you store new knowledge in your memory?

Martin: OK, that's reasonable. But what do you mean by knowledge?

Gabriel: What a question! Information, facts, that sort of thing . . .

Martin: OK – that works for stuff we can all agree on. Like the fact that paracetamol is a painkiller maybe?

Gabriel: Yeah, that's right.

Martin: So it's like a fact exists somewhere, and when you learn it, you make a copy of that fact in your memory, like copying a file onto your hard drive?

Gabriel: Now you put it like that, it makes it all sound a bit mechanical, so I'm not quite sure . . .

Martin: Good! Because that would mean that everyone's copy is the same. Do you construct knowledge the same way as everybody else in the same classroom? For example, at Half-Day Release, do you all take home the same messages?

Gabriel: I know I don't always see things the same way as other people – so I suppose that's because I'm constructing (to use your word) my own meaning, which will sometimes be the same as yours, and sometimes it won't?

Martin: Absolutely. And do you think this has any bearing on your work as a GP?

Gabriel: Yes – for a start, my patients won't necessarily make the same sense out of their problems as I do. A new diagnosis of diabetes might seem like an inconvenience to me, but might be more like a life sentence to the patient. Or a death sentence . . .

Martin: Indeed. And what about within the primary healthcare team?

Gabriel: That's true – different members of the team may see things differently – and perhaps that's one of the reasons some patients prefer one GP to another? Maybe patients look for a GP that seems to understand their view of the world?

Martin: Or at least they might look for a GP that recognises that they might have a different view of the world, and that it is just as valid as any other?

Gabriel: I like this relativism, it opens doors . . .

What does this conversation tell us?

- Teachers and learners are human beings!
- So are GPs, and their patients.
- All human beings are different. Constructivism[2] tells us that meaning is created uniquely, individually, by each of us (more on Constructivism in Chapter 10: Five Pearls of Educational Theory).

And where next? How about models?

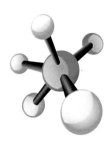

There are many models which attempt to describe the differences between us. And these definitely have their uses – but should all be viewed with a bit of constructive criticism. They can sometimes feel a bit like having a guide telling us about geological formations and glacial activity when we're walking up a mountain: it's an interesting perspective, but maybe we were just *experiencing* the mountain anyway?

 Red Alert: It's important to maintain an attitude of 'openness to difference'. Models are not the *truth*, and are only helpful in as much as they seem to provide meaning in a given situation. If the model doesn't 'fit', then it's not the right model for that time and place.

How can models help us?

- Models can help us understand our learners better. In so doing, we can construct teaching activities that blend nicely with their make-up.
- Models can help us understand ourselves better – for instance, why we teach in the way we do.
- Models can help us 'diagnose a stuck learning situation' – when things aren't going as well as you feel they should be.
- Models are exciting and interesting – and, therefore, can help us acquire exciting and interesting ways of doing (teaching) things.

So, what follows is a run-through of some of these models. It's not an exhaustive list, but there are ideas about where you can look for more detail, and this whole book is full of other models that will help. We're going to look at models that explore three areas:

1 our cognitive differences
2 our behavioural differences
3 our emotional differences.

For each of these models, try to figure out which style you think describes you and whether the suggestions which follow for that style would work for someone dealing with you.

A model that describes cognitive differences: Curry's Onion Model

In this somewhat 'aromatic' model,[3] Lynn Curry suggests that all the variables that affect the way we learn can be grouped into three strata, like the layers of an onion.

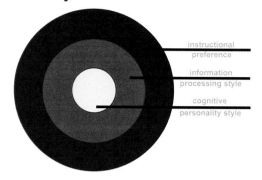

The innermost layer represents the **'cognitive personality style'**. In other words, our personalities affect the way we learn – the things that motivate us to learn. This is the most stable layer and is, therefore, less easily modified (you can't change a personality overnight!). The commonest method for looking at this layer is the Myers-Briggs Type Inventory[4] (more below).

The middle layer represents our **'information-processing style'** – in other words, the way new learning is processed, and there are several ways of processing information (styles). Once we've identified weak processing styles, we can then try to boost them by using various learning strategies. A common method of determining which processing styles are dominant within us is through learning style questionnaires like that of Honey and Mumford (H&M).

Learners also have a 'social interaction learning preference style' – where some individuals have a preference for learning through social interaction (like small-group work) while others prefer to work alone (or with someone in authority). This too would be represented by this layer of the onion but unfortunately is not measured by H&M's questionnaire. Instead, refer to work by Reichmann and Grasha.[5]

The outer layer represents **'instructional preference'** – which mainly talks about the environmental factors which can affect learning. Clearly, of the three layers, this is the one that is most unstable and, therefore, the one that we can influence the easiest. It includes things like temperature, light, sound, seating comfort and so on. Never underestimate the effect of this layer on the way learners learn. A test for assessing such individual instructional preferences has been developed by Dunn and Dunn.[6]

Myers-Briggs[4]

The Myers-Briggs Type Indicator (MBTI) classifies personality traits into four bipolar scales.

(I) Introverted	⇔	(E) Extroverted
(S) Sensing	⇔	(N) INtuitive
(F) Feeling	⇔	(T) Thinking
(P) Perceiving	⇔	(J) Judging

Permutations of these produce a matrix of 16 categories. The individual's place in the matrix can be correlated with the vocational direction they eventually take (as in their career pathways). It can therefore give a deeper understanding of an individual's approach to adapting and assimilating information. It can help us understand how they do things most comfortably and effectively and what we can do (in terms of our teaching) to make learning easier for them. Learn more at www.personalitypage.com/

Honey and Mumford Learning Styles

This model, developed by Peter Honey and Alan Mumford in the 1980s,[7] is frequently used by GP Trainers. In terms of Curry's 'Onion Model' (see previous page) it addresses the information-processing style. A learning style is the preferred way in which an individual likes to receive and process information. We can do two things when we work out our learner's learning style. We can alter our style and teach in a way that marries with their learning style (making learning easier for them). Or we can encourage them to engage with learning activities which work on their weaker style(s) in order to make them more 'all rounded' learners. H&M described four types of learning styles.

1 Activists – who welcome new ideas and use them straight away without question.
2 Reflectors – who like to reflect and consider the implications of new ideas first.
3 Theorists – who like to understand the logical basis behind new ideas first.
4 Pragmatists – who like to try them out and see if they work.

Each of these styles is important – one is not better than the other. Each of us has components from all of these four learning styles, but some are stronger in us than others. It's the overall combination which is important because that dictates the way we like to receive information best. For example, a Reflector-Theorist prefers to read and understand the anatomy of a shoulder joint before trying to learn how to examine it. However, the Activist-Pragmatist would probably just jump in there and give it a go. (By the way, you can tell an activist from a mile – they're the ones that don't bother with the instruction manual when they buy new gadgets or DIY furniture).

While it is good to be rounded in all four areas, having a strong preference for one or more of these four styles can confer additional advantages. But, unfortunately, some disadvantages too:

Style	Pros	Cons
Reflectors	Think things through very carefully before making a decision – they sit back and reflect from all angles.	But they can end up reflecting for so long that no decision is ever made – 'analysis to paralysis'.
Activists	Love getting involved and, therefore, come home with new ideas and then set on making things happen.	But because they 'jump in' without first considering things properly, they end up making rash decisions with bad consequences.
	What about Pragmatists and Theorists – can you work out their pros and cons?	

Anyway, back to the theory . . .

Honey and Mumford drew an association between their four learning styles and the four stages of Kolb's learning cycle.[8] In completing a cycle of learning, all the learning styles are required to some degree; this is why it's important to be rounded in the four styles. Read more about Kolb's learning cycle in Chapter 10: Five Pearls of Educational Theory.

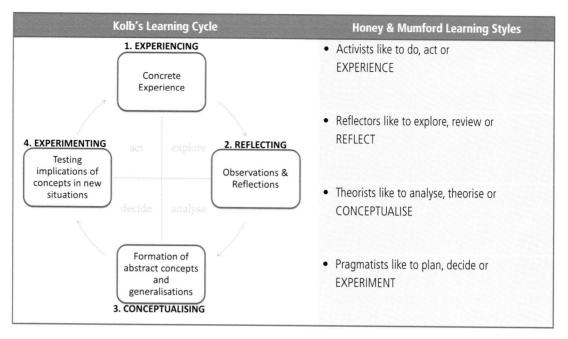

Kolb's Learning Cycle	Honey & Mumford Learning Styles
1. EXPERIENCING — Concrete Experience; **2. REFLECTING** — Observations & Reflections; **3. CONCEPTUALISING** — Formation of abstract concepts and generalisations; **4. EXPERIMENTING** — Testing implications of concepts in new situations (act, explore, decide, analyse)	• Activists like to do, act or EXPERIENCE • Reflectors like to explore, review or REFLECT • Theorists like to analyse, theorise or CONCEPTUALISE • Pragmatists like to plan, decide or EXPERIMENT

There is an 80-item Honey and Mumford's learning style questionnaire that is instructive and fun to do. It's available from www.peterhoney.com and gives an individual's degree of preference for all four styles. This is still only a preference, not a limitation. The point is that **effective learners are flexible, and can function, to a degree, in all the styles**. It is also worth considering that some types of learning will be achieved more effectively with some styles than others. For instance, the development of a practical skill is likely to be achieved more quickly using the Activist/Pragmatist style. Curry refers to this ability to adapt learning style to different situations as **'style flexibility'**, and suggests that the lack of it may be a cause of stress or failure in learning for some.

 Top Tip: Use your knowledge about learning styles to expand your repertoire of teaching strategies. Vary your teaching and learning activities: try to match the learner's style. If you're teaching a group, consider a variety of teaching styles to cater for the variety of learning styles in the audience.

Honey and Mumford's descriptors for their learning style preferences

Getting your head around learning styles is a bit complicated when you're just reading about it. It's better if you get hold of the questionnaire and try it out. In the meantime, here's a bit more description on each of the four styles.

Activists

Activists involve themselves fully and without bias in new experiences. They enjoy the here and now and are happy to be dominated by immediate experiences. They are open-minded, not sceptical. And this tends to make them enthusiastic about anything new. When one activity is dying down, they're on the lookout for another. They tend to thrive on the challenge of new experiences but are bored with implementation and longer-term consolidation.

Will often say: 'I'll try anything once.'

Reflectors

Reflectors like to stand back to ponder experiences and observe them from many different perspectives (the ones that often take the back seat in meetings and discussions – you might think they're uninvolved or disinterested, but you couldn't be further from the truth). By doing this, they collect data, both first hand and from others, and prefer to think about it thoroughly (observing all the different perspectives and implications) before coming to any conclusion. The thorough collection and analysis of data about experiences and events is what counts so they tend to postpone reaching definitive conclusions for as long as possible. Their philosophy is to be cautious. They tend to adopt a low profile and have a slightly distant, tolerant unruffled air about them.

Will often say: 'I'd like to think about it', 'We need to be cautious'.

Theorists

Theorists adapt and integrate observations into complex but logically sound theories. They think problems through in a vertical, step-by-step logical way. They assimilate disparate facts into coherent theories and will often go back to basic assumptions, principles, theories, models and systems. They tend to be perfectionists who won't rest easy until things are tidy and fit to a rational scheme. They like to analyse and synthesise. Their philosophy prizes rationality and logic.

Will often say: 'Does it make sense?', 'How does this fit with that?', 'What are the basic assumptions?', 'If it's logical, it's good'

Pragmatists

Pragmatists are keen on trying out ideas, theories and techniques to see if they work in practice. They positively search out new ideas and take the first opportunity to experiment with application. They are the sort of people who return from management courses brimming with new ideas that they want to try out in practice. They tend to be impatient with ruminating and open-ended discussions. They are essentially practical, down-to-earth people who like solving problems and making practical decisions.

Famous sayings: 'There is always a better way', 'How can I apply this to practice?', 'If it works it's good'.

Using learning styles in practice

Don't worry about the theory behind H&M too much; just play with it.

- Recognise that your own learning style(s) will strongly influence your teaching style.
- Be prepared to study and practise teaching methods which are not central to your 'comfort zone'.
- Recognise that trainees, as adult learners, will come with a variety of fixed concepts about learning. Therefore, use it with your learner as part of your introductory package, or induction. Use it to introduce a session on 'learning to learn'.
- In terms of teaching groups, it is probably best to cater for a mixture of learning styles. Develop plans which include activities that support different styles at different points in the overall program.
- Use it as a diagnostic tool if you feel your learner is 'stuck'. Maybe there's a learning style they need to develop to help them move on?
- Use it if you feel you are being judgemental about a learner: are your styles very different?

So where do I go next for resources on learning styles?

If you want to give learning styles a try, here are some leads.

- www.peterhoney.com – for the questionnaire.
- www.ldpride.net/learning-style-test.html – web-based, free, learning styles test.
- www.businessballs.com/howardgardnermultipleintelligences.htm – Gardner's Multiple Intelligences and VAK learning styles is something else we'd encourage you to read.

A model that describes behavioural differences: the Behavioural Style Identification Matrix
. . . the questionnaire and a fuller account can be found on our website

Each of us has a behaviour style which sits in our personal 'comfort zone' – the style we adopt most naturally when not under stress. This behavioural style dictates how we respond and assert ourselves in most situations. In the Behavioural Style Identification Matrix, there are taken to be four basic styles. They are often displayed on a 2x2 table and are given somewhat arbitrary labels, but don't be distracted by that . . .

The Axes:
RESPONSIVENESS (Y-axis)
People can **respond** in two ways: in a 'controlling' manner or in an 'emotive' way.

ASSERTIVENESS (X axis)
People can **assert** themselves in two ways: in a 'telling' way or 'asking' manner.

Using these two axes, the model produces four quadrants (see diagram right).

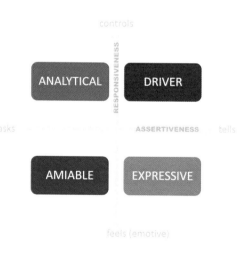

If we can work out which behavioural style our trainee has, we can then alter our behaviour in a way that engages them more readily with us.

Analytical, or processing style (e.g. John Major, Mr Bean)

Characteristics of Analyticals

- Pace: measured, systematic
- Voice: quiet, monotone
- Posture: formal, stiff
- Gestures: small, few
- Eye Contact: reflective, steady
- Face: fixed, unexpressive

Responding in a 'controlling' way, and asserting in an 'asking' way. Analyticals appear somewhat formal and conservative. You must have come across the type: they're often quiet, have a monotonous voice and appear formal and stiff with very few body gestures when they speak (but without the scariness of drivers). Their main priority is the job in hand, and the process to achieve it. Their pace is measured and systematic. They seek accuracy and dislike unpredictability and surprises (unlike the expressive). They prefer an atmosphere that encourages careful preparation and achieve acceptance through being correct, logical and thorough. Under pressure, an Analytical will withdraw into their own world, and avoid contact with the causes of stress.

To win over and work with an Analytical:
- ✓ Listen carefully: be formal, be quiet and let them put their point of view across.
- ✓ Be specific, organised and logical; use credible facts.
- ✓ Get down to business (and don't be late!)

Driver, or controlling style (e.g. Sir Alan Sugar, *The Dragons' Den* entrepreneurs)

Characteristics of Drivers

- Pace: fast, decisive
- Voice: clipped, monotone
- Posture: formal, forward
- Gestures: small, precise
- Eye Contact: intense, direct
- Face: fixed, immobile

Responding in a 'controlling' way, and asserting in a 'telling' way. Drivers are business-like and formal in appearance. Their main priority is the task in hand, and the results achieved. Their pace is fast and decisive, and their eye contact can be direct and intense. They prefer an atmosphere that encourages control of people and processes, and achieve acceptance through their productivity and competitiveness. Under pressure, drivers can become autocratic and dictatorial, which can make others feel apprehensive in their presence.

To win over and work with a Driver:
- ✓ Support their goals and objectives (i.e. show you're on their side).
- ✓ Demonstrate what your ideas will do, by when, and at what cost (i.e. results).
- ✓ Be organised, be factual and be succinct! (i.e. don't waffle).

Expressive, or enthusing style (e.g. Dawn French, Ainsley Harriot)

Characteristics of Expressives

- Pace: fast, spontaneous
- Voice: loud, fast, modulated
- Posture: relaxed, open
- Gestures: large, frequent
- Eye Contact: intense, but infrequent
- Face: very mobile, animated.

Responding in an 'emotive' way, and asserting in a 'telling' way. Expressives are those energetic, flamboyant people you know who are often the 'life and soul' of a party. Their tendency is to interact within relationships, and they dislike any loss of prestige. Their pace is fast and spontaneous: they hate boredom and routine. They try to create an atmosphere that encourages flexibility and achieve acceptance through sociability and creating a stimulating environment. Under pressure, an Expressive will go on the offensive or be sarcastic (i.e. becomes Driver-ish – so watch your step!).

To win over and work with an Expressive:
- ✓ Focus on your relationship with them (be sociable, energetic and have fun with them).
- ✓ Support their dreams and ideas.
- ✓ Show how you can help enhance their standing with others.

Amiable, or supportive style (e.g. Delia Smith, Marge Simpson)

> ## Characteristics of Amiables
> - Pace: slow, easy
> - Voice: soft, modulated
> - Posture: relaxed, informal
> - Gestures: large, but few
> - Eye Contact: warm, friendly
> - Face: open, animated

Responding in an 'emotive' way, and asserting in an 'asking' way. They're those quiet 'loveable' types that you feel like cuddling. They are motherly. Their preference is to maintain relationships and avoid confrontation. They're casual but conforming. Their pace is slow and easy. They prefer an atmosphere that encourages close relationships, and achieve acceptance through conformity and loyalty. Under pressure, an Amiable will submit or acquiesce.

To win over and work with Amiables:
✓ Be friendly and informal.
✓ Show interest in them personally (e.g. by listening and taking your time with them).
✓ Support their feelings.
✓ Give them time to make decisions (i.e. don't rush them).
✓ Show how our ideas will support their personal circumstances.

A model that describes emotional differences: Heron

One limitation of the preceding models (which focus on cognition and behaviour) is that they do not offer any role for emotions. Human beings, as well as thinking and acting, also do a fair bit of feeling, so it seems only right to have a model of learning that includes this part of our humanity.

John Heron[9] thought this too, and he introduced the term **'Whole Person Learning' (or holistic learning)** to draw attention to what was missing from other models. Heron is a hugely influential figure: a social sciences researcher who was involved in pioneering the ideas of holistic medicine, co-counselling, and humanistic learning. He said that holistic learning happened in a number of different ways:

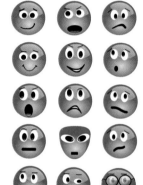

> ### Heron's Holistic Learning Model: whole person learning
> - Holistic learning can be used as an activity for learning about something else.
>   For instance, making paper planes as a way of learning about assessment.
> - Use holistic learning activities alongside other learning.
>   For instance, during a whole-day residential session, it may be necessary to do something in the afternoon to raise energy, like a dance, or physical game.
> - Use holistic learning activities to learn to be a whole person.
>   For instance, while learning about the consultation using videos, I may develop a new understanding about myself, and the kind of person I think I am.

He criticised Kolb (and others) for their experiential learning models, because he said they 'miss the depth of personhood, and its potential learning power'. He acknowledged the holistic nature of experiential learning – building as it does on the actual experience of an individual. However,

Heron asks: *'What is left out of this minimal model? What about intuition, psychic and spiritual capacities?'*

Heron's ideas on 'The Self' are complex and challenging, and are beyond our time, space and inclination here! But those who wish to explore further will find all they need in his 1992 book on the subject.[10] It is sufficient to say here that Heron feels Kolb (and others who promote experiential learning) is limiting his model, and missing out **emotion, intuition and imagination**. Certainly, in our experience, there are plenty of times when these are the most important aspects of our own learning, and in our facilitation of the learning of others.

**Having Heron and his model of holistic learning in our
mental toolkit can be a tremendous help.**

Conclusion

To maximise the effectiveness of your teaching, and of the learning you are facilitating:

Ask yourself:

1 Who is this learner? What do I know about him or her? What motivates him or her?
2 How can I find out more?
3 How does he or she like to learn?
4 What does he or she find difficult about learning?

Keep in the back of your mind:

1 The *value* of the learner's previous learning and experience.
2 How the context for learning influences the approach taken (if you're going to pass an MCQ, you've gotta learn some facts . . .).
3 The strengths of their learning style – while acknowledging that all styles are needed for a learner to be rounded and complete.
4 Don't forget about whole person learning or holism – keep a watch out for cues relating to emotion, intuition and imagination.

We think that trying to constantly be aware of difference **and uniqueness** in learners (different to us and different to each other) is the main message here. Using the models (like Learning Styles) can be a practical route in, but don't be too restricted by any one model.

A sample of resources on our website

● More on Honey and Mumford, Myers-Briggs, Behaviour and Social Styles.
● Transactional Analysis.
● Hermann's left and right brain thinking.

Please give us some feedback on this chapter to help shape it for the next edition.
Go to www.essentialgptrainingbook.com and simply click on the title of this chapter.

References

1 Grant J, Chambers G, Jackson G, editors. *The Good CPD Guide.* Sutton: Reed Healthcare; 1999.

2 Guba EG, Lincoln YS. *Fourth Generation Evaluation.* London: Sage Publications; 1989.

3 Curry L. Cognitive and learning styles in medical education. *Acad Med.* 1999; **74**(4): 409–13.

4 Myers I. *Myers-Briggs Type Indicator.* Palo Alto, California: Consulting Psychologists Press; 1978.

5 Reichmann SW, Grasha AF. A rational approach to developing and assessing the construct validity of a student learning style scale instrument. *J Psychol.* 1974; **87**: 213–23.

6 Dunn R, Dunn K. *Teaching Students through their Individual Learning Styles: a practical approach.* Reston, VA: Reston Publishing; 1978.

7 Honey P, Mumford A. *The Manual of Learning Styles.* Maidenhead, UK: Peter Honey Publications; 1982.

8 Kolb D. *Experiential Learning: experience as the source of learning and development.* Englewood Cliffs, New Jersey: Prentice-Hall; 1984.

9 Heron J. *The Complete Facilitator's Handbook.* London: Kogan Page; 1999.

10 Heron J. *Feeling and Personhood: psychology in another key.* London: Sage Publications Ltd; 1992.

PART FOUR

Teaching Groups of People

12

How Groups Work – the dynamics

MARY DAVIS – Associate GP Dean (KSS Deanery) & lead author
IAIN LAMB – Associate Advisor (SE Scotland)   **SHAKE SEIGEL** – TPD (Burton on Trent)

The term 'group dynamics' refers to the interaction between people in a group setting. In this chapter, we will look at what we mean by a group, how people in a group interact with each other and what can happen in that group that makes it function better for learning. To start off with, let's see whether belonging to a group is different from belonging to a team and whether it matters.

Am I in a group or in a team?

Most of us are part of several groups or teams, which have different functions, and where we play different roles. For instance, our families, at school, sports or other teams, at college, socially and so on. Each of these has its own ethos, sets its own norms, and we behave differently in each of them. But some of these are groups and some are teams and, yes, there is a difference and, yes, it does matter.

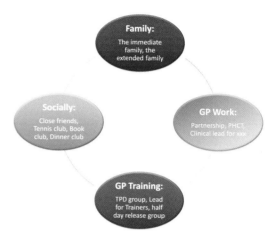

In a nutshell, a small group is a group of people meeting with a common purpose who feel a sense of belonging and exert influence on one another. Teams, on the other hand, have goals that are clear, and it's those goals that are the sole driving force. Roles and responsibilities of members in a team are more explicitly defined than those in a group. But there are other differences:

Teams (think of a football team)	Groups (think of a 'mother and toddler' group)
A team has a set of common specific performance goals.	A group also has a common goal, but it may or may not be performance linked.
These performance goals are usually externally set.	A group discusses and usually negotiates its own goals.
They are committed to those performance goals.	They are committed to each other.
The members are internally selected and organised based on their complementary skills.	The members are simply a collection of people with something in common or having a shared interest, e.g. GP trainees.
The members are coordinated usually by a leader. Members end up with specific roles.	Non-hierarchical structure. Members discuss and decide their own roles (they 'opt in'). They coordinate themselves.
Usually measured on their performance	Have greater freedom and creativity.
Atmosphere is more formal.	Atmosphere is more relaxed.
Learning takes place by pooling knowledge and skills.	Learning takes place by pooling *and sharing* knowledge, skills *and attitudes*.
Can result in pressure to conform to overall team opinion.	Individuals are more likely to express and be themselves.
Whole team is accountable when there is poor performance.	Individuals are accountable when there is poor performance.

Does that mean small groups are better than teams or vice versa? No, definitely not! If a task doesn't require joint working of people with specific skills, and people can be creative and as free as they want, then the small group might be best. However, if that task requires people with different complementary skills to come together, a team is most likely the best approach. In GP training (especially at Half-Day Release), we want to nurture the learners through their freedom to express themselves, interact with each other, and to be creative together. Small-group working is ideal for this because:

- the agenda can be socially negotiated
- members can offer mutual acceptance and support for one another's goals, and
- there is encouragement for life changes.

In small-group work, members discover the 'truth' for their own lives as well as achieving the group's common goal. And throughout all of this, there is a sense of shared ownership.

 Top Tip: When you are working with a group of people consider what kind of leadership is taking place. This is important because facilitating small-group learning is very different from chairing a *team* meeting. In a team meeting, there may be a defined task, and you might need to step in more to navigate the direction in which the discussion is going.

Both groups and teams come across similar issues. Things like:

- leadership and who influences what
- establishing the collective vision
- defining individual roles
- managing conflict
- providing and maintain support.

How these issues are handled depends on many different factors. In a team, this will be managed by the leader; in a group, the role of the facilitator is crucial, as we will see, but the whole group has a higher degree of ownership and responsibility for resolving the issues. The mode in which the collective are working therefore needs to be made explicit to them and you. For example, in a small group learning together, the direction of learning needs to be decided by the group.

 Top Tip: Clarify ideas, concerns and expectations: Members need to know what is expected of them so that they can then perform. The place to do all of this is shortly after the getting acquainted stage. For instance, they need to know that the group is responsible for its own effectiveness and that all members share equally in that responsibility. Members need to interact – we all have talents and expertise to share.

How do we learn in groups?

We know that adults learn best when they are *involved* in the learning process, and where *interaction* with other learners is taking place. But in groups, we know that there are additional ways in which learning takes place. Peer discussion results in the sharing of experiences and ideas with others. The facilitator or a group member may end up role modelling behaviour. And, finally, role play or rehearsing skills results in learning by doing. All of this leads to a greater level of competence – as defined by Miller[1] (more on Miller's Pyramid in Chapter 29: Assessment and Competence).

What can we learn in groups?

If the group has been set up so that the members can trust and be honest with each other, you will find that the members of a group can work and learn together to acquire all sorts of knowledge, skills and attitudes.

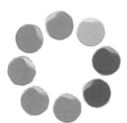

Knowledge	Skills	Attitudes
• Draw on *knowledge* brought from outside, pool it, and then go back to use it outside. • *Develop new ideas:* the sharing of different ideas can create a completely new, and sometimes unexpected, outcome.	• *Solve complex problems:* discussion of choices for managing difficult problems or ethical dilemmas. • *Rehearse skills* in a supportive environment: like communication, giving and receiving feedback and other interpersonal skills. • *Develop personal and professional skills:* for example, negotiation, time management and leadership.	• *Challenge behaviour* and be challenged and thence *change attitudes.* • *Raise self-awareness* as part of personal and professional development. • *Raise awareness* in terms of group dynamics, of the skills for working in other groups or teams and of the importance of a supportive environment.

We were working with simulated patients, and the patient described how difficult they found it to look after their aged mother. The GP trainee offered her the option of having her mother admitted to a home, and could not understand why the patient did not find this acceptable as he felt it would solve her problem. In the small-group discussion afterwards, other members were able to talk about how they too would find it very difficult to put their mother in a home, rather than looking after her themselves. The GP trainee who had done the consultation was surprised to hear the strength of feeling from some of the group members, and could see that he had made assumptions that the patient would have the same attitude to looking after their parents as he did.

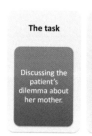

The task	Listening to the views of others	Reflecting on own attitudes and being challenged	Learning from the process (self-awareness)
Discussing the patient's dilemma about her mother.	Hearing other group members' views and attitudes.	How do I feel about putting my own mother in a home?	How do I get feedback? How receptive am I to it? How do I learn from it?

In this scenario, the GP trainee has learnt at different levels (see diagram left). Sometimes that learning (especially if it is around attitudes) isn't so obvious to learners at first.

Here's another scenario to illustrate the different levels of learning in groups:

A group decides it would be useful to talk about prescribing (after one of the members mentions a complaint they received about a prescribing error). Discussion follows where individuals discuss ways in which they reduce the risk of prescribing errors (like using the computer) and how they keep up-to-date with prescribing matters (*explicit learning*). The individual who received the complaint then went on to explain how awful an experience it was for her. This led to a discussion about how it feels to make a mistake and how to get 'back on track' (*related learning*). Finally, the group ended with a little discussion about how useful they found this session and a number commented how important it is to pluck up the courage to talk about these things and reflect on them, preferably with your colleagues (*learning about learning*).

The group dynamic

Dynamic: The energy or forces producing motion (*Oxford English Dictionary*).

A great deal can be learned by observing the group dynamic. If you sit back quietly in *any* group you will see certain patterns of behaviour emerge. For instance, there will always be someone who:

- starts off the discussion
- talks too much
- talks very little and sits quietly

- interrupts others or is always controversial
- jokes around (the group joker)
- and so on.

When I first ran a group, I thought there was no rhyme or reason why things happened or didn't happen. I had understood it was probably up to me whether the group sank or swam. It was a great relief to find out that there is such a thing as the *group dynamic*, and that most groups follow a pattern of behaviour, and as facilitator I could influence the group, but it was not only up to me. This liberated me, and enabled me to be more receptive within a group.

 Top Tip: As a facilitator you need not feel responsible for everything and everybody in the group; the group and its individual members have a collective responsibility. *'A sense of responsibility is inversely proportional to a sense of response ability.'*

What affects the group dynamic?

The way members of a group interact with each other (the group dynamic) depends on a variety of internal and external factors. Maslow[2] summarised them in his 'hierarchy of needs'. All of these things will affect the group's energy and this in turn will affect the progression of the group. Before you read Maslow's list below, you might like to read more generally about his hierarchy of needs first – which you can find in Chapter 10: Five Pearls of Educational Theory. Once you've read that bit, come back to this section.

Factors affecting the group dynamic

The individual members

- Their personalities: some members will be dominant and autocratic and others more quiet and shy. Read Chapter 11: Learning and Personality Styles in Practice.
- Their learning styles: the Activists in the group can end up 'running the show' while the Reflectors sit back quietly to reflect. There's a resource on our website called 'learning styles and the group dynamic'. Again, read Chapter 11.
- Their personal comfort: members need to feel physically comfortable, not hungry or thirsty.
- Their emotional status: while most of our personal and professional lives are hardly ever in a perfect state, individuals need to be in an emotionally stable position to work effectively.
- Their experience in previous groups: affects their general view of working in small groups.

The group

- The size of the group: 8–10 people is the ideal. Too small – not enough people to generate ideas and thoughts. Too large – a plethora of ideas, thoughts and discussions competing for attention, making it tricky to manage. The table below shows how complex the web of communications gets when the group size grows.

No. in small group	No. of individual communications	Facilitation
5	10	easy to manage
6	15	
7	21	
8	28	
9	36	
10	45	
11	55	
12	66	difficult to manage

If > 12 people, consider doing subgroup work. It's often difficult to establish/maintain trust in larger groups and cater for the needs of individual learners. Be careful, though, subgroups can result in a competitive attitude which sometimes can be healthy but other times not. And you'll also need to think about how the confidentiality rules apply between the subgroups.

- The stage of the group: the dynamic within a group depends on what 'stage of life' the group is at (more on this below).

The classroom environment

- Physical aspects: like room size, comfortable chairs and air conditioning. People will fall asleep if the room is too warm.
- Seating arrangements: sitting in a circle, in same-sized chairs, can make all the members feel included. It's important that every group member can be seen by all other group members.

The 'teacher'

- The position of the 'teacher': has a marked effect on the group dynamic. Who the facilitator positions themselves next to, and opposite, can be used for altering the dynamic.
- The skills of the 'teacher': the group dynamic is affected by your ability to engage with and motivate individuals to tackle their own learning.
- The facilitative style: the group dynamic is enhanced when the facilitator can alter their style of facilitation according to where the group is at.

 Top Tip: The best way to understand what affects the group dynamic is to consider the factors in terms of the individual group member, the whole group, the environment and the facilitator.

The stages in the life of a group

When groups have been observed, it has been seen that their formation follows a similar pattern (described as 'The Stages in the Life of a Group'). There are several models that describe these stages and while all groups follow these models, the way in which they do it, and the pace at which it happens, will always vary. There are three models which we have found particularly helpful in understanding the stages.

Tuckman[3]

Tuckman described group development in four stages before a group moves into the final fifth adjourning stage (where the group comes to an end).

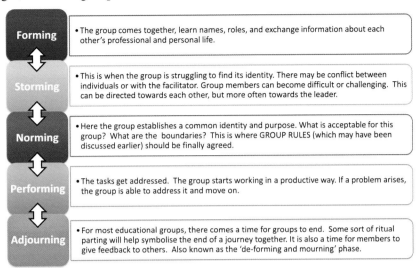

If you want to read more on what you can do as a facilitator at each of these stages, read Chapter 13: Teaching and Facilitating Small Groups.

A second similar model is this one (after Freeman)

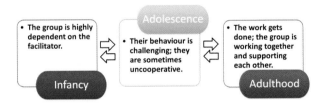

Freeman's model shows only three stages, but you can probably see which of these corresponds to those in Tuckman's. The only thing missing is the ending stage. The stage of adolescence (storming) has a marked counterpart in the home life of parents of teenagers, and can feel just the same! The style of the facilitator needs to reflect where the group is, but it can also enable or inhibit change. A group in 'infancy' will want the facilitator to make the decisions and lead, but if the facilitator stays in this mode for too long, the group will not move on. Similarly, if a facilitator disengages too soon (because he or she wants the group to become autonomous), the group will become anxious and disorganised.

Many years ago, I attended a workshop for learning group skills. The facilitator came in and sat down, and then said: 'Over to you.' The group members became very anxious and agitated. The group, who did not know each other, needed more direction initially, until they had got to know each other.

 Red Alert: These stages do not always result in a forward progression – sometimes groups can move back a step (hence the bidirectional arrows in the images above).

And another model – Heron's

A model with a slightly different slant comes from John Heron.[4]

	Winter	The ground may be frozen and the weather stormy: *Anxiety is high in the group, defences are up.*
	Spring	New life starts to break through the surface crust: *The group is beginning to trust each other; its life is under way.*
	Summer	There is an abundance of growth and the sun is high: *There is openness, risk-taking, working and sharing.*
	Autumn	The fruit is harvested and stored; the harvesters give thanks and go their way: *Time for reflection on learning and how it will be applied*

From Heron's model, the importance of Harvest Time (autumn) is stressed; it is important to make time for this stage in any group session. There should be time for members of the group to reflect on what they are taking away from their time together, and if they are not meeting again, to complete the ritual of parting (adjourning).

Why do these stages matter?

- All groups go through these stages. Knowing about the models helps you understand where the group is at; this can inform the facilitative approach you take.
- All groups go through a 'storming' or 'adolescent' stage. Some groups move through it swiftly but, in others, it can feel uncomfortable. Nevertheless, *it happens*. All you need to do is to be aware and recognise it when it happens. In that way, you won't be preoccupied with notions of whether the group is dysfunctional or whether you're doing a bad job of facilitating. Instead, it will encourage you to focus on how you might help the group through the 'storm'.
- When a group is challenged, it may respond by reversing its dynamic. This isn't necessarily a bad thing; going back a step can create powerful 'light bulb' moments.

EXAMPLE OF A GROUP MOVING BACK TO THE STORMING FROM THE PERFORMING STAGE

I was working with a group of GP trainees, who had seemed to be 'performing' for some weeks. We had asked an outside resource to come and talk to them about negotiation skills. The speaker started by telling them that she had previously been a hospital administrator, and had found doctors a difficult group to work with. The members of our group became distracted, disengaged and argumentative with the speaker. After she had gone, they were able to discuss this, and how they had felt challenged and put down by her, hence their behaviour, although they had not realised they were doing it at the time. From the discussion, the group learnt a lot about group behaviour and their own behaviour within a group, but unfortunately not as much about negotiation skills as they might have!

Top Tip: Storming is indiscriminate and may feel as if it is aimed at you, but you need to accept that *storming is a natural occurrence*. When it happens, it often results in greater understanding, reflection and learning, which will hopefully show in 'performing'. Storming is okay; embrace it.

Using the models to alter your facilitative style

If you are aware of the stage the group is at, you can use an appropriate facilitator style to match their position. Here are two models (both by Heron) which describe the different modes of facilitator style.

Heron's Three Modes of Authority and Power[5]	
Hierarchy: 'I decide' As facilitator, you need to take a degree of control, but with the participants' consent. You need to give some structure and framework to the learning. Groups need this when they first come together.	To be used at the stage of • Forming • Infancy • Winter
Cooperation: 'We decide' In this next phase of the group, there is more obvious collaboration, and negotiation of learning. The members are more confident and want to be involved in the decision-making.	To be used at the stage of • Norming • Adulthood • Spring
Autonomy: 'You decide' The group becomes more self-directed, and the members are able to work together without your guidance. The ultimate autonomy is for you to be absent from the group.	To be used at the stage of • Performing • Adulthood • Summer

Heron's next model describes six primary categories (or styles) of helping people (or facilitation). This model also helps heighten your sense of awareness about your own facilitative style and how to be more flexible.

Heron's Six Categories of Intervention	
Authoritative: *(the 'group leader' retains control)*	**Facilitative:** *(encouraging the group to take control)*
1 **Prescriptive** – giving advice/direction *'Okay, I think it's important that we talk about xxxx today.'*	4 **Cathartic** – expressing emotions (unexpressed emotion can block development and creativity) *'Mmmm . . . some of you seem quite reluctant to approach it in this way. Help me to understand how you feel.'*
2 **Informative** – providing information *'In such cases, one can normally do a number of things such as x, y and z. Let me tell you more about these.'*	5 **Catalytic** – exploring, 'drawing out' and eliciting self-discovery/problem-solving *'Okay, I can see your difficulty. Have you been in this sort of situation before? Can you remember a time when it went okay? Tell me more. Anything there that can help us here?'*
3 **Confronting** – challenging *'Do you really think it would be worthwhile talking about that?' 'I notice that you're avoiding talking about . . .'*	6 **Supportive** – validating, affirming worth and value of the other person, their qualities, attitudes and actions *'It sounds like you handled that in quite a mature and professional way. I can see it couldn't have been easy.'*

Actually, this model can be applied to *any* situation where you have to *help or interact with other people* (such as in the consultation when dealing with patients, or small-group teaching when

dealing with GP trainees). The model helps you analyse and decide what 'help' is required to maximise success in terms of effective training and building your relationship with them.

How can I move my group on through the stages?
This is covered in Chapter 13: Teaching and Facilitating Small Groups.

The Jenkins' Triangle – group task, process and support[6]
A group is always in a dynamic state, and moves around
within the area of the yellow triangle during its life. At any
one time, what is happening within the group will be somewhere within the triangle.

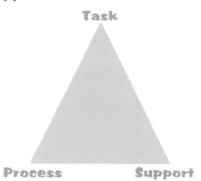

   TASK: This is the piece of work that the group has set
itself to do at any one time such as looking at communication
skills or working for an exam. This assumes that the group
has agreed on its task. There may be occasions when one or
more members of the group have a *different* task which may
interfere with the group getting on with the *declared* task:

> A group of GP trainees were meeting together, and the following week was their Clinical Skills Assessment
> exam. Although the teaching session was about communication skills, some of the GP trainees were
> very distracted and only wanting to learn about exam technique (i.e. not wanting to explore any of the
> consultations at a deeper level as they felt their needs were for 'quick exam tips'). This made it difficult
> for the other GP trainees who wanted to discuss the emotional aspects of the consultation.

PROCESS: This is going on between the members of the group all the time. It's to do with interactions between individuals, between subgroups, and with the facilitator. It's to do with feelings, and
is influenced by the social skills of the members.

SUPPORT: This happens when members make use of the environment to share experiences and
concerns, and get advice and feedback from the other group members, or just their empathy. This
will only take place in an environment where there is sufficient trust for support to take place, and
where it is encouraged in a non-judgemental way.

How does the triangle help us?
Try to be aware of the balance at any time in the group between *task*, *support* and *process*. If the
group is getting on with their task, and are supporting each other effectively, and are allowing each
other to express their ideas and feelings honestly, then the *process* is happening in a positive way.

 Top Tip: Periodically monitor your small group in terms of these three dimensions: task, process
and support. For each, it might be worthwhile revisiting Heron's Six Category Interventions to
see which facilitative style can help move things on.

When the process stops the group from dealing with the task, or makes them feel uncomfortable
about the level of support they are getting, you need to make an intervention to look at the *process*
that is happening, because it is preventing the other functions of the group. If you do nothing, the

group will end up becoming stuck in discomfort. The *process* issue may arise from something that has happened in the group, or from some external factor.

I was working with a group of Course Organisers (now called Programme Directors) and early on I decided we needed to make sure we had agreed on the group rules. I asked one of the group members to negotiate these. He misunderstood and instead just listed the group rules on a flip chart. Another member of the group was very annoyed that, as he saw it, these had been imposed on him, and said so to the person writing the rules. The group immediately felt very uncomfortable about the dissent that had arisen in a previously affable group. This had to be raised and discussed.

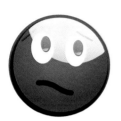

Another thing to watch out for is **when an individual brings their own process to the group** that is not related to the group activity. For example, if an individual has had a row with their partner at home that morning, or there are other major issues going on outside the group. Again, this will need to be acknowledged by the group, but may not need to be taken any further if the individual does not wish it. It is group business to know that the distress is not caused by them, but it is up to the individual to express the amount of support they need from the group, or whether they want to share the issue at all.

A member of the group was obviously distressed during a session about complaints. The rest of the group had observed this, and were getting quite uncomfortable. The facilitator sensitively acknowledged the member's upset: 'I can see that you are upset. Is there anything that we can do to help?' The member said that she had had a complaint in the past, which had been distressing, but it had been resolved successfully, and she did not want to discuss it today. She was happy for the group to continue its discussion, and did not want them to change the topic. The group expressed their sympathy, and could continue their discussion.

 Top Tip: You may find it a useful exercise early in the session to run a 'baggage check' – to see if anyone has some major issue they wish to share, but accepting that the session's agenda may need to be renegotiated by the group as a result of this.

There are various ways of running a baggage check:
1 Offer group members the chance to say something they want to leave outside for the session. Do this either as a round, with everyone saying something, or leave it open for individuals to opt in. *'Is there anything going on for any of you? Any burning or difficult issues that you'd like to discuss or simply get off your chest before we start?'*
2 Place a receptacle (e.g. wastepaper basket) in the middle of the group, and invite anyone to symbolically put into it something they want to leave outside the group. They can say as much or as little about it at the time. Make sure you offer them the choice of whether or not to reclaim what is in the bin at the end of the time together. Items put in the bin have included: the NHS, my partners, my house extension, my mother-in-law, my hospital appointment . . .

Don't forget about you – you also affect the group dynamic

The influence of your behaviour on the group is often more powerful than the other group members because of your position of being seen to be in authority (i.e. *not* authoritarian, not *an* authority, but *in* authority!).

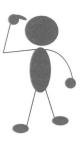

Take into account your own experience of groups, good or bad, and constantly check if that is interfering with the group activity. Be aware of your learning style (or preference) and remember that just because it suits you, it might not suit others. And if you're really serious about improving your skills at small-group facilitation, ask for feedback – from group members and colleagues.

As a small-group facilitator, you should:

- stay within the group rules, particularly regarding confidentiality
- be non-judgemental
- not show favouritism to any group member
- not discriminate towards any members of the group
- maintain trust with the group – being open and honest about your thoughts and feelings too
- remember that you are 'on show' all the time and, therefore, should role model behaviour even during coffee breaks.

In this chapter, we've covered the group dynamic, what affects it and what you can do to enhance it. We will look more closely at the specific skills required of the small-group facilitator in Chapter 13: Teaching and Facilitating Small Groups.

A sample of resources on our website
- Heron's modes and dimensions.
- How learning styles affect the group dynamic.
- When groups start fragmenting into subgroups.

Other chapters you may like to read
- Chapter 11: Learning and Personality Styles in Practice
- Chapter 13: Teaching and Facilitating Small Groups: especially the bit on: *'How can I move my group on through the Tuckman stages?'*
- Web Chapter: Troubleshooting Small Groups.

Please give us some feedback on this chapter to help shape it for the next edition.
Go to www.essentialgptrainingbook.com and simply click on the title of this chapter.

References
1 Miller GE. The assessment of clinical skills/competence/performance. *Acad Med.*1990; **65**(9): 63–7.
2 Maslow AH. A theory of human motivation. *Psychol Rev.* 1943; **50**(4): 370–96.
3 Tuckman B. Developmental sequence in small groups. *Psychol Bull.* 1965; **54**: 229–49.
4 Heron J. *The Complete Facilitators Handbook.* London: Kogan Page; 2009.
5 Heron J. *Six Category Intervention Analysis.* 3rd ed. Surrey: Human Potential Resource Group, University of Surrey; 1989.
6 Jenkins P, unpublished communication; 1989.

13

Teaching and Facilitating Small Groups

SHAKE SEIGEL – TPD (Burton on Trent) & lead author   **MARY DAVIS** – Associate GP Dean (KSS Deanery)
IAIN LAMB – Associate Advisor (SE Scotland)   **RAMESH MEHAY** – TPD (Bradford)

Before embarking on this chapter, we hope you've read the previous chapter. Some of the content in this chapter follows on from what is in there. Otherwise, some bits might not make sense to you. Let's start by looking at the role of the facilitator so that you're clear about *what* you're meant to be doing. We can then focus on *how* to do it.

The role of the facilitator

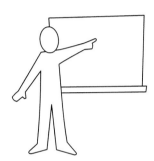

When people facilitate for the first time, they often default to 'expert mode': giving 'expert' advice straight away rather than opening the issue out to the rest of the group. It's not helped by the fact that when trainees in a group talk about cases, they usually look to the facilitator for an expert opinion too. However, try not to take the easy option of giving in to satisfying the content straight away. Facilitation is largely about looking after the group process. In this regard, remember that groups are more than just the sum of their parts; encourage them to *interact* and *learn creatively* with one another. Do this and you'll see what additional riches this *collaboration* brings to the table compared to what *any* expert could have brought alone.[1]

In small group work, an *expert* does this:

A trainee within a group: The patient was demanding antibiotics, and I became edgy and just gave in. I don't know what else I could have done.
Expert: What you should have done is explored his ideas, concerns and expectations. What did he think was going on and what was he worried about? How did he think antibiotics would help? In that way, you would have developed a better shared understanding.

In small group work, a *facilitator* does this:

A trainee within a group: The patient was demanding antibiotics, and I became edgy and just gave in. I don't know what else I could have done.
Facilitator: Mmm . . . I can sense your difficulty. Has anyone else in the group experienced anything similar? Does anyone have anything to offer in terms of what has and has not worked for them?

However, there's more to facilitating than just reflecting questions to the other members in the group. The Jenkins' triangle (introduced in Chapter 12: How Groups Work – the dynamics) talks of small groups being in a dynamic state of flux – constantly moving around within the area of the triangle. This means that the facilitator needs to keep an eye on three things. He or she will need to flexibly adapt between:
1 looking after what the group has to achieve (the *task*)

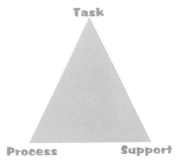

2 looking after how they go about achieving it (the *process*) and
3 looking after the individual group members (providing support).

Looking after the group task

Heron's tasks of the facilitator[9]

- **Prescriptive:** helps plan objectives, assessment and evaluation.
- **Informative:** makes sense of the meaning of what is going on in the group (in terms of task, process and the learning process).
- **Confronting:** confronts difficult issues; raises awareness about blocks to learning in the group – anxieties, ignorance and so on.
- **Cathartic:** releases emotions and feelings in the group (and helps facilitate them into a more positive emotional process).
- **Catalytic:** (a) helps the group structure itself to work together and (b) adds structure to the educational session by structuring learning experiences.
- **Supportive:** creates a climate in which people value and respect each other and their views.

Looking after the group process

Heron's modes of the facilitator[9]

1 **Hierarchical:** where the power is mainly with the facilitator who directs the learning process and does things for the group.
2 **Cooperative:** where the power is shared with the group by encouraging them to become more self-directing in their own learning. Although the facilitator shares his or her own view (which may be influential) it's primarily given to encourage others to express their views. The facilitator *helps* the group to make decisions, negotiate outcomes and collaborate in the direction of their learning.
3 **Autonomous:** where the power is mainly with the group – the facilitator respects the autonomy of the group. They have total freedom to exercise their own judgement and direction of learning. They require little assistance from the facilitator, if any. The facilitator is there simply to create space for autonomous learning. Don't confuse this with an abdication of responsibility – it's not. The facilitator needs to recognise a group that is mature enough to exercise full self-determination in their learning.

These three modes are all about who controls and influences the learning process within a group: is it the facilitator alone, the facilitator and group members together or just the group members alone? As a facilitator, you can employ all three modes to varying degrees as and when appropriate. The experienced facilitator is one who can *effortlessly* move from mode to mode in response to the change in group dynamics.

Providing group support

It helps for a facilitator to be Emotionally Intelligent (Goleman)[2] – a facilitator with high Emotional Intelligence is finely tuned into his or her own feelings and that of others. This helps them to pick up on emotions early and to help release them in a positive way. This in turn helps the group task and process to continue.

Being Emotionally Intelligent means:[2]

- **Being self-aware:** recognising your feelings as they are happening. Being positive and true to your real self can free you from responding to 'gut feelings' and can help you use your intuition creatively. Avoiding premature judgements and conclusions will help you hear others more effectively and thereby understand your impact on others.
- **Being self-regulating:** being able to handle your own feelings and emotions.
  Deferring judgements and 'parking' problems will enable you to 'go with the flow'. It will also help you express yourself more clearly (with congruency between your verbals and non-verbals) and in a way that honours the feelings of others.
- **Being self-motivating:** channelling your emotions in order to achieve goals.
  Striving to improve, attain high standards and a commitment to your goals will enable you to remain positive even in adversity so that you can take the initiative and seize opportunities as they present themselves. This can lead to high creativity and productivity.
- **Showing empathy:** tuning into another's emotions and needs.
  This puts you in a better position to help them with their personal development.
- **Having social competence:** being able to handle relationships with others.
  Sincerity is integral to social competencies, which underpin leadership and interpersonal effectiveness. This is also known as 'rapport' or 'connecting with others' – essential if you want to maintain and nurture relationships in groups.

 Top Tip: If you haven't already done so, we would urge you to read Chapter 12: How Groups Work – the dynamics. An awareness of group dynamic theories can help you anticipate what may happen in groups. This includes both the constructive positive dynamics as well as the unproductive negative ones.

Was that too heavy for you? Don't worry, the rest is easier. So, let's move on to the actual art of facilitation.

The art of facilitating

There are three stages to facilitating a group:
1 the Internal Stage
2 the External Stage
3 the 'Just Doing It' Stage.

Step One: The Internal Stage

This is about getting yourself ready to facilitate a group. We call this 'internal' as it deals with your personal internal focus: thinking about *yourself*, *your* own values and beliefs about education, *your* motivation and *your* capabilities for doing this job. If anything needs attention or changing, it requires you to 'go internal' and sort yourself out.

Key attitudes and behaviour of the facilitator

- You need to create a positive atmosphere in which individuals are motivated to learn.
- You must have a personal value that holds your learners in positive regard. Adult learning is always a learner-centred activity.
- Group learning is a collaborative process in which you need to encourage participation.
- The purpose of group learning is to help people learn in a way that is different to individual learning; *'It reaches the parts that other learning situations do not reach'.* You're there to help make that happen.
- The essence of adult education is for the learner to make sense and meaning of things for themselves; this is known as *constructivism*.
- Although members may have different views and opinions, everyone's contribution is important, and you are there to honour and protect them.
- That means you need to remain neutral and refrain (as much as you can) from evaluating people's contributions; let the group do that. **One of the key features which we feel makes the difference between successful and less successful facilitation is 'unconditional positive regard'**: warm acceptance and support of what a person says and does, without negative judgement (Carl Rogers).
- You have to 'walk the talk' which means acting out and demonstrating the above attributes by the way you facilitate.

Step Two: The External Stage

We call this stage 'external' because these are things external to you and things which can be done outside of (i.e. before) the session. There are two questions you should *try* and be clear about before facilitating a session.

1 **What is it that you are trying to achieve?** Some call this *Aims and Objectives*. Others call it *Intended Learning Outcomes*. We simply like to call it *The Purpose* or *The Agenda*.
2 **What educational methods will you use to help you achieve this?** Different educational methods are good at achieving different things and lend themselves differently to different types of learners. You will probably need to use a combination of methods.

Top Tip: The External Stage is represented in Chapter 6: Teaching from Scratch. If you are new to facilitating, we urge you to make time to read this chapter. As you become more experienced, you will realise that not all sessions need to be so rigidly defined. Experienced facilitators understand this; sometimes they'll set a loose initial agenda because the real agenda (and thus the educational methods) for some sessions can only be defined on the day as it evolves.

Doing these two things should help you formulate a lesson plan – a time grid which breaks the whole session down into manageable chunks, which details what is to be covered, when and via what educational method. However, at other times you may just wish to let the group run freely and creatively while maintaining a light touch on the task, process and support.

Some tips on the External Stage

- Write the three headings (aims, objectives and methods) onto your lesson planning sheet so that it forces you to answer the following questions for yourself:
  1 What is the aim or purpose of the session?
  2 What are the learning objectives (intended outcomes)?
  3 How will this happen and be facilitated?
- Remember to keep the Aims broad and succinct; 2–5 aims are usually sufficient.
- When considering Objectives answer the question:
  'What will the learners be able to do, or know, by the end of the session which they were unable to do, or did not know, before the learning session?'
- When considering Methods ask yourself:
  'Is the method fit for purpose – will it help us get what we are trying to achieve?'
  'How will we capture the learning points from each method?'
  'Overall, have I included a variety of methods to capture the diversity of learning styles that will be present among the learners?'
- On the lesson planning sheet, formulate a timetabled programme with estimated time scales for each section. Walk the timing through in your mind by imagining what participants will be doing and saying, and how long each activity or spoken bit may take. For instance, a group of 10 people introducing themselves with three items of information, such as 'name, current job and favourite pastime' might take around 20 minutes. A discussion (or debate) around an ethical issue might take 45 minutes. It's better to overestimate than underestimate.
- Pre-session information: is there any ground work information you need to send out to the intended audience before the session starts?
- Post-session information: is it worthwhile developing some sort of handout to summarise the session? What about evaluation forms to give you some idea of how the session went and how you might improve on it the next time around?

Some educational theories to help support the External Stage

The educational theories below are presented as good guiding principles.

Honey and Mumford's Learning Styles[3]

Activists	*'Doers'*	**Activists** like to learn by being involved; like doing things first and learning from it afterwards.
Pragmatists		**Pragmatists** like things that seem practically useful and are usually happy to give things a go.
Theorists	*'Thinkers'*	**Theorists** like to know the theory and evidence before embarking on something.
Reflectors		**Reflectors** like plenty of time to consider what has taken place and their learning.

How does this model help you? Knowing that different learners have different learning styles encourages us (as facilitators) to think about using a balance of different learning activities. Matching the educational methods we're thinking of using to these four learning styles is more likely to cater (and thus 'hook') the majority of learners. This usually has a positive effect on the group dynamic and learning outcomes. *See* Chapter 11: Learning and Personality Styles in Practice if you want to read more.

Entwhistle's Surface and Deep learning model[4]

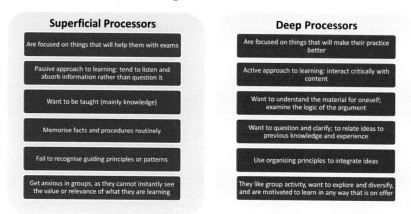

How does this model help you? For most GP training schemes, Half-Day Release intends to promote deep learning, yet at times it may be appropriate to approach something on the surface to meet a specific need.

Hermann's Left and Right Brain Inventory[5]

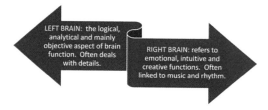

How does this model help you? This model reminds you to consider using learning methods that cater for both left and right brain descriptions within your objectives and methods.

Bloom's Taxonomy of Learning Objectives[6,7]

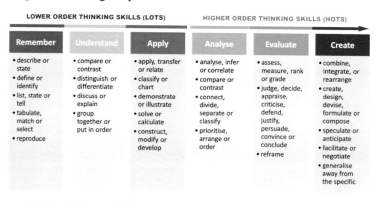

New Bloom's Taxonomy for the Cognitive Domain (after Anderson & Krathwohl, 2001)

New Bloom's Taxonomy: the cognitive domain (after Anderson and Krathwohl, 2001). The cognitive domain addresses knowledge structures.

Teaching Groups of People

How does this model help you? Bloom said that learning falls into one or more of three categories: learners either learn some new *knowledge*, a new *skill* and/or a new *attitude*. These three domains of learning are often referred to as the cognitive, psychomotor and affective domains. In each domain, there are different depths to which learning can take place. The diagram above is the taxonomy for the knowledge domain. A superficial learner will simply be able to recite something they have tried to *remember*. On the other hand, the deep learner will *analyse* that knowledge, *evaluate* it and use it to *create* new systems/processes/meaning. We hope you can see how this taxonomy encourages you to ask: '*At what level am I trying to pitch the intending outcomes?*' This particular diagram provides a list of action words (verbs) for the various depths of the knowledge domain. These verbs can help you formulate your learning objectives and outcomes. There's a similar taxonomy available for the skills (psychomotor) and attitudinal (affective) domains; you'll find them in Chapter 10: Five Pearls of Educational Theory.

Other theories in the previous chapter

Please read about these now before continuing. They're all in Chapter 12: How Groups Work – the dynamics.
1 Tuckman's stages of forming, storming, norming and performing.[8]
2 Freeman's ages of infancy, adolescence and adulthood.
3 Heron's 'seasons' of winter, spring, summer and autumn[9]
4 Heron's Six Intervention Categories.[10]

Step Three: The 'Just Doing It' Stage

We will split this stage into three equally essential elements in order to make it easier to understand and recall. Try to see the three elements as a set of bookends: the beginning and the end being the first and last bookend with the middle bit being represented by the books themselves. We've used this analogy intentionally – if you don't have good bookends, the books in the middle will fall.

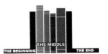

The Beginning (the first bookend)

How you start has a major effect on how the group functions later on. Here are some tips.
- **Make sure you arrive early** – with time to spare. That allows you to prepare the environment (like checking the seating arrangements), attend to any technical and catering requirements and get you mentally ready for the group work.
- **Greet people who are there before the session is due to start.** Be warm and friendly. Chat about anything. This will help build relationships, break down barriers, and hopefully result in them engaging without hesitation.
- **Arrange the seating in a circle** – so that there is no 'head' and that all participants can make eye contact with each other. We believe that the neater the circle, the more likely members will interact. Consider *seat-hopping*: periodically changing where you sit, especially if there are a number of planned breaks during the session. This encourages participants to sit next to someone new, which can help maintain dynamism about the group process.
- **Ensure the physical environment is adequate** – in terms of temperature, lighting, available space and air for group work.
- **Check that any materials required are there** – including a backup in case technology fails; for example, handouts in case projection fails.

- **Start proceedings in an upbeat and clear way** – you being positive and engaged will help set the tone and climate.
- **Consider a 'start-up' or game type activity** – rather than jumping straight into the main task. The purpose of this is twofold. First: to help people to get to know each other. Secondly: to get all participants to speak early in the session because it's then more likely they'll interact afterwards. A simple example is to start with a 'News Round' in which you ask participants to relay something about their lives and work that has happened since the group last met together. For a new group that has never met before, it will be a round of introductions. The way you do this is up to you. Clearly, the time you spend on the 'start-up activity' depends on how well established the group is; new groups that have not met before need more time: time building the group relationship is important if you want the group to function well. *See* our Web Chapter: 'Group Games' for more creative ideas.
- **Establish a 'learning contract' with the group early on** – this can consist of clarifying the aims and objectives, indicating what methods are planned, and clarifying what your role will be in the proceedings. It can also be an opportunity to say what is not on offer, and what will not happen, and what your role will not include.

Clarify your own role

Remind the group that you're there to manage the process rather than contribute to the content. Also let the group know that occasionally you might have to cut a discussion short if it is going off track: *'Sometimes, group discussions run off at a tangent, so I hope you'll agree to me bringing the group back to focus if that happens. Please don't be offended.'*

- **Group rules are best formulated at the first session**: get the group to come up with their own rules and map these out on a flip chart. If your group is to meet several times again, you might like to consider emailing the group rules out to them. You may also wish to revisit and review these later as the group norms.

Group rules

Group rules are important because they set boundaries for each member so that any behaviour or action(s) of certain individuals that is likely to affect the group dynamic adversely is kept in check. They also serve as a useful thing to refer back to when examining a dysfunctional group dynamic or an individual who is 'not playing by the rules'. In our experience, group dysfunction is more likely if you don't set group rules – even if the group is just meeting the once (e.g. at a conference). Make sure there is broad agreement on each rule and that one individual doesn't dominate the arena. Examples are provided below but it's important the group generates its own, in order to promote ownership.

Group rule:	Hopefully, the group will say something like:
Openness and honesty	*For everyone to get some meaningful learning, everyone needs to be open and honest.*
Confidentiality	*Anything of a personal nature that an individual reveals about themselves or a patient will not be disclosed to others outside the group. However, it is permissible to discuss non-sensitive learning material which may be beneficial for others to know (e.g. the actual learning outcomes).*
'Opt in or opt out'	*We realise some of us may have gone through some unpleasant experiences and that the material being discussed may evoke feelings that are still too raw. It is permissible for such an individual to 'opt out' of the session if he or she wishes.*
Respect and valuing all perspectives	*Each individual is entitled to have their own views. Although we are not here to destroy or devalue those views, it is permissible to challenge them in a constructive way.*
Owning your statements	*It is important that group members 'own' what they say rather than expressing it as a dogma. Therefore, members will try to use 'I' statements such as: 'I think that I would have done x, y and z' rather than 'One should have done x, y and z'.*
Constructive criticism and support	*All group members are here to support and learn from each other. Members must remember that constructive criticism is for the benefit of the recipient, not as a means for the giver to score points.*
Punctuality/time keeping	*Members who know they are going to be late should let someone know in the group in advance. We would also like to restart sessions promptly after tea breaks and so on so that we can finish on time.*
Preparation and commitment	*It's important for group members to share advance material and honour 'homework' commitments (i.e. doing the tasks we said we'd do). Otherwise, we will end up with a session that is less rich in content, less meaningful and less enjoyable.*
Mobile phones and bleeps	*We understand that people on occasions have to leave mobiles turned on for important calls. Please can members use the vibrating mode and let the group know in advance that they are expecting an important call. The individual concerned should then take the call outside the room.*
	Bleeps – can they be left with someone else?
Enjoyment	*If we can learn in an exciting, dynamic and fun way, we are more likely to engage positively with future sessions.*

And it is really useful to make this final group rule: *Responsibility for sticking to the group rules rests with all members of the group.* You should also agree how often the group rules should be revisited and revised if necessary.

A little more about the confidentiality clause

You will need the group to define, discuss and come to a consensus about the confidentiality clause so that everyone knows what is included, and has agreed to it. You will find that people have different understandings of confidentiality: does it mean *'Nothing said here can be repeated outside the group'*? Does it mean *information can be taken outside as long as it is totally anonymous*? For an educational setting, having absolute confidentiality may inhibit the 'extended' learning that might take place outside the group (through discussion and reflection with others from parallel groups). That's why you need to make sure that the definition is explicit and fully agreed if there is to be trust in the group.

Some rules about group rules

- Raise awareness of the need for group rules early on.
- Start introducing them sooner rather than later.
- Finalise them when the group moves on – at the performing stage.
- They may initially be proposed by you.
- They need to be agreed by the whole group.
- You need to revisit and revise them as the group goes along.
- You need to revisit them whenever a new member joins the group.
- Never leave them out.

The Middle (the book section)

This is the 'meaty' bit (apologies to the vegetarians). This is where you get going on the main task set out in your lesson plan and perform the art of facilitating. Facilitating is an art and here are some useful pointers.

General principles

- In general, be aware of your position in the group; try to keep one foot in the group and one on the outside observing and keeping some objectivity.
- Use a **multi-sensory** approach to learning activities: when setting tasks, try to use activities which engage the visual (e.g. flip chart, videos), auditory (e.g. discussions) and kinaesthetic (e.g. role play, practising) thinkers. This will also help you engage learners with different learning styles: activists and pragmatists tend to like role play while reflectors and theorists like to think, analyse and discuss.
- **Walk the talk**. If you're trying to instil certain attitudes, you must believe in them too (and your non-verbals will show you up if you don't!).

Ten points on the art of facilitating	
The basis of all facilitation is to 'look, listen and reflect'	
1 Act as facilitator, not as expert	Reflect things back to the group members as much as you can. Do *'spider webs'*: imagining lines of communication like strands in a spider's web being woven. Aim to reflect questions and comments away from yourself and across to as many other participants as possible and thereby weave the group's web. Get them to come up with ideas and solutions:
	• *'That's an interesting point. What do others think/feel about that?'*
	This is not to say that you can never give advice. Sometimes the group struggles and you'll 'know the answer' in which case impart your pearls of wisdom. The important thing is that you achieve a balance between facilitating and telling.
2 Encourage everyone to participate	It can take people a while before they pluck up the courage to talk. They may use an opening gambit like *'I'm not sure I'm going to put this very well . . .'* When it happens, appreciate their contribution to encourage them to relax and talk more:
	• *'Thanks for that Jaya. That's quite a helpful point.'*
	However, watch out for the 'dominant talkers' and the 'silent sitters'. Dominant talkers will need quietening down, and silent sitters will need gentle coaxing into the discussion.
	• To Dominant Dominic, you might say: *'That's an interesting point Dominic. Thanks for that. Shall we see what other people's views on that are?'*

Ten points on the art of facilitating	
The basis of all facilitation is to 'look, listen and reflect'	
2 Encourage everyone to participate (*cont.*)	• To Silent Sarah, you might say *'Thanks for that Dom. Let's see what other people make of that. Sarah, what do you think? Does that suggestion sit comfortably with you? Is there anything else you can suggest? . . . Mmm, that's sounds like a good alternative.'* Other ways to do this are discussed in our Web Chapter: Troubleshooting Small Groups.
3 Keep the focus	Those that go off at a tangent will need pulling back; that's part of your job. However, be careful of cutting people off too quickly – it can stop them from engaging again. • *'Can I just bring people back to what we originally set out to do? Can someone remind us? Would it be fair to say that the current discussion seems to be going off at a tangent from that? . . . Okay, let's get back to the task at hand . . .'* or • *'Do we seem to be getting bogged down with detail here? What do you think? How shall we move forwards?'*
4 Maintain a balance between task and process	This can be a difficult thing to do especially if the initial agenda needs changing. For instance, a group discussion might reveal an unanticipated learning need of greater priority than the one initially set at the beginning of the educational session. In such a case, you may need to change your plan completely – from the agenda (aims) to the content (task) and to the way you do it (the process). Be open about this and negotiate any change with the rest of the group.
5 CSS **Clarify**	If you're not sure you've understood what someone has said, it's likely others in the group also haven't. • *'Mmmm . . . I'm not sure I fully get your point Robert. Would you mind rephrasing it for me?'*
Signpost	When you notice a key learning point raised by someone in the group, signpost it to highlight it to others. • *'Before we move on, can I quickly highlight the importance of that last point that Hena has just made?'*
Summarise	Summarise themes as you go along. A verbal summary will engage the auditory learners while a flip chart will engage the visual ones. How about doing both? Summarising is important because it neatly 'packages' the learning points discussed up to that point before moving on. • *'Would someone like to summarise before we move on?'*
6 Be prepared to share *your* thoughts, *your* feelings and *your* needs with the group	If you're stuck in a dilemma, confused or simply not sure of how to proceed, share your thoughts and feelings and ask the group for their advice. Often, they'll point you in the right direction. Don't be embarrassed about this, and it does not mean your facilitation skills are inadequate. Remember, every person in the group (including you) is meant to be on an equal footing. How can you expect others to reveal their anxieties, weaknesses and difficulties if you're not prepared to share yours? • *'I think I'm a bit confused by that discussion. It seems like there's a few mixed messages, and I'm not sure what we're saying. Does anyone else feel the same way too? What shall we do to resolve it?'* Another example: Veering off towards a new but important learning area: • *'I've noticed that we've gone off track a little but, from what I sense, this discussion seems to be important and relevant to many of you. I'm wondering what we should do: do we stay on the original agenda or would you like to spend longer on this? If you decide you would, we might not have time for the other topics. However, for some of you, that might be okay. So, what would you like to do?'*

7 **Stay awake, be observant and mindful of the group's energy**	Continuously read and monitor your audience's energy levels. A few yawns, people becoming fidgety and others disengaging from the session means people need re-energising. Either it's time for a break, or you need to change tack – do things a different way.
	• *'Looks like some of you could do with a break. Is now a good time? How long shall we take to recharge ourselves?'*
	Most people will usually lose focus after an hour – so build in timely breaks.
8 **Watch for group dysfunction**	If a thorny issue comes up, respond in one of Heron's three modes: hierarchically (*'I see the group is avoiding the issue here'*), cooperatively (*'What do people think is happening at this point?'*) or leave it in autonomous mode for the group to address (or not). Take a break to allow emotions to settle down – most groups will then perform in a more productive way.
Watch for individual dysfunction	Some individuals will always want to fight for the group arena. They dampen the comments made by the person before them. You need to step in:
	• *'Thanks Dom for that. However, before we go onto that, can I go back to Sarah's point on xxx and see what people make of that?'*
Protect members	Discourage put-downs, remind people of group rules and **confront with love**.
	• *'Dom, before you carry on, can I just take a moment to remind you of the group rules: that we agreed every individual's viewpoint needs to be respected. I'd like to create space for both of you to contribute to things, so that we can work with each other.'*
9 **Maintain a positive educational climate**	If you ooze positivity and dynamism, it will rub off onto others. Add a bit of mild humour to 'lighten' the session and relax everyone. Value contributions. Show respect for people. Never denigrate even if someone comes up with something outrageous; instead, explore.
10 **Keep an eye on the time**	If you run late, the group's members will not thank you (many will lose focus anyway and become fidgety). So, if it's time to move on, move on. **You will need a watch**. If something 'meaty' comes up which would be inappropriate to cut short, seek permission from the group to continue.

 Another Top Tip: When you're talking to the group, try to make eye contact with all participants. *Be a lighthouse*: from time to time, sweep your gaze slowly across the group from side to side. Make eye contact with all participants slowly, in turn and in a relaxed yet definite way. This communicates your involvement, presence and commitment to involving all in the process. It is particularly useful if you happen to be the speaker at the time. It keeps everyone connected and awake.

The Ending (the last bookend)

This is the time to draw proceedings to a close in accordance with the initial contract you established with the group. It's also an opportunity to 'walk the talk' of reflective practice by reviewing the session in some form. Remember to stay with the agreed 'contracted finishing time'. Running overtime in the 'middle' section will diminish the time for 'The Ending'.

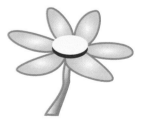

Make time in 'The Ending' for:
- **Summarising** the session in terms of the 'classic three steps'.
  1 Recalling what was anticipated at the outset.
  2 Briefly outlining what has actually taken place.

3 Summarising the final outcomes.

This needn't take more than a few minutes. And, of course, you don't need to do all of this yourself – get a group member or two.

- **Reflection** – ask the learners:
  'Was that session helpful?', 'In what way?', 'What bits had real meaning for you on a personal level?'
  Don't forget to put in your two pennies' worth.
- **Feedback** on how you ran the session. Think about some questions on your performance on which you'd like feedback (but you don't have to do this if you're not in a ready enough internal state to 'hear' the answers).
- **End on an upbeat note.** Leave everyone feeling good.

Facilitating the group through the Tuckman[8] stages?

If you've not read the previous chapter's introduction on Tuckman's group development stages, please do so now. Here are some ways in which you can move the group forwards towards Tuckman's performing stage – the stage where group members start working collaboratively *with* each other towards a *common* goal.

Facilitating the Forming Stage

The first stage – where groups come together. For groups to start working with each other, all the members need to get to know each other. Using all sorts of exercises at opportunistic points where they get to work in different pairs will help. When the group first comes together, use structured exercises, icebreakers or games, to speed up this *forming* stage.

EXAMPLE OF AN ICEBREAKER GAME

Each person writes a secret about themselves on a piece of paper. These are put into a receptacle, and each person takes one out. The group then mingles in the room, having to ask questions of each other to find out whose secret they are holding; they are not allowed to use the words on the paper to ask the questions. The exercise finishes with each person reading out their own secret.

Facilitating the Storming Stage

This is the stage where the group is struggling to find its identity and there is usually conflict between individuals or with the facilitator. Group members become difficult. The ***storming*** stage may be brief, or prolonged. It is important that you do not challenge the group, or become defensive. If you challenge you will prolong the storming phase; the discomfort you will produce can prevent the group from moving on. Try to accept what is being said, and even reflect on it in a non-judgemental way: *'It all feels a bit uncomfortable at the moment, I wonder if anyone else has noticed that too?'* Listen to what is being said and try to stay outwardly calm, even though this might be inwardly difficult. If you become defensive you will alienate the group, and produce 'sides'. If some of the member's project their 'storming' onto you, don't take it personally! You may want to take a break, and give yourself time to reflect on why this is happening.

Facilitating the Norming Stage

Here, the group establishes a common identity and purpose. You can help the ***norming*** stage by being open about setting the norms. What is acceptable to this group? If the group rules have already been discussed, this is the time to revisit, revise, and make sure that everyone has 'bought in' to them.

Facilitating the Performing Stage

In the performing stage, the group starts working in a productive way. In the ***performing*** stage, you will find that the group is running in a democratic way and is looking after its own dynamic. The group will, to a large extent, be in cooperative or autonomous mode and will be making decisions for themselves. Tailor your facilitation mode to where the group is at. For instance, as a group moves towards a cooperative mode, enhance it by asking for thoughts and opinions. Encourage them to problem-solve and take decisions. Heron's Six Categories of Intervention[10] may be useful here (if you're unfamiliar with Heron, *see* Chapter 12: How Groups Work – the dynamics). The interventions of being Confronting, Catalytic, Cathartic and Supportive may be particularly helpful and examples are given below of what you might say.

Heron's Modes of Facilitation – *examples of what you might say*

Confronting – challenging.
'Do you really think it would be worthwhile talking about that? Why? How will it help you?

Cathartic – expressing emotions. Unexpressed emotion can block development and creativity.
'I sense that some of you are quite reluctant to approach it in this way. Would I be right in feeling that? Help me to understand what's going on for you.'

Catalytic – exploring. 'Drawing out' and eliciting self-discovery/problem-solving.
'Okay, I can see your difficulty. Have you been in this sort of situation before? Can you remember a time when it went okay? Tell me more . . . what happened there?'

Supportive – validating. Affirming worth and value of the other person: their qualities, attitudes and actions.
'It sounds like you handled that in quite a mature and professional way. I can see it couldn't have been easy.'

 Red Alert: Even if a group is performing well, it can slip back into one of the other Tuckman stages at any moment. Look out for this and discuss it with the group if it happens.

When it's time for groups to say goodbye (Adjourning)

When good friends part, farewells are usually expressed. Similarly, it's important to acknowledge the end of a group's life cycle (particularly if they have been together for a while). Some members of the group may have something they want to say to the rest of the group, or to an individual, before the group disbands. You will probably have a few things to say yourself. If you're a little apprehensive about the closure, try an exercise to provide a little structure to the ritual of ending (see below). Whatever you do, provide a little time for closure so that people can move on. It can be as simple as a group hug or a group cheer. Hip Hip Hooray!

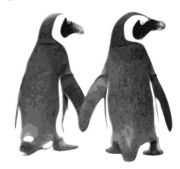

EXAMPLE OF AN ENDING GAME
I'd been facilitating the same small group of eight people for the last six months at Half-Day Release. A mixture of ST1s, 2s and 3s. It was our last session ever, and some would not be seeing each other again.

One of the TPDs gave me a closing game to try. I couldn't see what the big deal was and to be honest was a bit laissez-faire about it all. However, as the session drew to a close, I could sense emotions and see how important some form of closure was (just like you would ordinarily do with good friends). I retrieved the instruction sheet (which was now a scrawl of paper in my back pocket) which said:

- Give everyone a sheet of A4.
- Ask them to fold and tear the sheet into eight (roughly equal) strips.
- Write the name of one group member on each strip of paper (including the facilitator).
- On the other side, write one thing you value that the person has brought to the group over the last six months. Start the sentence with 'I want to thank you for . . .'
- Remember, the group facilitator is also a group member and will need to do this too.
- At the end, each member folds their strips and places each one under the corresponding chair of the person to whom it is addressed.
- Members can read their strips at the end of the session or in their own time elsewhere. There is no need to share this with the group.

Wow! This was powerful and perfect – people left on a high. I was amazed at some of the things they valued about me. Thing's I didn't even realise I was doing!

A sample of resources on our website
- Group Rules.
- Educational Theories which inform small group learning.
- The Facilitator's Emotional Intelligence.

Other chapters you may like to read
- Chapter 12: How Groups Work – the dynamics
- Chapter 10: Five Pearls of Educational Theory: especially Johari's Window
- Web Chapter: Troubleshooting Small Groups
- Web Chapter: Group Games.

Please give us some feedback on this chapter to help shape it for the next edition.
Go to www.essentialgptrainingbook.com and simply click on the title of this chapter.

References

1 Rogers C. *Client-centred Therapy: its current practice, implications and theory*. London: Constable; 1951.
2 Goleman D. *Working with Emotional Intelligence*. New York: Bantam Books; 1998.
3 Honey P, Mumford A. *The Manual of Learning Styles*. Maidenhead, UK: Peter Honey Publications; 1982.
4 Entwistle NJ, Ramsden P. *Understanding Student Learning*. London: Croom Helm; 1983.
5 Herrmann N. *The Creative Brain*. Lake Lure, North Carolina: Brain Books; 1990.
6 Bloom BS. *Taxonomy of Educational Objectives*. Boston: Allyn and Bacon; 1956.
7 Anderson LW, Krathwohl DR. *A Taxonomy for Learning, Teaching, and Assessing: a revision of Bloom's Taxonomy of Educational Objectives*. Harlow: Addison Wesley Longman, Inc.; 2001.
8 Tuckman BW. Developmental sequence in small groups. *Psychol Bull*. 1965; **63**: 384–99. The article was reprinted in *Group Facilitation: a research and applications journal*. 2001; **3**, and is available as a Word document at: http://dennislearningcenter.osu.edu/references/GROUP%20DEV%20ARTICLE.doc.
9 Heron J. *The Complete Facilitators Handbook*. London: Kogan Page; 1999.
10 Heron J. *Six Category Intervention Analysis*. 3rd ed. Surrey: Human Potential Resource Group, University of Surrey; 1989.

How to Teach Large Groups

JOHN LORD – Professor of Primary Medical Care (Univ. Huddersfield) & lead author
IAIN LAMB – Associate Advisor (SE Scotland) & lead author **RAMESH MEHAY** – TPD (Bradford)

What's so hard about teaching big groups?

Large groups are much harder to manage than small ones. Small groups, with up to 10 members, permit facilitation. This engages enough minds to create a whole that is larger than the sum of its parts, but not too many to affect the group dynamics. Chapter 12: How Groups Work – the dynamics and Chapter 13: Teaching and Facilitating Small Groups explore the group dynamics and facilitation of this size of a group. Much of what is explored in those chapters remains relevant to teaching large groups. However, the larger the group:

- the more impersonal it becomes – eye contact becomes more difficult
- the easier it is for individuals to hide or fall asleep
- the more the facilitator or presenter feels anxious
- the more difficult it is to get a response from the audience or group.

You've got to get some sort of interaction going. However, the problem is that members of the audience are often too inhibited by the fear of looking silly in public. If there is no interaction, you have sunk to the level of a lecture presentation, with its limited chance to influence or produce behaviour change. Engaging people in a fluid and responsive dialogue is important because it is likely to alter some of their thoughts and feelings, which in turn is more likely to change behaviour. Excellent facilitation skills can encourage a degree of interactive effective group work in a group size up to about 16. For groups larger than that, you need exceptionally high skills in presenting, teaching and facilitating. The extra challenge is to bring into the teaching of large groups, or lectures, some of the elements we treasure from small-group work. To meet the challenge, think opportunity rather than difficulty.

Set, Dialogue and Closure

With the potential for making a fool of yourself in front of a large number of people, attention to the basics really matters. Peyton *et al.*[1] provide a neat and memorable description of the three elements that you must cover in a successful presentation.

- **The Set:** what you need to think about beforehand
- **The Dialogue:** what happens during the event
- **The Closure:** how you finish off.

We are going to cover these as concisely as we can. That's not to say they're not important – it's just that we want to get onto the juicier stuff of engaging and playing with a large audience. We're pretty sure that you're thirsty for that too!

The Set
This is the preparation you need to do before the presentation. Acronym: **PALES:**[2]

PALES	
Purpose	• What does the group need from you? Consider doing a needs assessment. Don't forget to get set to provide learning for participants with different styles, interest and intent. • What do you want from the audience/group? Be explicit about what will be expected from the group.
Audience	• How much do you know about them? Are they a group with similar needs (e.g. doctors on a hot topics course wanting facts, guidance and handouts) or a diverse group (e.g. different professional groups with different levels of knowledge and needs)? • How much knowledge do they have? Is it possible to perform a short knowledge quiz at the start to help define main areas to focus on? (Doing the same quiz at the end is also a way of evaluating learning).
Logistics	• Timings • Room size vs audience size. • Room acoustics and so on . . .
Equipment	• Data projector, screen, laptop, flip chart and so on. • Workbooks and other provocation material (e.g. case studies, clinical guidelines or other items useful for provoking discussion). • Backup materials, feedback sheets.
Set-up	• Arrive early to check the room and equipment (electronics have a habit of playing up at the last minute). • Chair arrangement • Your presentation materials • Who is available to troubleshoot if there are problems?

The Dialogue
This is the content of what you want to happen and how you will do it.

> **Start on time**
> Although, with a large group, there are more chances of latecomers – so plan to make it easy for them to come in without causing disruption.
>
> **Introduce yourself**
> Be enthusiastic and passionate about this – yes, you do have to sell yourself by validating why you have the authority to speak. After all, would you want to listen to someone giving a talk on say 'Making Money on the Net' who's never touched a computer and was a pauper himself? Okay, perhaps if he said 'eBay was my idea!' you might just sit up in your chair a bit more. And remember that throughout you're acting as a role model as well as a teacher.
>
> **Explain your purpose and the context – 'hook' them**
> Outline what you hope to achieve – share your aims and objectives with the audience so that they can see 'what's in it for them'. You need to whet their appetite. You need to make them feel 'Yeah. I'm glad I'm here. I want some of that.' Not just 'Mmm, sounds interesting, let's see.' And there are a variety of ways you might 'hook' them.
> • Make sure your aims and objectives marry with what they want, and then deliver it with passion and style.

- Start with an interest-grabbing item, statement or picture.
- Keep the session active and dynamic – involve the audience, for instance, and reveal your personality.
- And . . . don't forget to re-hook the audience if you identify flagging interest.
- *See* Chapter 4: Powerful Hooks – aims, objectives and ILOs for more ideas.

Project your voice

To project your voice to a larger group, you usually need to stand, or at least sit in the BBC position – Bottom in the Back of the Chair.[3] This permits a comfortable stance in which you can breathe in fully with the diaphragm and let your abdominal muscles relax. You can then concentrate on the contraction of your abdominal muscles to produce volume when you speak. There's more about projecting your voice on our website. Remember to pause between statements to let key points sink in (it also gives you time to compose your next sentence). This pause needs to be longer, the larger the audience.[3]

Get the audience involved

Participants who speak early end up being comfortable with engaging in dialogue later on. It's the 'silent sitters' that you need to *gently* get going. The longer a person sits without saying anything, the less likely they are to do so later. It is worth making a special effort to get each of the participants to do something and to say something early on. However, participation requires more than just talking. Cognition needs encouragement too: e.g. *'Can you remember the last time you had to manage a patient with X . . . consider what went well, and what went badly. Talk to the person next to you about it for the next 3 minutes and then swap around.'*

The Closure

This is what you will do at the end – closing the session.
- Plenary statements; summarise what the group has achieved.
- List the unanswered questions/unresolved issues.
- End with a bang – people remember what they hear last. Often, this will be a summary or take-home message.
- Identify what level of evaluation you want. Is it just end-of-day forms to help with ongoing course development? Or do you want to know what gets taken into the future performance of participants?

 Top Tip: Summaries are essential for large-group learning. Summarising is a skill in itself. Take some time out now to see if you can summarise what you have learnt so far.

Playing with large groups – ideas for effective working

Before we give you some ideas on how you can add life and dynamism to your large-group session, it is important that you remember the following general rules of thumb.

1 Divide your event into several short components.
2 Ensure that these short components, together, provide a balance of different educational activities.
3 Incorporate as many *memorable* endings and beginnings into each of these components.
4 Inject some of *your* personality into *your* session (everyone has one!).

AN EXAMPLE OF DIVIDING A SESSION INTO CHUNKS, ADDING A BALANCE OF DIFFERENT EDUCATIONAL ACTIVITIES AND MAKING THINGS MEMORABLE

Because of reduced resources, a communications skills course that was usually run by four facilitators now had to be run by one facilitator for 32 GP trainees. The challenge was to keep it as interactive and interesting as before. The first module was to cover consultation models.

- Everyone spent 10 minutes writing down their ideas of what makes a good consultation. These were written on Post-its, which were stuck on the wall.
- The large group then needed to collaborate and arrange them into patterns and clusters that made sense.
- After this they were asked to line up against the wall in order of their date and month of birth (not year) and to do so without speaking or writing.
- They were then split into four groups of spring, summer, autumn and winter.
- Each group was asked to come up with their group's own consultation model.
- The four groups then had to negotiate a final model.

We went on to compare and contrast this with some of the standard formative models, including the requirements of the COT and CSA. Actually, the final model wasn't that dissimilar to the COT schedule – the group could see how it had been derived and how it 'made sense'.

Okay, let's move on to the different ways in which you can inject life into your large group session.

1 Divide and conquer

Subgroups: The simplest way of overcoming the problems of large groups is to divide them into small ones. It's best to divide them randomly so that participants get to 'know each other'. You can do this by

- Allocating participants to numbered subgroups. Go around the group giving each one a number 1,2,3,4, 1,2,3,4, 1,2,3,4 – then grouping together the 1s, the 2s and so on.
- Asking each participant to select a coloured strip of paper. The coloured strips would then sort people into Greens, Yellows, etc.
- Giving each participant a playing card. The playing cards have the advantage of allowing you to create groups by suit or by rank. For example, you can run the first activity in subgroups of hearts, diamonds, etc., and second activity by kings, jacks, etc.

 Top Tip: Each subgroup doesn't have to do the same task. You can allocate different tasks to different groups and later bring the whole thing together.

Subgroups can be asked to report to a combined large group plenary, or to share information in other ways. A member of the subgroup can be sent to visit other subgroups as an ambassador. The ambassador can be selected because they are the scribe, by a vote or by some arbitrary factor like height. The ambassador then explains to their new subgroup the achievements of their original group. As an alternative two small groups could be asked to combine to share information (snowballing). Clearly, for any of this to work, one must provide small groups with clear tasks and be explicit about the time allowance before they break up.

 Top Tip: If you want to go one step further, get the groups to self-select a group name – having a group name encourages group cohesion and adds dynamism through a bit of healthy team rivalry.

AN EXAMPLE

A group of 20 Trainers filled in Belbin team styles before a course. A Likert scale was laid out on the floor, and Trainers used this to move about as they went through the various team styles. After exploring differences, strengths and weaknesses, they were asked to form smaller groups that would provide a range of styles for when the group broke up for more interactive work. As an additional insight some of the Trainers worked together and found it useful to understand why there were some things they enjoyed doing together more than others.

Pairs/trios: Division into pairs or trios makes fairly sure that everyone takes part. If the group has never formed before, you can get the pair (or trio) to introduce each other to the rest of the group (it is easier for shy people to present their colleague than themselves). Groups of up to about 30 can work in pairs/trios and present back to the main group; above 30 it becomes too time-consuming for *regular* use. Trios work particularly well where there is a different function for each of the three members; for example, simulated patient, doctor and observer.

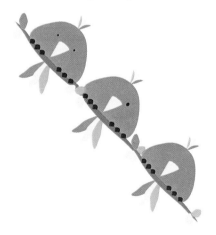

Working solo: Sometimes it helps to give participants a bit of personal space to enable them to internalise their learning. Give them 5–10 minutes where they can individually reflect. You could get them to write down some thoughts on Post-it notes. These Post-it notes can then be put on a wall for others to peruse. You can also cluster some of them together into thoughts, ideas and themes.

Top Tip: Issue each participant with a set of sticky red dots. They can then browse through other people's Post-it notes on a wall and place a red dot of approval on any ideas they particularly admire or with which they strongly agree.

2 Games

Games work well in small or large groups, but often it is harder to select a 'volunteer' from a large group. Some large-group facilitators implant a hypnotic suggestion, like *the person who is about to volunteer knows who they are*. However, there are other creative ways of getting people involved. For example, you could bring in some juggling balls. Anyone catching the ball has just volunteered. The best bit is that after performing their function, they can throw the ball at someone else, who will then have volunteered for the next bit! Alternatively, think about some sort of competition or game between subgroups or teams. Please take a peek at our Web Chapter: Group Games for more creative ideas. Alternatively, there are a number of books available – try typing something like 'group training games' into Amazon just to kick off with.

3 Quizzes

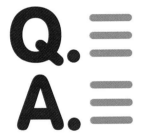 These work particularly well with larger groups and most large groups love them. One of the best 'audience response' kits around is QWIZDOM,[4] though there are others, e.g. 'Turning-Point'.[5] You convert your PowerPoint presentation to QWIZDOM format, and you give the group members a 'Who Wants to be a Millionaire' type of handset. Each slide gives a new question, and you can see on screen how many participants have selected an answer. Then the facilitator can show what proportion (but not who) has voted for each answer. Check with the venue where you are presenting. Do they have such equipment available? More and more local postgraduate centres do.

Some of you may feel at this point that you can't be bothered with all this fancy new techno wizardry. We personally believe that you should be more open and more willing to play. After all, if you've agreed to do any sort of presentation, then you've also agreed to putting the effort into it. Just like a Maitre d' ensures the service in his feeding house is of top form, you need to do the same with *your* service to *your* audience (who, don't forget, have taken time out, and most likely paid some sort of fee, to come and see you).

 Red Alert: Dear technophobe, you have to come out of your comfort zone and just play with some of this stuff; it's designed to be simple.

4 Using videos/DVDs

Videos are powerful training tools because they show you how something is done rather than just talking about it. And they're multisensory by nature – touching on our visual and auditory senses but having a significant impact on our feelings (as many cinematic films do). Videos can be paused for thought or rewound back to highlight particular points. For instance, videos have been successfully used up and down the country with Trainers to help calibrate their assessment skills for the COT – and often in quite large groups too.

5 Brainstorming

With a large group, a plea for suggestions can be met with silence often because the level of self-consciousness increases the larger the group. Here are some tips for 'waking up the dead'.

- First state the obvious to relax them all: *'Can I remind people that all suggestions are welcome. Can I also ask you to refrain from judging or discussing them until all suggestions have been received? We need to get them down on paper first. Is that okay?'*
- Divide them into pairs or trios and give them, say 5 minutes, to discuss and come up with a list of suggestions. Then, just ask them to shout things out – it's surprising how well this seems to get over the problem.
- Alternatively, divide them into subgroups and give them a bit more time.
- Finally, if one part of the audience seems to be more vocal than another, walk towards the silent side and ask: *'So, what do people from this area think?'*

Collating the information from brainstorming (or at the plenary) can be difficult if the main group is too large for everyone to see the flip chart or whiteboard. Here are some suggestions.

- Don't write too much on the flip chart or whiteboard, but what you do write, write in large letters.
- Use a laptop, data projector and mind-mapping (or spreadsheet) software to collate the data. You need to be a pretty good typist to be able to do this, but the good thing is that you can save the results. If there are two of you, one can facilitate while the other types.
- Get people to jot things down on Post-it notes and then stick them on a wall for the group to peruse at their leisure.

6 Problem-solving

Presenting cases to large groups for them to problem solve generally works very well. Participants could even be allowed to bring along their own cases for discussion. But for problem-solving cases to work, you must give the audience time to digest the material and time to think about their approach. You could get them to work initially alone and to form pairs or subgroups later in order to contrast and compare.

> **EXAMPLE**
> Participants were asked to think about a given case using an ethical framework. Once they formulated some individual ideas, they were then asked to pair up and start exploring solutions. Following this, the ethical conundrum was opened up to the large-group – there were clearly two markedly opposing views. Members of the audience were invited to form two small self-selected debating groups which 'fought it out' (in a friendly way), and the large group asked to vote at the end.

7 Using the humanities

There are many ways the humanities can be used to stimulate large-group interest and discussion.

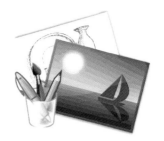

- Film or TV clips can be used to cover a huge range of topics, and these are increasingly accessible through DVD or YouTube. You might want to show a scene and break the group up into sub-groups that are asked to look at the clip from alternative points of view – for example, through the eyes of different characters. For such clips to be educationally useful, you need to set some specific questions or discussions about them beforehand.

EXAMPLE:

One of our communication skills sessions was about initial greetings and building rapport. We played a short clip of Sir Lancelot Spratt ('The Doctor' Movie Collection) on a ward round which led to an interesting discussion on the bedside manner! We then went onto play another video clip but in silent mode to focus on non-verbal communication. Asking for comments on what the audience thought went on was most fun.

- Pictures like this one can be used to discuss perception (do you see the young woman or the old woman?). By the way, look on our website for a PowerPoint on some other wonderful illusions (it's called Double Vision).
- A painting can also be projected through PowerPoint. This could be used in the traditional way to provide an interpretation of a medical or social scene.

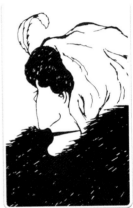

However, if you find all this arty stuff a bit woolly, don't blankly discard it from your repertoire of educational methods. Read this:

The aim of the training session was to help build our skills at giving feedback. It's interesting what the facilitator did. She presented a painting from an amateur artist and asked us to observe carefully the painting and then write down some points that would help the artist develop. It was interesting to see how different people framed feedback on the same perspective differently. The artist was more accepting of some responses than others. We then went on to explore what is was about those more accepting ones that made them that way. Overall, a very interesting and fun way of learning about feedback. It certainly made me question the way I do it presently.

- Short poems or pieces of prose can be read out to touch people on an emotional level. You could get members of a large group to write three-liner poems on Post-it notes to stick on the wall for people to read later. Again, we cannot stress how you don't need to be 'arty' or brilliant at 'English' to use this stuff. And you don't need to link poems to the main educational content either. For example, how about using it for evaluation:

Using the same evaluation form repeatedly gets a bit boring. I'm sure the punters don't particularly care for it either. So, for my session, I wanted something that would encourage the audience to think rather than scribbling a scrawl in a desperate move to get home. And this is what I did . . .

I asked them to evaluate my session by writing a three-line poem in the following format.
- I see . . .
- I hear . . .
- I feel . . .

Some of the most useful feedback I've ever received!

The poem on the right has been used successfully with a large group of trainees as a way of exploring what names we should use with patients.

Names
She was Eliza for a few weeks
When she was a baby –
Eliza Lily. Soon it changed to Lil.

Later she was Miss Steward in the baker's shop
And then 'my love', 'my darling', Mother.

Widowed at thirty, she went back to work
As Mrs Hand. Her daughter grew up,
Married and gave birth.

Now she was Nanna. 'Everybody
Calls me Nanna' she would say to visitors.
And so they did – friends, tradesmen, the doctor.

In the geriatric ward
They used the patients' Christian names.
'Lil' we said, or 'Nanna',
But it wasn't in her file
And for those last bewildered weeks
She was Eliza once again.

Wendy Cope
NAMES comes from Wendy Cope's collection
Two Cures For Love published by Faber.

For more depth, *see* Chapter 17: Using the Creative Arts.

8 De Bono's Six Thinking Hats

Sometimes large group discussions can be sabotaged by more opinionated members who:
1 skew the discussion in a certain way
2 stop a balanced discussion from happening
3 can be quite destructive in nature
4 stop others from engaging.

One way to tackle this is to use De Bono's six thinking hats.[6] It's already covered in detail in Chapter 5: A Smorgasbord of Educational Methods, and there are additional resources on our website.

9 Lectures

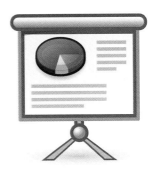

Sometimes the sheer size of a very large group, the requirements of the organiser, the arrangement of the furniture, lack of breakout rooms, or other features of the venue may force you to adopt a lecture format. All is not lost: there are still some advantages to lectures in presenting new information to a large number of people.[7,8] The important thing is to break the presentation up into small chunks, with interludes in which the audience has activity. Possible interludes might be:

- Working in pairs to discuss something. Beware: collating the results becomes very time consuming with audiences over 100. In such circumstances, the interaction of hearing replies from the pairs may sometimes have to be foregone.
- A self-marked quiz.
- Physical props.
- Demonstrations (with audience assistance).

 Top Tip: Have you ever seen the 'Christmas Lectures at the Royal Institution'? If not, record the next set (at Christmas time, of course!). They are exceptional at demonstrating how to deliver a lecture in the most engaging of ways. There are short sections of presentation, physical props and interludes of demonstration or experiment where participants come out of the audience to assist.

And then there are the Edinburgh fringe stand-up comedians who really know how to milk the audience: *'Anyone here from . . .', 'Hands up all the GPs', 'Stand up all the nurses', 'What do you do?'*

 Top Tip: There's a whole host of different methods detailed in Chapter 5: A Smorgasbord of Educational Methods.

FAQs – frequently asked questions

Using a co-facilitator

If you're lucky enough to have a co-facilitator or co-presenter, divide the management of group activities between you both. This also breaks the event into manageable chunks; a technique used elegantly on television by newsreaders and *The Two Ronnies*. The dummy of the pair can monitor the group and chip in, e.g. *'I don't think everyone understood that – could you rephrase that?'*

Hecklers

Very large groups and particularly large lectures seem to be more prone to hecklers – those people who ask awkward questions either to make themselves look good or just to try to trip you up.

- Rule one – don't be scared of them. Hecklers are as frightened as you are.
- Rule two – don't bite back; that just adds fuel to the fire. Remain calm, collected and be nice. Eat humble pie if you need to. The audience are more likely to side with the nice person than the aggressive one and may even come to your rescue.
- Rule three – be honest. If you don't know, say so rather than fudging something. If you fudge, the heckler will pick up on that and ruin your life even more.
- Rule four – think about *gently* challenging the heckler back. Heckler: *'So how do we know that it is effective? Where's your evidence that it works?'*; You: *'Yes, you've brought up a good point. The evidence is a bit scanty but in the light of limited options would you agree it's worth a shot?'*

Conclusion

Ultimately, you have to run large groups in the way that suits you and your personality. If you can tell good jokes fine – but if you can't don't. If you like games use them but only at the right times. All three of us (the authors) are happy to show our own failures to put people at ease.

The final pearl of wisdom we'd like to give you is to relax! Nothing is likely to be as bad as it was for Iain to be the first medical student in Edinburgh to have a case history videoed. His video was shown to 230 people, while he sat in the front row between two eminent professors. Feedback was dramatic and instant: the whole row of chairs started to shake and vibrate to the sound of laughter. Oh Pendleton – where were you when you were really needed?

A sample of resources on our website

- De Bono's Hats.
- Heron's Facilitator Modes and Dimensions (as applied to large groups).
- A PowerPoint called 'Double Vision'.

Other chapters you may like to read

- Chapter 4: Powerful Hooks – aims, objectives and ILOs
- Chapter 6: Teaching from Scratch
- Chapter 5: A Smorgasbord of Educational Methods
- Chapter 12: How Groups Work – the dynamics
- Chapter 13: Teaching and Facilitating Small Groups
- Chapter 16: Presentation Magic.

Please give us some feedback on this chapter to help shape it for the next edition.
Go to www.essentialgptrainingbook.com and simply click on the title of this chapter.

References

1 Peyton J, editor *Teaching and Learning in Medical Practice*. Rickmansworth, UK: Manticore Europe; 1998. pp. 193–207.

2 Clark D. *A Trainer's Toolbox of Templates*. Available at: www.nwlink.com/~Donclark/hrd/templates/templates.html

3 Houseman B. *Finding Your Voice: a complete voice training manual for actors*. London: Nick Hern Books; 2002.

4 www.qwizdom.co.uk

5 www.turningtechnologies.com

6 De Bono E. *Six Thinking Hats*. 2nd ed. London: Penguin Books; 2000.

7 Bligh DA. *What's the Use of Lectures?* 2nd ed. Exeter: Intellect Books; 2002.

8 Bligh DA. *What's the Point in Discussion?* Exeter: Intellect Books; 2000.

PART FIVE

Taking Centre Stage

15

How to Run a Course

ALLYSON HORNER – Scheme Manager (Durham & Tees Valley) & lead author
RAMESH MEHAY – TPD (Bradford)

So, you've got a course or conference to organise; here's how to make it relatively painless and fun! In this chapter, the focus is on the organisational aspect of putting a course together rather than on defining the aims, objectives, the content and the methodology. For the latter, you should read: Chapter 4: Powerful Hooks – aims, objectives and ILOs, Chapter 5: A Smorgasbord of Educational Methods and Chapter 6: Teaching from Scratch.

Why should you listen to us?

Because we've organised many courses to date, and what we've written about is based on our experience and the common themes that emerge time and time again; you're in good hands. And we're going to tell you some secrets, some tips and some things other books wouldn't dare to tell you.

Here's a checklist of what you need to do

Here's an overview of what sorts of things you need to pay close attention to. We know it looks a bit boring or laborious but by breaking this up and looking at the various chunks in turn, we hope you will feel less anxious, find it more manageable and a bit more exciting.

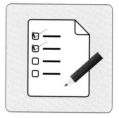

Checklist for planning an event/course	
• Budget	• Group leaders/facilitators
• Size of the event	• Group lists
• Know your audience/participants	• Equipment
• Venue	• Advertising
• Location	• Registration
• Dates	• Evaluation

The budget – how much money have you got?

Do you want to end up in County Court through bad debts? We're sure you don't: so start off by checking and double-checking the budget for your event. To work out how this compares with what you'll actually need, use the template below. It's available from our website as a more useable electronic Excel form for download. Excel will tot up the maths for you.

Costing sheet for organising an event/course		
(a) How many people do you expect to attend?		
(b) What's the venue's delegate fee?[1]	£	
• Multiply (a) by (b)		£
(c) How many people require overnight accommodation?[2]	£	
(d) How many days is overnight accommodation required?[2]	£	

Costing sheet for organising an event/course		
(e) What's the accommodation rate?[2]	£	
• Multiply (c) by (d) and by (e)		£
(f) How many people require a special menu?[3]		
(g) What's the rate of a special menu?[3]	£	
• Multiply (f) by (g)		£
(h) What's the total cost of all rooms required for all the days?[4]		£
(i) What's the total cost for the hire of additional equipment?[5]		£
(j) What are the photocopying and printing costs involved?[6]		£
(k) Costs of folders, pens, name badges and any other incidentals		£
(l) Do you have an estimate of the advertising costs?[7]		£
(m) What's the total cost of the fees and expenses for the facilitators?[8]		£
(n) Guest/celebrity after-dinner speaker's fee[9]		£
(o) Your fee for organising the event. If there is more than one of you, enter the total amount.[10]		£
(p) What's the total cost for others involved in organising the event?[11]		£
(q) What's the cost of any 'thank you' gifts?[12]		£
TOTAL COST:		£

Notes:

1 The delegate fee is the venue fee per person attending for things like refreshments and lunch. There are usually two rates.
   - Day delegate – coffee, lunch, tea and one main room hire included.
   - 24-hour delegate – usually, coffee, lunch, tea, dinner, overnight, breakfast and one main room hire. This can (if required) start at different times of the day, i.e. dinner, overnight, breakfast, coffee, lunch, tea depending on your needs and timing of your event.
2 Accommodation fees only apply if your course is residential. If so, use the 24-hour delegate rate.
3 Special menus are for people who have allergies or particular religious requirements. You must make sure you ask about this in your booking form. It's usually provided at no extra charge by the venue but some will include the additional cost of a specially selected conference dinner.
4 This relates to the room required for delivering the presentation and any break-out rooms.
5 Hire equipment such as a data projector: it's better (and cheaper) to bring your own if it's not free! Even so, check with the venue first as they may charge you anyway, or not allow non-PAT tested equipment to be used on their premises.
6 Such as any handbooks that accompany the course.
7 For some courses an email flyer will do but for others, to capture a wider audience, consider using a variety of advertising methods such as ads in mainstream journals and/or A4/5 flyers.
8 This includes travel expenses. Some will require overnight accommodation too (or accommodation the night before).
9 Celebrity after-dinner speakers can charge a hefty amount. It's better to use someone who fits in with the theme of your event: like your local Postgraduate Dean.
10 This is your fee for organising the event and the fees of any other co-organisers.
11 This includes others who you've cajoled into helping you out: maybe the VTS administrator, your Practice Manager and so on.
12 Sometimes it's important to acknowledge the value and hard work put in by organisers, speakers and guests. That's what thank you gifts are for – things like flowers, a bottle of wine, and so on.

How to select your venue

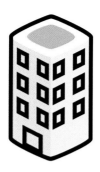

This depends on your budget; it's no use having dreams of using The Carlyle in New York, or The Dorchester in London, if your budget is limited. Anyway, do you want to suffer the same fate as our Members of Parliament in 2009 and have your expenses plastered all over the media?

Do bear in mind that hotels often offer special rates for 'local government' organisations (yes, the NHS is classed as government so you can get excellent deals). Hotels like accommodating government bodies because they settle their bills and come back in the future. Therefore, they're more likely to offer special deals – so ask! If at first approach there aren't any special deals, be un-British and haggle: don't be afraid to ask for reductions. Most venues expect this anyway, especially the larger hotels. If you don't ask, you don't get.

As a guide the following are average costs (2011) for a 3- or 4-star hotel:
- £150 for 24 hours includes bed and breakfast, mid-morning coffee, sideboard lunch, afternoon tea, three-course dinner – and the hire of one meeting room.
- £45 – day delegate rate includes tea/coffee and pastries on arrival, tea/coffee mid-morning, two-course sideboard lunch and afternoon tea, plus hire of one meeting room.

I have recently negotiated this type of deal to £25 per person – see what I mean?

AH

Other things to do

Book as early as you can – you might find your rate is protected even if the event is into the next financial year. And bear in mind that weddings are now held almost every day of the week, not just weekends, so you need to plan ahead. Even local Postgraduate Centres can get booked up for months or years in advance, so be quick!

- **Ask for sample menus:** especially check special dietary options; there is nothing worse than a vegetarian delegate being offered the same meal, three days running! And also enquire about food provisions for those with particular religious beliefs: at a recent event, all the sandwiches (vegetarian, ham and other sandwiches) were mixed together. You can understand the upset caused to some of our vegetarian and Muslim attendees (it's totally unacceptable). If your event is a one-day affair and the menu seems expensive, ask about outside catering. Hotels might not agree, but your local town hall is likely to be more relaxed about it.
- **Ask for the wine list:** check the cost of pre-conference dinner aperitifs. You might be better off asking for a fruit punch rather than sherry. A word of caution: alcohol *with* meals must be paid for by delegates; government bodies (especially healthy ones!) cannot be seen to be promoting alcohol consumption.
- Any hotel worth its salt will (if you ask), provide contacts of **previous customers** with similar events. Give them a bell and ask about their experience and recommendation.

Caveat emptor: buyers beware

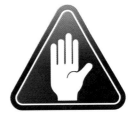

- **Negotiate:** hotels are in business to make money, and they're experts at adding in hidden costs. *I once had a fairly heated discussion with a hotel general manager who tried to convince us that it was reasonable to charge £63 for one flip chart in each group room. Six groups meant £378 for flip charts! When it was pointed out his hotel stood to make over £25 000 for the event, we were provided with free flip charts.*

- The larger hotel groups, such as Marriott, De Vere and so on, tend to require **credit agreements** for hire of their facilities. This can be fine if you are settling your account through the SHA, i.e. one large organisation to another, but if you are organising an independent conference such as the APCE annual event, you may be asked to apply for a credit agreement. I have successfully persuaded hotels to charge a larger deposit and then allow settlement of the final account on departure, thus avoiding the need to provide credit references, banker's references, etc.

- **Don't overestimate the numbers attending.** If in doubt, give a smaller number and risk having to turn people away than be left with a large bill for accommodation you did not use. Hotels will likely have empty rooms anyway so it's much easier to ask them to add to your requirements than reduce numbers dramatically.

- **Check arrival and departure times** with the hotel and ask about facilities for storing luggage. Check what time the bedrooms will be ready: remember, if your conference starts at 10 am bedrooms may not be available until 2 pm. Likewise, if your conference closes at 2 pm, most hotels require rooms to be vacated by noon: where do delegates leave their luggage?

- **Check arrangements for parking:**
  - Are there sufficient spaces?
  - Is car parking free?
  - Is it secured?
  - Disabled parking?

- Ask the venue for your own **designated registration table** – not too far away from the hotel reception if the course is residential, but far enough away to be separate. This avoids delegates standing with suitcases around their feet while others are trying to register for the conference. If your conference is residential, you may need to keep this in place and manned for the duration of the event as a 'help desk' for queries.

- **Check your invoice** – it's amazing how 'extras' creep into the final bill. Do you really want to pay for a delegate's *News of the World*, in-room raunchy film or phone calls to children backpacking in Australia?

Location

When you choose a venue, make sure it is convenient for transport links; especially if you're organising a national conference or course, where delegates will be travelling from far and wide. While the

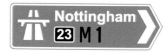

Outer Hebrides and Shap are beautiful and wonderful scenic places, no one's going to come if it's a one-day course, three hours to get there by train followed by a 20-minute walk.

Location

Ideally, try to pick a venue that is no more than 30 minutes from a:
1   main trunk road or motorway (like the A1, M1, M6, etc.)
2   main-line train station
3   local airport.

If a lot of people will be coming by air or rail, you may wish to consider organising a mini-bus pick-up at selected arrival times. These costs will need to be added to your budget.

 Top Tip: When you have picked a venue, be sure to get the official address (including postcode) and ask them for a map of their location (or locate one on Google Maps). The map (with address *and* postcode) should be sent to all attendees and facilitators. Many people use a navigator to get to a venue these days, and that's why the postcode is crucial. Otherwise they will end up lost, become all flustered, arrive late and all of this will affect the event in a negative way. One or two unfortunate ones might become so frustrated that they end up in an accident. *Please use the postcode!*

Size of the event

I have organised events ranging from a 10-person study day to the UKAPD Conference and the Northern Deanery Trainers conference of around 120+. Who said size doesn't matter? It's utter rubbish. Believe me when I say size *does* matter!

AH

For a start, a hotel manager's eyes will positively glisten at the thought of filling the hotel for three full days. It also gives you more power to haggle for better deals. In essence, it's a win–win situation for both of you. However, more people mean more organising. If you are an administrator reading this chapter, you need to liaise with the educator lead for the event. If you're the educator lead, make sure you are clear about your aims, objectives, the content and methodology (format of the session). Methodology is particularly important: splitting a large group into small-group working is a highly effective way of learning. But, the more small groups you have the more breakout rooms you will need and that adds to the cost.

Dates

Do not organise an event at these times:
1 At the start of the academic year – there are simply too many things people have to do

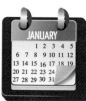

2 During the school holidays – even if your target audience would like to come (because the colleagues they need to cover them will be on holiday)
3 During special religious holidays – like Christmas, New Year, Ramadan, Eid al Fitr and Yom Kippur. An interfaith calendar can be found at: www.interfaithcalendar.org/

So when is a good time?	
March	*March is generally a good bet. But do it before Easter (which occurs sometime after 21 March).*
British Summer Time (BST)	*British Summer Time (BST) is usually in force from the last Sunday in March till the last Sunday in October. But remember, avoid the Easter period.* *BST is good because the weather is lovely, people feel good, and they generally want to get away and refresh their other parts.*
Autumn	*Autumn begins 22–23 September, and ends 21–22 December. But try to hold your event in early autumn before the weather turns and the dark nights set in. An interesting course or conference in the autumn is something to look forward to after a summer holiday.*

 Top Tip: When organising any event, check the calendar of events of any big organisations to which your intended audience belong (such as the deanery and RCGP). You need to make sure your event does not clash with other events like deanery recruitment, ARCP panels and other workshops. This is particularly important if your event is big, like a national event, with a UK-wide audience.

Other points
- You really need to think and plan in advance. Everyone has other demands on their time. So plan ahead, try to give facilitators a year's notice if this is a national event; if it's a local event, you can get away with six months.
- You must consider how long you need for your event. Will a study day suffice, or is this a three-day residential event? Will people turn up for a weekend event? Sometimes you have to be prepared to go the extra mile to encourage attendance.
- And, of course, sometimes you have to be flexible:

Some years ago I was involved with the organisation of a Northern Deanery Trainer Conference. It was held from Friday evening through to Sunday lunchtime in a local hotel. There were 120 Trainers, some with partners, children and dogs in tow. Clearly, the programme they were expecting consisted of a cosy couple of days. However, the programme we devised included a mock MRCGP exam – MCQ, MEQ and oral. Mutiny was threatened, but once everyone got down to it and realised it was planned to be educational and fun, anxiety levels reduced. Partners and children were bussed to York, a tour of the Jorvik Museum arranged, tea was taken with a local Lord and Lady in the Manor; dogs were walked; early dinner and magicians organised for children, nannies provided etc. It is still talked off fondly as one of the most successful conferences ever, even though the fire alarm went off midway through the conference dinner on the Saturday evening, and we spent a chilly hour in the carpark!

AH

Once you've got your date finally agreed – then go for it!

Advertising

Advertising or marketing is instrumental for success. Take boy-bands, for instance. There are loads of boy-bands out there who can sing but the ones who make it are the ones who have managers that are masters in the art of marketing. Their voices have little to do with it.

Similarly, to 'pull' your potential applicants, you need to do three things:

1 find a very effective advertising method – consider more than one
2 develop a really powerful advert
3 send the ad out in a timely way.

The advert

Don't just think about A5 paper flyers: how about an electronic advert (either a Word attachment or the body of an email itself) or an ad in a mainstream journal/magazine or maybe a mixture of these? Emails are particularly good if you can get your 'contacts' to cascade them down to your intended audience, and it costs nothing.

Things to put in your advert

- Who you are: Northern Deanery GP Educators, APCE, etc.
- What you are organising: GP Educators Annual Conference, CSA Prep Course, etc.
- Who your target audience is: e.g. primarily aimed at newly qualified GPs.
- Get a few powerful 'hooks' in there: why they should attend and what's in it for them?
- When you're holding this event.
- Where you're holding the event.
- Cost of the course.
- How they can apply and the closing date.
- Contact details for further enquiries: ideally, an email and/or website.
- Jazz the flyer up.

Whichever advert you choose, it needs to contain powerful hooks to show the recipients what's in it for them. A powerful advert should not be overloaded with text but should be short and to the point. Add colour and pictures to get people to want to pick it up and read it. Instead of a boring title such as: *'Health and Work'*, opt for something snazzier like: *'Sick Notes – feel sick no more!'* There's a lot more about powerful hooks in Chapter 4: Powerful Hooks – aims, objectives and ILOs. Take a look at the A4 flyer on our website.

The booking form

It's good if you can reserve part of the flyer to serve as a booking form, but if you can't, enclose it as a separate document. Five weeks before the event, tot up the numbers attending – this will give you a rough guide to the size of your event. Let the venue know of this number as it will serve as the minimum they will charge you. Four weeks is usually the deadline for reductions in numbers.

When devising your booking form, make it clear that unless booking forms are accompanied by the cheque, no firm reservation will be made. In addition, be sure to have a little paragraph detailing your cancellation policy. Can you afford to reimburse the full cost?

Cancellation policy

- Full reimbursement (minus an admin charge) if cancelled >2 months before the event.
- 50% reimbursement if cancelled 1–2 months before the event.
- No reimbursement if cancelled <1 month before the event.

As you start seeing booking forms coming through, set up a spreadsheet to help you keep a list of who's coming. This should include things like: Title, First Name, Surname, Address – split into five columns, Home Phone, Work Phone, Mobile, Email, Deanery/region/scheme – depending on your delegate group, Special Diets, Paid – enter the amount paid. A downloadable Excel spreadsheet template is available from our website. You can add columns for choices of workshops (e.g. if you're running a course on the RCGP ePortfolio, you might have one group doing CSA, another doing WPBA, COTs, and so on). Furthermore, add a column for networking event choices (e.g. walking, tour of art gallery, tour of the local heritage site and so on).

And while you're constructing and adding data to your spreadsheet, one thing we urge you to do is to get the spelling of names right as you add them to the spreadsheet. People might not say it, but they will feel offended or insulted if their name badge isn't spelt correctly. And the reason why we say get it right on the spreadsheet is because that will form the reference point from which you will produce other materials for the course like group lists, name badges, named packs, dinner place cards and so on.

If the event is self-funding, ensure that cheque or Bankers' Automated Clearing Services (BACS) payments are recorded as they arrive, and pay these into your account, say, once a week. At the same time, receipts of payments should be sent to the delegates so that they can claim back any funds as necessary or for their tax records.

Top Tip: Liaise frequently with your contact at the venue; don't keep them in the dark. Send them copies of the programme, group lists and the entire delegate list as often as these change. If you have any special requests – let the venue know as soon as you can. *And* when working out numbers from a spreadsheet of attendees, remember to subtract one; spreadsheets are always one row out due to headers.

Speakers and group leaders

Speakers and group leaders

- Make sure your speaker(s) are notified in writing (email or letter) of the date, time, venue and what you expect them to speak about. At the same time, send them a map and a timetable so they know exactly how long they have.
- Ask if they need any equipment, photocopying of handouts or anything else.
- Be explicit about facilitator fees, expenses reimbursed, staying for lunch, dinner and overnight accommodation.
- Brief them about the event: in particular, who the audiences are, their needs and a discussion around the type of educational methods that might prove most effective. You may need to encourage them to be interactive.

Speakers must be introduced and thanked: make sure that you know who is doing this. There is nothing worse than the mumblings and mutterings of four organisers standing up to do the same job!

Top Tip: We've had a number of speakers and facilitators who've got stuck in traffic, been held up by a late train or suddenly taken ill. Don't be left with your pants around your ankles – have a contingency plan! The British weather is also unpredictable so bear this in mind – do you really want all your delegates snowed into the hotel for a week!

Group lists and name badges

Group lists: If you are working in small groups, sort your groups before the event. Don't do it too much in advance; maybe when the booking forms are no longer trickling in. It's ideal to circulate group lists in advance, but remember you will get cancellations and late arrivals, which will mess the whole thing up. You may end up with one group of 10 and one group of 4 – be prepared to juggle.

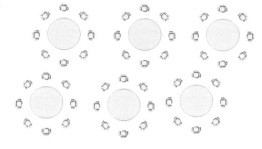

Brief your group leaders so they know which group room they are in and where it is; you won't have time to go rounding up stray sheep! Make sure they have a group list in their room and, preferably, one stuck on the door of the room so any late arrivals can check before they walk through the door. On the day, give a copy of your final group list to the venue reception – if they need to find Dr Thingymajig when nobody is around, they will know at least which room to go to.

Name badges: These are important because people cannot be expected to remember a whole mass of new names. Name badges help you to relate how a person calls himself or herself to the way it is written (aids memory and recall). And it becomes embarrassing if you have to ask someone for their name seven times throughout a two-day event.

As mentioned earlier in this chapter, get the spelling of names right. How would you feel if your name is Mrs Dianne Rudd, but your name badge says Mrs Dyno Rod? Okay, so we've exaggerated than one, but you get our drift. And just because a person is from a different country and has an unusual name (to you!) doesn't justify any spelling errors on your part (besides, *your* name might sound weird to them). Names are personal and sensitive things and spelling them incorrectly offends people, even if they don't say so. Inaccurate spellings also give off a vibe about you: not only of your administrative and organisation skills, but also (in the case on non-English names) an impression of how you embrace culture and diversity.

You can colour code name badges, so if you are running several workshops the colours will show which group a delegate is in, i.e. if a delegate is sitting in a group wearing a yellow badge and everyone else's is blue – guess what, wrong room, wrong workshop! If you are running a sequence of workshops mark name badges with colours in order – remember people get flustered, lose their normal logical thought processes, and it will save you having to give directions every hour! For example: Red = ARCP panels workshop; Blue = CSA workshop; Green = Equal Opportunities workshop.

Equipment

Make sure you have everything you need by checking the requirements of speakers and group leaders. For instance:

> ## Equipment
>
> - Laptop with PowerPoint, and mouse.
> - Overhead projector and transparency films/pens.
> - Flip charts and pens – make sure the pens work.
> - Slide projectors – yes, sometimes still needed.
> - TV/DVD/video and extension leads.
> - Microphone – you may have a very quiet-voiced speaker, or one with a cold!

Don't forget the spares: bulbs, fuses, memory stick, CDs and possibly even a screwdriver.

The applicant's pack

There are things you need to send to the applicant before they come to the event (directions, for instance) and there are things that can be given out when they arrive. That means there are two packs you need to arrange: pre-course material and the course material.

Pre-course inventory	The course inventory
This needs to go out well before the start date of the course and even earlier if there is pre-course homework that needs doing.	*The contents of this pack, which is usually dished out on the first day, is mainly determined by the structure of your event, such as:*
<ul><li>Hotel directions, map and parking.</li><li>The programme – especially detailing refreshment and comfort breaks.</li><li>A résumé – detailing each speaker and their job experience and education.</li><li>Group lists and allocations to activities.</li><li>Pre-course homework.</li><li>Other important information – like suggested clothing for activities and cancellation fees.</li><li>Dress code – If it's formal tell your delegates 'you will need to bring tux or ball gown'. For a walk on the moors: 'You will need comfortable stout footwear, waterproofs, etc.' It is embarrassing to turn up in a tux when everyone else is in jeans.</li></ul>	<ul><li>Course material and handouts.</li><li>Group lists and allocations to activities – for the same reasons as above.</li><li>The programme again – in case they've left it at home.</li><li>Spare paper – to make notes (+/- a pen).</li><li>Evaluation form.</li></ul>

Top Tip: If your event involves a variety of workshops where the attendees will attend more than one, consider printing the material for each workshop on different-coloured paper. In the example used earlier, the material for the CBD workshop might be printed on pink paper; that for the COT workshop on yellow and so on. In that way, if the course pack becomes voluminous, delegates will have no problem locating the relevant material at a glance.

Registration

Ask, beg, borrow or steal someone to help you on the day. If numbers are large, it's likely you will need two or three helping hands. Be prepared. Here are some top tips.

- Keep smiling and wear comfortable shoes.
- Prepare your register in alphabetical order and display it on the reception table.
- Have several pens available – someone will sign in and walk off with the pen!
- Consider blank name badges – so they can write their own name and in whatever style they wish. Will might want to be called Bill and Elizabeth might prefer to draw a flower on hers and write the name Lizzy. It saves you a job.
- Unless they are already inserted into delegate folders:
  - have programmes ready
  - have group lists ready – highlight the group leader and the group room so people know where they are going or who to follow.
- Ask for a plan of the venue and stick it on a flip chart near the registration table – saves those on the conference registration desk doing impersonations of human windmills, or acting as tour guides.
- If residential, leave the accommodation check-in to the venue – the experts.
- Have a few spare delegate folders, copies of programmes, etc. – delegates lose things!

For many years I have carried a 'Black Bag' to conferences and courses. It's a large bag containing:	
<ul><li>Blu tack – *not to be used on expensive flock wallpaper, unless you want a decorating bill!*</li><li>Sellotape – *caution as above*</li><li>Drawing pins – *only for pin boards*</li><li>Scissors</li><li>Stapler, staples and paperclips</li><li>Pens, pencils, eraser, highlighter pens, OHP and flip chart pens</li><li>Spare lined and plain paper</li><li>Spare shorthand notebooks</li><li>Flip chart pad</li><li>Ruler</li></ul>	<ul><li>A USB memory stick</li><li>Writable CDs</li><li>Spare name badges – *in case of spelling mistakes*</li><li>Tissues</li><li>Kitchen paper towels – *for cleaning screens*</li><li>Paracetamol</li><li>Elastoplasts – various sizes</li><li>WD40 – *cleans white boards too!*</li><li>Screwdriver and pliers</li><li>Spare cables – mains and projector to laptop</li><li>. . . And last but not least – spare socks!*</li></ul>

*A request was made to me for this on the Friday night of a weekend conference when a delegate had forgotten to pack socks. I went home that night and raided my husband's supply. It probably won't surprise you that I am often found with a laptop, data projector, TV, DVD player and a floor stand in my car boot or draped around my neck! AH.

On the big day

- **Keep calm!** Get there early – there are always things which needed organising, dealing with at the last minute, e.g. fielding phone calls from lost delegates, speakers and caterers; projectors which just refuse to function, etc.
- **Keep smiling** as your delegates are likely to be more nervous or anxious than you are. Unknown venues, unknown delegates – people need a friendly welcoming face!
- **Housekeeping:** it is vital that whatever event you are organising, you or another organiser brief all delegates at the introduction and welcome, on what to do if the fire alarm goes off, where people have to gather, etc. And do remember to take the register with you – the Fire Brigade will not be impressed if you have no idea who is at your event and unaccounted for. Boy Scouts' motto – 'Be Prepared'. If the fire alarm is regularly tested on a Friday, the day of your course, the venue should brief you about the differences between a test and the real thing.
- If there are any other housekeeping issues you need to address, now's the time before your flock all disappear into their groups or become so involved in your event, they forget everything.

Evaluation

Everyone wants feedback when they have been involved in organising or taking part in an event. The delegates may also be interested in global feedback. Evaluation might be necessary to justify your expenditure. Besides, it's always useful for your PDP.

After a heavy one or two days, people won't feel like writing and even worse will fill in evaluations without much thought if it looks complicated: so keep it simple! The form itself should contain items relating to the organisational component as well as the content and methodology. By that we mean things like:

Evaluation

- The suitability of the venue
- The meals
- The helpfulness of venue staff
- The information given before the course
- The material given on the course
- The organisation of the course
- The helpfulness of the organisers and administrators.

You can include an evaluation form in your delegate pack and ask delegates to leave this with you as they leave or take it with them and post it back. Alternatively, you can circulate it via post or email a week or so after the event, giving delegates time to reflect. Having tried many ways we feel the most effective is to include the feedback sheet in the delegate folder and ask delegates to complete it before they leave. Feedback sheets taken away to be completed later tend to end up being ignored, as do emails after the event: people move on. Once you've got all the feedback forms, hand them over to the administrator who can then collate the results to make them more meaningful prior to distribution. There are a variety of downloadable evaluation forms on our website and even more under the web section for Chapter 28: Reflection and Evaluation.

Top Tip: If the course is a single day, the feedback sheets can be circulated and filled in over the last tea break. That way there is less rush at the end of the day, and you are likely to get more forms with useful information.

At the end of the event

The end of the event

- Issue any certificates of attendance for delegates if necessary.
- Give out any 'thank you gifts' to facilitators/group leaders/speakers.
- Write to the venue thanking them for their help and pay the bill promptly.
- Write to the speakers and group leaders thanking them for their time and efforts.
- When the collated feedback is ready, check it over to make sure there isn't anything too harsh and inappropriate: remember feedback is about helping people not destroying them. Then distribute (usually via email).
- Reflect on the event collaboratively with your fellow organisers: what went well and what could be done differently the next time around. If the venue was successful, you may want to go back.

Relax, reflect and plan your next venture! Oh, and don't forget to thank anyone else who helped you, including the person who supplied the spare socks!

A final note on how to use your administrator

If you've been nominated as a course organiser, one key person who will help make the task easy and a complete success is the administrator. Running and organising courses is usually second nature to them: so contact them as soon as possible. If you haven't got one, get one! Brief them as much as possible about the event. Delegate as much as you can and then continue to keep in contact with them regularly. The administrator is your key to a successful hassle-free course without a headache!

> The course secretary is invaluable, unless you can type and use a word processor, have your own personal photocopier and vast supplies of copy paper, a prodigious memory and lots of spare time.
> 'A secretary whose time is always respected will perform miracles in an emergency.'
> Patrick McEvoy, *Educating the Future GP: The Course Organiser's Handbook*[1]

We couldn't have put it better ourselves! Before we close, we'd like to wish you every success for the event you're reading this chapter for.

A sample of resources on our website

- Conference Flyer, Programme, Booking form, Group list – examples.
- Conference Attendance Register.
- Conference Costings tool.
- Conference Evaluation Form.

Other chapters you may like to read

Please give us some feedback on this chapter to help shape it for the next edition.
Go to www.essentialgptrainingbook.com and simply click on the title of this chapter.

Reference

1 McEvoy P. *Educating the Future GP: the course organiser's handbook*. 2nd ed. Oxford: Radcliffe; 1998.

16

Presentation Magic

CLARE WEDDERBURN – APD (Wessex Deanery)   JOHN LORD – Professor of Primary Medical Care (Univ. Huddersfield)
RAMESH MEHAY – TPD (Bradford)

> Ultimately, presenting is a means of communicating thoughts and ideas to individuals within an audience.

Introduction

This chapter is mainly written to offer a *'how to do it'* guide for those new to presenting. However, it doesn't stop there: we also provide alternative suggestions and tips for more experienced presenters and possible methods of coping with problems as they arise.

 Top Tip: Did you know that only 20% of our communication is verbal? That means more than three-quarters of the communication which takes place in any presentation is actually non-verbal (like the use of voice, facial expressions, posture and gestures).

Presenting is often daunting. Appearing confident and making a good impression is more difficult when you are nervous. Audiences tend to judge the speaker before they judge the content of a presentation. They absorb a variety of visual and auditory information, observing you and your visual aids, while listening to your voice. From these *few* pieces of information, every member of the audience forms an opinion within a *few* minutes of you starting your presentation.

The audience will draw their own conclusions from the simple things you say and do.

- Are you confident?
- Are you relaxed?
- Are you using eye contact?
- Are you standing still or walking around?
- Is your opening sentence punchy and attention grabbing?
- Are you familiar with the content of your talk?
- Are you reading directly from notes, or slides?

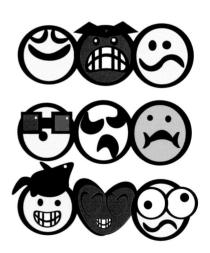

If you behave confidently, your audience will respond positively, regardless of how you feel inside. Believe it or not, audiences want you to do well! Listening to an effective speaker is a pleasure and allows them to be able to relax, listen and take in your message. To present effectively, **the opening lines of your presentation need to be polished, positive and said with conviction**. If you need time to warm up so that you are at your best, do so in the car or in an empty room before the audience arrives.

What does the audience remember?

Question: If you were to stand up and speak for 20 minutes, using supporting visuals and without handouts, how many points or ideas do you think the average member of the audience would walk away with?

Answer: 7 points or ideas![1,2]

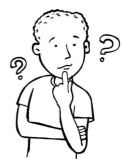

In the absence of any control from you, the memorable points might be: that you were wandering around in a distracting way, you were wearing a shirt that they didn't really like, and if you are lucky, they might remember something about the content of your presentation. With this in mind, as a presenter, you need to be aware that it is your responsibility to control what the audience remembers. However effective you are as a presenter, you can only really communicate three ideas to your audience.

Planning and designing your presentation

Objectives

Before you decide what you want to say, consider your objectives.

> ## Aims and objectives
> - Ask yourself: why am I speaking and what is the purpose of my talk?
> - What is it that I want the audience to take away with them, at the end of the presentation?
> - Am I trying to inform, educate, influence or motivate?

A presentation can only have a handful of objectives: what do you want the three 'take home messages' to be? For more, *see* Chapter 4: Powerful Hooks – aims, objectives and ILOs.

Audience

> ## The audience
> - Who are they? Are they homogeneous or a multidisciplinary group?
> - What is their level of expertise, knowledge and experience?
> - Do I know any of the members of the audience and in what capacity?

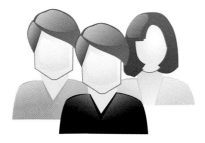

Asking yourself these questions will ensure that you pitch your presentation at an appropriate level. If there is doubt about the knowledge or expertise of your audience, you could ask them questions at the outset of your presentation. This would give you some idea as to whether you need to adjust your talk as you go along. It's not ideal but sometimes necessary. If you can find out about your audience before you prepare your talk, it makes for a smoother and less stressful presentation!

Venue

Preferably, check out the venue before you start. Otherwise contact who-ever is in command of the event, well in advance, so that you know where you will be giving your presentation. Always plan to arrive with plenty of time and make sure that any equipment is there, and that it works! There is no point designing your presentation in a way that relies on specific auditory acoustics, if they are not feasible at that particular venue. For 'big' presentations, things like lighting, windows, air conditioning and room temperature are key to helping you know how best to deliver your presentation. The time of day is also a consideration. Have you ended up with the after lunch 'graveyard slot'? In which case you will need something to keep your audience awake!

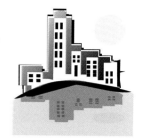

> ## Venue essentials
> - Where are you speaking?
> - What size is the room – small and cramped vs large and spacious?
> - What are the acoustics like?
> - What are the seating arrangements?
> - Is there a podium or platform?
> - Is there equipment available: a data projector, flip chart or DVD?
> - Is there internet access?

Presentation/teaching plans

When you have a clearer picture of the design of your presentation, we strongly recommend you map this out onto a 'presentation plan'. Presentation plans can help you to:
- reflect and decide whether your presentation is balanced
- quickly check on things that could potentially sabotage your day
- keep on track.

 Top Tip: You can read more about presentation or teaching plans in Chapter 6: Teaching from Scratch. There's an example in that chapter for you to look at too. Downloadable teaching plan templates are available from our website.

What to say

There are three main stages to a good presentation:[3]
1. An introduction or **'Set'** – why you want to say things.
2. The main part or **'Dialogue'** – what you want to say.
3. A conclusion or **'Closure'** – what you want the audience to do or to remember.

The introduction (the Set)

Aim for an opening statement, thanking the organisers for inviting you, and letting the audience know why you enjoy this subject, and why you think it will be important to them. If you have not been introduced, then your audience may also need to be told why you have the temerity to address them, or what qualifies you to speak on the subject.

Then outline the purpose of your talk, and how long you intend to speak for. If there will be a handout, tell them now: it will save them having to make notes and thus help them devote their attention listening to you. Give your audience a breakdown of the specific areas you will be discussing (bulleted headings are helpful when preparing your introduction). Decide when to take questions, either during or at the end of your talk; tell your audience this at the outset so that they know how to behave.

The main part (the Dialogue)

The main body of the talk should consist of three or four key points only. Use bulleted headings for these key areas and then flesh out what you intend to say from there. Write drafts in spoken English, using simple familiar words. Avoid technical jargon and acronyms and keep the sentence construction short. Above all keep what you say simple. Decide on your role:

1 Is it to impart information as an expert (often a difficult and dangerous position)?
2 Is it to guide your audience as you would a colleague?
3 Is it to discuss issues in relation to your own experience (often a safe place to start)?

 Red Alert: Humour is fine, especially at your own expense; the audience may warm to your humility. Be careful, though: no jokes based on race, religion, culture, sex (in both senses of the word) or sexual orientation. Cartoons may work, but only tell jokes if you're a natural. If in doubt, don't tell any!

The conclusion (the Closure)

Emphasise the key take-home messages. Think about the specific learning points and ensure these are highlighted both verbally and in any visual aids or handout material. Your audience will otherwise only recall a few facts from your presentation!

Ways to present

There are many ways to present information; here are some of the more popular ones.

Speak off the cuff

We feel this requires considerable skill, experience and confidence. If you intend to speak off the cuff, ensure you have notes or diagrams of your key messages to refer to, should you dry up and forget what you were going to say!

Notes or cue cards

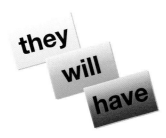

This is a popular way to speak at larger events. It provides a natural way of giving your presentation with the prompts available to refer to on cards. We find it helpful to write drafts out on A4 paper initially and then transfer key words, sentences or diagrams onto the cue cards. If you plan to do this, ensure the cards are either numbered or clipped together. Avoid reading them word for word, as this will result in a stilted, awkward talk, and your audience will not remain attentive for very long!

Flip charts

Flip charts are a great way of encouraging an interactive talk. They are an excellent tool for gathering the audience's opinion or existing knowledge, but a poor way of presenting yours. However, it may be the only medium open to you to provide graphical responses to questions or suggestions from the audience. Do not use flip charts if your writing is illegible and only do so if you have suitable coloured pens that work (check beforehand). Avoid using flip charts if you are speaking to a large audience, as it is unlikely that those sitting at the back will manage to read your scrawl.

The overhead projector

This is being used less and less these days because of data projectors: but that doesn't mean because it's old it's useless. In some venues, it may be all you've got and may be a better alternative to a flip chart, as at least people in the back row might be able to read from it! Do make sure that the equipment works and do be prepared for equipment failure. Always plan to be able to deliver your presentation effectively without the overhead projector, if the worst-case scenario occurs.

Overhead projectors

- Obtain new overheads. Old ones look messy as scratches and smudges magnify when projected.
- If you are typing your overheads, use at least font size 20 point, with roughly four words per line.
- Print in black and white and photocopy onto new overheads.
- Beware of using coloured pens in handwritten overheads, especially red and yellow, which are more difficult to read.
- Always number your sheets: it will keep you organised.

 Top Tip: Using overhead projectors: put a table next to the projector for your overheads. Face the audience, not the screen, and don't read directly from the visuals. Don't cover and reveal your text line by line – it is irritating for the audience.

The data projector and PowerPoint

The first thing we'd like to write about is **PowerPoint mania**. PowerPoint in itself is an excellent tool for making presentations but many people seem to think the best way of delivering *any* session is through PowerPoint – and it's not. For example, a skill is often better taught through demonstration and practice, not via PowerPoint! Unfortunately, people aren't listening and blocks of texts seem to be encapsulated in megabytes of PowerPoint junk. And because so many people have jumped onto the PowerPoint bandwagon, it's resulting in lazy teach-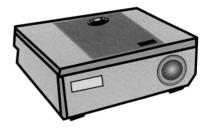

ers, lazy learners and is minimising the learning experience. Sometimes, the audience is so fixed on the slide rather than the speaker, they switch off, failing to hear what's being said. Don't just go with PowerPoint when you're asked to do a presentation; consider other methods like flip charts – better still, consider using a variety of tools.

If you're still reading, you've probably decided on PowerPoint! Okay then, let's help you by looking at the practical side of things. First check that a data projector will be available, you have the right connectors, and that there is a PC to use (or take your own laptop). Print out your entire presentation to paper so that you know which slide is coming next before you press the advance key. Print using the format 9 slides to a page.

Slides

- Aim for one main message per slide. Remember the **4 by 4 rule** (4 words per line and 4 lines per slide).
- Carefully consider the font. Arial, Garamond or Times New Roman can be easily read, while fancy fonts often project poorly.
- Aim for a font size of 30–40 point for key messages. While most data projectors can display fonts as low as 6 point, small sizes are only useful for page numbers or background items like your name or institution.
- Keep colour, font and point size consistent throughout your slides.
- Avoid using red font as it projects badly.
- Avoid animated graphics – they will only serve to distract.

 Top Tip: Bring your presentation on a simple memory stick. Be careful of complex sticks with security locks or U3 programs; they may fail to operate on the venue computer. And most NHS computers only allow you to use NHS-issued USB sticks – check with your organiser. And if you've got the latest version of PowerPoint, consider saving your presentation in a previous version (e.g. as a .ppt rather than a .pptx file) in case the host computer has an older version of the software. Finally, be prepared to deliver your talk without the data projector, if you have to.

Layout: Slide layout is important. PowerPoint has many wacky backgrounds. They may look fun, but can distract from your talk and often make the text difficult to read. Plain backgrounds are usually best. If you think you are going to end up apologising for a slide, because it is too busy or complicated, or it doesn't project well, just don't use it.

Text: If there is too much text on a slide, seriously think about reviewing it to see what can be cut out. 'Chunking' the information, by getting a chunk of text to reveal itself with each click, can help your audience to assimilate the information. Avoid flying text or fancy fading in and out of words; the same goes for using sounds as words appear on the screen: this distracts the audience from the content of your presentation.

Remember too that it is difficult for the audience to comprehend two grammars at once. For example, you speaking a sentence and the audience reading the same text are two different grammars. You are unlikely to speak the text aloud at the same rate that your audience reads the written text, and this mismatch will severely limit their understanding. Instead, speak the text aloud first (from memory), and then hit the forward button, to display the words you have just spoken. In this way, reading from the slide will help consolidate what they have just heard.

Pictures and photos: Photographs, drawings, cartoons and diagrams can be amusing and can be used to inject humour into your talk. They can also be distracting. It's better **if pictures are relevant** because they then help visually to consolidate the point you are trying to make. Actually, a single, simple picture, without any text, can provide a thought-provoking backdrop to something that you describe in words. And before we forget, beware of clip art. Often, it does not capture the concept as well as a photograph. Many people in your audience may be familiar with some of your clip-art images from other presentations, thus rendering yours as unexciting.

Live Internet links and demonstrations: Stills captured from the Internet are more *reliable* than live demonstrations. To copy a Windows screen onto a PowerPoint slide:

1 Hold the ALT key and Print-Screen key together.
2 Now use CTRL-V to paste it into your slide.
3 If you wish, crop out sections that you do not need.

If you must link live, the stills can serve as a useful backup. Do remember to check if the venue has Internet access if you intend to do this.

 Top Tip: Avoid using a laser pointer. The laser light wobbles and every tremor of your nervous hand is amplified upon the screen. If you feel that a laser pointer will help you to navigate around a particular slide, *stop!* Your slide is overcomplicated; it needs trimming down. If you have to point out specific bits on a slide, it is better to go up to the screen and point it out with your hand.

Time planning: Aim to allow about 40 seconds per slide. Therefore, a 10-minute talk might encompass roughly 12 slides, but if you're presenting for an hour, that doesn't mean you can use 72 slides – you'll bore them to death! In the case of the latter, try to break up the PowerPoint with, say, an interactive discussion, a relevant video clip or some other learning activity. If you are asked to deliver a 10-minute talk, be strict with your preparation and do not use more than 12 slides. Time the first practice delivery of your talk: if it overruns, remove some less important slides and time it again. There is nothing more irritating than a speaker who overruns, and an audience that stops listening to what you are saying and starts to clock-watch instead. Keep it succinct and to time!

Video and recorded sound: These items are notorious for going wrong on the day for a number of reasons (usually technical), and if you are a novice presenter, consider avoiding them. Otherwise, you can play a CD before your session starts (as the audience walks through the door) and/or interrupt (say) your PowerPoint or speech with a few video clips. If you're experienced you could even *embed* a video into PowerPoint (search Google for instructions).

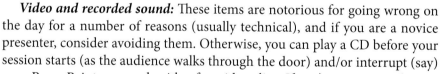

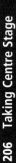

Video

- Be certain that you know how to find the clip you want, and when to start and stop it.
- Check the equipment before you start your presentation (including sound) and make sure you know how it works.
- If part of your presentation involves looking at video material that you have asked some members of the audience to bring, make sure you have briefed them properly.
  - What format: VHS, mini-tapes, DVD, etc.
  - If VHS: make sure they've set it to the right point *before* they come.
  - If mini-tapes: they must bring their camcorder and appropriate leads.

 Red Alert: Just because a video clip plays on your computer does not mean it will at the venue. Videos can freeze on the first frame, display jerkily, appear in black or white, or without synchronised sound. Recorded sound is less of a problem. The best thing to do is to go down and check these things out on the equipment at the venue.

Effective delivery

Effective delivery

- Practise delivering the whole presentation in front of a mirror.
- Try to speak naturally and try to stand comfortably.
- Pace yourself to avoid racing and consider your intonation.
- Emphasise key words and phrases, repeating the key main points, summarising slides as you go along.
- Smile, ensure good eye contact and avoid distracting mannerisms.

Stance

There are two important components to stance:

1 how to stand when you are standing still
2 how and when to move.

Whenever you deliver a key point, make sure you are standing still. Visual signals are generally more memorable than auditory ones. Things said while moving will therefore tend to be lost to the audience, who are focusing on your movement. However, that doesn't mean you can't use arm gestures and so on. Stand with your feet about a hip-width apart, evenly weighted; too wide and it looks aggressive, too close and it feels unstable!

Moving around is essential to any effective presentation: it energises an audience, can help to motivate them and adds a sense of dynamism to your talk. It probably takes less than 3 seconds to walk from one side of an audience to another, so aim to stop talking as you walk, pause and deliver your message, before moving again. Try to avoid pacing backwards and forwards, or turning your back on the audience. Swaying from side to side, playing with money or keys in your pockets can irritate your audience and distract their attention from the content of your talk.

Arm gestures

Used well, gestures are your **most powerful tool after your voice**. They must be relevant and purposeful to give impact to your talk. Gestures can add focus and a visual punctuation to your presentation. To use them effectively, you first need to establish a resting position for your hands.

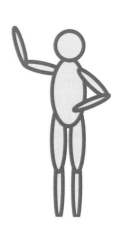

Hand position: a bad hand position can give the wrong impression. So consider starting off with your hands hanging loosely by your sides, clasped gently together above your waist or in an open position, relaxed, as if you were holding an orange.

The gestures: Much of the impact in a presentation comes from the use of **asymmetrical** movements and being aware of the three-dimensional space around you. Symmetrical gestures, where both hands make the same movements at the same time, can also be effective but if used repeatedly can bore the audience and lack impact in terms of effective communication of a concept or idea. Therefore, as a general rule, consider dropping one hand momentarily, while you make a gesture with the other, before bringing both hands back to the resting position.

Now consider the size and shape of the gesture. Gestures begin at the outer edge of your body line and go outwards from there. They are driven from your shoulders, not your elbows, and should be large enough to encompass the people sitting at the outer edges of your audience. If you are talking to six people, a narrow span of gestures is fine; if you're talking to 600 people, the gesture will be considerably larger. Gestures need to flow expressively and the shape of your gesture is dictated by what you are trying to illustrate. It takes practice and confidence to use them well, but don't be afraid of trying them out; you can only get better with repeated practice.

Eye contact

Effective presenters simulate the kind of eye contact that people use when talking one to one between friends. This consists of a definite steady attention on the other person, alternating with short breaks, where there may be no eye contact at all. Rather than presenting to an audience, imagine you are having a series of short one-to-one conversations with individuals. Look randomly from one part of the audience to another, pausing to give steady eye contact to one individual, before moving your eyes on. If you have a large audience, mentally divide them into blocks and rest your eyes on one individual, provide steady eye contact and then move your eyes onto another individual in another block. Hold your eye contact for the duration of a thought, or until there is a natural break in the rhythm or subject that you are delivering. Your eye movements will then appear natural and will quite likely correspond with your breathing pattern. This will make it seem less threatening and make individuals **feel like** there's been some one-to-one personal contact with you.

Voice

There are four easily controlled variables to voice, which are important in presenting:

1 Pitch	2 Volume	3 Silence	4 Pace

Effective presenting has a theatrical quality. Using a full range of these variables can emphasise the key points in your presentation, by providing momentary impact. By slowing down, pausing or lowering the volume of your voice, you create interest in your talk and create an impression of confidence and control. It's a bit like a long-distance car journey. A totally straight motorway drive for 3 hours will be monotonous and tiring. However, the same motorway, but with occasional bends here and there, stop-off points and things to see along the way, will be more entertaining and less likely for you to need matchsticks to prop your eyes open!

The *power and tonal quality (pitch)* of your voice depend upon using your abdominal muscles to maximum effect. The ideal is to take breaths in using your diaphragm, allowing your tummy to expand at the same time, while keeping your shoulders and chest relatively still. Then speak with this awareness of increased tension in your abdominal muscles. When you have made one point, take a breath in, allowing your abdomen to expand again. This pause allows the audience to take in your last sentence, and gives you time to think about your next sentence.

Varying the *volume* of your voice at certain points in your 'speech' can highlight the key points or considerations you wish to impart. If you're worried that you have a soft voice, check with an assistant whether you can be heard at the back of the venue room. Alternatively, ask if a microphone is available, figure out how to use it and where it is best to stand, if it's not a mobile one.

If you find that your voice dries up, or you start feeling a choking sensation, try maintaining a neutral stance of the body and neck. If you stretch out your larynx, by having your head too extended, or if you compress your larynx because of the muscle tension in your neck, the quality of your voice will deteriorate.

Silence is an exceptionally powerful tool too. If it is used appropriately it allows the audience to consider the implications of what you have just said or to alert the audience to an important key message to follow. It gives variance to your talk. Silence can be used in your introduction, within the flow of your presentation or when answering questions.

Pace: You can have the best presentation in the world with the funkiest PowerPoint slides, but if you get the pace wrong, your presentation will be a disaster. Speech needs to be clear and spoken at a steady pace. The content of your talk may be obvious to you, but you need to allow your audience time to assimilate what you are saying and to understand any new concepts or ideas. Don't speed up unnecessarily. Allow time to pause, give your audience time to read chunks of text and use silence where appropriate. Nerves tend to affect how we speak, usually speeding up our diction. A gabbled presentation won't do you or your audience justice. Pace comes down to breathing. Try to maintain reasonably deep breaths. Shallow breaths, which just use your diaphragm, cause a rise in pitch and pace. If you feel this happening, use your abdominal muscles and inspire deeply before speaking. Sometimes it helps to place a hand on your abdomen and feel yourself breathing. Try this at home when you are practising your talk and feel the differences in your breathing as you change the pace of speech.

Top Tip: If you want to learn more about effective delivery, get a couple of DVDs from some of the great motivational speakers like Anthony Robbins and Paul McKenna to see how they do it. If you want to look specifically at posture and behaviour, turn the sound off and watch the DVD at double-speed.

Closing the session

This is a very important stage of your presentation. It is your opportunity to remind the audience of your main points with a summary, then answer questions or unresolved issues, and distribute a feedback form.

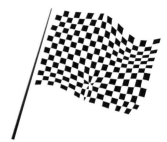

Summarise

At the end, thank the audience for attending and for paying attention. Give a summary of why your talk needed saying, what you have said and what you want your audience to remember or do as a result of attending, i.e. the key take-home message.

Question time

Listen carefully to the question then repeat the question out loud to the audience. This allows everyone in the room to be able to hear what is being asked and also gives you a few more moments of thinking time to mentally compose your response. You may want to reflect the question back to the audience, to get their opinion or thoughts (always worth doing especially if you feel stuck).

Feedback

Make sure you have enough feedback questionnaires for the numbers attending. Distribute them at the conclusion of your presentation. Ask for their opinion on both the *content* and *delivery* of your talk. A feedback questionnaire should include *some* of the following.

Feedback

- Was the content relevant to your work? If not, which areas?
- Was it pitched to your level?
- Which bits did you find most helpful? Why?
- Which bits did you not find helpful? Why?
- Is there anything you feel should be included or concentrated on next time?
- What should I do less of next time?
- Is there anything I do that irritates you, or that I should avoid in the future?
- As a result of this presentation, what will you do differently in your practice?

Top Tip: There are different types of evaluation forms available from our website. However, not all feedback has to be written. You could ask the audience for a few verbal responses. Alternatively, get them to respond in the form of a human bar chart. More ideas in Chapter 28: Reflection and Evaluation

IT'S IMPORTANT YOU ASK FOR SPECIFIC AND DESCRIPTIVE FEEDBACK . . .

'I really hope you have found today's session useful and enjoyable. Please would you pay a bit of attention to filling these feedback forms for me. I would like to know how I can do this session better the next time around, and I can only do that with your help. So, when you get these forms, try to be specific and descriptive. For instance, rather than saying 'that bit was great', tell me exactly what made that bit great. The same goes for what you didn't like *but* in addition give me a suggestion as to how I might do it differently. Does that make sense?'

Feedback is the breakfast of champions.[4] You cannot better yourself if you don't ask for feedback. If you want to become a master at presenting, you must get feedback to define what it is that you do well and what it is that you need to work on. All of this means that you need to be 'internally ready' and be willing to 'receive' the answers to the questions you ask. This is not an easy thing to do, but it gets easier with time.

A sample of resources on our website
- Some FAQs on Giving Presentations.
- Presenting well without nerves with NLP magic.
- Teaching plan templates with examples.
- Useful shortcut keys for PowerPoint.
- A collection of evaluation forms.

Essential reading
- Frank MO. *How to Get Your Point Across in 30 Seconds or Less*. Corgi; 1987.

Other chapters you may like to read
- Chapter 4: Powerful Hooks – aims, objectives and ILOs
- Chapter 6: Teaching from Scratch
- Chapter 8: Teaching Gems
- Chapter 13: Teaching and Facilitating Small Groups (many same principles apply)
- Chapter 14: How to Teach Large Groups.

Please give us some feedback on this chapter to help shape it for the next edition.
Go to www.essentialgptrainingbook.com and simply click on the title of this chapter.

References
1 Miller GA. The magical number seven, plus or minus two: some limits on our capacity for processing information. *Psychol Rev.* 1956; **63**(2): 81–97.
2 Baddeley AD. *Human Memory: theory and practice.* Hillsdale, New Jersey: Erlbaum; 1996.
3 Peyton J. *Teaching and Learning in Medical Practice.* Rickmansworth, UK: Manticore Europe Ltd; 1998. pp. 193–207.
4 Blanchard K, Tate R. *Feedback is the Breakfast of Champions.* Available at: http://howwelead.org/2009/08/17/feedback-is-the-breakfast-of-champions/ (accessed 21 February 2010).

PART SIX

Special Areas of Training

Using the Creative Arts

ROGER HIGSON – TPD (Northallerton)   ELAINE POWLEY – retired. Ex Course Organiser (Scarborough)
JOHN SALINSKY – TPD (Whittington)   MARION LYNCH – Associate GP Dean (Oxford Deanery)

What's this all about?

Teaching the knowledge, skills and attitudes it takes to be a competent general practitioner in 21st-century multicultural Britain is a daunting prospect, despite now having a curriculum to work to and well-defined competencies to achieve. One of the reasons is that much of what is important lies in the 'white space'[1] between the lines. (See our website for a fuller explanation of white space). Such white space makes the rest of the curriculum visible, but it is never mentioned itself. There is more to illness and disease than can be recognised, reduced and categorised through a biomedical lens. This is the humanity of medicine: what people are all about, why they feel the way they do about life, why and how they respond to these feelings, to other people, their families, friends and local communities and the events that have formed their view of reality.

Life for many patients is a pretty catastrophic happening, or at least it has got that way, by the time they come to see us. How can we possibly get our trainees to understand these important facets of being human? How can we teach them about fear, anger, jealousy and other destructive emotions? Many experienced GPs, in their search for the truth about a patient, are of course aware of and understand the influence and impact of these events through a lifetime of dealing with people and their 'messy' lives. How can this wealth of experience be captured and distilled into a moment? What is needed is a different way of looking at the experience of illness and medical intervention.

A very good and exciting way is to call upon the experts at describing human behaviour. Writers, artists, playwrights, film makers, poets and music makers have the means of capturing and portraying life at its most painful. They have the ability to analyse, diagnose and portray the many kinds of pain that arise within us or are inflicted on us, including the pain of existence.

What we plan to cover

Narratives	Literature	Art and image (including sculpture)	Film and poetry

We will show you how these can be used to enhance teaching and learning; but first we need to lay down some guiding principles.

How to structure a session using an arts resource in easy stages

In their book *The Arts in Medical Education: a practical guide*, Powley and Higson[2] lay the ground rules for teaching with the arts. You will see that the structure is very simple and easy to apply.

How to structure an arts session

1 Have a **clear educational aim**.
2 **Design the exercise** to enable trainees to experience the ideas and feeling you are trying to elicit.
3 **Select a resource** appropriate for the exercise.
4 **Achieve engagement** – present the material in a stimulating and creative way.
5 **Facilitate responses**.
6 **Apply** what has been explored to personal and professional development.
7 **Evaluate** the exercise.

Narratives: the stories patients tell

All patients have a story to tell, in which they try to make sense of their lives and what's happening to them. The telling about events gives meaning to experience. Using patient narratives can even be thought of as harnessing their own creativity. Reflection using these stories can expose contradictions and challenge the GP to look at situations from new perspectives, thereby gaining additional insights to facilitate new ways of responding.

The narrative approach, advocated by Launer,[3] brings patient care, reflection and GP education together. Such educational activity can reach the attitudes and behaviours other approaches cannot reach. It can move mindsets,[4] and help trainees cope with uncertainty.

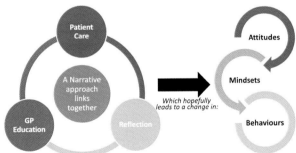

HERE'S A *NARRATIVE* EXERCISE WE HAVE USED

- Programme Directors explained complexity theory (handout available on our website) and then outlined the aims of the project, using simple rules in line with complexity approaches.
- Each trainee, on discussion with the Trainer and practice, chose a patient with a long-term condition (LTC) with whom they could work on the project.
- They then gave a camera to the patient they had selected and asked them to take pictures of the people who looked after them.
- The patient returned the camera to the trainee, who then created an illustrated narrative of the patient's life by making a poster using the photographs and minimal text.
- The posters were designed individually, printed professionally and then displayed to Trainers and peers as a narrative of the patients' lives (rather than a case presentation), using a story approach to sharing of pictures and personal learning.

- Facilitation included challenging assumptions made by trainees about patients and allowed for reflection throughout the group discussion.
- Learning was evaluated through open discussion and a reflection log in trainees' ePortfolios.
- Consent was gained from all those who took part in the project. Where the photographs were to be displayed was made clear to all from the start.

 Red Alert: It is crucial to note that patient involvement in GP education must not be a burden to the patient. In this example, families and neighbours were happy to be involved and some wanted their posters back.

What was learnt?

The project created a space where the role of the GP could be explored. Trainees created a safe learning environment where they explored their own prejudices and assumptions.

- The trainees acknowledged that in order to understand the patient perspective and therefore provide excellent care, *'you need to be involved to get the insight into their needs'* (GP trainee). They recognised that unconscious judgements biased their interpretation of patient behaviour.
- They became aware of the insignificance of the GP in some posters and the significance of family, friends and neighbours unrecorded in any care pathway or patient notes.
- Reflection and discussion using photographs taken by patients allowed trainees to gain an understanding that a patient's expectation of how their LTC was managed was as individual as the trainees.
- They realised that they were all different and knowledge was not universal – when it came to mapping aspects of the exercise to GP competencies:
  - Holism to one GP trainee was the whole team involved in care, to another it was a patient's whole life.
  - Community Orientation to one was the GP coordinating care through the Multi Disciplinary Team (MDT), to another it was the patient coordinating their care through networks, possibly including the MDT.
- Holism and Community Orientation domains can be displayed and discussed with patients, peers and partners and then reflected on individually in portfolios.
- Mindsets can be made visible through the design of the posters and discussion of the process and content. When such mindsets are made visible, they can be acknowledged, challenged and if appropriate changed.
- The posters highlighted that sometimes what cannot be explained can be displayed.

The final verdict

We hope you can see how this educational activity:
1 explored and explained complexity
2 brought the patient into GP education
3 reached parts of the curriculum which are otherwise difficult to access, and
4 explored the impact of personal belief systems on the interpretation of the patient's story.

The process and discussion provide a new experience for the trainees. Through this new experience, they develop new language and therefore new thoughts. Such activity not only builds their capability to connect with patients, it also builds language capital. Together this builds their communication skills, perhaps their ability to share decision-making and develop the skills needed to come to an understanding with people. By expanding language, thoughts and insights, they may begin to *'recognise the value of what is left out or neutered by the authorised biomedical narrative forms'*.[5]

 Top Tip: Try to formulate exercises which look at things from the patient's perspective. Other examples of narrative exercises for you to try are described by Powley and Higson.[2]

Literature: read any good books lately?

John Salinsky is an acknowledged expert on the use of literature in GP trainee teaching and is well known through 'The Green Bookshop' in the 'Education for Primary Care' journal. He will now give us a 'how to do it' tutorial using a series of questions and answers.

Q. What is the point of trying to teach literature to trainee doctors (and nurses)?

A. GPs (and nurses) spend much of their time listening to patients and trying to understand them. I believe that the classics of literature have more to teach us about the human condition that any number of textbooks. The great writers have insights into human relationships, which are powerful and memorable. They are able to create characters that become a permanent part of the reader's inner world. Speaking for myself, I find that when I am in the surgery, a patient will frequently remind me of a character from Dickens or Tolstoy. This recognition of an old friend from literature helps to make me:

- more tolerant of eccentricity
- better able to cope with negative emotions, and
- quicker to find something likeable in a difficult personality.

To put it another way, it increases my capacity for empathy. That has to be good, doesn't it? I wanted to share this discovery with my trainees, and my experience has been that they appreciate the inclusion of a study of literature in the teaching programme.

Q. What else might literature do for GPs?

A. Doctors are deprived of a proper education in literature by the narrow specialisation of our education system. They may never open a 19th or 20th-century novel because they are afraid it will be too difficult. As a result, they are in danger of missing out on an important source of **pleasure and spiritual refreshment** for the rest of their lives. Serious reading encourages an interest in **language and narrative**, which also fosters better understanding of what our patients are saying. The close reading of a text can be as revealing as the close study of a patient. Finally, discussing a great book and analysing its layers of meaning helps to develop **clarity of thought and expression**.

Q. Wouldn't you have to be an expert in literature to facilitate it?

A. *No*, that might be a disadvantage. The key ingredient is to enjoy reading literature yourself. Having an enthusiast to help you run the session is a bonus.

Q. Do you use extracts or whole books?

A. *Always whole books!* In my view, the proper appreciation of literature requires reading the whole thing. Long books can be a bit daunting for some of our trainees, and it's true that they have lots of other work to do. So, in our course, we prescribe a mixture of long and short books with more time given to read the long ones.

Q. What sort of books?

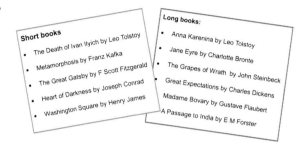

Short books
- The Death of Ivan Ilyich by Leo Tolstoy
- Metamorphosis by Franz Kafka
- The Great Gatsby by F Scott Fitzgerald
- Heart of Darkness by Joseph Conrad
- Washington Square by Henry James

Long books:
- Anna Karenina by Leo Tolstoy
- Jane Eyre by Charlotte Bronte
- The Grapes of Wrath by John Steinbeck
- Great Expectations by Charles Dickens
- Madame Bovary by Gustave Flaubert
- A Passage to India by E M Forster

Q. What about modern books?

A. Yes of course, we include them too. But only if they are really well written 'literary' novels rather than 'popular' novels.

> **Modern novels**
>
> - Engleby by Sebastian Faulks
> - Saturday by Ian McEwan
> - The White Tiger by Aravind Adiga

Q. What's the difference?

A. Briefly, a popular novel may tell a good story and be very entertaining. It may even be very moving. However, a literary novel has greater depth. You may want to read it more than once, and you find new things in it with each reading. Its language is likely to be more poetic, more evocative of sights, sounds and emotions; more revealing about its characters' states of mind.

Q. Shouldn't we give our learners novels with a strong medical theme?

A. Not necessarily! In fact, in some ways it's better if they are not medical. The aim is to give the learners a new and effective way to tune in to all aspects of human life and relationships. Nevertheless, a story about a doctor or a patient may be a good way to begin, as the learners will feel they are on familiar territory. A good example is Tolstoy's *The Death of Ivan Ilyich*, a short novel that deals with the subjective experience of coming to terms with death. In any case doctors are so important to us that they are constantly creeping in at the margins of most novels, even if they are not given a starring role.

Q. OK. Suppose I want to give literature a try. How do I start?

A. I'll tell you what we do in our course to give you an idea.

- Before the beginning of the term, the Programme Directors choose our 'set book'. We listen to suggestions from the trainees, but we veto the kind of best-seller that is not written to a high literary standard. We go mainly for classics, which the trainees might otherwise never read or even know about.

- Then we buy a shipload of books from Amazon and give everyone a copy. This literal 'ownership' of the book is much appreciated.
- Towards the end of the term, we have a session of 90 minutes devoted to discussing the book.

Q. How do you facilitate a good discussion?
A. We supply some notes, which consist of a brief introduction to the book and its author, followed by some open questions for discussion. The trainees can use this as a guide while they are reading. When the session starts, we usually divide the trainees into three small groups. We may ask each group to look at the book from a different angle. For instance, with Jane Eyre, we asked each group to look at one of the three sections into which the book is divided: beginning, middle and ending. With Kafka's story *Metamorphosis*, the groups looked at: (1) The story as literature, (2) The medical metaphor (in which Gregor's transformation into an insect can be regarded as the onset of a chronic illness), (3) The relationship between the story and Kafka's own life. There is no single way to do it. There is no such thing as 'correctness' in using the arts in medical teaching. One of the joys is to be able **to think widely and creatively and incorporate new ideas in your teaching**.

Q. How do you actually structure the discussion?
A. The small groups have about 45 minutes for their discussion. Each group elects someone to take notes and feedback. We then get together and each group representative reports on its discussion with comments from other members. Finally, we have a general discussion which can range more widely.

Themes to use in the discussion of a book

- Characters: liked and disliked
- Similarity to patients
- Can you feel empathy for a flawed or dysfunctional character?
- How people see themselves
- Hidden aspects of personality
- Relationships between lovers, parents and children, friends, enemies
- Power relationships and exploitation
- Performance of the doctor characters
- Ethical conflicts
- Styles of writing
- Metaphors.

 Top Tip: If you'd like to give literature a try, why not start with Tolstoy's novel, *The Death of Ivan Ilyich*. To help you, there's a guidance sheet on our website. This details some specific questions that we have used when discussing this book.

Q. I bet they don't all read the book!
A. Quite true, they don't. Some will read the whole thing. Some will have gotten about halfway or a little more. Some will have read only a few pages. And a few will not even have started. We are not discouraged, and we emphasise that **everyone will get something out of the discussion session**

no matter how little they have read. Our hope is that, after the discussion, those who have read a little will be interested enough to read more. The fact that they have a copy of the book means that they may take it down from the shelf at any time in the future and start reading it, with our discussion in mind. This is a long game.

Q. Do you do any evaluation? How do you know whether your sessions are enjoyed or merely tolerated? Do people learn anything?
A. Here's some feedback we had from the session on *The Death of Ivan Ilyich*.

'I really enjoy the book discussion sessions – in fact, they're my favourite VTS sessions. However, it is quite frustrating when half the group hasn't read the book. I think there is still quite a barrier to reading books that are perceived to be difficult or old-fashioned. Some people feel that their lives are too busy for books, which is such a shame.'

'I think Ivan Ilyich was a worthwhile read because Tolstoy is such a talented writer – it's a privilege to read his work. I can't say I enjoyed the book, but that's not to say I didn't value it. That's because of the nature of the subject and characters. I think considering what may have inspired authors to write is a fantastic way of stoking up our curiosity in other people's lives.'

'I was able to feel the characters' experiences and also to be an observer who is invited to reflect on those "big issues". I found the discussion really enhanced my appreciation of the book and provoked lots more thoughts. I'm certain that reading and discussing the book had an impact on me and will inform how I deal with such patients in the future.'

'I didn't get round to reading the book but I enjoyed the discussion. I am definitely going to read it now and thanks for giving us all a copy.'

So, there you have it. Looks easy doesn't it? Why not give it a go.

 Top Tip: Always read the book thoroughly yourself and make notes. *Be prepared*!

The visual arts – how we see things

It is now time to think about what happens when we look at something (or somebody), and to consider how to use visual images such as pictures, photographs and sculpture in GP training. Artists have the ability to observe, capture and record what they see. **Art is a sort of shorthand which endeavours to portray everything about a moment in a single image.** The artist has the need to express their reaction to things and people around them, tell stories, and create an explanation of a feeling. We can then relive what they have expressed by looking at their paintings, which are a permanent record that can be returned to time after time. Trainee GPs need to understand as much as they can about human behaviour and how people, including themselves, respond to situations perhaps outside their normal environment. **Your aim is to facilitate their emerging ideas and observations that the artworks have released, and then help them look at applying this in everyday medical work.**

How do we teach using art? To help trainees use art to understand the chaotic world as presented to them in the surgery, there are three basic principles to apply:

General principles for teaching using the visual arts

1 Looking at pictures helps to develop **observational skills**. Observation means looking in detail, and then describing what is seen and interpreting that image. We learn so much by just looking at our patients and their immediate environment and relationships. We are alert to visual clues and cues and subconsciously record their facial expression, what they are wearing, their general demeanour and any manifestation of, for example, old age, infirmity or illness. This **skill** can be practised by looking at pictures and photographs, which are, in effect, a 'stilled narrative'. So a basic question to ask is:

    'What do you see?'

2 Images usually provoke **feelings and emotions**, i.e. our inner response to what we see. The interpretation of art is essentially subjective – it is the observer's response which is important. Trainees experience feelings when confronted by all sorts of events. They often need help in recognising them and reflecting on them (their learning logs have helped in this regard). The next question to ask is:

    'What does the image make you feel and how do you respond to those feelings?'

3 Trainees want all their learning to be **relevant to their work**. So the next challenge is to bring them back into their world. Ask:

    'How can what you have seen, how you have felt, and your response be applied to your everyday life as a GP?'

A specific example – a visit to an art gallery

You will have near you an art gallery, or art museum. They make wonderful classrooms. Take a group there; leave them individually to wander and look, choosing a painting to talk about to the rest of the group, when you gather again.

Before the visit	During the visit
How are you going to direct their visual thinking, and what are you hoping to achieve? It is often a good idea to have a preliminary discussion about visual thinking – when we describe events or hear the description of an event we have a vivid mental picture, we 'see' the narrative.	You will find that as the group looks at a painting that one of them has chosen, individually they will have seen different things in it. Here are three basic questions that they can think about as they look at the art: 1 What do I see and feel? 2 How do I respond to that? 3 What can I learn from detailed observation that is relevant to me and my work? Then get them to think themselves back in their surgeries and ask: 1 What do you see and respond to in the consulting room, as you are listening to a patient's narrative? 2 What visual cues and information do you acknowledge and give value to in your diagnostic deliberations?

Think about using art resources for topic teaching in the medical curriculum

Trainees need biological knowledge about an illness and its effects, but also need to understand something about the experience for the patient of the illness, their beliefs and expectations. Looking at a painting depicting, for example, old age, or a sick child, can extend the trainee's holistic comprehension of disease states. Use the following three basic questions to facilitate and aid this understanding:

1　What do you **see and feel**?
2　How do you **respond** to that?
3　What can you learn from detailed observation that is **relevant to you and your work**?

Trainees are used to the idea of images in the form of X-rays and CT scans, which relay information about structures. They give value to what they see, comprehending as a result more about the patient's illness. Images in works of art can provide another dimension as a resource for information gathering and thus good patient management.

How others see us or what patients see

Doctors are often portrayed in art. Artists paint doctors who have treated them.[6] Look at this BMJ article (Park MP, Park RHR. The fine art of patient-doctor relationships. *BMJ*. 2004; **329**: 1475–80) to see: Goya's portrait of Dr Arrieta, Van Gogh's portraits of Dr Rey and Dr Gachet, and Munch's portraits of Dr Jacobsen.

EXERCISE: WHEN DOCTORS ARE PORTRAYED IN ART

Get trainees to look at some pictures where doctors are portrayed in art. Discuss the following:
1　What do these pictures tell us about how we are seen as doctors?
2　How is the doctor–patient relationship depicted?

Artists may also depict medical scenes, catching the drama of the event, the colours and shapes and faces, and **in looking at such works we can step outside the frame**, see the whole and perhaps get a better knowledge about ourselves. These pictures may give insights into the physicians' role in society. One of the most famous pictures is Sir Luke Fildes' painting entitled *The Doctor* (1891) – which you can see at www.tate.org.uk. It shows a doctor attending a sick child and demonstrates the importance of *'just being there'* – illustrating care and compassion. Other examples can be found in *Medicine and Art* by Alan and Marcia Emery.[7] Explore these pictures with your trainees and see if they gain any insights into themselves as doctors or into the very practice of medicine itself.

Self-portraits – doctors and patients as actors

Consider these questions with your trainees:

SELF-PORTRAITS 1

1　How do doctors choose to represent themselves to their patients and colleagues?
　　As a profession, especially in general practice, where our interaction with our patients is one to one, we are looked at all the time. What image of ourselves do we choose to project? How do we dress? How do we behave? What body language do we use?
2　Conversely, how do patients try to tell us things about themselves by the way they dress, talk, or behave?

Numerous artists have painted self-portraits, and these are a wonderful teaching resource with which to explore these concepts. The Phaidon art book of *500 Self Portraits*[8] is a good starting point. Get the trainee to pick a few from these and look at them one by one then use the simple questions to start a discussion about the resulting ideas.

SELF-PORTRAITS 2

1   What do you see and feel? What is the artist trying to say?
2   How do you respond?
3   What can you learn about yourself? (i.e. If you were the artist, how would you paint yourself? What image would you show?)

Help! I just don't get this art thing!

Many readers will be daunted at the prospect of using resources with which they are uncomfortable and out of their depth! **Of the many books on art and art appreciation, John Berger's book *Ways of Seeing*[9] is a great starting point**. This book demystifies art appreciation and really does explore how we look at and interpret things. Another common worry is how on earth you find pictures to use. The answer to this is to visit art galleries either in reality or virtually on the Internet. There are many wonderful exhibitions in galleries in the UK and abroad.

 Top Tip: Using the visual arts – anyone can do it, just stick to simple rules. And it's not about art appreciation. It's about using the art to understand our lives.

Sculpture – shapes and textures

This might be considered by many trainees to be a rather 'too exclusive' an art form to have any relevance to clinical medicine. However, it can be demystified by careful facilitation and reassurance that the exercise is not one of 'art appreciation'. (The exploration of negative feelings can itself be a useful learning exercise – see the section on using film). Using sculpture as a teaching resource provides a further opportunity for exploring the process of seeing (observing), interpreting and responding. **Sculptures have the added dimension of ambiguity** – they demand attention, awaken curiosity and pose the question: *'What does this mean?'* This is highly resonant with our daily experience in the consulting room. How do we make that connection?

Teaching using sculpture

Task the learners to look and touch the sculptures and think about the following metaphors.

* What they see when they look at a sculpture:
    * What is the sculptor (patient) trying to tell me and how?
    * *What do the sculptures (patients) make me feel?*
    * *How do I respond?*
* What they feel when they touch a sculpture:
    * What information are they acquiring through their hands/fingers? (Clinical medicine is much less 'tactile' these days; this important sensory information gets forgotten.)
    * *Are they happy touching the sculptures (patients)?* (May unearth cultural differences).

The exercise can be made more exciting by giving the groups cameras on which to record their experiences and then present their findings to the whole group as a narrative. A group visiting the Yorkshire Sculpture Park viewed Barbara Hepworth's sculptures entitled *The family of Man* as a representation of the members of their own practice teams and used this as a basis to explore the question of hierarchy and power within the team.

Top Tip: With sculpture, never forget the tactile bit!

Using film – a trip to the movies

Film (seen on DVD or in the cinema) is now an established teaching resource in both under-graduate and postgraduate medical education. Film is a comfortable and familiar medium that readily engages most trainees. When used as clips, they only demand a short attention span. They usually provoke good discussion, with assessment of values, and of self if the scenes have a strong emotional content.[10] Films can be used to:

- explore doctors' behaviours: illustrating both good and bad communication skills
- illustrate patients' narratives: giving insight into the patient's perspective of healthcare, i.e. what it is like to be on the receiving end of medical care (two French films: *The Officers Ward* and *The Diving Bell and the Butterfly* are filmed as if the patient is holding the camera)
- portray the psychosocial aspects of medical care and illustrate compassion and empathy
- illustrate different cultures
- explore humour
- explore the use of metaphor (see also poetry section) and symbolism
- teach analytical skills, e.g. how film-makers have achieved a particular effect
- develop skills of observation: to look at what is on the surface and what lies underneath (e.g. body language and tone of voice may contradict the story being told).

 Top Tip: Film clips are often better than whole films.

How do we teach using film?

As with all teaching, the environmental setting must be conducive to learning.

Teaching with film

1. Start with the classroom

Select a room which is:
- Adequately ventilated, free of clutter and quiet.
- Has video/DVD/projection equipment all working nicely – check this before the session!

2. Have a clear aim

- A clear educational aim like *looking at communication skills with adolescents*.
- A clear idea of why an arts resource will be the most effective way of delivering the session. You should be using it as a way into feelings, perceptions and ideas of the group about a particular topic.

3. Find and select a resource

- Think about its relevance to the personal and professional development on the topic that you plan to explore. In particular, think about:
  1. Diversity of human behaviour and personality
  2. Culture and environment
  3. Life events
  4. Communication
- Think about what responses it might engender.
- Think how you might awaken insights and foster enthusiasm in the learner.

4. Design an exercise using the chosen film clip

- Be creative and imaginative. Develop exercises which:
  1. *Encourage reflection* and
  2. *Focus on feelings, beliefs and ideas.*

5. Define the task and achieve engagement

- **Caution:** some films provoke an unexpected emotional response. Remember that trainees will themselves have had traumatic experiences in the past and watching a film can bring extreme emotions to the surface. Should your intro to the film carry a health warning?
- If showing an extract, give a brief 'the story so far . . .' Do not reveal what you want the learners to perceive for themselves.
- Try to present the material with enthusiasm and passion. Otherwise engagement will not occur. Remember that some participants will take time to awaken to the idea and usefulness of creative arts in medical education before they go into action. In contrast, others may show an immediate response and engage in it effortlessly.
- Guide the learners and get them thinking along these lines:
  1. *What did you see?*
  2. *What did you hear?*
  3. *What did you feel?*
  4. *What did you think?*
  5. *What impact does all of this have on your practice?*

6. Facilitate responses (*Many people find that this is the difficult bit*)

- When the extract/film finishes, there is usually total silence as people are still absorbed in the film. Don't worry – just wait a bit while everyone comes back to the present. (Use your consultation skills to cope with the silence.) This is a very important moment.
- Start with a non-specific open question on first thoughts.
  — *'Does anyone have any thoughts on what you've just seen and heard?'*
- Ask more specific questions.
  — *'What is it about?'* This is a non-threatening way of questioning their understanding.
  — *'What does this do for you?'* This begins the exploration of feelings and emotions.
  — *'What does this remind you of?'* This promotes discussion of the learners' own previous experience that the film may remind them of and new intuitions.
- Ask what elicited these replies – *'What was the film-maker trying to portray?'*
- When emotions and feelings are being expressed, encourage reflection.
  — *'I'm wondering what it was in the film that made you feel so strongly about what you've just said.'*
- Encourage and rehearse suggestions. If the film has doctor–patient interaction, try saying:
  — *'If you were the doctor, how would you have approached this situation? Pretend that I'm the patient – what would you say?'*
- While you are doing all this don't forget to read your audience:
  — Look out for verbal and non-verbal cues (just like in a consultation).
  — Acknowledge feelings but remember to clarify their meaning where necessary.
  — Develop any ideas or themes that are produced.
- Unexpected responses – don't forget that the group may sometimes produce ideas which you may not have even thought of. You must work with what you are given, and such ideas should not be ignored just because they don't follow your agenda. You might say:
  — *'That is new to me. You're taking me down a path I had not seen. Tell me more.'*
- Encourage reflection on the application of what they have just seen, and discuss its relevance to their own learning and to situations they encounter with real patients.
  — *'So what insights has this given us in our work with patients?'*
  — *'What differences will all this make to the way we work with patients?'*

7. Feedback and evaluation

Try to get some feedback (this obviously applies to any teaching session!). Ask for:
- Comments about the teaching session itself – the contents, the resources used, the quality of presentation, the style of the teacher and group work.

- Reflection about the personal experience of the learner – the overall feelings, opportunities for active participation, discovering learning needs, any changed perspectives, their own development, insights gained and relevance to the work.

You may want to encourage them to do this in a narrative way (e.g. a reflective diary). Feedback is also useful for the learners in that it helps them to consolidate and summarise the learning: **to give meaning to the experience** from the session they have just undertaken.

Which films are suitable educational resources?

The answer to that question may be any film, as most are about human beings/human behaviour and that is what we are trying to teach! They don't have to be about doctors.

RESOURCES WHICH LIST SOME USEFUL FILMS

- Memel has written a comprehensive how to do it tool, with examples and synopses of films to use.[11]
- Cinemeducation: a comprehensive guide to using film in medical education[12] is another useful resource when looking for film material to illustrate a range of medical conditions and encounters.
- Powley and Higson[2] also give some suggestions about films to use for particular topics and include a worked example using 'An Angel at my Table'.
- The New York University Medical School Literature, Arts and Medicine Database[13] is a wonderful online topic searchable database of humanities resources including film.
- Read 'Sight and Sound' magazine – which gives a synopsis of every film and DVD release.
- Read film/DVD reviews in the media.
- Television programmes about doctors (the medical 'soaps') are another resource that can be used to explore medical 'behaviours'.

Examples of films

- *The Death of Mr Lazarescu* (significant events and professionalism)
- *The Diving Bell and the Butterfly* (communication skills, disability and empathy)
- *The Piano* (communication skills)
- *Officers' Ward* (the patient perspective and communication)
- *The History Boys* (teaching and learning).

What about taking trainees to the theatre?

Film is perhaps the most accessible and universal arts resource to use in medical teaching. And it lies within most trainees' comfort zones. Equally valuable but requiring more bravery and organisation is a trip to the theatre – to see live drama being acted out on stage. Take them to see:

Examples of theatre

- *Macbeth* with its multi-layered themes of trust and betrayal, fear, greed and power, madness vs badness, and guilt.
- *King Lear* to learn about dementia and families.
- *Henry V* to find out about leadership.

And that's just Shakespeare – nearly all plays, like films, are about being human and that is what our trainees have to learn. This seems a good moment to repeat the following:

For a successful educational session using any arts resource

1 Have a **clear educational aim**. *What are you trying to achieve? It's usually about finding a way into feelings, perceptions and ideas of the group about a particular topic.*
2 Think about the **responses** it might engender.
3 Make it **relevant**. *All GP trainees want something they can map to a curriculum topic or competence.*

Poetry – is this a step too far?

Working with poems allows us to consider how closer attention to words can improve our understanding of the views and experiences of others, which may be very different from our own. They also help us to consider our emotional experiences and even public events, which have marked people's lives. In addition, analysing poems is useful for thinking about the language within a consultation, which often contains ambiguity, with hints of the patient's emotional experience, and is sometimes expressed as a metaphor. The interpretation of poetry demands imagination and insight. Poetry finds the form of words to tell of events we cannot measure, and which are difficult to explain or understand.

Does poetry therefore have a place in GP trainee curriculum?

Salinsky[14] worries that there is no proof that the appreciation of poetry or painting make people better doctors; the end points of using poetry as a teaching resource are hard to get hold of. Foster[15] has identified relevance to personal development and professional practice by enabling discussion of emotional issues and enabling empathy, which will enhance doctor–patient relationships.

Here's a good starting point . . .

'What is poetry?' or 'What constitutes a poem?'

There is really no answer to this question, but skilfully managed discussion can demystify what at first sight is a daunting subject. RS Thomas's poem 'Don't ask me . . .'[16] could be used to help the discussion if you get stuck. Be aware that many trainees will have had very little experience of reading poems and may have been quite put off at school.

How to run an educational session using poetry (*Foster,*[15] *Powley and Higson*[2])

1 Before the session – three set-up questions

1. Are the poems to be selected by the facilitator or by the participants? If the latter it is always a good idea to have some in reserve!
2. Should the poems be read aloud during the actual session?
3. Have you made several copies of each poem available to distribute?

2A At the start of the session – survey the learners' starting point

Ask participants:
- about their previous experience of poetry
- how they feel about this session
- whether anyone has ever written any poetry
- what they consider is the relevance of poetry in their education, e.g. which curriculum heading(s) or competence(s) might be covered.

2B At the start of the session – give trainees reassurance

Make the following points:
- The session will not be about literary criticism.
- No prior poetic knowledge is needed.
- There is no right or wrong way of reading or listening to a poem. Any poem can be interpreted in more than one way. Poetry, like much of art, is subjective.
- It is all about individuals' response to the poems which is important.
- Reading poetry should give pleasure. It should not be a penance.

3 The trainee guidance sheet

a Read the poems, either to yourself or out loud, and several times – it often aids understanding.
b Use imagination if bits are unclear.
c Ask yourself these questions:
- *What is it about? (getting started)*
- *Whose voice are you hearing?*
- *What feelings/emotions does it evoke in you?(exploring emotional response)*
- *What images or memories does it evoke?*
- *What metaphors does the poet use?*
- *What is the poet saying?*
- *What is the meaning of the poem or of certain lines or phrases?*
- *What do you like about it?*
- *Is there anything in the poem which helps you see something in a new light?*
- *Are there any echoes in the poem from your own experience?*
- *What is enjoyable about the poem?*

4 The facilitator guidance sheet

a Ask why they think the poem has been chosen.
b Watch participants for non-verbal cues.
c Use prompts, which amplify the questions you have already suggested above.
d Follow up with open questions to elicit expansion of ideas and reflection on personal feelings.
e Have some additional questions, e.g. about the meaning of some words in a particular poem; why a poem works or is difficult, in case the discussions get stuck.

In all this, two points above all are worth emphasising:
- Metaphor* often appears in patient narratives.
- Attention to a patient's individual words/phrases can lead to clearer insights into their thoughts, feelings and emotional states.

*A metaphor is a literary figure of speech that uses an image, story or tangible thing to represent a less tangible thing or some intangible quality or idea. It comes from the Greek word metapherin meaning 'transfer'. Examples: 'you are my **sunshine**', 'he **broke into** her conversation', 'he was dressed in a **loud** checked shirt'. A simile is slightly different. Both similes and metaphors link one thing to another. A simile usually uses 'as' or 'like'. Example: 'your eyes are like the sun', 'he lives like a pig'. Mixed metaphors are best avoided – the awkward use of two or more different metaphors at the same time. It creates conflicting images in the reader or listener's mind, reduces each metaphor's impact, and generally causes confusion (www.englishclub.com).*

Any suggestions for sourcing suitable poems?

The choice is huge. There are many anthologies available as well as poetry websites. It is probably best to start with poems about medicine (the first two in the resource list below). It is always a good idea to ask trainees to bring poems of their own choosing but guide them to bring ones which are interesting, moving, uplifting, intriguing, amusing, profound, challenging, affirming, insightful or ambiguous. And don't forget, poems can of course be used in topic teaching. Examples include teaching about old age, body image, disability and adolescence (cited by Powley and Higson[2]).

FINDING GOOD POETRY
A good starting place are two collections:
- 'The poetry cure' – a themed collection of poems, edited by Julia Darling and Cynthia Fuller[17]
- 'Playing God, poems about medicine' by Glenn Colquhoun,[18] a GP in New Zealand.

There are also online resources to tap into:
- The Poetry Society[19]
- The Poetry Archive[20]
- Academy of American Poets[21]
- Favourite Poem Project[22]
- Poem Hunter[23]
- The New York University Literature, Arts and Medicine Database[13]
- Poems in the Waiting Room[24] (a charitable organisation which publishes fold up cards of poems for patients to read and keep – worth looking at the website for some interesting commentary on poetry).

And if you are still stuck you can always get Google to search for you!

Writing poems
This really might seem like a step too far, but doctors can surprise themselves that they can write poems. Powley and Higson[2] demonstrated this with a group of Trainers. Many of the four-line poems written provided powerful expressions of anxiety, inadequacy, vulnerability and emotional fatigue, which many doctors experience but are often reluctant to express. Feelings which can be dangerously buried can be brought to the surface in a poem which would/could not have been otherwise confronted and expressed.

More recently Albardiaz[25] asked trainees to write haiku (a three-line poem with 5, 7 and 5 syllables in corresponding lines, which is complete in itself and stating the heart of the matter) as an evaluation of the Half-Day Release course. These again highlighted the stresses doctors face and led to discussions on patient-centred care. It was also hoped that such writing would improve linguistic skills.

Maggie Eisner[26] describes a useful poetry writing exercise. This is quite a good exercise to do in a large group (to get a good variety of responses, although they don't all have to speak).

EXERCISE: I SEE. I HEAR. I FEEL
Set-up
- You will need a flip chart and pens and paper for everyone, and Post-it notes.
- Take care how you introduce it as telling them they are going to write poetry will make some of them feel like switching off, and raise the anxiety levels of others.

Step 1: Ask the group to get into pairs
Probably just with the person sitting next to them unless you can see a good reason for doing it a different way. Make sure they all have pens and paper.

Step 2: Ask them to think and write about a clinical encounter
- Think of a recent interesting patient encounter.

- Write the clinical note about it which they would put in the hospital notes or practice computer.
- Tell their partner all about what happened in the encounter (probably about 5 minutes each way).

Step 3: Writing the 'I see, I hear, and I feel' poem
Write the following phrases on the flip chart:
- I see . . .
- I hear . . .
- I feel . . .

Then explain that they are going to write about the consultation in a different way.
- Choose either their point of view or that of the patient.
- Write a poem with at least 3 lines, beginning with the 3 phrases on the flip chart.
- They can have as many lines as they like, but each line must begin with one of the 3 phrases.
- *Emphasise that 'I feel' should not be used in the sense 'I think'.* It should refer either to what you feel with your *emotions* or perceive with your *senses* ('I feel anxious', 'I feel cold' – not 'I feel the patient may have a connective tissue disorder').
- When they've composed the poem, transcribe the final version onto a Post-it note.
(Probably 10–15 minutes)

Step 4: Sharing what they've written
- Ask if anyone is willing to read out their poem. They may also like to read out the clinical note about the consultation.
- Ask the group to all stick their Post-it notes on the flip chart or on a wall.
- Give everyone time to look at the poems.

This is a variant of a narrative prose writing exercise in which the patient's medical record is taken as the starting point for thinking of the records we keep on patient encounters from their point of view and how it is very possible to gain insight into that encounter by writing from a different perspective. Two examples of poems written are shown below.

I see a young man who looks older than his years . . .
I hear a cry for help which has so far been ignored . . .
I feel uncertain and concerned.

I see beauty and elegance . . .
I see anxiety and fear . . .
I see vulnerable and damaged . . .
I hear maturity but insecurity . . .
I hear hopes and dreams for the future . . .
I hear fear of doctors and men . . .
I feel angry
I feel responsible
I feel sorrow.

Many of the poems express the uncertainties and anxieties felt by doctors (and experienced by patients), which might otherwise have remained unsaid. Those written from the patient perspective are a powerful vehicle for **demonstrating empathy**. The exercise can be a very useful starting point to discuss that we all have feelings and emotions, which may be unlocked as part of our response to what happens during a consultation.

 Top Tip: Poetry is relevant and helps to understand metaphor and language in the consultation.

What to do when trainees *don't* want to engage in a session using the arts?

Some participants will be concrete thinkers – but we think that the arts are very good at breaking up the concrete. They will state they can't see the relevance of the session.

- *'I can't see why watching a feature film has anything to do with medicine.'*
- *'I mean it's just someone's idea, and it might not have been like that at all.'*
- *'It's a waste of time when there is so much else to get my head around and learn.'*

These responses are often a defensive reaction on the learner's part to an **unknown world**. Try to see it from their perspective. Whenever any of us does anything new for the first time, it usually feels uncomfortable (remember your first driving lesson?). And we like to revert to our 'comfort zone' (*'Thank goodness that first driving lesson's over'*). What might at first seem like a failure of imagination, a lack of curiosity, a lack of desire to see an alternative view or being preoccupied with the facts they are accustomed to using may just be a reflection of wanting to revert to their comfort zone. The facilitator has to penetrate sensitively if they wish to change such attitudes. Such attitudes are worth changing – they form that 'blind spot' of Johari's Window where you know it's good for them, although they can't see it . . . just yet.

How can the facilitator deal with this, and not get stuck?

The following approaches may help the 'dissenter' to start thinking laterally and to the facilitator by appreciating that person's learning needs.

1 Recognise your own sense of exasperation at this apparently blinkered naive thinking and neutralise your feelings.
2 Do not getting caught up in the confrontational and aggressive nature of the learner's statement by responding in a similar fashion.
3 Get them to see the value of **new** methods by using their previous experience of something **new**. *'You said you're having some difficulty finding any relevance of this new creative stuff to your work. It is an interesting point to consider. Can I ask you to consider something which you had to do for the first time that was also unfamiliar? How did you set about that? Was it worth it? So you didn't just abandon it then?'*
4 Engage other group members – get them to offer their thoughts and opinions. Use them to provide insight into the different ways of learning and how many things can be done in a number of ways, but with the same outcome.

Conclusion and caveats

We hope that these ideas will encourage you to cast away caution and have a go at teaching with the arts. Reluctance is usually based on the notion that, as teachers, we do not possess the knowledge and expertise to do this sort of teaching. We have given you some pointers about finding resources but most of us at the very least do read books and watch films, either on television or at the cinema.

Some of you will have noticed teacher-centredness about the choice of arts resources, but it is good practice to encourage trainees to suggest and bring their own resources to this sort of teaching. Most of the books, poems, films and art mentioned in this chapter are firmly rooted in Western culture and may not always seem so relevant to doctors from other cultures despite the universality of human suffering. Having resources from other cultures can only provide further enlightenment.

However, what we have described works and is enjoyable to do. Watch Alan Bennett's play *The History Boys* (film version is available on DVD) and see how the eccentric Mr Hector takes teaching and learning onto a different level by breaking out of the conventional mould. Be bold; light the fire under the knowledge pot of learning.

A sample of resources on our website
- Diversity through images.
- Notes on *The Death of Ivan Ilyich*.
- An Explanation of White Space.

Other chapters you may like to read
- Chapter 30: Quality – how good are we? – especially the qualitative vs quantitative debate.

Please give us some feedback on this chapter to help shape it for the next edition.
Go to www.essentialgptrainingbook.com and simply click on the title of this chapter.

References
1 Maletz MC, Nohria N. Managing in the whitespace. *Harv Bus Rev.* 2001; **79**(2): 103–11.
2 Powley E, Higson R. *The Arts in Medical Education: a practical guide.* Oxford: Radcliffe Publishing; 2005.
3 Launer J. *Narrative-based Primary Care: a practical guide.* Oxford: Radcliffe Publishing; 2002.
4 Gosling J, Mintzberg H. Management education as if both matter. *Management Learning.* 2006; **37**(4): 419–28.
5 Morris DB. Narrative medicine; challenge and resistance. *TPJ.* 2008; **12**(1): 88–96.
6 Park MP, Park RHR. The fine art of patient-doctor relationships. *BMJ.* 2004; **329**: 1475–80.
7 Emery A, Emery M. *Medicine and Art.* London: Royal College of Physicians; 2003.
8 Bell J. *500 Self Portraits.* London: Phaidon Press; 2000.
9 Berger J. *Ways of Seeing.* London: Penguin; 1972. p. 7.
10 Champoux JE. Film as a teaching resource. *J Management Enquiry.* 1999; **8**(2): 240–51.
11 Memel D, Raby P, Thompson T. Doctors in the movies: a user's guide to teaching about film and medicine. *Educ Prim Care.* 2009; **20**: 304–8.
12 Alexander M, Lenahan P, Pavlov A. *Cinemeducation: a comprehensive guide to using film in medical education.* Oxford: Radcliffe Publishing; 2005.
13 http://litmed.med.nyu.edu
14 Salinsky J. Commentary: art for whose sake? Some thoughts about poetry in the curriculum. *Educ Prim Care.* 2007; **18**: 683–4.
15 Foster W. Should poetry be included in the curriculum for specialty registrars? *Educ Prim Care.* 2007; **18**: 712–23.
16 Thomas RS. *Residues.* Tarset: Bloodaxe Books; 2002.
17 Darling J, Fuller C. *The Poetry Cure.* Tarset: Bloodaxe Books; 2005.
18 Colquhoun G. *Playing God.* London: Hammersmith Press; 2007.
19 www.poetrysociety.org.uk
20 www.poetryarchive.org/poetryarchive/home.do
21 www.poets.org
22 www.favouritepoem.org/poems/index.html
23 www.poemhunter.com/poems/
24 www.poemsinthewaitingroom.org
25 Albiardaz R. Using haiku poetry to evaluate the GPVTS and develop linguistic skills. *Educ Prim Care.* 2009; **20**: 314–15.
26 Eisner M. Poetry writing exercise. Personal communication; 2010.

18

The Simulated Patient – your walking, talking learning tool

FIONA DUDLEY – Patient Simulator, Facilitator, Lecturer & Trainer (Univ. Leeds & Hull-York Medical School) & lead author
MIRIAM HAWKINS – Patient Simulator and Facilitator (Patient Simulated Resource Centre, Yorkshire)
EMMA STORR – Clinical Lecturer in Primary Care (Univ. Leeds)   **MARY DAVIS** – Associate GP Dean (KSS Deanery)
MAGGIE EISNER – TPD (Bradford)

Why spend time on simulation?

Working with simulated patients to explore consultations and develop trainees' skills can reach parts other teaching methods don't. For instance:

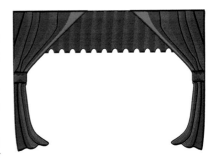

- It's **interactive and dynamic** – low risk of boredom or losing someone's attention. And it impacts deeply on people as it focuses on human interaction.
- It's **collaborative** – the group members will bounce ideas off each other, thus encouraging cross fertilisation of ideas.
- It tackles a **variety of learning domains** – knowledge, skills and attitudes (and it is an exceptional way of developing each).
- It's about **'doing'** in contrast to just 'talking' about something (cf. Miller's Pyramid in Chapter 29: Assessment and Competence). As a result, the trainee will process the experience on many different levels (and it is therefore more memorable than a lecture):
  - ✓ emotionally – I've had a real experience with another human being
  - ✓ intellectually – I have had the opportunity to discuss and analyse what happened
  - ✓ contextually – I know this was not 'real life', but my learning is deeper because I have experienced this as real life.
- If done the right way, it can be **fun!**

However, as it is such an immensely powerful way of working, it should be treated with great care! It can shatter confidence as quickly as it can build it. The facilitator, the simulator and the group need to work together to ensure it is a positive experience for all. We're going to provide you with some basic guidelines and tips to make your sessions with simulated patients safe and beneficial, educational and enjoyable. Let's make it easy by breaking it down into six steps.

1 **Preparation and Planning** – getting your environment, personnel and paperwork in order.
2 **Initiation** – getting to know the group.
3 **Setting the scene and the agenda** – being explicit about the learning objectives.
4 **The Act** – actually doing it; the performance.
5 **The Epilogue** – facilitating the learning after the 'act' is over.
6 **The Review** – getting feedback on the whole process.

STEP 1 – Preparation and Planning

 Top Tip: It's really important to prepare the session if you want things to run smoothly. If you don't, things become chaotic; you and others will get all flustered making the session hard work and a negative experience for all.

Getting ready

- **Prepare the room:** things like seating arrangements, flip charts, working pens etc.
- **Make sure you have all the relevant paperwork** and that the right people have the right paperwork (more on this below).
- **Check your scenarios:** are there any features in the scenarios which may need discussion with the group beforehand? Are there any gaps in your own knowledge? Are there any discrepancies between the scenario and the simulated patient that you need to flag to the group before they start, such as age or physical appearance?
- **Remind yourself of any learning objectives** so you can help navigate the session in the right direction.

The paperwork

You should have copies of:

- The **simulator's brief** – which gives instructions to the patient simulator.
- The **practitioner's brief** – which sets the scene for the person/s carrying out the consultation. (Not always necessary – especially if you plan to brief them verbally.)
- **Medical notes** – a brief summary of the clinical record for the practitioner. (Not always necessary.)
- Facilitator's **notes** – to make sure as much potential learning as possible is achieved.

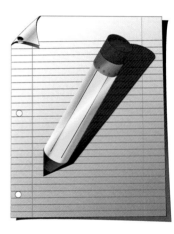

You should ensure that:

- The **simulated patient** is sent, in advance if possible, their own brief as well as that of the trainee, plus medical notes and any additional material you feel is appropriate.
- The **group** knows what information is in the trainee's brief: either handed out or read out during the session.
- The **facilitator**, in case it's not you, has a copy of everything.

STEP 2 – Initiation

There are many ingredients in the simulated patient session which can help or hinder its success, but one of the most vital is the group itself. The better you know the group, the easier it is to use the skills and personalities within it. You should **always take plenty of time with a group** you don't know to get to know each other and make them feel at ease.

Initiation

- How well do you and the rest of the group know each other?
  Do you need to start off with introductions and an ice-breaking game?
- Are there any difficulties within the group dynamics you are aware of?
- What is their experience of working in this kind of way?
  'How many of you have worked with simulators before?'
  'Those of you who have, what has been your experience so far? Be honest.'
- What are their expectations of this session?
  'What are you all expecting this session will do for you? Do you have any concerns?'

STEP 3 – Setting the scene and agenda

After talking about the case and the process, define the agenda.

Setting the scene

- What's going to happen:
  'Today we're going to be involved in an exciting session where you'll learn some skills that will be invaluable for the rest of your life. It involves an actor who will behave as a patient, and it will give you an opportunity to practise some of your consultation skills rather than just talking about them. 'It's important to see this as a group learning activity. That means you will all be having a turn in the "hot seat". I will need a volunteer to start proceedings, but someone else can take over at any point.'
- Explain that it is an opportunity to learn, not a threat, and alleviate any fears or concerns identified in step 1.
  'Remember, this session is an opportunity for all of us to learn from each other – about the different ways of handling a challenging consultation. It's not about humiliation or trying to impress anyone so please don't feel threatened. Just have a go, do what you normally do and play around. Besides, it's better to make mistakes here in a safe environment than with real patients. Don't you agree? What does everyone think?'

Setting the agenda

- Introduce the case: get someone to read out the scenario and information on the practitioner's instruction sheet.
- Set the aims/objectives and group rules (for more about aims and objectives read Chapter 4: Powerful Hooks – aims, objectives and ILOs; group rules in Chapter 13: Teaching and Facilitating Small Groups).
- Briefly discuss the rules of feedback (covered in Chapter 7: The Skilful Art of Giving Feedback).
- Explain what is expected of them: clarify what the person in the 'hot seat' has to do and what the observers will do; tell them to equip themselves with pen and paper.
- Give them a 'get out' clause: *'If you're finding things too stressful in the hot seat don't worry – just raise your right hand in order to step out. If the case itself brings up an issue that is personally difficult for you right now, simply say that you'd like to sit this one out. Is that more comforting to know?'*
- Discuss how they're feeling at this point: tease out any further fears/concerns and put them at ease.
- Ask for a volunteer.

Additional notes

- **Introducing the case:** The amount of information you give about the session will largely depend on your objectives and the nature of the scenario. It helps to have the doctor's brief and the patient's brief on separate sheets of paper.
- **The aims, objectives and group rules:** The group rules are to protect the learners from destructive feedback (*see* Chapter 13: Teaching and Facilitating Small Groups). The aims and objectives will help focus the session on their learning needs. Encourage ownership of the session by getting the group to set their own ground rules at the beginning. Encourage them to identify their own learning needs too. If one trainee is to carry out the entire consultation, it is helpful to ascertain what that individual would like feedback on. Map these on a flip chart for all to see and to return to after each consultation or in the plenary.
- **What is expected of them:** Other than the person in the hot seat, give all the others observational tasks to do. Although a little prescriptive, it can be a useful way of ensuring the rest of the group is actively involved. Ask them to equip themselves with paper and pen in order to jot down relevant observations during the consultation. This can be done in a structured fashion where they note down specific behaviour or words (= *'what they see or hear'*) or, alternatively, be left free to decide what they want to give feedback on.

- **Asking for a volunteer:** Only do this once your group has warmed up to you and each other. If no one comes forward, one way to move things on may be to treat their embarrassment like that of the patient who wants to discuss an embarrassing problem – the more comfortable and matter of fact you can be, the easier it becomes for them. Stress that everyone in the group is working together to explore the issues within the consultation and that the trainee carrying out the consultation is simply playing their part in the team effort. Re-emphasise: *'this is not about impressing people but just having a go and learning from it'* and that *'it's okay to make mistakes: we're only human after all'*. Whenever possible use humour to relax the situation. If finding a volunteer still seems tricky despite all your best efforts, another tactic is to say something like *'I'm just going outside for a minute to talk to the simulator. While I'm doing that, can the rest of you decide among yourselves who would like to have a go first and to set the room to how you'd like it.'*

⚠ **Red Alert:** Try not to use the word role play. For some reason, it has become a term that makes trainees shiver and withdraw. Instead, use something less formal, like *'Let's try that out.'*

STEP 4 – The Act or Performance

There are a variety of ways in which you can run the actual simulated consultation (covered later). Generally, let the session run a little while. Try not to stop it prematurely. One of the reasons for stopping it might be to communicate with the simulated patient.

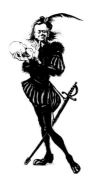

- You might want them to play the character slightly differently.
- You want them to increase/decrease the challenge.
- Perhaps some essential clinical detail is not coming to light.
- Because the scenario is heading down the wrong path and won't fulfil the group's objectives.

It may be possible to do this using your body language (using signs you might have discussed and agreed to beforehand). However, if you do have to talk to them outside the room, explain to the group what you are doing in order to avoid increasing their anxiety further. The other reason for stopping the scenario is if the trainee seems to be in significant struggle or distress. In which case, bring the session to a temporary halt and see the box below.

If the learner in the hot seat is struggling . . .

1 Ask them what difficulty they are having.
2 Ask them where they are trying to get to in the consultation.
3 Get the other group members to problem-solve.
4 Ask the trainee if they feel they'd like to try the suggestions offered or would like one of the others to 'have a go'.

Top Tip: During patient simulation sessions, it is important that the facilitator remains in the driving seat. Do not be frightened to discuss this with the simulated patient.

STEP 5 – The Epilogue
(Epilogue – a section or speech at the end of a book or play that serves as a comment on or a conclusion to what has happened.)

The Epilogue

- Start with the role-playing trainee – *'How was it for you?'*

If they respond in the negative, get them to spell out why they think this is. Get them to focus on words and actions (behaviour). To ensure balanced feedback, get them to reflect on some of the good things they felt they did. Not only does this increase their morale, but it also provides learning points for the other group members.

- Invite the other trainees into the discussion

'Would you like to hear what some of the other group members thought about that?' This is best done once the trainee has spoken or has brought up a specific point.

- Invite the simulator into the discussion

'Shall we see what the patient thought about that?' The purpose here is to check whether a trainee's perception holds true or not.

- Revisit the agenda you set at the start

Revisit the aims and objectives and see if you have covered what the group/individual wanted specific help with.

- Provide a summary of the learning that's taken place

You don't have to do this all by yourself. Ask each member for a key learning point.

- Check everyone's feelings

Throughout the process and at the end, look after people's feelings; especially, those who have been in the hot seat. If you're concerned about an individual, take them to one side after the session and help them get back on track. Finish the session as thoughtfully and sensitively as you began – all participants should leave feeling positive about the experience.

STEP 6 – The Review
This is about getting feedback on (1) your facilitation so that you can become better (i.e. your professional development) and (2) how to run the session better the next time around. You can do this formally (using written evaluation sheets) or more freely via a general discussion (*see* Chapter 28: Reflection and Evaluation).

- Ask the group whether they found the session useful and **tease out** what particular bits.
- Ask them if there were *'any bits not so helpful'* – again tease out the specifics.
- Finally, ask them how they felt you performed as a facilitator.

Top Tip: Reflect on the session with the patient simulator too. Ask whether they had any issues in relation to: the scenario, the organisation, the group, the subject matter and your style of facilitation. They get to experience a wide variety of facilitation styles and techniques and are well placed to advise you.

The different ways you can facilitate the consultation

There are several ways you can run the actual simulator–trainee consultation. Which method you choose depends on the learning objectives you set with the group.

1. Straight through session

You may feel it best to run the consultation from start to finish, using one interviewer, with no breaks. This may be for many reasons: perhaps the aim of the group is to look at the structure of the consultation, or an individual wants to practise time management.

2. Pausing (or Stop-Start)

This is where the consultation is used much like a video, in as much as it can be paused, restarted, replayed or fast-forwarded. It's good for practising specific skills or specific phases of the consultation. **Before the session, talk about who can stop the session, how they do it and why they might want to.** It may be paused by the trainee carrying out the interview, you as facilitator or by a group member should you decide that is appropriate. It is rarely helpful for the simulated patient to stop the session.

The trainee might pause the session if:
- they seem unsure where to go next in the consultation – they may ask for help from the group and then carry on, or nominate someone else in the group to continue the consultation
- they are struggling and need some suggestions from the group
- they've said/done something regrettable and would like to rewind and try it in a different way.

A member of the group may pause the session if:
- they have an idea or an alternative way of managing the situation – either for the learner or themselves to try out.

You, the facilitator, can pause the session if:
- you feel the trainee is struggling and needs some help from the group
- you wish to change the trainee carrying out the consultation
- you have identified a learning point you would like to highlight and discuss further
- you feel the consultation is going down a route which is unhelpful
- you wish to talk to the simulated patient about playing the role slightly differently
- you wish to create a whole new scenario in response to the needs of the group.

Restarting
- When a consultation has been paused, you will need to think how you will restart it. It is important that everyone knows exactly where to restart. This may be at the point it was paused, at the beginning or at some significant point within the conversation.
- It may be useful to ask the trainee to summarise to the simulated patient what has happened in the consultation so far, or you may ask the simulated patient to repeat a certain phrase said in the previous consultation to get the ball rolling again.

3. Rewinding

You can rewind the consultation back to any point. You may wish to:

- take it back to the beginning to see how a different approach could change the outcome
- take it back to a challenging moment to explore some alternative approaches
- give the trainee the opportunity to try out suggestions they have had from the group
- give another group member a chance to carry out the consultation.

In contrast to video, when one rewinds and replays a simulated consultation, one is not just restricted to replaying it exactly the same way – it can be played differently according to the needs of the group.

4. Fast forwarding

You can also fast-forward to a later point in the consultation. This may be useful if the group wants to focus on management planning rather than history taking. Maybe the consultation is going round in circles, and you feel it would be better to make some assumptions and move it on in order to get to the nub of the case. You can also fast-forward to a follow-up consultation – useful if you want to explore the effects of the initial consultation, or to explore a developing problem.

5. Hot seating

There are many other ways simulated patients may be used, most of which cannot be fully explored here. However, we will describe one very useful technique called 'hot seating'. In hot seating the simulated patient sits in front of the group members, who are then able to pose any questions they like. The simulated patient will answer these 'in role neutral' (i.e. in role but without any of the emotions which may be inherent in the situation). They will be very honest and open in their answers. For example, a drug user may admit to an intention of selling their benzodiazepines, or a very shy person may confess their real feelings about their husband. Hot seating can be used at the beginning of a consultation, during it or at the end. Clearly, hot seating adds to the artificiality of the situation, but it can be used creatively to move on a consultation.

Use it at the beginning if:

- the focus is on a later part of the consultation, and the group needs to get a quick history
- the simulated patient is playing a frequent attender or long-standing patient, who is supposed to be known to the trainee. The group can build the bones of what is already known and form a relationship/picture of the patient
- the group wants to know some background information that the patient might not be willing to reveal to the role-playing trainee.

Use it during the session if:

- a trainee has been interviewing for some time, but the salient points remain elusive
- a scenario has become very emotional, but some elements still need to be discovered.

Feedback

Giving feedback is the **most powerful and important part of the session**. If you do it badly, the session can shatter confidence at a breakneck speed. We have listed some salient points about giving feedback below. However, you can find everything you ever wanted to know about feedback in Chapter 7: The Skilful Art of Giving Feedback, and there's more stuff on our website.

- **Always ask the trainee who has just consulted how they feel it went first.** After that, you can start bringing in the feedback from others.
- **Ask the group how they would like feedback** – and make sure the simulator is aware of the feedback method chosen.
- **The facilitator's role in feedback:** there are an infinite number of things on which feedback can be given. If you are working effectively, you should not have to think of these as the group will be coming up with their own ideas. Your main role will be to *structure* the contributions of

the group, and perhaps to *summarise* them at the end. However, it may be appropriate to contribute some observations of your own, especially if you are faced with an unresponsive group.

- **Involve the patient simulator** in the feedback process. However, some simulated patients will not have received the same quantity and quality of training on feedback as you. You may need to give some sensitive and constructive advice.
- **Make sure all feedback given is specific and descriptive.** To be told we are lovely may make us feel all warm inside, but it doesn't really give us anything to replicate or further develop. It is only by being given specifics that we can go away and think about them and work on improving them.
- **All feedback should be honest – but not brutal.**

 Top Tip: Liven up the feedback process by encouraging the group to check out their assumptions and ideas with the simulated patient: *'That's interesting; shall we see if the patient felt the same way?'*

Frequently asked questions

What's wrong with the word 'role play'?

 How many times have you said, *'Let's do a bit of role play'* only to find the trainees squirm, grumble or moan? Exactly! For some reason, the term 'role play' is not well received. However, if you just do it without signposting it as 'role play' or by saying, *'That's interesting. Okay, pretend I'm the patient, and let's go back to that point where she said . . .'*, trainees engage without realising that they're doing role play! Instead of the word role-play use something like 'rehearsal', 'practice' or 'simulation'. Alternatively, just say, *'Let's try that out'*.

I'm worried that the group members might all go quiet on me.

You need to fill the group with **reassurance** *and* **enthusiasm**. Reassure them about:

- the prospect of 'performing' in front of their peers or colleagues
- seeing it as an assessment; in the UK since 2010, GP trainees will have encountered patient simulations as part of their assessment for recruitment
- a previous bad experience of simulation in medical school or GP recruitment
- it being completely new to them (especially those trained outside the UK).

Setting **group rules** will show them that there are boundaries not to be crossed and this in itself will be very reassuring (For more on group rules, *see* Chapter 13: Teaching and Facilitating Small Groups.) In terms of enthusiasm, you need to hook them in (see the box below).

How do I brief the simulated patient?

The primary function of your simulated patient is as a learning tool, but it is important to remember they are a human one! Just as a carpenter would sharpen their chisels before working with them, so must you *prepare your simulated patient **before** the session.* Although all simulated patients should have received general training, they work broadly and will not necessarily have an understanding of the specific requirements of your organisation, your learners or your session. Therefore, it's important that you take the time to familiarise them accordingly. The better your communication with the simulated patient, the more likely it is that they will provide you and the group with the material you need and the easier it will be to work as an effective team. If there are *points crucial to the scenario*, it is as well to reiterate them before the session; for example, emphasising the *negative responses* to some medical history questions. So, if the clinical diagnosis is anaemia, you may wish to highlight the importance of answering depression screening questions in the negative to avoid misleading the trainee.

> ### Briefing the patient simulator
>
> - The aims of the session.
> - How you plan to run the session. One trainee? Straight through/Stop-Start/Replay.
> - About the patient simulator's role:
>   What level of emotion do you want? A scale of 1–10 can be helpful for the degree of emotion and can be changed during the session.
>   What type of emotion you are looking for? Do you want, e.g. cold anger or loud aggressive anger? Do you want tears or shocked silence?
>   How challenging do you want it to be?
> - What the trainee/group are like:
>   How confident/skilled the individual trainee in the hot seat is.
>   What level of training/experience the group members have.
>   What the group dynamics are like: lively group? Treacle waders?
> - What you want them to do when the group discuss stuff? Leave? Stay? Freeze? Join in?
> - How you want them to give feedback? (more about this later)

Red Alert: Although you may be very clear about what is expected of a GP trainee, not all patient simulators will know. Always tell them what level of training and experience the group members and the individual in the hot seat have.

What do I do with the simulator if I pause the session?

Your options are pretty straightforward. They may:

1 **leave** the room (still in role) and wait outside
2 **stay** in the room and 'freeze' (i.e. look down and detach themselves from proceedings yet still remain in role), or
3 **join** in the discussion.

If they leave the room:	If they stay in the room:
• They will not hear the discussion and so will restart the consultation with no bias. • It will take slightly more time as they have to leave, and you will have to go and call them back in, explaining what you would like them to do next. • It's more realistic.	• They will hear the discussion and may adapt their reactions accordingly. This may be helpful or not. An experienced simulator should not have any difficulty with staying in the room and maintaining their role. • It will be slightly quicker as the simulated patient will know exactly what is expected of them in the next part of the consultation, and will already be in the room. • It makes the situation seem even more artificial.

It's rarely useful for the simulated patient to join in the discussion at this point, because it raises issues of whether they stay in or out of role. It's usually easier to give time later for their opinions in feedback and it gives them the opportunity to collect and organise their thoughts.

Should I use simulated patients 'in role', 'out of role', or 'in role neutral'?

It is important that everyone knows whether the simulated patient is 'in role' or not, and it is your job as facilitator to make this clear. Trained simulated patients should be capable of giving feedback 'in role', 'out of role', and 'in role neutral' (where the simulated patient stays in role but without the emotions of the actual scenario). It is up to you to decide which is most appropriate for the given situation. This will depend on the nature of the session, the scenario and the character the simulated patient is playing. **As a general rule it is most effective for them to feedback both in and out of role:** in role first and then add anything out of role. This may need to be adjusted if, for example, they have been playing a very emotional patient, where feedback out of role may be more useful. Here's how you can signpost whether you're requesting feedback in role or out of role:

● 'in role' – use the patient's name and refer to the patient in the second person
'*Mrs Carmichael, how did **you** feel when the doctor mentioned the situation at work?*'
● 'out of role' – use the actor's real name and refer to the patient in the third person.
'*Angela, how did **the patient** feel when the doctor mentioned the situation at work?*'

And that's all there is to working with simulated patients. Remember to have fun! Don't forget to check out our website, which hosts a whole array of resources just for you.

A sample of resources on our website
- Organising a simulated patient session.
- Instructions for simulators.
- Instructions for the amateur simulator.
- Instructions for the facilitator.
- A Kiwi Approach to Simulation – Safe and Effective Clinical Outcomes (SECO) clinics.

Other chapters you may like to read
- Chapter 13: Teaching and Facilitating Small Groups
- Chapter 7: The Skilful Art of Giving Feedback.

Essential reading
Fiona has her own book out:
- Dudley F. *The Simulated Patient Handbook: a comprehensive guide for facilitators and simulated patients.* London: Radcliffe Publishing; 2012.

Please give us some feedback on this chapter to help shape it for the next edition.
Go to www.essentialgptrainingbook.com and simply click on the title of this chapter.

19

Multiple Trainee Practices – a rough and ready guide

JO BUCHANAN – Deputy Director (Yorkshire & Humber Deanery) & lead author
RICHARD WATTON – GP Trainer (Sheffield)

Introduction

Some of you reading this chapter may be thinking: *'I've already got one trainee, and that's more than enough thank you very much.'* But read this:

> 'It's been fun. I have enjoyed training more in the last year and a half than I ever have.'
> GP Trainer whose practice hosts 4–6 trainees at any one time with two Trainers.

What are you waiting for? Read on . . .

Definition of 'multiple trainee practices'

- Do you want to feel like this?
- Make the work in your practice more interesting?
- Work in an exciting practice environment which is a constant source of intellectual stimulation?
- Be surrounded by keen young learners eager to take on new tasks?
- And increase your practice income at the same time?

For the purposes of this chapter, which is primarily concerned with GP training, we will define a multiple trainee practice as one which trains more than one GP Specialty Trainee (GPStR) at a time. Most of our discussion will be around this concept of multiple training, though we also refer to a practice that has developed a broader concept of multiple training, which includes other professionals.

Why do we need multiple training practices?

In the current climate, we need to train more GPs, and that means developing more training places in general practice. There are a number of reasons for this:

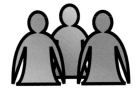

- People are living longer, meaning there will be a need for more medical care.
- The focus of ongoing care for many medical conditions is shifting into the community.
- After training, more and more doctors are going part-time and so more are needed to replace the current generation of full-time GPs, who are retiring.
- There is a move to extend GP training to five years to prepare trainees better for the role of a general practitioner.
- There is a growing need for general practice to offer training placements for foundation trainees, trainees from other specialities and medical students.

To increase training capacity, we need to:

1 Develop new training practices and
2 Encourage existing training practices to accommodate more trainees (what this chapter will focus on).

But whatever the driver behind increasing capacity we have to ensure that one thing remains a top priority: that we maintain a high quality of GP Speciality Training.

What's so great about taking on more than one trainee?

Multiple training can be good for you, your practice and the trainees themselves.[1] Let's look at each in turn.

You, the Trainer

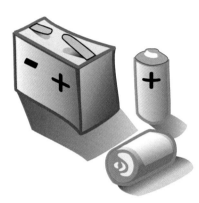

- **It can recharge your batteries**

  Established training practices usually have a body of motivated and enthusiastic Trainers. Even so, in some practices, things may have become a bit 'humdrum'. Taking on multiple trainees not only strengthens existing practice but recharges one's batteries if they're running a bit low.

- **You'll learn lots too**

  As the facilitator of a group of trainees who are actively and dynamically learning from each other, you will learn lots of new things too; clinical knowledge, for instance. It is therefore an *effective* and *effortless* way of keeping up to date. You'll learn group facilitation skills – which are invaluable for practice meetings, learning time events and other small-group working.

- **It helps you with benchmarking**

  Having a group of trainees in a practice enables both you and the trainees to benchmark performance. Trainers have said that it is also easier to spot someone who is struggling and sometimes the more experienced trainees can help them.

- **It adds variety to your work**

  If you're currently doing 8–9 sessions of weekly clinical work, that will need to change if you're committed to multiple training. Multiple training cannot be done by squeezing things into your already hectic timetable – it needs time that is devoted and protected. For instance, you can't clinically supervise four trainees if you're to do a surgery alongside them. Something has to give – you will probably end up doing 5–6 clinical sessions. Imagine the variety in your work timetable other than seeing patients all the time.

247   Multiple Trainee Practices – a rough and ready guide

- **It's incredibly satisfying**
  The reward of seeing young enthusiastic learners develop is an incredible source of personal satisfaction as is the relationship you form with them and the gratitude they show you along the way.

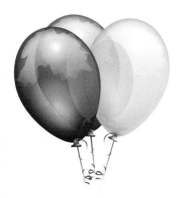

The practice

'You can get multiple trainees to do things together – things that would be a bit risky to do on their own. For example, the PCT asked us to do an in-house session on planning for a flu pandemic. We gave it to them, and they did it really well, but it would have been a lot to give to one individual. That was a big advantage.'

- **Your practice will become dynamic and lively**
  Having multiple trainees in your practice will change the atmosphere and ethos: adding a new dimension to it. There will be the intellectual stimulation of being surrounded by young doctors who are generally eager to learn. Your partners and other practice members will benefit as well as you. We have seen this happen.
- **Your practice will become an active 'learning organisation'**
  Learners bring with them new ideas on medical care that not only keeps you up to date but also benefits the patients by keeping the practice in touch with the latest medical developments. They can bring with them ideas about practice systems to help things run better (and safer) for patients.
- **More appointments and meet that QOF target on access – at last!**
  Multiple trainees can increase the total number of appointments you have available on any given day. The effect will obviously depend on the experience level of the trainees and the length of their appointments. It would be unusual for multiple training not to be beneficial in terms of appointments offered: helping to meet access targets.
- **More money**
  In a practice with multiple trainees, the total training grant can be a significant source of income.

Trainees

'Sometimes it's easier to catch one of your colleagues and get their opinion on something than it is to find your Trainer; not something you are desperately worried about, just something you want an opinion on. It's less threatening. We use each other quite a lot, without thinking about it.'

- **Less isolation and more support**

  No matter how friendly you try to be, trainees in single-trainee practices miss the hospital camaraderie. Trainees in multiple practices say they feel less isolated.

- **It promotes working in collaboration**

  The future of general practice is moving towards practices working together. Multiple training allows peers to interact and learn from each other. However, this won't happen miraculously – it is down to the Trainer and the Practice Manager to set up systems to enable this to happen. Senior trainees, for example, can lead tutorials for less experienced colleagues or take them on visits. This enhances the teaching skills and confidence of the senior doctor (a competency requirement for MRCGP). It provides a less threatening learning environment for the novice trainee. Doctors learn more easily from their peers than their assessors – fact!

- **It provides for the 'Hidden Curriculum'**

  The term 'Hidden Curriculum' was coined by sociologist Philip Jackson in 1968.[2] He argued that what is taught in schools is more than the sum total of the curriculum. He said that in addition to the things that are *formally* taught, schools provide a *socialisation process* where students pick up additional messages through the experience of being in school. A modified version of Meighan's[3] definition may help you to understand this better: the hidden curriculum is something which is *not* taught by any teacher; it is the stuff learners learn by being in a learning organisation but which may not be explicitly taught: like an attitude to learning. The amount of informal or peer learning that occurs among a group of learners is under-appreciated. In multiple trainee practices, this takes place anyway as they discuss their experiences. It is very satisfying to see a group of trainees 'talking the talk' of professional practice. As a Trainer, your role is to provide the environment where this can take place by:
  - ✓ providing a common room or library where they can sit and chat
  - ✓ producing timetables and work patterns that structure the day in order to facilitate informal contact
  - ✓ modelling this behaviour yourself – of 'readiness to reflect' on experience with your colleagues in front of and with the trainees.

- **Helps trainees benchmark themselves**

  Finally, having a group of trainees enables them to see and reflect how well they are doing in comparison to their colleagues: a powerful motivator for inducing change!

Multiple training – things to watch out for!

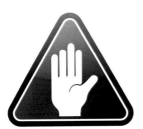

There would seem to be few disadvantages to multiple training for the learners. However, it is possible that **individual learning needs are lost sight of in the needs of the whole**. The learners may have a **less nurturing relationship with you** as Trainer if you have commitments elsewhere. You need to take actions to avoid these risks, and a key part of the timetable should be to offer protected time each week for 1–1 contact between Trainer and learner.

Multiple training takes time. If you and the practice are not prepared to *carve out* time for it, it is not for you. Furthermore, the **practice needs to be sufficiently flexible** to adapt the training programme to cater for individual needs as they are discovered. You will need to **create time for 1–1 activities**. The practice needs to understand that this is part of the deal.

Multiple training needs space. Trainees require consulting rooms. You need a common room and a library or study area. Most practices do not have this space. With goodwill multiple training can still take place, but it is not easy. There have been grants available to extend the training capacity of general practices and provide more facilities. Even so, this might not be enough or your practice building may not lend itself to extension.

The burden of teaching can only be taken if the **Trainer significantly reduces his or her clinical commitment**. The patients may benefit from seeing clever young trainees but they probably will want to see the old family doctor they have grown to trust over the years. More supervision and availability of juniors mean fewer appointments for you. You may see this as a positive thing for yourself, or you may not. We train our trainees to practise family medicine and appreciate the values of *continuity of care*, but in setting up the training programmes, we remove ourselves from the front line and reduce our own availability to patients. This is a tension you need to be aware of. However, many other GPs are now choosing to have portfolio careers and work as GPs with Special Interest (GPwSI) outside of the practice. If you are training multiple trainees, **you are essentially working as a GPwSI within the practice**.

The ingredients for a successful multiple training practice

You have a think first. This will only take 5 minutes: Get a piece of paper and jot down what you think the essential ingredients are and then compare your list with ours below.

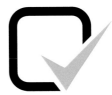

- **Commitment from the whole practice to the concept.** This cannot work if you are the only Trainer, and the others aren't particularly interested. It is essential to establish a 'whole practice' ethos towards multiple training.
- **Good organisation.** A high degree of organisation is necessary to manage multiple trainees with multiple training needs. For example, there needs to be absolute clarity for the learners about the supervisory arrangements on any given day.

- **Adequate Time.** There needs to be a balance of 1–1 and joint activities in the week for each learner. Practice Managers are good at making this happen.
- **Flexibility.** The training timetable may need to change to adapt to the individual needs of learners. Practice Managers are good at building day-to-day rota flexibility.
- **A good Practice Manager.** Spend some time with your Practice Manager; get them to adopt the same vision and enthusiasm for multiple training as you.

Where are you and your practice in relation to these? This will tell
you whether you're ready or not to take the plunge.

What the practice needs to know . . .

In the past, the Trainer was often an isolated figure in the practice as far as education was concerned

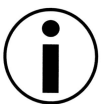

and training went on with variable levels of support from partners. This is changing, with training being seen as a practice activity rather than down to any one individual. This practice approach is incredibly important for taking on multiple trainees. Everyone needs to sign up and commit to it.

Non-training partners have to be supportive of the time commitment you and the other trainers will need to give to it. They too need to get involved – your practice will have many learners, and everyone has to be prepared either to supervise formally or at least to be available to discuss problems. The key to

multiple training is to integrate learning into the everyday workings of the practice. Having multiple trainees can help your practice become a 'learning organisation' (in contrast to an organisation with individual learners).

Implications for other practice staff
- Your Practice Manager will find that he or she has to sort out the administrative and organisational problems of several learners, not just one.
- The receptionists have to accommodate the needs of an ever-changing team of trainees and balance the wishes of the patients to see the doctors they know with the need for trainees to gain experience.
- The other doctors need to accept that you, as the nominated Trainer, will end up seeing fewer patients. Hopefully, this will be counter-balanced by the number of patients the trainees are seeing. Make this clear and have a talk about it right from the start. Otherwise, you will start getting annoying and demotivating comments, like *'How many patients did you see today?'*

Top Tip: Periodically (and opportunistically), remind the practice of the extra significant amount of service provision from multiple trainees and the additional benefits of having a group of bright, enthusiastic young people around.

'The practice feels different; it feels more up to date . . . They make the place very lively, they have different needs.' 'It keeps the practice and the partners fresh.'

Now for the nitty-gritty: the practical bits

Organisation
This requires a sophisticated level of organisation: room allocation, timetabling and arrangements for supervision. Choose a specific member of your administrative team who is responsible for this.

Responsibilities
The responsibility for training of the GP trainee should rest with the nominated Trainer, and it is essential that the trainee is clear who this is. The trainees can be a mix of full-time or part-time, foundation doctors or GP trainees at different levels of experience. Each training partner can be responsible for one or more trainees. It is difficult to be responsible for more than three learners, particularly given the number of assessments that need to be completed, but the number will depend on the arrangements in your own practice. Recent changes to the ePortfolio now make it easier for others to input into support and assessment.

Induction
Induction can be a challenge in August when the need for clinical staff to take annual leave coincides with an influx of new learners. Induction needs careful planning: if you're already a GP training practice, you'll have an induction system in place that you will be able to build on. The main difference is the complexity inherent in increasing numbers. The changes required will be organisational, so get your Practice Manager involved when tweaking the induction programme you already have.

The differing levels of previous experience need to be taken into account. You will have to ask yourself how much time you want to allocate in the induction to each learner. An F2 who is only spending four months in the practice will not need to spend more than a week getting to know the systems and individuals in your practice and local community. A GP trainee who is to spend a year in your practice may need a more in-depth induction that could last two weeks.

In August, you may need to consider using locums to ensure that the needs of the patients are met while clinicians spend time with the new learners. Do remember, though, that the learner must never be under the sole supervision of a locum. Some features of the induction can be delayed until later if needs be (such as sitting in on a practice nurse's diabetic clinic).

Timetabling and supervision

Once induction is over, a routine needs to be established that integrates the needs of the learners with the supervising capacity of the partners, and the service needs of the patients. As a Trainer you have to be prepared for your surgeries to be interrupted. The more trainees you supervise the more interruption you may get, and you will need to be expected to see fewer patients to accommodate this. Your partners and the Practice Manager need to understand and accept this. Consideration also has to be given to the mix of the learners. Three new F2 doctors would be too much to supervise and still hold a surgery. However, three ST3 GP trainees may not interrupt the Trainer at all. If the combination of the numbers of trainees and their level of experience is such that you cannot consult well, you need to drop your surgery altogether and be allocated the role of Clinical Supervisor alone. Here, you will be available just to field enquiries from the learners (who will be doing a significant amount of service provision). You should also encourage the trainees to help each other out towards the end of their surgeries: whoever finishes first helps out doctors who may be running late, by offering to see their patients. This encourages the right attitude to teamwork and by making everyone finish at the same time helps debriefing to happen on time.

Debriefing

Debriefing is the core activity of GP speciality training and time needs to be available for each learner to reflect on his or her experience of consulting with patients. The culture should be such that your learners feel free to discuss any urgent matters during surgery and to reflect on the others afterwards. The debrief doesn't have to be straight after surgery. You may wish to schedule it for later in the day, for example, at 2 p.m. for a morning surgery.

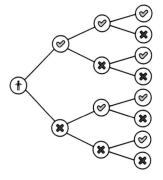

You can arrange to have individual or group debriefs: we suggest having a combination during the week – it works well! The group debrief enables learners to learn and bounce ideas off each other. It builds their confidence in teaching skills, and in medicine as they realise they do have knowledge and skills to bring to the discussion. The level of intervention of the Trainer will depend on the knowledge and skills of the learners, particularly the senior trainees. You will find that most trainees like the group debrief and like learning from each other. They do not feel as threatened as they can in a 1–1 setting – not surprising as there will be more of them than there are of you.

Some tips on group debriefing and facilitation

- **Listen and reflect** – the same skills you use in consulting.
- **Ask about urgent concerns or problems** that need sorting first.
- **Don't solely ask about problems.** Shift the focus to a wider look at training issues.
  - *'Did anyone have any really interesting cases today?'* or
  - *'Does anyone think they did anything really well today?'*
- **Move away from being the expert.** Model the idea that no one, particularly in a generalist situation, can know the answer to everything. Make it clear that it is okay not to know something providing they identify and tackle their learning needs.
- **Get them to problem-solve for themselves.** Don't rush in and give 'answers'. Help them build the skill of 'looking for information when you don't know it'.
- **Get them to work collaboratively.** Open out issues to the rest of the group. Get them into the habit of learning from each other. *'Can anyone else offer ideas?'*
- **Some questions do need to be answered directly.** Learners find it very annoying if everything is reflected, and nothing answered directly.
- **If the group discussion is going well, leave it alone.** If they are working well without much input from you – let them carry on. Do not feel that you have to say something to justify your role. You are not there to teach, you are there to ensure they learn.

Read Chapter 7: The Skilful Art of Giving Feedback.
Read Chapter 13: Teaching and Facilitating Small Groups.

The quiet trainee (the 'silent sitter')

Bringing someone into a discussion because they haven't said much needs doing sensitively. There may be all sorts of reasons for a trainee being quiet.

- They may just be quiet because they are a good trainee with lots of things to say normally but today, on this topic, they simply have nothing to add. If so leave them alone.
- You may sense the quietness is a result of personal issues around what is being discussed or something else in their life. Think about dealing with this separately on an individual basis later. Alternatively, if you think the trainee will be okay with this, engage in a general discussion on how personal issues can influence us in the consultation.
- They may always be quiet, in which case encourage them to say more. However, be wary of drawing attention to their shyness by directing questions to them just because they are quiet.

The talkative trainee (the 'dominant dictator')

A talkative trainee can stop others having their say and thus limit the breadth of discussions. Use the same skills you use with talkative patients and sensitively calm them down. Do not make them feel humiliated – remember, we said calm them down not put them down; a talkative person can be just as insecure as a quiet one.

- Thank them and ask for someone else to comment. *'Thanks for that Krishna. What do others think?'*
- Thank them and look to someone who you know can counter-balance them. *'That's a really interesting start to the discussion Mark. Kamal, what's your view on this?'*
- If you need to move things on, explain the need to do so. *'I'm sorry to cut the discussion short Anita but in order to fit in other people's issues, we need to move on. Is that okay?'*
- If the dominating behaviour is a recurring problem, deal with the particular trainee on a 1–1 basis. *'Rajinder, some of the things you say in group discussions are really interesting, and I value what you bring to the discussion. The problem I am having is getting some of the others to engage. So, I wonder if you could help me with that by . . .'*

If the debrief is working, leave it alone. If it isn't, do not be afraid to steer it just as you would a consultation. **It's very important that in debriefs trainees learn the facts of good safe patient management.** The group debrief is an efficient vehicle for learning/teaching facts, and if it is facilitated correctly trainees learn a whole host of other things. They learn to use their colleagues when they're not sure what to do. They develop self-confidence by realising they have more skills than they think. They learn to respect other people's opinions. They learn to cope with uncertainty and realise that, sometimes, there just are no answers. All these things will make them better lifelong learners, better GPs and better people in general.

Tutorials

'Group tutorials are brilliant. For example, last week we did something on ethics, and it was quite a deep session. In fact, I thought you could only achieve such depth on a 1–1 basis!'

The point of the tutorials should be understood and may need to be highlighted. It is not for the teacher to impress the learner or for the learner to impress the teacher. Rather, it is for the learner to walk away from the tutorial with something they will remember that will help them in consultations not just for the next few days but maybe for the rest of their life. This is more likely to be achieved if the subjects are prepared in advance, active participation in group discussion takes place and ideas are shared. Follow-up work may be given. All this reinforces the learning.

Many of the principles for 1–1 tutorials hold true for multiple trainee tutorials:
- the tutorials should be planned in advance
- time should be set aside and protected
- attempts should be made to identify learning needs, and the tutorials designed to fill in the gaps.

Planning joint tutorials is not an easy task. It can be difficult to integrate the different learning needs of learners with varied levels of experience. Even then it is not easy because often different learners are in the surgery at different times. All we can say is that, in practice, there is usually sufficient overlap for these things to be reconciled. Encourage the trainees to plan their own educational programme (of course, with guidance from you). Consider a mixture of joint and individual tutorials. Get them to lead and teach each other – teaching based on cases, for instance. This will help them build their teaching skills. Learners will have a range of abilities in this area. Encourage those who lack teaching expertise to give it a try. They'll soon realise that others feel less intimidated and learn more readily from their peers.

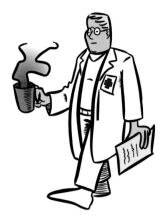

Teamwork

Effective primary care depends on good teamwork. The single trainee in a practice has to learn how to integrate with the primary healthcare team. This is also true for multiple trainees. In addition, multiple trainees form their own team. You need to help them turn this team into some kind of partnership – where they don't just work with each other but work for each other (like in a real GP partnership). For example, encourage them to help each other out during surgeries, especially if one of them is struggling or running behind. Promote the idea that surgery is not over until everyone's surgery is over. Finishing surgery together also allows everyone to meet over coffee and encourages more informal team building (and thus strengthens the partnership). The habit of meeting together and discussing work and the stresses of the day is a good habit to get into. It's a valuable lifelong work ethic to instil.

CASE STUDY – THE WHITE HOUSE SURGERY

This practice, serving an area of Sheffield with high levels of deprivation, has trained multiple trainees for many years.[4] The practice is participating in a project funded by the strategic health authority which will look at the ability of general practice to expand the training not only of medical students and doctors but of nurses and other disciplines such as physiotherapists and social workers too. The training will be multidisciplinary and will aim to increase respect between disciplines and give a greater understanding of roles and build up teamworking skills. The emphasis will be on integrated learning. Learners, wherever appropriate, will be used to teach other learners in their own or different disciplines. It is looking at the training capacity of a single practice.

These are exciting times for training and by establishing multiple training in practices and using the whole team as a training tool you are training the professionals of the future. Also, doing it in general practice helps defend us from the threats that exist from privatised healthcare and geographical models of attachment.

> ## Key messages for a multiple trainee practice
>
> 1 A Trainer who wants to have multiple trainees needs to redefine the ratio of education to practising medicine in their working week. If you're not prepared to do this, it is not for you. The practice has to understand and accept this too.
> 2 The practice needs to be very well organised. Your Practice Manager is the key and needs to be as enthusiastic about taking multiple trainees as you.
> 3 Your practice needs to have sufficient flexibility to adapt the training programme in response to new educational insights about the learner as they are discovered.

Please give us some feedback on this chapter to help shape it for the next edition.
Go to www.essentialgptrainingbook.com and simply click on the title of this chapter.

References

1 Buchanan J, Lane P. Grouping GP registrars in practice placements. *Educ Prim Care.* 2008; **19**(2): 143–50.
2 Jackson PW. *Life in Classrooms.* New York: Holt, Rinehart and Winston; 1968. p. 177.
3 Meighan R. *Sociology of Educating.* UK: Taylor & Francis Group; 1981.
4 Watton R. The training capacity of general practice. *BJGP.* 2005; **55**(514): 402.

Understanding and Teaching about Diversity

MAGGIE EISNER – TPD (Bradford) & lead author
ARUN DAVANGERE – recent GP Trainee (Sheffield), now salaried GP (Worksop)
JON CHADWICK – TPD (Scarborough)

What do we mean by diversity?

It is important to get away from thinking that we (whoever we are) are the norm, while other people are diverse. Effective diversity education must begin with asking people to look at themselves.

An essential concept is that everyone's identity is made up of a variety of different dimensions. It is a dangerous oversimplification to think that any human group (women, teenagers, working-class people, Muslims) is homogeneous, or that any individual could be defined by their membership of a single group. In addition, people's membership of human groups changes throughout their lifetime, as does the relative importance of each dimension in their identity.

There are many dimensions of diversity, some immediately apparent and some hidden. The iceberg model[1] illustrates this (see diagram right).

Which dimensions are easily discernible (above sea level) and which are hidden will vary with the situation a person finds themselves in as well as at different stages of their life. They may consciously choose to show some aspects of their identity and conceal others. The question of how people choose to define their identity is explored by Gary Younge in his recent book *Who are We – and should it matter in the 21st century?*[2] which raises questions such as 'If Obama was raised by his White mother, why is he the first Black president?'

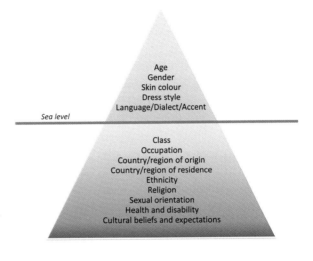

Where does diversity fit into general practice education?

Promoting Equality and Diversity is a subsection of the Personal and Professional Responsibilities section of the RCGP curriculum. Many GP educators think of Equality and Diversity training as a box to be ticked before the annual Training Recruitment round, mostly involving regulations and good practice on equal opportunities in employment. Others dismiss the entire topic as a matter of 'political correctness', currently fashionable but of no real significance. We hope to show that the complex, dynamic subject of human diversity is more important, more interesting and broader than you may have imagined.

In this chapter, we define the promotion of diversity as the recognition and valuing of differences between people, and the creation of a working culture and practice which recognise, respect, value and harness difference – for the benefit both of organisations and of individual patients and trainees.

Recognising and harnessing diversity benefits organisations because cultural and other differences between people mean they have different ways of thinking and acting. If these are acknowledged and respected in a team, its members can contribute a variety of perspectives, leading to greater creativity and more successful outcomes.

Understanding diversity is at the heart of general practice because GPs constantly encounter patients, staff, colleagues and others who differ from them in age, gender, background and many other dimensions. It is at the heart of GP education because GP educators teach learners who differ from themselves in many ways.

A qualitative research study in the Midlands in 2007[3] showed that when professionals try to meet the needs of patients of ethnicities different from their own, they struggle with uncertainty and apprehension. They feel ignorant about cultural differences and are anxious about being culturally inappropriate, causing offence, or appearing discriminatory or racist. Although they are trying to do their best, their uncertainty makes them feel disempowered and creates hesitancy and inertia in their practice. These findings confirm that educators of health professionals need to understand and teach about diversity.

We also need to understand that patients, colleagues and trainees may experience discrimination, harassment or oppression because of any of the dimensions of diversity.

The scope of this chapter

We aim to provide *guiding principles* rather than detailed 'recipes'. The chapter includes examples of educational materials to help GP Programme Directors and Trainers recognise and work with differences between them and their trainees and patients, and to help trainees learn to recognise and work with differences between them and their practice teams and patients.

In this area, as with many other aspects of general practice, educators need to facilitate the development of attitudes and skills rather than conveying knowledge. This means mostly using *experiential* educational methods.

Starting to teach about diversity

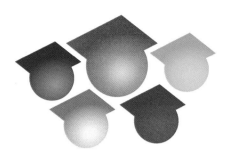

Perhaps our most important resource is the diversity within the group. It is often very helpful to work with mixed groups of educators and trainees. This immediately increases diversity in terms of age, generation, medical experience, life experience and status. Because of the changing demography of trainees, it also increases it in terms of gender, ethnicity, social class and religion. Trainees usually welcome learning about diversity in groups which include educators, but facilitators need to bear in mind that educators may feel uncomfortable and even threatened because they are not accustomed to being at the same level as the trainees.

Effective diversity education starts with getting people to look at themselves. A useful introductory tool, which works well in groups of up to about 20, is the Name Game.

THE NAME GAME

Each participant is asked to tell the group their *full name and the origin and meaning of each part of it*. The group learns about the diversity in their backgrounds as well as their names.

In a group of apparently homogeneous white British Trainers, the names may tell the group about non-English origins, perhaps Scottish or Irish, possibly Catholic or Protestant, often also something about the class background of their family.

Arun Krishnamurthy Davangere – 'Davangere is a place in India where my ancestors came from, Arun means sun and Krishnamurthy is the name of a Hindu god. In India, like in Britain, the surname can indicate the profession of one's ancestors – a Sastry or a Jois will have ancestors who were priests, while a Shetty is the descendant of a businessman.'

A trainee from a Chinese family in Singapore told the group that he had been given names meaning Ambition and Prosperity, but he would like to give his own child names meaning Contentment and Happiness.

Margaret Claire Eisner – 'Through my surname, I can tell the group that my parents came to Britain as Jewish refugees from Central Europe. My first name, Margaret, is common in British women born between about 1940 and 1960 and reminds me how important my generation is to my identity, as well as the fact that my parents chose an English name to help me fit in. At 17 I shortened it to Maggie as a symbol of adolescent rebellion and identification with the informal youth culture of the 1960s.'

The iceberg model (shown at the beginning of this chapter) can also be used interactively: learners can be asked to think about their own position on all the dimensions, and which are above and below 'sea level' in their own case. Discussing their own position with a few others helps to raise awareness of the diversity within the group.

 Top Tip: Many other stimulating exercises and training materials can be found in Joe Kai's education pack *Valuing Diversity*[4] available from the RCGP.

Understanding stereotyping

Stereotyping is labelling an individual with characteristics which you believe are typical of the group they belong to (e.g. young people, English people, women, Muslims, homosexuals, football fans). Stereotyping may help us make sense of the world and recognise patterns, and may have value in interactions with both learners and patients. However, problems arise when we forget to question the assumptions we make.

 Red Alert: Stereotyping people into groups can be dangerous because:
- you may be wrong about the characteristics of the group
- the individual's identity may have many dimensions, of which that group is only one
- you may have assigned them to a group to which they don't belong.

A useful exercise to help us understand stereotyping, and accept that we all do it, is the flashcard exercise.

THE FLASHCARD EXERCISE

This works best in facilitated groups of about six, selected for maximum diversity (of age, gender, ethnicity etc.) within each group. Each group is given a set of flashcards which each has either a short description or a picture of a person, e.g.:

- woman in a headscarf
- man who smells of cigarette smoke
- woman who shouts at her children
- older man who gives the impression that he knows best
- couple where the man does all the talking
- young man in a baseball cap who doesn't make eye contact with you
- Asian man with state-of-the-art mobile phone
- man with shaved head and tattoos
- woman in wheelchair.

(You can download my flashcards from the website if you don't want to create some from scratch.)

The participants are asked to turn over one card at a time and discuss their immediate reaction to it. Who could the person be? How would they make you feel (if you saw them in the street, or as a patient)? How would this affect the way you responded to them?

The facilitator should encourage participants to give their immediate reaction, not what they think is the acceptable response, and should help the group to see different interpretations of the description or picture and to challenge each other rather than get into cosy agreement.

The exercise, and subsequent discussion, should help participants understand how some stereotyping is inevitable and may even sometimes help a busy GP find an appropriate approach to a patient, but that we should be aware of our own assumptions and should question them.

Race, ethnicity and culture

None of these concepts is well-defined, and they are often confused with each other. The concepts of ethnicity and culture overlap, so that it is almost impossible to give clear examples.

- **Race** usually refers to the categorisation of people into groups based on various sets of inherited characteristics, including skin colour, facial features and hair texture. Most present day anthropologists consider that the term reflects a socially constructed idea rather than a scientific truth.

- **Ethnicity** refers to identification with a social group on the basis of a shared heritage (real or assumed) of common ancestry, history, kinship, religion, language, territory, nationality or physical appearance.
- **Culture** refers to the values, norms and traditions which affect how individuals of a particular group perceive, think, interact, behave and make judgements about the world. Culture is dynamic, fluid and constantly changing.

Cultural competence (the ability to interact effectively with people of different cultures) is a term which can be applied to institutions as well as individuals. It is a mistake to imagine that cultural competence is simply a matter of acquiring knowledge about other people's cultures. In relation to individuals, it includes:

- *awareness* of how one sees the world through the lens of one's own cultural values and beliefs
- *attitude* towards cultural differences
- *knowledge* of different cultural practices and world views
- *skills* in cross-cultural interaction.

This diagram (adapted from an article in the Student BMJ[5]) shows the interdependence of attitude and knowledge.

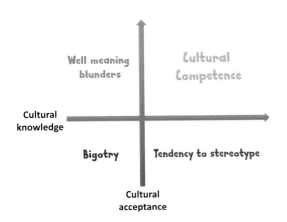

By 'cultural acceptance' we do not imply passive, uncritical acceptance, nor any suggestion that one's own culture is of less value than the other person's.

Living in a different culture

It is important for GP educators and GP trainees to develop an understanding of how it feels to live in a different culture, in relation to both our colleagues and our patients. Films and novels provide excellent material for this, and a list can be found in a document called 'Using the Arts in Diversity Teaching' on our website. The simulation game BaFa BaFa can also provide powerful experiential learning.

BAFA BAFA – A CROSS-CULTURAL SIMULATION GAME

The game is suitable for 12–40 participants and takes 2–3 hours.

After an initial briefing, two cultures are created. The Alpha culture is a relationship-oriented, hierarchical culture with different roles for men and women, very friendly as long as its unspoken rules are not broken. The Beta culture is a highly competitive trading culture, non-hierarchical and with no social rituals. After the participants learn the rules of their culture and begin living it, observers and visitors are exchanged. The participants experience the alienation and confusion which comes from being different. The resulting stereotyping, misperception and misunderstanding provide material for discussion.

The full set of materials and instructions is available in the UK from Wessex Training (www.wessex training.co.uk).

Cultural dimensions – a tool to understand cultural differences

The work of Geert Hofstede, a Dutch anthropologist, can help our understanding of both patients and trainees from different cultures. His website[6] is a useful resource.

He rated 58 nationalities on five dimensions, as follows.

- **Power Distance (PD):** the extent to which less powerful members expect and accept unequal power distribution. High PD cultures usually have centralised, top-down control but this is accepted by followers as well. Low PD implies greater equality and empowerment.
- **Individualism versus Collectivism:** In an individual environment, the individual person and their rights are more important than groups that they may belong to. In a collective environment, people are born into strong extended family or tribal communities, and these loyalties are paramount.
- **Masculinity versus Femininity** focuses on the degree to which 'traditional' gender roles are assigned in a culture; i.e. men are considered aggressive and competitive, while women are expected to be gentler and be concerned with home and family.
- **Uncertainty Avoidance (UA)** defines the extent to which a culture values predictability. UA cultures have strong traditions and rituals and tend toward formal, bureaucratic structures and rules.
- **Long-term versus Short-term Orientation** is the cultural trait that focuses on how much the group invests for the future, is persevering and is patient in waiting for results.

Hofstede's work helps us understand the influence of hierarchy, individual or group thinking, male and female perspectives, the ability to cope with uncertainty and how patient we are. All these issues are relevant to our work as trainers.

Cultural differences within the UK

As well as differences between countries, it is worth drawing attention to the considerable cultural differences between the different nations and regions of Britain, as well as between different classes. Doncaster PCT produced a glossary of local medical terms 'to assist doctors who do not speak English as a first language', available on the Internet.[7] Some of the South Yorkshire terms puzzled us even after many years as GPs in other parts of Yorkshire.

Among the innumerable aspects of language which vary across the UK between regions, classes and generations, one example is the names and times of meals. A traditional working-class Northerner would eat *tea* between 5 and 7 p.m., often as the main meal of the day. The midday meal would be called *dinner*, while *supper* would be an extra meal (anything from tea and biscuits to fish and chips) eaten late in the evening. In the South of England, especially for people from a higher class background, the midday meal is more likely to be called *lunch* and the evening meal either *dinner* or *supper*, usually eaten between 7 and 9 p.m. *Tea* in the South (but mostly for an older generation) may mean *afternoon tea*, a cup of tea with scones and cakes. And all formal meal times are much less common in younger people who tend to eat whatever they feel like, whenever they feel hungry.

 Top Tip: Kate Fox, a social anthropologist, explores this theme in the chapter on Linguistic Class Codes in her provocative and witty book *Watching the English: the hidden rules of English behaviour*.[8]

Some key health and cultural issues for UK minority ethnic groups

As we have already made clear, it is not appropriate to adopt a 'cookbook' approach to social groups, specifying their characteristics and giving learners the impression that understanding diversity is a matter of acquiring *knowledge* about other people's cultures. However, as long as we remember that **cultures are dynamic and multifaceted** and that **individuals have complex multidimensional identities**, it may be helpful to offer some broad illustrations. Interactive presentation of these issues in an educational course can be useful.

Comparing 'Eastern' cultures with the UK, we are likely to find:

- greater respect for elders
- families are seen as more important than individuals
- marriage is highly valued
- there are distinct roles for men and women
- the mother-in-law (husband's mother) is an important figure in the family
- families are bigger and sons are valued
- mental illness carries more stigma
- there are taboo subjects, such as termination of pregnancy, sexually transmitted diseases and domestic abuse
- the UK-born generation are very different from their parents
- there is cultural conflict for the UK-born generation.

Refugees and asylum seekers:

- are a very diverse group
- may have very complex health needs
- are likely to have different health beliefs and expectations of the healthcare system
- may be separated from all or some of their family
- post-traumatic stress is very common
- experience significant additional stress from their reception in the UK.

Doctors working with them:

- shouldn't underestimate the value of small welcoming gestures
- should try (even harder than usual) not to make assumptions about the patient's life history and socioeconomic, political and educational background
- may need support because they will hear very distressing stories
- may find it very hard to get old health information
- may need to allocate longer consultation times
- should provide extra reassurance about confidentiality.

Comprehensive information and support for health professionals available from
Health for Asylum Seekers and Refugees portal: www.harpweb.org.uk

Another useful approach is small-group discussion of clinical scenarios with cross-cultural aspects, such as the following:

CLINICAL SCENARIOS WITH CROSS-CULTURAL ASPECTS

A 15-year-old girl from a traditional Muslim family is brought to see you by her mother, complaining of abdominal pain. You examine her abdomen and think you can feel a 16-week pregnancy. How can you manage this situation? Later, she says, *'My father will kill me.'* How do you respond?

One of the few non-European families at the practice is that of the owner of a local Chinese restaurant. His widowed mother has come to live with them. She speaks no English. She presents with a cough and 'pain all over'. A chest X-ray and subsequent CT scan show bony metastases. Her son rings you saying that a radiotherapist has asked him to discuss the diagnosis with her, so they can have informed consent for palliative radiotherapy. He feels that such a conversation would be shocking and cruel to her. What do you do?

A 55-year-old Bangladeshi woman has been on your list for a long time. She has ischaemic heart disease, mild diabetes and bilateral cataracts. She is a frequent attender, and usually brings you a small gift of home-cooked food. Since her husband died, she has been living alone and receiving an incapacity benefit. She has two daughters in distant cities in the UK, both with their own families. She has a son in Bangladesh, who has repeatedly been refused entry into the UK. She attends one day asking you to write a letter saying that he is needed in the UK to care for her. How do you react?

Trainees from minority ethnic groups

Today's GP trainees include many from minority ethnic groups. Some are International Medical Graduates (discussed in Chapter 21: Supporting GP Trainees Who Graduated Outside the UK) but others are the British-born children of immigrant families, mainly of South Asian origin.

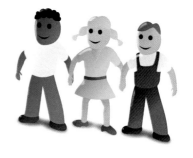

Having trainees from a wide variety of backgrounds makes a GP training scheme more lively and interesting, enabling the group to learn from a variety of perspectives and to experience diversity at first hand. However, it is useful for educators to be aware of issues which may be raised for these trainees.[9] These include the following.

- They may experience a sense of conflict between their home culture and the UK medical culture into which they have moved. A colleague from an Indian family pointed out to me that he never felt 'half British and half Indian' but flipped back and forth between an Indian identity at home with his family and a British identity when out with his peers (*see* discussion of 'double consciousness' in Chapter 21: Supporting GP Trainees Who Graduated Outside the UK). Others might have the opposite experience, feeling too English to be comfortable with their traditional extended family, but too foreign to really fit in with their English colleagues. These issues are well illustrated in the film *Yasmin* and several other novels and films (listed in 'Using the Arts in Diversity Teaching' on our website).
- Their families will have been through the disruption of immigration, and may have experienced financial and social disadvantage.
- Some come from traditional family structures, which contrast with the more individualistic 'Western' way of life. Some trainees from immigrant families may have had a much more sheltered upbringing than those from UK families. One important issue is that unmarried women

trainees from immigrant families may well have had no sexual experience, making it difficult for them to discuss and manage patients' sexual health problems.

- Some have considerable responsibility for their extended families and, because of the prevalence of ischaemic heart disease and diabetes in South Asian families, may find themselves caring for ailing parents at an earlier stage in their careers than most trainees from British families.

Language and communication
Consulting with patients with little or no English
Almost all GPs will consult occasionally with patients with limited or no English. Many in urban areas will do so several times a day, and in some practices the majority of patients will be in this category. Trainees are often very aware of their educational need for skills in this area. The material which follows is based on courses we have run in Yorkshire.

EXERCISE EXPLORING LANGUAGE BARRIERS
At the start of the session, participants are asked which languages they speak and whether they speak each one fluently, enough to get by, or just a few words.

No language: The learners work in pairs. Each is given a simple medical problem and a little background information, e.g.
- You've had a cough for 2 weeks which has been keeping you awake. You are short of breath on exertion. The cough is productive of green phlegm. You feel quite feverish and ill. You are afraid you might have TB.
- You have a painful left knee since playing football with some friends last week. You are particularly worried about this as you have just got a job in a factory which involves standing up all day.

They then role play doctor and patient, using no spoken language or written words at all, to see how much mutual understanding can be achieved and what means they use for this.

Limited language: Using the information obtained earlier, the facilitator pairs the learners so that both speak the same foreign language but only 'enough to get by' or 'just a few words'. They then role play doctor and patient again with different scenarios, this time using only the foreign language.

Outcomes: The learners experience how much can be conveyed non-verbally, and also how difficult it is to communicate in a foreign language and how powerless both patient and doctor can feel without a common language. The facilitator can use a flip chart to summarise the discussion. This can lead to a summary of resources which can be used in consultations with language barriers.

SIMULATED CONSULTATIONS WITH LIMITED LANGUAGE
These provide memorable and powerful learning, and are an essential part of the courses we have run. The principles are the same as any other simulated consultation (see Chapter 18: The Simulated Patient – your walking, talking, learning tool) but the bilingual simulators should be specifically trained. It is useful to include at least four situations:
- a patient with limited English and no interpreter
- a family member interpreting
- an 'ad hoc' interpreter such as an untrained practice receptionist, or casual acquaintance of the patient
- telephone interpreting.

We do not include scenarios with *professional* face-to-face interpreters, as these are so rarely used in day-to-day general practice. However, in exceptional circumstances, especially with patients with mental health problems, it may be invaluable for a GP to book a professional interpreter in advance and reserve a double (or, preferably, triple) appointment.

As in real life, more time should be allocated for these simulations than for those without language barriers. If there are enough resources (rooms and facilitators), groups of four participants are ideal. The practical aspects of the telephone interpreted consultation are important – it is best to use a speaker phone so the group can hear both sides of the consultation, and organisers need to remember to allocate a room for the telephone interpreter.

Either before or after the simulation session, it may be useful to present ideas about ways to manage these consultations. Some of these are summarised below.

Consultation tips for basic English

- Speak clearly, slowly, calmly (don't shout).
- Pause between sentences (chunk and check).
- Simplify English.
- Simplify the grammar – short, simple sentences.
- Avoid idioms and colloquialisms.
- Avoid jargon and technical terms.
- Simplify consultation structure.
- More closed questions than you would usually use.

- Offer alternatives to check that Yes means Yes (e.g. 'is the pain worse when you sit? Or when you stand?').
- Consider using pictures and diagrams.
- Consider using mime (but some gestures are not universal and some may offend).
- Remember your own expressions and body language.
- Check understanding.
- Don't overload.

Resources doctors can use in limited-language consultations

- Simplified language ('basic English')
- Paraverbals – loudness, tone, manner of speaking
- Non-verbals – body language, gestures
- Sign language
- Drawings and diagrams (prepared, or drawn by either doctor or patient)
- Leaflets in foreign languages
- Internet resources:
  asylum seekers' health portal: www.harpweb.org.uk
- Translated leaflets:
  www.patient.co.uk
  www.mind.org.uk/information/BT.htm
  www.healthinfotranslations.com
- Interpreters – telephone (e.g. language line), professional face to face, informal interpreter (e.g. family member), ad hoc interpreter (e.g. practice staff member).

Joe Kai's education pack *Valuing Diversity*[4] includes a DVD with enlightening examples of consultations with interpreters.

 Top Tip: The e-learning for Healthcare website, free to all primary care professionals and educators in the NHS, includes useful modules on consultations involving language and cultural differences.[10,11,12]

Consultations with interpreters
These raise the same issues as other three-way consultations:
1 Who is in control?
2 Risk of consultation becoming two-way, excluding the patient or possibly the doctor.
3 Always try to look directly at the patient and address your questions to them.

Here are some points to consider:

Consulting with interpreters

Family or friend of patient
- May be the only option or may be the patient's preference.
- May be planned, or may be arranged at short notice.
- Confidentiality issues with relative or member of patient's community.
- Embarrassment when discussing intimate health problems.
- Interpreter may have poor language skills.
- Interpreter may not understand their role.
- Complex – like presence of relative in any consultation.
- Interpreter may also be finding the situation difficult.

Family and friends – consultation tips
- Careful introductions – who are they? What is their relationship?
- Are patient and translator comfortable with the situation?
- Assess translator's level of English.
- Doctor may need to use 'basic English' tips with the translator.
- Be directive with the translator.
- Explain what you want to happen, and why.
- Ask for direct translation of everything you and patient say.
- Acknowledge a relative's dual role – perhaps ask for relative's point of view after you have asked for patient's, and ask relative to translate this back to patient.
- *Consider* offering appointment with an alternative interpreter (e.g. telephone service).

Using practice staff members as translators
- They may have not have had any training.
- They may not understand their role as a translator.
- Check their level of skill in the foreign language.
- Explain confidentiality to the patient.

Professional interpreters – good practice
- Beforehand – check who employs them, how well they are trained, their code of conduct (esp. confidentiality).
- Check that *language* and *dialect* are correct for the patient.
- Pre-consultation discussion: orientate interpreter and recap confidentiality.
- Check specific knowledge (health-related language).
- Clarify pronunciation of names.
- Allow interpreter to introduce self to patient, explain role and confidentiality, check they are acceptable interpreter.
- Encourage interpreter to check patient understands, ask you to clarify if necessary.
- Debrief with interpreter afterwards.

Telephone interpreters

- Generally – very accessible, many languages, expensive, interpreter may not be in UK.
- Unlike face to face – feels unfamiliar, may make it harder (or easier) to deal with sensitive issues, harder to use diagrams, harder to have help while examining, very hard to arrange continuity of an interpreter over several appointments.
- Before you phone – identify organisation and language needed.
- At start – introduce self to the interpreter, check language and dialect, explain the situation.
- Non-verbal communication remains very important (yours and the patient's).

Cultural aspects of communication

It is impossible to consider the use of language in isolation from culture. Cultural issues will inevitably form part of the simulation scenarios and should of course be included in the discussion. A very useful resource illustrating culture-related linguistic patterns in consultations with patients from different language backgrounds is the video *Doing the Lambeth Talk* produced by Celia Roberts at King's College, London. *To order your copy contact Dale Burton at dale.burton@ londonDeanery.ac.uk or phone 020 7866 3123 or write to Ms Dale Burton, 2nd Floor, London Deanery, Stewart House, 32 Russell Square, London WC1B 5DN.*

Doctors whose first language is not English and who have graduated in medicine outside the UK will have particular difficulty with linguistic and cultural aspects of communication. *See* Chapter 21: Supporting GP Trainees Who Graduated Outside the UK for an exploration of this issue, with discussion of the concept of 'linguistic capital' and suggestions how to help this group.

Social class

The power of the class system in the UK should never be underestimated. In the GP education context, it has several implications.

- Trainees from less privileged backgrounds may feel less confident in the medical world. This may affect their interactions with their colleagues, their consultations and their performance in examinations (*see* Chapter 21: Supporting GP Trainees Who Graduated Outside the UK).
- Social class stereotypes may also affect their interactions with patients. Some trainees may view unemployed people who live on Council estates as 'chavs' and assume that they are unintelligent and will not want detailed health information, or understand or act on it.
- Some trainees struggle to understand the concept of poverty of ideas, poverty of expectation or spiritual poverty in areas of high social deprivation, and may assume that anyone, whatever their background and circumstances, could access education or become upwardly socially mobile if they tried hard enough.
- Others may view more affluent patients as 'posh' and feel irritation rather than empathy when they seek reassurance about apparently trivial problems.

Gender and parenthood

The gender balance in medicine has changed dramatically. In the 1960s the proportion of women in UK medical schools was about 20%, whereas it is now about 70%. Today's generation of women doctors are unlikely to experience the level of sexism experienced by those who trained a few decades ago. It is no longer the norm for young doctors (male and female) to complete their training before starting a family.

However, both GP educators and trainees continue to make many assumptions based on gender, and trainees of both sexes may feel disadvantaged or discriminated against because of their gender or parental status or both. Some examples for possible discussion are listed in the box below:

> The group of trainees decides to organise study sessions at 5 p.m. after the Half-Day Release course. Those with small children to collect from a nursery feel excluded, and ask the Programme Directors to revise the educational programme so that all educational activities take place in normal working hours.
>
> A male trainee requests a change of working hours because he has to drop his children off at school. His female trainer, recalling the sacrifices she has made to ensure her family life never impacted on her work, is horrified and asks why he can't employ a nanny as she did.
>
> A senior male partner in a training practice refers to all women colleagues and staff as 'girlies'. At a practice away day including the female trainee, he teases the women about how long it took them to get ready for the day and then suggests to the men that they go off and have a beer.

Sexual orientation

The website of the Gay and Lesbian Association of Doctors and Dentists (GLADD)[13] states that *'although the law has changed, both in terms of legal protection at work and in terms of civil partnerships, there is still much to be done in terms of promoting a culture of acceptance of gay and lesbian people within and by the medical profession. Although many of our members have not experienced any problems as a result of their sexual orientation, many have faced substantial challenges, and it can be an isolated and lonely time.'*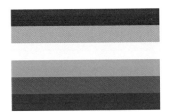

It is important when running educational events to be aware that participants may include gay and lesbian doctors, and to be careful what you say. Older GP educators, themselves educated at a time when homosexuality was more hidden, occasionally forget this. A gay colleague told me how unsettled he felt at a training course where, at lunch, he overheard the facilitator whisper 'Watch your backs, boys' when he saw a feminine-looking male waiter.

On the other hand, younger GP educators brought up in the UK in the last 20 years may forget that not all the trainees will share their liberal approach – you may need to protect your gay and lesbian trainees from exposure to their colleagues' attitudes. For example, a colleague told me about a light-hearted awareness-raising exercise including little scenarios for the participants to comment on. A young woman trainee picked one which said: *'Someone tells you that your best friend is gay (they saw him kissing another bloke in a gay club). But he hasn't confided that to you yet.'* She responded: *'Well, that's just not natural, is it?',* making my colleague feel concerned about how at least one group member, who he knew was gay, would be feeling.

The issue of heterosexual bias in language should not be dismissed as 'political correctness'. Problems occur when the words used are unclear or have been associated with negative stereotypes. For example, because the word 'homosexuality' has been associated in the past with deviance, mental illness and criminal behaviour, it is better to use 'same-sex relationships' or specific terms such as 'gay men', 'lesbians' or 'men who have sex with men'. The Committee on Lesbian and Gay Concerns (CLGC), founded in 1980, has produced a report on heterosexual bias in language, which is the basis of a PowerPoint available on our website.

Key issues relating to gay and lesbian patients are summarised below.

In general, gay and lesbian patients:
- Have experienced a huge change in public attitudes in the UK in the last 40 years, but may still live with prejudice.
- Are diverse in terms of age, class, etc.
- Vary a lot in how much they define themselves by their sexuality.
- May have had bad experiences with health professionals, e.g. not having a same-sex partner recognised in a hospital as their next of kin, or having had consultations with GPs who assume they are heterosexual.

Doctors working with them need to:
- Avoid assuming that all their patients are heterosexual.
- Learn phrases to use in the consultation which don't assume that everyone is heterosexual (e.g. *'Do you need contraception?'* rather than *'What contraception do you use?'*).
- Show acceptance, create rapport and then take a detailed sexual history if clinically indicated.
- Understand health issues for gay and lesbian patients, e.g. understanding that whether a lesbian patient should have a cervical smear depends on her sexual history (if she has never had sex with men, she is at low risk and a smear may be technically difficult and quite traumatic – but heterosexual experience, willing or unwilling, will put her at greater risk and make it more important to consider having a smear).

Doctors from countries where homosexuality is less openly accepted and less visible are:
- Likely to be less familiar with these issues.
- Less likely to recognise the 'non-verbal cues' of dress and behaviour by which some gay and lesbian people express their sexual orientation.

Educational methods for raising awareness of the needs of gay and lesbian patients include simulated consultations as well as arts materials such as the film *If These Walls Could Talk 2* which deals with lesbian bereavement. Sexual health issues affecting gay and lesbian patients can also be included in clinically focused education sessions.

Religion

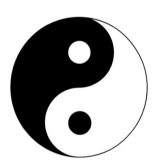

This is an area of great diversity, and one where great sensitivity is required. The population of GP trainees includes a wide spectrum of religious belief and lack of it. There are huge differences between fundamentalists and liberals in the *same* religion, and also between those with a religious world view and those with a secular one.

Material is available about the major religions and healthcare,[14,15,16] but our most important educational aims in this area are to raise awareness of the breadth of the religious spectrum, and to help learners understand how religion may affect attitudes to health and healthcare.

As usual, it is useful to start with the experience of the group of trainees:

RELIGION – AWARENESS-RAISING EXERCISE

In a group which has already got to know and trust each other, it can be very effective to sit in a circle and ask each person to tell the group about their own religion and what it means to them. Alternatively, it may be appropriate to start the session with an exercise in pairs.

Facilitation needs to be sensitive. It may be better to allow people to speak 'as the spirit moves them' rather than to go round in turn. The facilitator may choose to discourage discussion, so that each person has a safe space to say things which may be very important to them. Some people in the group may choose not to speak.

What is learnt will, of course, depend on the composition of the group. Participants may learn the range of reasons people feel attached to their religion, such as a sense of belonging, community or identity, a moral code to guide them or a spiritual path. Some may be devoted to religious practice, while others emphasise beliefs and principles. Some participants may describe rebellion against a narrow or prescriptive religious upbringing. Others may have developed a strong religious sensibility as young adults, after a secular or liberal upbringing. Those to whom religion is very important may learn that they should not assume that secular or agnostic people lack moral values.

When planning educational events, it is useful to be aware of religious restrictions on food and drink which may affect participants, perhaps making some trainees feel discriminated against or excluded. Examples of things to *avoid* include:

- offering a bottle of wine as the only prize for winning a clinical quiz
- labelling the food at a buffet lunch as 'meat', 'fish' or 'vegetarian' but not differentiating the meat into chicken, pork, beef or lamb
- making a shared meal a centrally important part of a course held during Ramadan (when Muslims fast during daylight hours)
- choosing the pub or bar as the venue for informal networking after a course.

A presentation of the range of cultural aspects of religion affecting patients' health beliefs and attitudes to healthcare can be a useful introduction to discussion of the trainees' experiences with patients:

Cultural aspects of religion affecting health beliefs and healthcare	
Family life • Importance of extended family • Gender roles • Contact between the sexes (this may include doctor and patient) • Attitudes to marriage	**Sexual issues** • Attitudes to sexual behaviour • Menstruation taboos • Attitudes to contraception and to termination of pregnancy • Attitudes to assisted conception • Attitudes to homosexuality
Attitudes to illness • May be seen as God's will, or as punishment for sin • Mental illness • Inherited disorders • Physical illness	**Diet** • Dietary restrictions • Fasting • Alcohol, smoking and drug abuse
Death and bereavement • Attitudes to death • Attitudes to suicide • Attitudes to withdrawal of 'futile' life prolonging treatment • Attitudes to euthanasia • Attitudes to post-mortem examination • Funeral customs • Mourning customs	**Childbirth** • Birth customs • Infant circumcision • Religion-specific naming • Breast feeding • Attitudes to disability • Attitudes to adoption and fostering

Disability

Disability is a dimension of diversity which is often overlooked – both in teaching and in recruitment and employment.

Teaching about disability

Disability is defined as the end result of mental, physical or sensory impairments or long-term ill health which can limit functional ability. It is easier to teach about it if the group of trainees includes someone with a disability. If it doesn't, it can be useful to ask the group to reflect on what they know of the experiences of any friends, colleagues or relatives who have a disability.

Other useful resources are the organisations and agencies which support people with disabilities, such as local services for the visually impaired or the Royal National Institute for Deaf People (RNID). Trainees' awareness of disability issues can be raised very effectively by an articulate speaker who is, for example, blind, deaf or a wheelchair user. Some agencies have also developed exercises enabling the participants to experience something like the disability; for example, wearing glasses which create tunnel vision.

 Top Tip: The website of the Partners in Practice project, a collaboration between the University of Bristol, the University of the West of England and the Peninsula Medical School, is a useful resource for training health professionals to work with disabled people as patients.[17]

Supporting trainees with disabilities

The BMA, which provides support for doctors with disabilities[18] states that doctors and medical students who are disabled or who have impairments often have a difficult time. As well as having to come to terms with their condition, they also face problems in their career. Inflexible working patterns, poor contingency cover, and colleagues who are 'sympathetic until it affects them' often add guilt to an already difficult situation and leave ill or disabled doctors wondering whether they can continue working in a position that makes little allowances for their health needs. There are no figures on the number of disabled doctors in the UK or the distribution of disabled doctors among the different specialties.

GP educators will find their local Occupational Health Department a source of valuable help and guidance on how best to support trainees with disabilities. The quotations below are taken from 'A Celebration of Disabled Doctors'.[19]

General practice has evolved as an organised and unique specialty reflecting the change in training over the last few years. Recruitment and training are now competency based, tested by standardised tools and therefore more objective. Support for trainees with disabilities is still variable, depending on how willing the individual NHS trust is to accommodate disability.

I strongly believe that disabled doctors bring a personal understanding of suffering from a disease or condition which helps maintain the doctor–patient relationship and provide role models to other talented disabled individuals who may give up pursuing professions which they could do with some determination and adequate adjustments.

Saima Salahuddin, GP trainee with Ehlers Danlos syndrome

I think each disabled doctor, like any doctor, should be taken on their own merits and judged on ability rather than by their disability. Having said that, I think many disabled doctors may be more resilient than their peers and have greater determination, having had to fight harder throughout their lives at every point to prove themselves. They might also bring a different and personal perspective and insight into treatment, coping strategies, and management of patients with disabilities.

Katherine Thomas, salaried GP with hearing impairment

Learning disability

Perhaps because having a learning disability precludes training as a doctor, this is an area for which we show particularly low awareness. The RCGP curriculum provides some good resources for teaching sessions. Asking trainees if any of their family members or others in their circle of acquaintance suffers from a learning disability can be a helpful opening to a session discussing healthcare for this neglected group.

Age

Established GP educators often observe that today's doctors show less professional attitudes, and may even stereotype them as 'the youth of today'. Jean Twenge, a psychologist at the University of San Diego, California, has coined the term 'Generation Me' for today's students, and carried out extensive research throwing light on this area.[20] She has identified four major areas of change in today's medical students in the US:

- high expectations which may not be realistic
- a sense of entitlement which includes expecting plenty of leisure time
- an increase in mental health problems
- changing study skills, with IT competence but reduced ability to obtain information from long texts.

Understanding these generational changes may help GP educators plan their teaching appropriately, and help them avoid developing negative attitudes towards modern trainees.

Age can also be an issue for trainees. Their attitudes to older patients may be tinged with ageism, sometimes uncomfortably apparent to ageing GP educators. This can lead them to ignore clinically important issues for older people. For example, they may need reminding that their 'elderly' patients may be driving, drinking alcohol, taking illicit drugs or being sexually active.

Another relevant attitude to ageing is the respect for elders which is built into non-Western cultures. Trainees from non-Western families may feel particularly uncomfortable asking personal questions or giving advice to older patients, especially those from a similar cultural background.

Patients sometimes tell trainees that they look too young to be a doctor. Although GP educators may wish they were so lucky, the trainee may need support and advice if they feel undermined and unable to behave with appropriate authority.

Dress

People (doctors and patients) may consciously use dress to express their identity; even where they are not conscious of it, the way people dress is a signal to others of aspects of their identity.

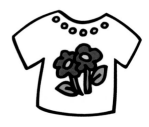

Sometimes dress can raise issues in the training scheme or the practice. For example, both GP educators and older patients may feel unsettled by young doctors who look scruffy, dress scantily or have visible tattoos or piercings. Some doctors choose to dress in ways reflecting their culture or religion; in some GP practices and hospitals, their distinctive clothing may surprise staff or patients and perhaps lead them to make unjustified assumptions. Occasionally, GP Programme Directors may be called on to intervene in cases where a doctor's dress, chosen for religious reasons, is in conflict with the hospital's dress code (for example the 'bare below the elbows' policy).

Promoting diversity in practice

Promoting awareness and acceptance of diversity has organisational implications. There may be training needs for both clinical and administrative members of practice teams.

Organisational points for the practice and the training scheme

Names: do the practice receptionists routinely ask patients of all religions for their 'Christian' name (rather than their 'first name')?

Forms of address: asking trainees to be on first-name terms with their teachers is seen by doctors brought up by British families as welcoming and friendly. However, doctors from countries (such as India and Pakistan) where there is more respect for elders and particularly for teachers may feel very uncomfortable with first names. This may also apply to the children of immigrants from those countries. (*See* Chapter 21: Supporting GP Trainees Who Graduated Outside the UK.)

Food and alcohol: practice or training scheme social events in pubs are not likely to be welcoming to Muslim doctors (or others who don't drink); educational events involving catering should take account of likely dietary restrictions.

Time off for religious observance: this needs to be discussed within the practice or training scheme, made explicit at Induction, and applied fairly to everybody.

Educational games: games where participants touch each other are unsuitable for groups with participants from cultures where physical contact between unrelated people of different sexes is discouraged. In Bradford, we abandoned an ice-breaking game where participants were supposed to stand on chairs in a circle and rearrange themselves in order of their dates of birth, after two Muslim women explained that the physical contact was unacceptable and another woman, 24 weeks pregnant, said she thought she shouldn't be climbing on chairs. My colleague saved the situation by asking these three to help him facilitate another game.

Educational programme timetable: if you have a significant number of trainees of any particular religion, avoid timetabling important educational sessions during religious holidays. Be careful what you schedule during Ramadan, as trainees who are fasting may be less alert and responsive than usual; it is helpful to provide a pleasant space for them to relax during breaks when other participants are eating and drinking.

Group discussion of the following organisational scenarios can make the subject of diversity more alive and less abstract.

PRACTICE ORGANISATION SCENARIOS

- At a practice meeting, you propose that *asylum seekers and others with language problems should be offered double appointments*. One of your colleagues objects, saying that this is unfair to all the other patients who might like a double appointment. What are the implications?
- The Practice Manager comes back from a Diversity course and says that she would like to implement a *Zero Tolerance of Racism* policy. What might this mean?
- The practice (which has three male partners and one woman) has advertised for a new partner – at interview, a shortlisted applicant tells you that she is a *practising Catholic and is unwilling to see any patients for contraception*. How do you react?
- You are *planning a new Health Centre*, at last. What features would you like to include in order to meet the needs of all the diverse groups who use your practice?
- (for white British doctors) A patient opens the consultation by saying, *'I'm glad you're not one of those foreign doctors'*. How do you feel, what do you say?
- A woman comes to see you with a cervical smear reminder letter; she hasn't had a smear for about 10 years. She says she is a *lesbian and does she really have to have a smear test*? How do you respond?
- Your trainee complains to you that, at the end of a dysfunctional consultation, a *patient has been racially abusive*. He insists the patient should be removed from the practice list. How would you respond?
- One of your office staff tells you that she is thinking of resigning because of *repeated sexual comments from one of your partners*. What issues does this raise and how would you respond?
- A locum from a minority ethnic group who is working in your practice complains to you that a *receptionist is treating him unfairly* and giving him excessive numbers of patients to see. He feels that her attitude is racist. The receptionist tells you that she is simply giving him the same workload as the rest of the partners, but considers him unpleasant and work shy. What steps do you take?

Using the arts for diversity teaching

There are many books and films which deal with cross-cultural situations and help to illuminate the issues in this chapter (*see* Chapter 17: Using the Creative Arts). Participants can be invited to read novels (some will, some won't) and films can be shown on educational courses.

 Top Tip: A collection of books and films to teach about diversity can be found in a document called 'Using the Arts in Diversity Teaching' on our website. We will periodically update this document as we find more.

Equality, diversity and the law

GP educators who are interested in diversity and have developed cultural awareness should have no cause to worry about the legal aspects of this subject. However, training in equality and diversity is mandatory for those involved in recruitment procedures. Excellent training resources on race discrimination and other relevant legislation are available on line via:

- BMJ Learning[21]
- Doctors.net[22]
- E-learning for Healthcare.[23]

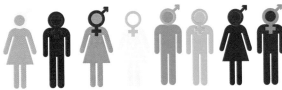

Getting it right

Finally, we would like to emphasise that this is an area where there are no right answers, you can't know everything and people will not always agree. We will all make mistakes, which provide the raw material for the most powerful learning. The most important things are to be open-minded and to enjoy the fact that all of us – educators, trainees and patients – are different in innumerable ways.

A sample of resources on our website

- Using the arts in diversity teaching.
- Exploring stereotypes – flashcards exercise.
- Avoiding heterosexual bias in language (PowerPoint).

Other chapters you may like to read

- Chapter 21: Supporting GP Trainees Who Graduated Outside the UK
- Chapter 17: Using the Creative Arts.

Further reading

- Beavan J, *et al. Promoting Equality and Valuing Diversity*, Module 3.4. Available at: www.e-lfh. org.uk (accessed 10 December 2010).
- Helman CG. *Culture, Health and Illness.* 5th ed. London: Hodder Arnold; 2007.
- Kai J, editor. *Ethnicity, Health and Primary Care.* Oxford: Oxford University Press; 2003.
- Morrison T, Conaway WA. *Kiss, Bow or Shake Hands: the bestselling guide to doing business in more than 60 countries.* 2nd ed. Avon, Mass: Adams Media; 2006.
- Younge G. *Who are We – and should it matter in the 21st century?* Glasgow: Viking; 2010.

Please give us some feedback on this chapter to help shape it for the next edition.
Go to www.essentialgptrainingbook.com and simply click on the title of this chapter.

Acknowledgements

Many thanks to my chapter buddies, Jon Chadwick and Arun Davangere, to the colleagues who kindly offered comments and amendments on draft versions: Juliet Draper, Miriam Hawkins, Ben Jackson, Joe Kai, Amar Rughani, Shake Seigel, Emma Storr and Veronica Wilkie, and to Iain Lamb for contributing the section on Geert Hofstede's work.

In addition, I would like to thank everyone who has helped me develop ideas about diversity, including my parents Conrad and Gisela Eisner who came to the UK as refugees from Central Europe in 1939, my patients in North London, South London and Bradford, the trainees on the Bradford GP training scheme, and the trainers and trainees who have participated in our diversity seminars. For the work on consulting with patients with limited or no English I am indebted to Sarah Escott who first developed the simulation work, and to our team of bilingual patient simulators.

References

1 Kreps GL, Kunimoto EN. *Effective Communication in Multicultural Health Care Settings*. London: Sage; 1994.

2 Younge G. *Who are We – and should it matter in the 21st century?* Glasgow: Viking; 2010.

3 Kai J, Beavan J, Faull C, *et al*. Professional uncertainty and disempowerment responding to ethnic diversity in health care: a qualitative study. *PloS Medicine*. 2007; **4**: e323. Available at: www.plosmedicine.org

4 Kai, J. *Valuing Diversity*. 2nd ed. London: RCGP; 2006.

5 Cohen D, Desai M, Leinster S. Medicine in a multicultural society. *studentBMJ*. 2001; **9**: 357–8.

6 www.geert-hofstede.com (accessed 20 May 2011).

7 http://regmedia.co.uk/2006/04/24/glossary_for_international_recruits.pdf (accessed 6 December 2010).

8 Fox K. *Watching the English: the hidden rules of English behaviour*. London: Hodder; 2005.

9 Bass D. Where the wild winds blow. *J Balint Soc*. 2007; **35**: 38–42.

10 Kai J, Beavan J. Cross-Cultural Communication. Session GPS_02a_007 in Module 2, *The GP Consultation*. Available at: www.e-lfh.org.uk (accessed 10 December 2010).

11 Kai J, Beavan J. Health Inequalities. Session GPS_02a_008 in Module 2 *The GP Consultation*. Available at: www.e-lfh.org.uk (accessed 10 December 2010).

12 Kai J, Beavan J, Wright. Language Barriers. Health Inequalities. Session GPS_02a_009 in Module 2, *The GP Consultation*. Available at: www.e-lfh.org.uk (accessed 10 December 2010).

13 www.gladd.co.uk (accessed 10 December 2010).

14 Sheikh A, Gatrad AR, editors. *Caring for Muslim Patients*. 2nd ed. Oxford: Radcliffe; 2008.

15 Thakrar D, Das R, Sheikh A, editors. *Caring for Hindu Patients*. Oxford: Radcliffe; 2008.

16 Spitzer J. *Caring for Jewish Patients*. Oxford: Radcliffe; 2003.

17 www.bris.ac.uk/pip/project-info.html (accessed 10 December 2010).

18 www.bma.org.uk/equality_diversity/disability/disableddoctorsandmedstudents.jsp (accessed 6 December 2010).

19 www.bma.org.uk/equality_diversity/disability/disableddoctors.jsp (accessed 6 December 2010).

20 Twenge JM. Generational changes and their impact in the classroom: teaching Generation Me. *Med Educ*. 2009; **43**: 398–405.

21 *Discrimination in the Workplace: what it is and how to prevent it*. Available at: http://learning.bmj.com (accessed 6 December 2010).

22 E-learning module *Equality and Diversity*. Available at: www.doctors.net.uk (accessed 10 December 2010).

23 Beavan J, Gill P. Equalities legislation. Session GPS_03-4_002 in Module 3.4, *Promoting Equality and Valuing Diversity*. Available at: www.e-lfh.org.uk (accessed 10 December 2010).

Supporting GP Trainees Who Graduated Outside the UK

MAGGIE EISNER – TPD (Bradford) & lead author   JON CHADWICK – TPD (Scarborough)
ARUN DAVANGERE – recent GP Trainee (Sheffield), now salaried GP (Worksop)
AMAR RUGHANI – APD (Sheffield)

The NHS has always included a significant proportion of doctors whose medical training was outside the UK. General practice would probably be unsustainable without them. The majority of current overseas GP trainees are from the Indian subcontinent, but others come from Africa, the Middle East, South-East Asia and both Western and Eastern Europe.

When any trainee arrives at a new training scheme or practice, educators aim to welcome them, be interested in them, understand them and help them to maximise their potential. This is a more complex task with those who trained outside the UK. This chapter aims to help educators understand the issues and challenges involved and to offer a repertoire of ways to respond positively.

European medical graduates

The term International Medical Graduates (IMGs) strictly applies to those doctors whose primary medical qualification is from a medical school outside the UK and the European Union (EU). Doctors who trained and have worked in the EU have similar residence and employment rights to UK doctors. In other respects, however, they share many of the same challenges as IMGs. Currently, EU doctors are not required to demonstrate proficiency in English, and language can present a particularly significant problem for them. Most of this chapter can be applied to both groups, although much of the illustrative material is drawn from work with trainees from non-European countries.

How may the situation of IMGs differ from that of UK graduates?

The UK medical and social cultures are different from those the IMGs are used to. Their own experience will determine which aspects are most significant for them, but there are many articulate accounts of their impressions.

'This was my first trip to a foreign country. I came with little money and no friends or relatives in Britain. . . . For someone who has always been "one of us", it is impossible to imagine the feeling of being "the other" that engulfs you soon after arrival in a new country. The deafening silence of the countryside, the palpable discomfort at meeting a stranger's gaze, astonishment at everyone's attempts to hide behind a newspaper in the London tube, inability to react to the smile of a stranger that never quite reaches the eyes and the early awareness of racial stereotypes are all disconcerting experiences. You are torn between the need to make human contact and a greater need to hide.'

Swaran Singh. Personal View. *BMJ*. 1994; **308**(1): 1169

'The way that doctors and staff talk to each other in this country is different. I'm not sure what is "the right way". For example, what are acceptable topics of conversation? I always seem to be meeting new people but how should I break the ice?'

Respondent to S Yorks GP training IMG survey, 2009

'I'm not always sure that people are interested to find out about my background and why I think and believe in the ways that I do.'

Respondent to S Yorks GP training IMG survey, 2009

Journey to GP training: Before they can practise medicine in the UK most IMGs, but not EU doctors, have to take a demanding English test, the International English Testing System (IELTS) followed by a two-part medical examination set by the Professional and Linguistic Assessments Board (PLAB). After this, they are often advised to undertake an unpaid clinical attachment with a hospital consultant. While preparing for the exams and during the attachment, they are not able to undertake paid medical work. UK immigration regulations have changed frequently over the last few decades and immigration status is often a source of background worry for IMGs, especially when arbitrary changes in the regulations make them feel understandably distrustful and insecure.

Life-stage: On average older than the majority of GP trainees, IMGs may be at a different stage in their personal lives, perhaps with an established family. Their spouse may be another IMG doctor working in a distant area or, on the other hand, may not have a work visa and be stuck at home all the time. They are likely to be far from their extended family, friends and medical colleagues. This may make them feel isolated, particularly in contrast to many of their UK-trained colleagues who may be on a GP training scheme with people they have known since medical school.

Familiarity with the NHS and general practice: They are likely to be unfamiliar with the NHS and with UK general practice, both professionally and from personal experience. Unlike UK graduates, they will have no childhood memories of visiting the GP. Family members in their home country, even less familiar with UK general practice, may be disappointed with their career choice.

Role within a team: They may have had considerable medical experience in their home country and/or in UK hospital practice. In both these situations, they may be used to the doctor being the head of the team. In a more democratic multidisciplinary team, they may feel they have lost their role, and may experience an uncomfortable sense of disorientation. Our impression is that this may more often be a significant issue for male doctors, as women may be more used to accepting a non-leading role in social situations.

Educational culture: Their primary medical training will probably have differed from UK training in several ways. It is likely to have been more didactic and more hierarchical, with educators respected for their position rather than their expertise. The educational culture may have been one in which it is difficult to admit to making a mistake, which may mean that the learner 'loses face'.

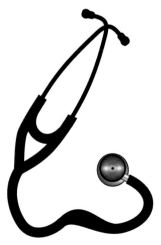

Communication skills training: IMGs are unlikely to have had any formal communication skills training, and many of the methods of teaching and assessment current in the UK, such as small group discussion, video and simulated consultations, will be unfamiliar. However, the extract on the following page presents a persuasive case against assuming that our methods are superior in every way to those used in their home countries.

STUDENTS FROM DIFFERENT CULTURAL BACKGROUNDS[1]

One thing we are sure you will have noticed in your institution or from your reading is that stereotypes are attached to students from different cultural backgrounds. One of these stereotypes is that students, particularly those from Asia, are rote learners. Yet many studies have shown that these students score at least as well and sometimes higher than Western students on measures of deep learning. You may also have noticed how there seems to be a disproportionate number of these Asian students who receive academic distinctions and prizes! This apparent 'paradox' – adopting surface approaches such as rote learning but demonstrating high achievement in academic courses – has been the subject of much investigation.

What is emerging is that researchers have assumed that memorisation was equated with mechanical rote learning. But memorisation is not a simple concept. It is intertwined with understanding such as when you might rote learn a poem to assist in the processes of interpretation and understanding. Thus, the traditional Confucian heritage way of memorisation can have different purposes. Sometimes it can be for mechanical rote learning. But it is also used to deepen and develop understanding. The paradox of these learners is solved when memorisation is seen as an important part of the process leading to understanding.

Racism: Although the UK is a relatively tolerant country, IMGs may experience discrimination from patients, colleagues or both. Some patients in general practice express antipathy to 'foreign doctors'. At a recent GP conference for GP educators, we heard about a hospital consultant whose policy is not to allow any IMG GP trainee attached to his unit to see patients independently, but only to 'shadow' other doctors.

Refugee doctors

Question: How many refugee and asylum-seeking doctors do you think there are in the UK?

Answer: In 2008 there were nearly 1200 refugee and asylum-seeking doctors registered with the BMA, with the actual numbers in the UK thought to be nearer 2000.[2]

Refugee doctors differ from IMGs in a number of ways.
- Most IMGs have chosen to come to the UK; refugee doctors have not.
- Some IMGs have community or family networks in the UK; refugee doctors do not.
- They are more likely to have had longer career breaks out of medicine.
- They come with social and psychological issues related to their experiences in their own country and in relation to their enforced flight.
- They experience further difficulties created by the UK asylum system.

These differences mean that they have additional needs to those of other IMGs. Some deaneries, especially in London, have organised special projects for refugee doctors.

 Top Tip: The BMA provides support for refugee doctors[3] and a useful guide is produced by the Jewish Council for Racial Equality.[4] More information is available from BMJ Learning[5] in a module written by Emma Stewart, a lecturer in human geography at the University of Dundee's Centre for Applied Population Research. As part of her thesis she investigated forced migrants living in the UK and discusses the main problems encountered by them.

IMGs and the MRCGP

Failure rate in the Clinical Skills Assessment (CSA) examination in 2008		
UK graduates	*EU graduates*	*Graduates from outside Europe*
8.4%	*28%*	*46%*

These failure rates in the CSA exam, which currently only assesses English-speaking consultations, are quite alarming. There are similar, but less marked, differences for the Applied Knowledge Test (AKT). This situation has been recognised as a significant issue by many GP Training Schemes[6,7] as well as by the RCGP. From December 2010, Celia Roberts (Professor of Applied Linguistics at King's College London) and Kamila Hawthorne (Clinical Senior Lecturer at the Department of Primary Care and Public Health, Cardiff University) are undertaking a two-year research project to identify the particular challenges posed for IMGs by the CSA and to develop an analytic framework for examiners, Trainers and candidates.

 Red Alert: GP educators should be aware that this may be the first ever experience of examination failure for IMGs, who often have a distinguished record of academic achievement in their home countries.

Some insights from social science

Celia Roberts has studied the disadvantages faced by linguistic and ethnic minorities in interaction with institutions. It is a complex area involving issues of language, ethnicity, culture and class. She quotes from the work of Pierre Bourdieu, a 20th-century French sociologist who developed concepts including *habitus*, *social capital* and *cultural capital*, to shed light on how a person's position in society is determined by factors in addition to their economic status.[8]

- **Habitus** refers to the system of dispositions (ways of standing, speaking, walking, feeling and thinking) which position a person within the social structure. Habitus is a product of early opportunities and constraints, including socialisation within the family. It reflects a person's social and cultural capital.
- **Social capital** refers to personal resources based on group membership, relationships and networks of influence and support.
- **Cultural capital** refers to the forms of knowledge, skills, education and other advantages which give a person their status in society.

One aspect of cultural capital is *linguistic capital*, the mastery of language and non-verbal communication central to a person's self-presentation. It is gradually acquired during childhood, in education and during professional training. Medical linguistic capital is central to consultation skills. Doctors, like other people, develop patterns of speech and non-verbal communication in everyday conversation; these will blend unconsciously into professional communication in the consultation. Doctors who graduated overseas are the least likely to have developed this particular type of linguistic capital, but other groups may also have difficulty with it – for example, those who came to the UK for their undergraduate training, as well as UK working-class and ethnic minority groups. Those whose habitus includes the dominant linguistic capital are more likely to feel like 'a fish in water', communicating with 'unconscious competence' in their familiar environment. Communication in the consultation will come more naturally and comfortably to them than to others.

The sociologist WEB du Bois was the first African-American graduate of Harvard in 1890. He coined the term *double consciousness*. This refers to the way in which a person may compartmentalise their mental life, maintaining distinct cultural spheres in which their personal, private and emotional self, perhaps related to their family and cultural origins, is kept separate from their public, professional self. Many doctors are occasionally aware of this phenomenon within themselves – a sense that their true self is not the competent professional whom they appear to be, and a fear that they might be 'found out'. It is frequently experienced by those who do not belong to the dominant culture, such as IMGs and UK working-class and ethnic minority doctors.

How does this affect CSA performance?

- The ability to use one's linguistic capital to the full is reduced by any stress, including that generated by the exam situation.
- Simulated consultations put additional pressure on those with less linguistic capital, who have less 'feel for the game' and who may never have experienced role play as a means of learning or assessment either at school or in medical training.
- Candidates with less linguistic capital may 'over-model', so that their consultations appear formulaic (in the same way as when a waiter routinely asks you in a restaurant *'Are you happy with your meal?'*) There is a gap between knowing the model and being able to apply it in practice. For example, the trainee may have been told to develop a more patient-centred approach, but may not understand how to express it in the consultation.
- Candidates with less linguistic capital will also have more difficulty understanding the nuances of what is expected of them in consultations involving sensitive issues such as death, bereavement and sexual behaviour – both in the CSA and in real-life consultations. They may understand that they are supposed to find out what the patient thinks, but don't know how.
- They may also find it difficult to interpret the expectations of them expressed in both the CSA positive indicators (e.g. 'responds to needs and concerns with interest and understanding'), negative indicators (e.g. 'treats issues as problems rather than challenges') and feedback statements, which may be couched in too general terms to be practically useful (e.g. 'does not identify or use appropriate psychological or social information to place the problem in context', 'does not use explanations that are relevant and understandable to the patient').
- The 'double consciousness' of IMG and other minority candidates adds another dimension of difficulty. For example, the inner experience of anxiety about being assessed, and worry that they may be 'found out' may be at odds with an expected performance involving the expression of empathy and sensitivity.

Stereotype threat

The term *stereotype threat* refers to the risk of confirming, as self-characteristic, a negative stereotype about one's own group. This term was first used in 1995 by Steele and Aronson[9] who showed in several experiments in US colleges that Black students performed more poorly on standardised tests than White students when their race was emphasised. However, when race was not emphasised the Black students performed better, reaching the same standard as the White students. The results showed that performance in academic contexts can be harmed by the awareness that one's behaviour might be viewed through the lens of racial stereotypes.

Red Alert: We should take care that our knowledge of the higher MRCGP exam failure rate of IMGs does not lead to negative stereotyping and a self-fulfilling prophecy of failure. There is a useful US website where this concept is explored, with suggestions for minimising the problem.[10]

The IMGs' perspective – lessons from Sheffield

In 2009, Sheffield GP Training Scheme conducted a survey of educators and IMGs to look closely at the issues affecting them. The full results, as well as a summary of both the findings and suggestions for educators, are available on the Yorkshire and Humberside Deanery website.[11] Unless otherwise specified, all the quotations in this chapter are drawn from the survey.

Language and communication

As suggested by Celia Roberts' work, there is no doubt that this is the biggest single issue causing difficulties for IMGs. This has been confirmed by the responses to the Sheffield survey, by a focus group of Bradford IMGs, and by many informal conversations with both IMGs and educators.

Communication difficulties may be related to:

- Language, including colloquialisms, pronunciation and regional accents.
- Style of English, e.g. the somewhat literary, old-fashioned English widely spoken in India, in contrast to modern British English.
- Use of language, including humour, understatement and irony.
- Non-verbal behaviour, which varies markedly between cultures, e.g. physical distance ('personal space'), touch, eye contact, posture, gestures, facial expressions.
- Paralinguistic features of speech which differ between languages – these include emphasis, pace, intonation and volume.
- Features of conversation structure, such as turn-taking and use of silence.
- 'Manners', i.e. cultural rules about greetings, politeness, saying 'no' or expressing anger.

This idea that *language is more than just words* is very helpfully explored at greater length in a guide from the SE Scotland Deanery.[12]

'British people often don't demonstrate much emotion, so the cues are subtle. I sometimes get these wrong – and sometimes I don't know that I am doing so.'

'I'm not used to having to explain things. Back home, most patients would accept my "authority" without question.'

'Patients use humour, which I don't always understand. It makes me nervous about using humour myself.'

A recent letter to the *British Medical Journal* illustrates that the difficulties are not confined to communication with patients:

I was a specialist registrar (SpR) in medical microbiology. My consultant and I were discussing a complicated case of an elderly man admitted to the surgery ward. I had earlier asked the surgery SpR to hold off antibiotics and instead monitor the patient. My consultant thought otherwise and wanted antibiotics started. 'I would speak to him,' he said, as he finished the conversation. I assumed that my consultant had decided to speak to the surgery SpR himself to start antibiotic treatment and so I did nothing. I later realised that 'I would' had meant 'You should'.[12]

If educators only do one thing for IMGs, we should help them to develop their communication skills by attending to all the factors which make this area particularly difficult for them. There are practical suggestions later in the chapter. However, before deciding on our approach, we should listen to the voices of the IMGs themselves:

Holistic care

'Back home, I know the social structure very well, particularly what is expected from the various members of an extended family. For example, the elderly often have a significant say in what goes on, the younger members less so. Therefore, I'm not used to thinking about or checking out how patients are supported by their families. Perhaps I just assume that families offer support?'

'If I did ask about psychosocial factors or family support back home, patients would be perplexed or even insulted that I assumed the possible lack of support.'

'I don't know how people interact with each other over here. What are their expectations of each other? What is it permissible to talk about? What are the taboos? What are the different social classes and what practical difference does this make for my work as a doctor?'

'I also don't know the work culture, what employers and employees expect from each other and what the implications might therefore be for my work as a GP.'

Managing medical complexity

'My focus back home was more medical. I'm not used to thinking in terms of a multi-layered problem with a mix of psychological, social and cultural factors.'

'Back home patients are usually younger, cases more acute and very much less protocolised.'

'Back home, I can't assume that my patients will return to me, so "continuity of care" doesn't attract the same emphasis.'

'The medical strategies I use have often been more limited by resources. Medical care is sparse and has to be reserved for the most important cases or patients who can pay for it. I'm therefore not used to the idea of patient choice or to the range of the choices that are available in the UK.'

Patient expectations

'Sometimes I'm very amazed at what people come to see the GP for. Back home, if you were upset and your dog died, you wouldn't dream of going to see the doctor.'

Bradford IMG trainee, 2010

'In other cultures, patients may expect a concrete solution, e.g. "problem identified, prescription/treatment given" – not "advice/education/wait and see" which to them would seem negligent on my part.'

'Some patients *choose* to see me (a non-UK trainee) because they think I can give them what they can't get from the British doctors. Sharing the same language is an obvious reason, but also doing tests/ giving prescriptions/referring quickly to a specialist. Maybe also they don't want to be involved in making the decisions?'

Involving the patient in the management plan

'There is a major cultural barrier here. Back home, I am expected to take responsibility and dictate the plan.'

'A patient-centred approach sometimes feels to me like a doctor-absent approach. I ask myself, "Why am I here in this consulting room?" – I don't feel like I'm doing my job.''

'Back home, patients may seek alternative help because there is no NHS and occasionally because they believe in other types of healer (examples – shaman, witchcraft, quacks, abortionists). This makes me as a doctor feel that I have to protect my patients. When I "instruct" patients, it is partly driven by wanting to keep them out of harm's way.'

Safety netting

'I'm comfortable with the idea of reducing patient risk. However, I don't have the additional driver of reducing risk to myself caused by patient complaints or medico-legal problems. Therefore my ability to reduce risk overall, e.g. through the safety net, is less developed than it needs to be.'

'In my country, you still have to safety net – but instead of medico-legal problems, it may be relatives beating you up or torching your hospital if things go wrong!'

Former IMG trainee, now a GP Trainer

Ethical issues

'UK GPs respect and encourage autonomy. But in many other cultures being paternalistic is thought of as being kind. "I will take care of your medical problems."'

'Some ethical approaches don't translate. For example, end of life care is different and back home it would not be acceptable to stop active intervention in terminal care. I therefore wouldn't discuss it because if I did it would be unethical. However, over here, I might be thought unethical if I didn't discuss it! Therefore, I might be interpreted as being unethical in a new culture when, in fact, I have ethical reasons for my behaviour according to my own culture and reasoning.'

Working with colleagues

'The work culture in the UK is likely to be very different – I'm not really sure.'

'For example, back home, doctors have the main responsibility and are expected to take the lead. I would treat other members of the team with respect, but they are not meant to be "equal".'

'The way that doctors and staff talk to each other in this country is different. I'm not sure what is "the right way". For example, what are acceptable topics of conversation? I always seem to be meeting new people but how should I break the ice?'

'People here always want us to call them by their first names. They say it will make everyone feel more comfortable, but it makes me feel very uncomfortable. For me it would be disrespectful to call my teacher by their first name, especially if they are older than me. In my culture this goes very deep, from 5000 years ago – it is in the Vedas (the ancient Sanskrit scriptures of Hinduism).'

IMG GP, a recent trainee

'When I'm on a committee and have an important point to make, I sometimes feel that if the other members don't understand what I am trying to convey, they will just nod their head and move on. It is much more helpful if they ask me to clarify what I'm saying by asking, "Do you mean . . .?." Perhaps it would help if practice staff were aware of this, as well as GP educators.'

Former IMG trainee, now a GP Trainer

Teaching methods

'Back home, I'm used to being taught mostly through being told.'

'I look up to my teachers (who are also my elders) and would not be expected to challenge them. It makes me really uncomfortable when expected to do so. This shouldn't be misinterpreted as meaning that I am not "tough" or lack the ability to think for myself. I'm simply trying not to be rude or disrespectful.'

'When I'm "lost", I expect my teacher to guide me. Therefore, when I get non-directive feedback which tries to help me find my own way by using my own experience, I feel confused and frustrated. I therefore prefer feedback to be more explicit and targeted, allowing me to clearly see the problem. Also, I need more opportunities to practise and be informally reassessed so that I can boost my confidence by seeing that I'm improving.'

'For my UK colleagues, they have the culture and communication that allows them to engage in this form of discussion much more easily than myself. For me, it just adds another layer of confusion when I'm already grappling with understanding a new culture and it feels very demotivating not to be able to live up to what my teachers expect of me.'

'I definitely don't feel empowered by having autonomy and being told to be self-directed. Back home autonomy comes when you are older, not at my stage of life. There, I am not expected to be independent, which includes being self-directed in my learning.'

'At home, I receive guidance on what to learn, not how to learn. In addition, my programme of learning is planned and timetabled for me. My job is to turn up and to diligently apply myself to learning what my teachers require of me.'

'People expect me to exercise autonomy and self-direction over here, but I need help with getting over the cultural barrier to doing this. I also need practical help/facilitation on how to do it.'

'Maybe more than my UK colleagues, I feel very vulnerable especially early on in training and there is a real need to boost confidence at this stage. Criticism needs to be balanced so that I can see that I have some strength as well. Maybe in some ways, my own culture is an asset? I certainly feel so, but people haven't in the past tried to understand me so that they can see this.'

What should schemes, educators, practices and Trainers do?

Many GP educators struggle with the idea of confronting explicitly the fact that IMGs are likely to face more challenges, and present more challenges to educators, than UK graduates. There is a feeling that this may stigmatise them. Perhaps this belief that it would be embarrassing to show someone up, so the best thing to do is to say nothing, reflects a distinctly British (or English) cultural style.

However, in our experience, most IMGs are very keen to learn, and are happy if special efforts are made on their behalf. The spirit in which this is done is crucial – there is a world of difference between *People like you have a higher failure rate in the exams so you will need extra teaching* and *We understand it must be very difficult to work as a doctor in a foreign culture. We would like to welcome you, and wonder how best we can help you.*

The suggestions below were generated by our own experience in the GP training schemes in Yorkshire and Humberside, as well as a guidance document from Scotland.[14] Some are responses to the IMG perspectives expressed in the Sheffield survey. Not all of them will be applicable everywhere, but we would like to encourage you to try some of them and find out which suits your particular situation and your particular trainee or group of trainees.

Suggestions for Trainers and practices

Some principles

- It's essential to start early! It is always important to **know learners as individuals**, but never more so than when they originate from a different culture, and it is difficult to remedy this at a later stage if problems have developed.
- **Beware of making unsupported assumptions** – for example, assuming that a particular aspect of a trainee's behaviour is part of their personality when it is a cultural characteristic, or vice versa.
- All training schemes, educators and training practices should be aware of the general **challenges faced by IMGs** – it may be appropriate to address this at deanery level, at Trainers' Workshops or at practice meetings.
- It may be appropriate to provide **training for educators in understanding general issues of culture and diversity**: how cultural factors enter into language and communication at every level (*see* Chapter 20: Understanding and Teaching about Diversity).
- It is important to **respect the IMG trainees, to understand their point of view, and not to view them as a problem**. It can be destructive to attempt to force change in culturally determined behaviour – change, if required, should be facilitated and supported.
- Like other trainees, IMGs in difficulty may need **multifaceted support** (from Trainer, Educational Supervisor and Training Programme Director).
- To teach consultation skills to IMGs, **Trainers need to have excellent basic skills for consultation skills** teaching to build on.
- Whether working with an individual IMG trainee or with a group, **use consultation principles:** start by building rapport, then identify their ideas, concerns and expectations, then bring in the content of the session.

The training practice

- Reflect on the **practice culture** and whether it can be made more welcoming (*see* Chapter 20: Understanding and Teaching about Diversity).
- Think in advance about **issues which may cause discomfort** such as forms of address, dress codes, having time off work for religious observance. Devise rules which can be applied to everyone working at the practice.
- Consider a training event to **raise awareness among practice staff** of the issues affecting IMGs.

Starting well – general

- **Ask the trainee about their name** – which name they would like to be called by, and exactly how to pronounce it, *and* talk to them about how they would prefer to address you (*see* 'Forms of Address' in Chapter 20: Understanding and Teaching about Diversity).
- **Get to know the trainee as an individual** as early as possible and show interest in their cultural background. If you prefer a formal method, the Kiddy Ring[15] is structured and comprehensive.

More equal and democratic is for both Trainer and trainee to make a timeline of their lives, perhaps illustrating key events with drawings, and then discuss them together.

- Consider **inviting them to your home** as Trainers used to do in the 1970s – a powerful signal of welcome and an opportunity for the trainee to see a non-patient example of UK home life.
- Plan a **team social activity** early in their time at your practice.
- Encourage them to **go out or sit in with different team members**, to enable them to understand their roles.

 Top Tip: Tell IMGs about a very informative resource for international visitors to the UK set up by Leeds University Staff Development Unit[16] and another, produced by the UK Council for International Student Affairs, with helpful advice about culture shock.[17]

Starting well – education

- Have an early tutorial on the **role of the GP** in the NHS, patients' perceptions and expectations of their GP, and the help-seeking behaviour of the practice's patients.
- Assess their English (speaking, listening, reading and writing) and make a plan together to address their **language needs**.
- Explore their **learning style and educational background** in order to plan your approach to their training.
- **Discuss and explain the educational methods** you use – reassure them that there is no need to 'prove' their extensive medical knowledge, and focus on helping them understand the need to learn in a way which is relevant to general practice. It may be helpful to explain the theoretical basis of experiential learning (e.g. Kolb's learning cycle).
- Always **provide more feedback** than you would with a UK trainee, to give encouragement and build confidence, and to identify learning needs.

Things to encourage IMGs to try

- **Self-assess on the GP competencies** early in their GP post, and understand what they mean.
- Recognise and practise **patient-centred consultation skills** (ICE, looking for cues, sharing options) as early as possible in their GP post.
- **Be curious about patients' lives** and ask about them during the consultation.
- **Observe consultations** by experienced colleagues.
- Remember to **learn from their mistakes** rather than just feeling embarrassed by them.
- Get involved in the **informal aspects of practice life**, such as chatting with the reception staff, or practice outings.
- Get more familiar with **colloquial English**, possibly watching TV soaps, e.g. *Emmerdale* for Yorkshire trainees, or *East Enders* in London; perhaps the *Archers* on Radio 4 for gentler styles of speech. Discussing them (and possibly also articles in the local paper) with the practice's reception staff will help develop team relationships as well as improving everyday English.

 Top Tip: Encourage IMGs to try to get involved with UK social groups – for example, a sports club or a parent-and-toddler group.

Teaching sessions in the practice

- Plan tutorials about the **cultural and linguistic aspects of consultations in sensitive areas**, including: care of the elderly; death, care of the dying and bereavement; sexual behaviour, sexual health, sexual orientation.
- Plan **tutorials on ethics and professionalism**, sharing dilemmas and areas which might be dealt with differently in different cultures.
- Offer extra support in dealing with **'non-medical' consultations**.
- **Joint surgeries** are helpful, both being watched and watching. If the trainee is being watched, consider involving the patient in the discussion. Feedback and suggestions for change should be specific, perhaps related to a consultation model. When the trainee is watching, give them specific things to watch (e.g. what cues did you pick up? How does the trainee think you were feeling?)
- Use **video and role play** extensively. It is very helpful for the Trainer to role play the patient and encourage the trainee to rehearse different approaches to parts of a consultation which have appeared problematic on the video.

 Top Tip: Providing appropriate explanations for patients is particularly challenging for IMGs. One suggestion is to have a 'lucky dip' hat full of conditions to explain (plus, perhaps explore risk and break bad news); the trainee draws one out, has 5 minutes to think about it and then has to explain the condition clearly.

A CASE STUDY FROM SCOTLAND

I support Trainers who identify they have a trainee in difficulty, and Dr S's female Trainer asked for advice very early on.

Dr S trained abroad in a very teacher and doctor-centred university. Much of his training has been theoretical and lecture and book based. He has experience of working with patients in structured protocol-led ways and never had communication skills training. The university was not in his own country and was taught in his third language. English is his fifth language. His post is in a rural town and neither he nor his wife knows anyone in Scotland. He is insightful, delightful and naturally empathic but very anxious and introspective.

These are the main things he found helpful.

- Being treated as an individual and having his ideas, concerns and expectations explored.
- Learning about transactional analysis and adult-to-adult communication. This also helped him explore the unusual situation for him of having a woman as his Trainer.
- Doing a Honey and Mumford learning styles questionnaire, having a discussion about adult and deep learning, and developing his style of learning to become experiential.
- Doing a Belbin teamwork questionnaire and identifying his strengths and weaknesses and then being asked to reflect how his Belbin style affected his work in the PHCT and how it would impact on his contributions to practice meetings. Indeed, he identified the partner most like him and explored what stresses this led to for them in GP.
- Learning to be patient-centred with lots of use of the video for formative work and joint surgeries with all partners. And, with peers, to practise and practise in various role plays. He found it useful to think about Mehrabian's research and the suggestion that 7% of communication is what is said, 38% how it is said and 55% non-verbal. He looked and listened to his videos to identify what he got and what he missed.

- The Educational Release Programme was excellent and gave him lots of different perspectives.
- Having extra sessions provided for a group with similar needs, with facilitated discussion, role play and use of actors.
- Acknowledging the need for plenty of directive feedback so that he could explore his agenda of needs.
- Having previously had very little feedback he initially found it difficult and benefited from explicit discussion about challenge and how it differed from bullying.
- Having his Trainer as the mentor during his hospital posts, some of which were stressful. There he no longer felt like an individual. He experienced confusion about his religion, and he found he and similar colleagues were often labelled as being the same even when they came from different countries and had different religious beliefs.
- And crucially he took responsibility for his own journey to understand the culture he wanted to work in and valued that this was possible while he was able to retain the right to be who he was.

We celebrated his exam pass appropriately and well.

Iain Lamb, Associate Advisor (SE Scotland)

Other approaches to understanding your trainee's cultural background are discussed in Chapter 20: Understanding and Teaching about Diversity. You may find Geert Hofstede's work[18] on cultural dimensions useful.

Suggestions for GP training schemes

What is feasible and appropriate will vary greatly between schemes, depending on the size of the scheme and the proportion of trainees who are IMGs. Below are some examples from our experience.

A medium-sized scheme with 15% IMGs and a tradition of teaching across the ST years

Include sessions targeted specifically at trainees who qualified outside the UK (i.e. both IMGs and EU graduates) to help them identify and address their own concerns. These sessions should be additional to the general educational programme so that they do not feel they are missing out on anything other trainees are receiving.

Depending on what the group wants, the sessions could include the following.

- Looking at video resources on consultation skills designed for this group.
- Discussion (and role play) about ways to talk to patients about sensitive subjects (such as sex and death).
- Discussion about aspects of UK culture which have puzzled or surprised them.
- Discussion focusing on the less straightforward MRCGP competencies (holistic care, medical complexity, ethics, fitness to practice).
- Other consultation skills practice.

In Bradford, our group of IMG trainees (across the three training years) told us that they valued the group support and felt less embarrassed in front of a group they perceived as their peers. They had developed increased confidence for consultations about sensitive issues, and they found the specific language and cultural points we had covered very useful.

A large scheme with a moderate proportion of IMGs
- Consider running CSA practice sessions for the IMGs in ST3, working in small groups of trainees from different countries, facilitating each other.

A small scheme with a high proportion of IMGs
- Intensive consultation skills teaching for all the trainees early in training, focusing on the aspects which create particular challenges for IMGs.
- Consider starting in their first year, even if they are not yet in a GP post.

Support in hospital posts during GP training
- Our consultant colleagues are not always aware of the issues surrounding IMGs, may stereotype them and may not be respectful of them as individuals.
- It is helpful if Programme Directors and Educational Supervisors provide opportunities for IMG trainees to discuss issues in their hospital posts with them. It is important to explicitly encourage the trainee to do this – they may need to feel they have been given permission.
- If you run sessions on GP training for hospital Clinical Supervisors, it is valuable to include information on IMG issues.

Cross-fertilisation
Trainees from other cultures are a very valuable resource for a training scheme (*see* Chapter 20: Understanding and Teaching about Diversity). All participants will benefit from educational sessions in which different cultural perspectives are presented and discussed. Examples of cross-fertilisation sessions in which trainees from other cultures are invaluable:
- ethical issues
- professionalism
- health beliefs in different cultures
- health-seeking behaviour in different cultures
- different ways of organising health services
- families and how they work.

How to help trainees to develop patient-centredness
(from SE Scotland Deanery)
- **Think conversation rather than consultation:** For example: 'Pair up and have a 10-minute conversation about music and at the end feed back what you have learned about your colleague.'
- **Only ask questions:** 'Bring cases and pair up. You each have 10 minutes to find out as much as possible about your colleague's case and are only allowed to ask questions. Then brainstorm the best questions.'
- **Only listen:** 'Prepare a scenario with both clinical and psychosocial elements and present them to your colleague for 5 minutes. Your colleague is then allowed to ask clarification questions (only). At the end, they then summarise what they have heard and how it made them feel.'
- **ICE:** 'Bring cases where you have identified a patient's *ideas, concerns and expectations* and discuss how it helped you develop a shared management plan.'
- Look at a video with the aim of looking at **cues, psychosocial understanding and non-verbal communication**; discuss how you knew whether or not the patient was happy.

The joy of working with IMGs

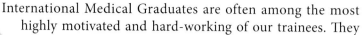

International Medical Graduates are often among the most highly motivated and hard-working of our trainees. They offer us a new perspective on our own culture, and rewarding insights into many cultural, social, linguistic and ethical issues.

When the practice and GP educators work together as a team to support IMGs, and when the Training Scheme creates an atmosphere of openness where all trainees feel that their perspectives will be heard, respected and valued, working with IMGs can be one of the most enjoyable and fulfilling aspects of GP education.

'I was apprehensive when I was asked to take on an "inter-deanery transfer" trainee with very poor AKT results. When I met him, I found him committed and hard-working but very demotivated – both from the exam result and from his last practice, where he had come to dread going in to work.

It's almost a year now, and we have a good relationship. He has pushed me as much as I have pushed him: being his Trainer has taught me how important it is for an educator to understand a learner's background and identity, how the Trainer–trainee relationship (like all relationships) needs constant nurturing, and how I mustn't become complacent about my teaching methods because different learners need different approaches. For example, recently we spent an entire tutorial practising the inflexion and other tonal qualities of particular phrases – I've never done that with a trainee before.

Working with him has stimulated me to think differently and expand my repertoire of educational methods – more than any other trainee I have had to date. I've seen an improvement in all dimensions of his knowledge, skills and attitudes too – whether this is enough to get him though AKT and CSA, I cannot say for sure. However, one thing is for certain (and he would agree with me) – we have had an enjoyable and enlightening training journey together. Of course, it's been hard work, but he has been one of the trainees who has given me most pleasure.'

GP Trainer, Bradford

A sample of resources on our website
- Culture and language.
- Helping IMG trainees at all levels.
- Guidance for Trainers with IMGs by NHSE Scotland.
- IMG Survey by the Yorkshire-Humber Deanery.
- Role modelling.

Other chapters you may like to read
- Chapter 20: Understanding and Teaching about Diversity.

Please give us some feedback on this chapter to help shape it for the next edition.
Go to www.essentialgptrainingbook.com and simply click on the title of this chapter.

Acknowledgements

Many thanks to my chapter buddies Jon Chadwick, Arun Davangere and Amar Rughani, and to the colleagues who kindly offered comments and amendments on draft versions: Ben Jackson, Sudhir Krishnan and Celia Roberts. In addition, I would like to thank everyone who has contributed to the ideas in the chapter, especially my mother Gisela Eisner who came to the UK as a refugee doctor in 1939 and worked for our health service for more than 40 years. I am particularly grateful to the IMGs on the Bradford scheme who have been involved in our seminars for both trainees and Trainers, and to my Bradford TPD colleagues.

References

1 Newbie D, Cannon R. *A Handbook for Medical Teachers*. Dordrecht: Kluwer Academic Publishers; 2001.

2 Refugee doctors' database statistics, June 2008. Available at: www.bma.org.uk/international/refugee_doctors/refugeedoctorstatsjune2008.jsp (accessed 10 December 2010).

3 www.bma.org.uk/international/refugee_doctors/index.jsp (accessed 10 December 2010).

4 www.jcore.org.uk/downloads/rdoct6.pdf (accessed 10 December 2010).

5 Refugee doctors; how they can help you. Available at: http://learning.bmj.com/learning/search-result.html?moduleId=5000070 (accessed 10 December 2010).

6 Knight C, Knight R. Diversity: what is behind the CSA failure rates? *Med Educ.* 2009; **20**: 397–400.

7 Remedios L, Deshpande A, Harris M. Helping international medical graduates to success in the MRCGP. *Med Educ.* 2009; **21**: 143–4.

8 Bourdieu P (translated by Raymond G and Adamson M). *Language and Symbolic Power.* Cambridge: Polity Press; 1991.

9 Steele CM, Aronson J. Stereotype threat and the intellectual test performance of African Americans. *Pers Soc Psychol.* 1995: **69**: 797–811.

10 www.reducingstereotypethreat.org (accessed 10 December 2010).

11 www.yorksandhumberdeanery.nhs.uk/general_practice/IMGs (accessed 10 December 2010).

12 Henley A, Schott J. Language is more than just words. In: Henley A, Schott J. *Culture, Religion and Patient Care in a Multi-ethnic Society: a handbook for health professionals.* London: Age Concern; 1999.

13 Bal A. English as she is spoke. *BMJ.* 2010; **341**: c3882.

14 Lamb I. Guidance for Trainers of International Medical Graduate trainees. 2010. Available at: http://gpst.mvm.ed.ac.uk/resource/655

15 In: Lamb I, editor. *Educational Tools for Dealing with Trainees with Difficulties.* p. 37. Available at: http://gpst.mvm.ed.ac.uk/resource/655

16 www.internationalstaff.ac.uk/living.php (accessed 10 December 2010).

17 www.hw.ac.uk/registry/resources/ISA/UKCOSACultureShockGuidanceNote2006.pdf (accessed 10 December 2010).

18 www.geert-hofstede.com (accessed 10 December 2010).

22

Interprofessional Learning

JUDY MCKIMM – Dean & Professor of Medical Education (Univ. Swansea) & lead author
PRIT CHAHAL – TPD (Nottingham) & lead author   RAMESH MEHAY – TPD (Bradford) & lead author
RICHARD PITT – Associate Professor and Director of Interprofessional Learning (Univ. Nottingham)
IAIN LAMB – Associate Advisor (SE Scotland)   GLYNIS BUCKLE – Head of GP School (Oxford Deanery)

Introduction

Several public inquiries, often around safeguarding children, have highlighted the failures of health professionals and others (e.g. the police, social workers) to function in healthy teams. These inquiries have highlighted poor communication, cultural barriers and prejudices between professional groups leading to the tragic situations that result in intense media attention. In response to these

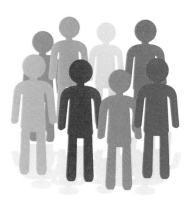

reports, many undergraduate curricula and virtually all specialty schools and colleges have included elements of interprofessional learning (IPL) in their respective curricula.

Primary care is uniquely placed to promote the ideals of interprofessional learning and collaborative practice as it represents the first place where most individuals seek help with respect to their emotional, physical and psychological needs. The culture of multiprofessional team meetings is well established, and many primary care clinicians are already engaged in both undergraduate and postgraduate medical education. In this chapter, we explore what IPL really is and some practical pointers towards doing it.

Definitions

> Interprofessional education occurs when two or more professions learn *with*, *from* and *about* each other to improve collaboration and the quality of care.
>
> CAIPE 2002[1]

In practice, interprofessional learning and interprofessional education (IPE) basically mean the same thing. We will use both terms throughout this chapter. The Centre for the Advancement of Inter-Professional Education (CAIPE) uses the term to include all such learning in academic and work-based settings before and after qualification, adopting an inclusive view of 'professional'.[1]

What's all the fuss? Why IPL?

Most of us don't just interact with other doctors in our day-to-day working lives; we interact with loads of other different health professionals. **If we are all ultimately going to be working together, doesn't it make sense to be learning together?**

And as patients live longer, many end up having complex needs (e.g. the diabetic who also has heart failure and asthma, whose mobility is declining and is living alone in a high rise flat). It's beyond the capacity of one person to sort out all those needs. IPL makes us aware of our professional boundaries and personal limitations and encourages us to seek help from other professionals when necessary in the best interests of patients.

More and more hospital care is moving out into the community where patients are managed by several different health professionals, making the case for IPL even stronger. Despite the role overlap between professions, we continue to work in a fragmented way – doing the tasks that each of us thinks we need to do rather than working *together* on the *whole* patient. IPL does several things.[2,3,4]

- It helps us develop more awareness about our own identity and roles.
- It increases our knowledge and understanding of other professional groups.
- It encourages us to develop a sense of teamwork which encapsulates trust and respect.
- It promotes a more unified approach to patient care, which will hopefully optimise service provision.

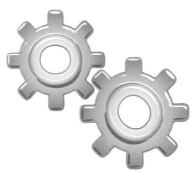

When lots of different healthcare professionals are involved in the care of a patient, it can be a bit like 'too many cooks spoiling the broth'. IPL refocuses us and places the patient at the centre of learning: encouraging all of us to acquire the relevant knowledge, understand health promotion, promote disease prevention and formulate management plans in the context of the *whole* individual, their family and society. Through optimising care, IPL makes your working life easier, yields savings and, most importantly, improves the quality of care being provided.

AN EXTRACT FROM A PAPER BY HEADRICK *ET AL.* (1998):

Schön wrote that what practitioners most need to learn is what professional education seems least able to teach. He pointed out that much of professional education rests comfortably on the 'high ground', where manageable problems lend themselves to solution through the application of research based theory and techniques. Unfortunately, the problems of greatest concern tend to lie in the 'swampy lowland' of messy, confusing problems that defy technical solution. Broadening our vision of continuing medical education to include continuing professional development in the context of interprofessional collaboration and practice improvement may help doctors and their professional partners find answers to the swampy problems most important to the health of their patients and communities.[5]

Isn't it the same as multiprofessional education?

No it's not! Multiprofessional education (MPE) is where students or professionals learn alongside one another – not from each other! For example, sitting side by side in lectures where they are passive recipients of facts with little interaction. The primary objective is to teach (usually in an economic way) rather than sharing practice and improving patient care.

Boyd and Horne[6] say that MPE is *'A collection of health professionals who independently contribute their particular expertise in parallel to each other, with minimal interdisciplinary communication'.* Parsell goes further, saying that: *'Interprofessional approaches to learning are essentially about the* integration and synthesis *of knowledge to solve problems or explore issues. Conversely, "multiprofessional" or "multidisciplinary" approaches entail bringing together different perspectives to solve the same problem.'*[7]

Some concerted attempts to promote interprofessional learning across deaneries currently exist. These include using GP practices as multi-professional learning organisations (MPLOs). The structure and organisation varies from single, often large practices to a collection of smaller practices. Many of these already have a history of taking medical and nursing undergraduates and foundation doctors and GP trainees. Additionally, multidisciplinary team meetings are informally attended by student midwives and health visitors attached to their respective mentors. The leap to becoming a MPLO is therefore not that great for existing Teaching and Training practices who have offered additional attachment to, for example, pharmacy undergraduates, social care trainees, paramedics, physiotherapists, counsellors and so on. However, the leap from MPLO attachments to meeting the criterion for IPL experience within the GP practice is a greater challenge that demands a higher degree of commitment and organisation at all levels of schools and practice. Nevertheless, MPLO is a start.

There is a great document on our website called 'Setting up a Multi Professional Learning Organisation' – but remember, this is not the same as true IPL.

So, are our multidisciplinary team meetings IPL or not?

So many people confuse multidisciplinary teams (MDTs) coming together in an event as being the same as IPL – they are not. We will give you two examples to illustrate this point.

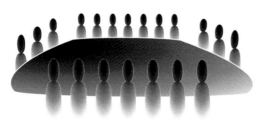

Many of you will be familiar with hospital departments where different health professionals come together to discuss patients. Often, the lead clinician dominates with a few updates provided by the senior nurse while others usually sit down and just listen. The finale is usually a mini-lecture on a clinical topic given by a trainee. This is not IPL.

Now let's look at the inter-specialty referral pathway typical of most hospitals. The second consultant comes in and does his or her bit, wanders off and occasionally comes back to review the patient. Other than what is written in the notes, is there ever much contact between the two consultants? Do they meet up to discuss the patient? Yet on a logical level it seems ludicrous not to be working together in a truly collaborative way on a patient whom you're both looking after.

Neither of these is IPL. People who believe it is either don't have a full grasp of the principles behind IPL and how it works or that their departments are so busy that they end up implementing it in a 'quick and dirty' sort of way. In IPL, each group contributes and works *together* in complementary ways. The groups question, explore the case and suggest ways of making things better *together*. There is no hierarchy. **IPL is not about all of us working as one big fat team but rather sub-teams (that retain their professional identity) coming and working *together* to provide seamless healthcare.**

What's in it for the punters?

The benefits of IPL

- Leads to a change in our negative attitudes and perceptions.
- Remedies failures in trust and communication between the various professions.
- Gets us to work collaboratively in a way that effects change, improves services and implements or refines policies (collaborative competence).
- Promotes the sharing of knowledge.
- Provides opportunities to experience areas of work outside our own remit.
- Helps us cope with problems that exceed the capacity of any one profession.
- Eases our stress, improves our confidence in dealing with difficult situations and enhances our job satisfaction.

Modified from Barr, 2005[3]

 Top Tip: In essence, IPL is collaborative *learning* to enable collaborative *practice*.[2,3]

IPL – what it is and what it is not

IPL is not different professions coming together to teach each other. Common core lectures do not constitute IPL. IPL is more than different professions just sitting in the same 'classroom' together. IPL is about learning *from* and *about* each other, not just *with* each other. It's about 'joined up thinking and education': learning and working together in complementary ways *which results in better patient care*. When patient care improves, everyone is a winner. It's a bit like a ticking mechanical clock: for the clock to work, all the different cogwheels need to work together in a harmonious and 'profitable' way.

The intent of interprofessional education is not to produce khaki-brown generic workers. Its goal is better described by the metaphor of a richly coloured tapestry within which many colours are interwoven to create a picture that no one colour can produce on its own.[5]

Or as Dr Edgar Meyer puts it:
IPL is a bit like '. . . salad and not soup', in other words it is about professions complementing each other to provide better services, not about everyone doing the same task.[8]

And IPL is green and organic!

IPL is organic (as opposed to strategic). If you don't understand the difference, it might help you to know that those directives that come from PCTs (for example) are usually strategic. Let's compare the two.

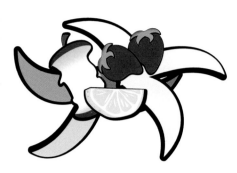

1 A strategic process is usually driven 'top down' – by which we mean that someone at the top of the ladder (the 'Master') tells the rest of us (the 'workers') what to do. IPL is organic and is usually driven 'bottom up' because those at the front line know what is needed through their everyday experience.
2 Strategic processes are usually national whereas IPL is local: the group decide to form and act; no one tells them to do that.
3 Strategic processes are management led but IPL is led by its constituent professions and often on an 'opt in' basis rather than being coerced.
4 Strategic processes are generally long term but an IPL group and activity only form to work collaboratively on a specific task. When that task is done (i.e. results in improved patient care), there is no longer a need for them to remain together. They can then disband and form/join other IPL groups to work on other tasks to improve patient care.

Isn't IPL just the latest fad? Where's your evidence?

While the theoretical arguments are compelling for promoting IPL, what is the evidence that there is any benefit? At the end of the day, the whole point of IPL is to result in:
1 an improvement of patient experience and/or
2 an improvement of services.

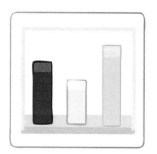

The Cochrane Collaboration proposed that in order to judge the effectiveness of IPL, randomised controlled trials must demonstrate one of the above two outcomes. So far there have been no good studies that have met all of these rigorous criteria. This has been used by critics to imply there is no good evidence that IPL is of any benefit. In reality the *qualitative* evaluation methods used to judge the impact of IPL do not lend themselves to rigorous *quantitative* analysis amenable to randomised controlled studies. Yet many do meet recognised standards of qualitative methods used in educational research.

Reviews of the literature have been carried out by the Inter-professional Education Joint Evaluation Team of some 107 evaluations that met a modified albeit rigorous version of the Cochrane criterion. These reviews do confirm the benefits of IPL. However, the majority of these evaluations were from outside the UK and from countries with different healthcare systems such as the USA.[3] More high-quality UK-based studies are needed to affirm the benefits of IPL to educationalists and health policy makers. Many are now under way. More research is also needed to determine whether 'learning together' during basic training will result in better 'working together' in practice. But one thing is for certain – poor collaboration between professionals has been highlighted as a contributory cause to some really big critical events like the Victoria Climbie and Bristol case inquiries.[10,11] Read those reports and you'll understand why we're passionate about IPL.

Principles of IPL

The principles of effective IPL

- It works to improve the quality of care.
- It focuses on the needs of service users and carers.
- It involves service users and carers.
- It promotes interprofessional collaboration.
- It encourages professions to learn with, from, and about one another.
- It enhances practice within professions.
- It respects the integrity and contribution of each profession.
- It increases professional satisfaction.

This is detailed further in our web document 'Principles of Interprofessional Education'.

Facilitating IPL

IPL has been described as good educational practice, with a 'twist', in that learners come from different professional groups and need to be actively involved in the learning process.[12] Your skills as a facilitator are vital to the success of an IPL activity. Just because members from different professions show a willingness to work together does not mean that they will function well or be effective. The facilitator is the crucial link.

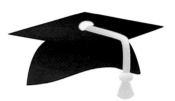

Attributes of the good IPL facilitator

- Good communication skills.
- Good facilitation skills.
- Good at managing different people and professions.
- Being able to manage conflict.
- Being able to keep people 'on track'; bring them back to focus if they go off.
- Monitors the environment (to protect members and to promote collaboration).
- Has empathy, humour and passion for the process.

Setting up an IPL group

- Before embracing any type of IPL session, make sure you (as the facilitator) have a good grasp of the key principles behind IPL (see box above). Otherwise, it will become a session of *shared teaching* rather than the *facilitation of shared learning*.
- Involve all participating departments in planning and preparation – it shows members that their departments value the process (which motivates them to engage).
- Make sure that the topic(s) selected will meaningfully involve all professions.
- Recruit a diverse and equal mix of professionals (i.e. a good balance).
- Timetabling – choose a time and place which makes it possible for most people to attend most of the time.
- You may need to secure adequate funding somehow.

Top Tip: You need to acquire knowledge of the professions and the current issues facing them in practice. You also need to be aware of their cultural and training differences and of their own personal prejudices and limitations.

The first IPL meeting

Going through these points at the start with the group will ensure everyone is on the same wavelength, and understands what is expected of them and each other.

- Discuss the **purpose of IPL** – to hook them in.
- Remind people: they are to **learn** *from* and *about* **one other** not just *with* one other.
- Set some **group rules – respect, honesty, openness** and so on (*see* Chapter 13: Teaching and Facilitating Small Groups for more on group rules).
- Start activities where they **get to know one another**.

 Top Tip: When getting people to know each other, we mean on a human and professional level. Include activities where they learn what each other's jobs actually involve. This might be an ice-breaker or a team-building game. *See* our Web Chapter: Group Games. Please do not dismiss the importance of becoming comfortable with each other – it's one of the keys to successful IPL.

Talk specifically about the following.

- **Respect for each other:** traditional barriers need breaking down; ask people to set their prejudices aside for a moment and try a more neutral stance.
- **Everyone plays an equally important role** in the care of the patient. Therefore, everyone is on an equal footing and the absence of hierarchy should enable individuals to feel more comfortable with questioning, sharing and learning together. Others should not behave defensively in responding because the remit is to understand and learn, not to accuse.
- Thus, everyone needs to **be open and honest** – otherwise it becomes superficial and meaningless. This may mean exchanging secure for insecure feelings. Remind them that you will be there to manage any conflict, and that you're there to protect them.
- Everyone can **learn something from each other** – each one of us has different skills, knowledge and expertise and as a learning unit 'we are educationally wealthy'.
- **Good communication** between all members is essential. The more communication there is the more likely enhanced team interactions are likely to develop.
- **Responsibility** – everyone needs to participate for it to work, and everyone needs to do 'their bit'. In addition, remind them of their duty to protect one another should they witness anything 'going off'.

The facilitation process

 Top Tip: The aim of IPL facilitation is to get members to continuously reflect and (if appropriate) question their personal views. It is the dissonance between these two things that will reshape their beliefs, identities and behaviour.

There are two reflective cycles you can use to facilitate the process – one based on that of Kolb[9,14] and that of Gibbs.[15]

The CIPP reflective model

Kolb (1984) and Driscoll (2000)

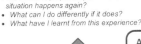

CONCRETE EXPERIENCE
something that has happened in your clinical experience

• What happened?
• What did I see?
• What was my instinctive reaction?
• What did I do?

REFLECTIVE OBSERVATION
analysing the experience

• What did I think?
• How did I feel at the time of the event?

ABSTRACT CONCEPTUALISATION
making sense of the experience: finding meanings, justifications and rationale for your actions

• Why did I feel or think in the way that I did?
• What am I thinking now?
• How am I feeling now?
• What were the effects of what I did (or did not) do?
• What could/should I have done or thought differently?

ACTIVE EXPERIMENTATION
planning for future experiences: formulating new understanding and ways of acting

• Do I need to prepare myself in case a similar situation happens again?
• What can I do differently if it does?
• What have I learnt from this experience?

Both models essentially do the same thing and it really doesn't matter which you use.

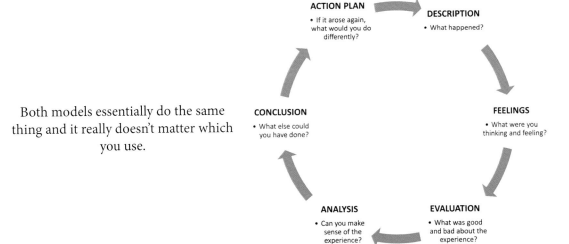

ACTION PLAN
• If it arose again, what would you do differently?

DESCRIPTION
• What happened?

FEELINGS
• What were you thinking and feeling?

EVALUATION
• What was good and bad about the experience?

ANALYSIS
• Can you make sense of the experience?

CONCLUSION
• What else could you have done?

General facilitation tips

Please read Chapter 12: How Groups Work – the dynamics and Chapter 13: Teaching and Facilitating Small Groups. Both of these chapters will help you understand the nature of groups and help you with IPL facilitation. As a facilitator, you need to keep an eye on three things: (1) the task, (2) the process and (3) support. Here are some tips for each:

Task

- Help the group **decide on an area that has meaning and relevance** to all the different professional groups: it has to be engaging, motivating and something which will have a real-life impact.
- Help the group to set **goals, which are clear, realistic and shared**. Consider task-orientated goals based on the needs of the patient – they're more likely to be attainable and measurable.
- The session should **incorporate members' concrete experiences and their reflections** on that experience. Use real-life clinical problems and consider patient involvement in the sessions (extremely rewarding and keeps the event grounded).
- Towards the end of each session, **match specific interesting tasks to the individual professional groups** and their working environments. Otherwise, it will be difficult for them to transfer that learning to their work, and they'll disengage.
- Arrange a **follow-up** meeting.

Process

- **'Hook' members into IPL** – if you show passion and an infectious form of enthusiasm for IPL, others will catch it too. Revisit reasons why members have 'opted into' the group in the first place (hopefully voluntarily).
- Remember that you are there to **facilitate, and not to lecture**. Promote interaction and discourse between the various professions. **Get members to open up** – to share their thoughts and feelings.
- **Challenge any stereotyping and negative views.** Older and more experienced members are more likely to hold traditional and prejudiced views about other groups than younger ones; they need careful handling.
- **Watch for conflict**; facilitation isn't about stopping it but managing it (through stimulating discussion and debate) in a way that is creative, constructive and helpful in terms of professional and personal development (termed 'constructive friction' by Freeth[4]). These 'fierce conversations', if well managed, can provide real learning edges for participants as views are challenged.
- Encourage **interprofessional problem-solving and that decisions need to be made collectively** by the group. In that way, each group will be motivated to do 'their task'.

Support

- **Provide support at all times.** Continuously monitor the 'micro-culture of the classroom' to make sure it is one which is safe, encourages openness (people feel at ease to say what's on their minds), demonstrates equality and respect.
- **Manage the power relationships** between the different professional groups. Remind people that all groups are equal and play an equally important role in the care of a patient. You yourself must avoid any sense of hierarchy or promotion of one profession over another.

And it's important to get the facilitation right

A General Medical Council (GMC) consultation in 2006 felt that 'poorly designed *interprofessional learning could harm collaborative interactions and polarise attitudes*'.[16] Howkins and Bray[17] say that a good IPL teacher is one who *facilitates* learning that is 'accommodative and transformative' rather than 'cumulative and assimilative'.

Educational methods which work well with IPL

Problem-based learning (PBL) lends itself particularly well to IPL. There's more about PBL in Chapter 5: A Smorgasbord of Educational Methods. However, there are other methods:

Educational methods for IPL	
<ul><li>Problem-based learning</li><li>Case studies</li><li>Debates</li><li>Joint professional shadowing or visits to a patient</li><li>Role play – re-enacting scenarios (get the group to formulate the scenario)</li><li>Task-orientated games/activities</li><li>Exchange placements with different professions</li></ul> **Modified from Barr *et al.* (2005)[3]**	I know earlier on we said to try to avoid lectures and didactic methods, but the key thing is to use a balance of activities (with varying levels of interaction). So, lectures or doing combined e-learning are fine providing: 1 These less interactive methods are necessary for the task to proceed (e.g. brushing up everyone's knowledge). 2 There is a balance of other activities.

Promoting IPL in GP training

- Acknowledge hierarchies and **stereotypes within your workplace**. Discuss further with your trainee.
- Challenge the **trainee's negative views and stereotypes** of other professions as you hear them. Find out why the trainee has said this. What is it based on? What is their experience so far? Is it real or perceived? Is it their view or that which they have 'caught' from someone else?
- Get trainees to **shadow real teams** to see how professions work with one another.
- Build into your curriculum or learning programme **topics like ethical issues or end of life care** – which can only be satisfied through interprofessional collaboration.
- Expose the trainee to **clinical situations like joint home visits and joint clinics**, where one has to learn and share experiences with both patients and other professions.
- Look for **teachable IPL moments both formally and informally**. Raise awareness by asking questions opportunistically and signpost the IPL theory as you go along. For example, when a trainee presents a case (e.g. CBD or something more informal), ask them how they might learn from other professionals about the patient's journey.

  'So, what did the Health Visitor say about the child and family? . . . Oh, it hadn't crossed your mind? Okay, do you think the Health Visitor could provide you with helpful information in this scenario? And is there anything you and the Health Visitor could work on together to achieve a more desirable outcome?'

- **Walk the talk** – be a role model. Your attitude and behaviour needs to be in keeping with respecting and valuing the input of other professionals. Just verbalising this is not enough. You've got to say it with conviction and through observable behaviour (for example, at the next palliative care meeting).

Troubleshooting IPL

The problem	The prophylaxis or remedy
Members not showing signs of interest or engagement.	• Spend some time deepening their understanding of what IPL really is. Get them 'hooked' into it. Whet their appetites. • Hook them by teasing out meaningful and relevant objectives right from the start. • Planned activities have to be interesting to all, relevant and rooted in clinical practice. • Match tasks to the individual strengths of different professional groups. • Make sure the overall aim is centred on solving a real problem (in terms of service delivery) rather than just an open discussion or chit chat.
Different members clashing because of their historical rivalries, culture differences or professional stereotypes. The 'us and them' culture. Groups showing signs of territorialism ('fighting' to maintain their professional identity).	• Set some ground rules on behaviour. • Explore people's feelings and apprehensions at the start. Acknowledge them and seek the opinion of others in the group. Hopefully, this will reassure people. • Promote a positive regard for difference, diversity and individuality. • Remind people of the things that unite them all: that they are all here because (1) they want to learn, (2) they are passionate about it, and (3) they all want to do the best for patients. • Some members of a professional group will have strong views about their roles and the boundaries of their professions. Some of these boundaries may be appropriate but others may need challenging. The key is to challenge without destroying their professional identity. The facilitator should welcome, acknowledge and respect such professional differences and such tensions should be used opportunistically to promote mutual understanding.
The process is fragmented and seems to be falling apart.	• You have probably set too many objectives: better to focus on one objective or task which matters to all of the people involved.
Different groups of people speaking a different 'language' and jargon (e.g. the doctors' speak making the social workers feel small).	• A group in greater numbers can end up dominating a session and using their own lingo. For IPL to work, you must try to get strong representation from each professional group. • When jargon is used, encourage the person to explain what they mean (shows other individuals that they aren't the only ones that don't understand – and that it's okay).

The problem	The prophylaxis or remedy
Some people becoming dominant (over-talkative), with others remaining silent and hardly saying much at all.	• Often, those in greater numbers as a group will talk forever! However, those scared of losing their professional identity may purposefully steal the limelight too (in other words, dominance can be a sign of insecurity). • You may need to revisit the constituency of the group to get a better representative balance. • Reassure members about their professional identity and convey the message that each and everyone is *equal* and as *important* as the other. • Encourage the quiet members to share their different knowledge and experiences. • You may need to (subtly) encourage the dominant group to listen to the views of others.

Let's see what you've learnt from all of this . . .

Let's say you work in a GP practice where there is a high A&E attendance rate. The PCT have asked you to look into this and try to reduce it if you can.

1 *How would you normally go about this?*
2 *Having read about IPL, how might your approach be different to the usual?*

    1 Most practices would hold a *practice-based* problem-solving discussion (among nursing staff and doctors) which would then lead to action points.

    2 What IPL is saying is that it is premature to engage in problem-solving and formulating plans without involving all the appropriate stakeholders in a truly collaborative and supportive way. That means getting the A&E department involved (the doctors, nurses and admin staff there), as well as your own. Even better if you can get the right patients involved too. IPL is a bit like a jigsaw puzzle – where each group retains its own identity but works together in a perfectly fitting way to produce a complete picture at the end.

Real examples of promoting IPL

No matter how much you talk about it in theory, it is not always easy for GP trainees to realise just how many different people and healthcare disciplines can be involved in the care of just one single patient (let alone the practice population as a whole). This can be particularly true for a patient with a chronic disease or comorbidity. The following examples[18] are ways of making them more aware of this:

EXAMPLE 1: THE PATIENT PATHWAY

The GP trainee was asked to talk to his Trainer and to identify a patient (well known to the Trainer) whose care involved at least three other healthcare professionals. The next time that patient came to the surgery the GP trainee was to ask the patient if they would be prepared to help them get a better understanding of the role that people other than doctors played in their healthcare by taking photographs each time they received care from someone else (so long as the someone else was happy to do this). If the patient agreed, they were given a disposable camera and asked to return it to the GP trainee when they felt they had taken enough photographs. The GP trainee then had the photographs developed and met with the patient so that the patient could provide a brief narrative to go with the photographs. The GP trainee then presented his work to the primary healthcare team. The final stage was to ask the GP trainee to reflect not only on what he had learnt about working with other healthcare professionals but also what he had learnt through undertaking this activity, e.g. the importance of consent, presentation skills, project management and even the patient's clinical condition.[18]

Although this was a time-consuming exercise the GP trainee had a far greater appreciation of the role that other health professions (and family and friends) played in the patient's care. The rest of the healthcare team also had a better understanding of what each other had to offer a particular patient. In addition, the patient really seemed to enjoy being part of the educational process.

EXAMPLE 2: MIND MAPPING

At a Half-Day Release session, the GP trainees were asked to think of a chronic illness, e.g. diabetes, hypertension, asthma, etc. and with the patient at the centre to draw a mind map of everyone who over a period of 12 months (assuming no acute emergency) was likely in some way to play a part in this patient's care. They were then asked to write a couple of sentences outlining what they thought each of these people contributed. They were then asked to go back to their practice and find out how accurate their mind map was. Finally, at the next day release session they were asked to reflect on how accurate they had been and whether there had been many omissions or misconceptions about the role that others played (some admitted to forgetting how important admin and reception staff can be in supporting others to play their role).

This is also a good exercise to do if you have learners from different disciplines. Just ask them to compare their mind maps and then explore with each other any differences.[18]

Closing statement

IPL should be seamlessly integrated into a training programme rather than as an 'add on' here and there. It should seep throughout the curriculum, throughout teaching and learning and throughout the assessment process: Biggs' process of constructive alignment.[19]

Research shows that trainees least value the 'soft components' of learning like team working, negotiation and interpersonal skills and prefer harder core areas like knowledge. This is because it is the harder core stuff which tends to get assessed and, as we all know, it's the assessment which drives their learning. IPL currently remains part of the hidden curriculum and will remain hidden unless we assess it using markers such as attitudes, beliefs and team working (the MSF tool being a good example). If we fail to constructively align IPL, learners will continue to devalue it.

'We are all lifelong students learning together.'

A sample of resources on our website
- CAIPE's Principles of Interprofessional Education.
- How to Set up a 'Multi Professional Learning Organisation'.
- Wenger's Communities of Practice (excellent document).

Other chapters you may like to read
- Chapter 12: How Groups Work – the dynamics
- Chapter 13: Teaching and Facilitating Small Groups.

Useful websites
www.caipe.org.uk – subscribe to the *Journal of Interprofessional Care*
www.eipen.org
www.interedhealth.org
www.sheffield.ac.uk/cuilu

Please give us some feedback on this chapter to help shape it for the next edition.
Go to www.essentialgptrainingbook.com and simply click on the title of this chapter.

Acknowledgements

Some of the material in this chapter is derived from the following sources (to whom we are grateful).

- An e-learning module on IPE written by Judy McKimm and Dulcie Jane Brake, available at: www.faculty.londondeanery.ac.uk/e-learning (which we strongly urge you to look at).
- Linda Headrick's paper on 'Continuing medical education, interprofessional working and continuing medical education' in the BMJ (1998).

References

1 Centre for the Advancement of Interprofessional Education (CAIPE). Defining Interprofessional Education. Available at: www.caipe.org.uk/about-us/defining-ipe/ (accessed 29 April 2011).

2 World Health Organization. *Framework for Action on Interprofessional Education and Collaborative Practice.* Geneva: WHO; 2010.

3 Barr H. *Interprofessional Education: today, yesterday and tomorrow;* 2005. Available at: www.health.heacademy. ac.uk/publications/occasionalpaper/occp1revised.pdf (accessed 29 April 2011).

4 Freeth D. *Interprofessional Learning.* Edinburgh: Association for the Study of Medical Education; 2007.

5 Headrick L, Wilcock PM, Batalden PB. Education and debate, continuing medical education, interprofessional working and continuing medical education. *BMJ.* 1998; **316**: 771–4.

6 Boyd M, Horne W. *Primary Health Care in New Zealand: teamworking and collaborative practice.* Auckland: Interprofessional Learning; 2008.

7 Parsell G, Bligh J. Interprofessional learning. *Postgrad Med J.* 1998; **74**: 89–95.

8 Meyer E. Cited in Report on the Conference on Interprofessional Learning, Leeds, 20 May 2008, General Social Care Council. Available at: www.gscc.org.uk/Publications (accessed 20 August 2010).

9 Kolb DA. *Experiential Learning: experience as the source of learning and development.* Englewood Cliffs, New Jersey: Prentice-Hall; 1984.

10 Laming H. *The Victoria Climbie Inquiry: report of an inquiry by Lord Laming.* Cm5730. London: The Stationery Office; 2003. Available at: www.victoria-climbie-inquiry.org.uk (accessed 29 April 2011).

11 Department of Health. *Learning from Bristol: the report of the Public Inquiry into Children's Heart Surgery at the Bristol Royal Infirmary 1984–1995.* London: The Stationery Office; 2001.

12 McKimm J, Brake DJ. *Interprofessional Education.* 2009. Available at: www.faculty.londondeanery.ac.uk/e-learning (accessed 29 April 2011).

13 Holland K. Interprofessional education and practice: the role of the teacher/facilitator. *Nurse Educ Pract.* 2002; **2**: 221–2.

14 Driscoll J. *Practising Clinical Supervision: a reflective approach.* London: Balliere Tindall; 2000.

15 Gibbs G. *Learning by Doing: a guide to teaching and learning methods.* Oxford: Further Education Unit, Oxford Polytechnic; 1998.

16 General Medical Council Education Committee. *Final Report: strategic options for undergraduate medical education;* 2006. Available at: www.gmc-uk.org/strategic_outcomes_final_report_jun_2006.pdf_25397182.pdf (accessed 29 April 2011).

17 Howkins E, Bray JA. *Preparing for Interprofessional Teaching: theory and practice.* Oxford: Radcliffe Medical Press; 2007.

18 Buckle G, Gregory S. UKCEA Bursary. *A comparison of multi-professional education in General Practice Vocational Training between Canada, Denmark and UK – what lessons can we learn and how can we apply them?* 2005.

19 Biggs J. Enhancing teaching through constructive alignment. *Higher Educ.* 1996: **32**: 347–64.

PART SEVEN

The Consultation

23

Road Maps for Teaching on the Consultation

RAMESH MEHAY – TPD (Bradford) & joint lead author   ADRIAN CURTIS – TPD (Bath) & joint lead author
LUCY CLARK – TPD (Bradford)   JULIE DRAPER – Author (Skills for Communicating with Patients), retired GP (Cambridge)
LIZ MOULTON – Author (The Naked Consultation), Deputy Director (Yorkshire & the Humber)

What we're going to cover

This chapter tells you *how* you can help your trainee *develop* consultation skills (the second bit of the diagram on the right).

Although not essential, prior to reading this chapter you might like to refresh your knowledge about consultation models (the first bit of the diagram on the right). To help you, we've created a *web* chapter called Consultation Models.

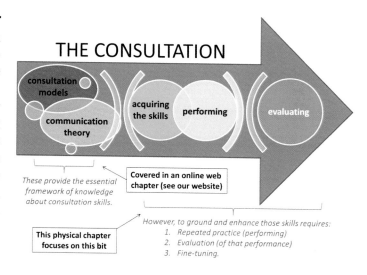

THE CONSULTATION

consultation models

communication theory

acquiring the skills

performing

evaluating

These provide the essential framework of knowledge about consultation skills.

Covered in an online web chapter (see our website)

This physical chapter focuses on this bit

However, to ground and enhance those skills requires:
1. Repeated practice (performing)
2. Evaluation (of that performance)
3. Fine-tuning.

Why teach consultation skills?

Is there a need to teach consultation skills in general practice when hospital doctors don't and manage to do just fine? Unlike hospital clerk-ins, we only have an average of 10 minutes for the consultation in general practice. It's important that we use this little time as effectively as possible. In addition, Maguire and Pitceathly[1] suggest that:

Doctors with good consultation skills:

- Identify patients' problems more accurately.
- Patients are more satisfied with their care.
- Patients leave the consultation with a better understanding of their condition.
- Patients are more likely to adhere to treatment.
- Patient anxiety is lessened.
- There appears to be increased well-being and satisfaction for the practitioner.

If you still need convincing, get a copy of *Teaching and Learning Communication Skills in Medicine*[2] – it is jam-packed with all the evidence you need as well as generally being a good book.

To make things even easier to follow ... We've split this chapter in two sections. Section 1 deals with the theoretical (but important to know) bits. Section 2 is more pragmatic and looks at what to do with ST1s, 2s and 3s on a practical level.

SECTION 1: The theoretical side of things

As a newbie, how do I teach on the consultation?

You cannot teach effectively on the consultation if you don't have the appropriate knowledge about consultation skills. *Skills for Communicating with Patients*[3] is a good book for helping you with this. Once you've got the knowledge, teaching effectively on the consultation depends on five things (see diagram right). Let's look at each in turn.

> 1. Understanding the **basic principles** of skill acquisition
>
> 2. Your **attributes** as a teacher
>
> 3. Your **teaching style**
>
> 4. The **teaching media** you use
>
> 5. The **facilitation method** you use

1 The basic principles for acquiring any skill

. . . even learning how to tie your own shoe laces!

Let's go back to when you first started to learn how to ride a bike. What was **solely** responsible for your success?

- Was it being *told* 'how to ride a bike'?
- Was it being *shown* how to ride a bike?
- Was it being made to *do it* that was responsible?

You will probably agree that it was a *combination* of all these things: repeated practice interjected with instruction and being shown. This is the basis for teaching any skill: **instruction–demonstration–repeated practice** all woven into one another. Repeated cycles of this interaction help fine-tune a skill and move the learner from conscious incompetence to unconscious competence (*see* Chapter 29: Assessment and Competence if you're unfamiliar with these terms). However, this isn't the 'whole answer' to acquiring a skill – there are a few other essential bits you need to understand too.

1 **Micro-skills teaching:** Complex tasks need to be deconstructed into more manageable constitu-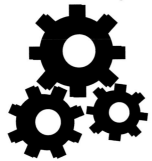ent parts (micro-skills). Each of these can then be taught and learned before being reconstructed and put together as a whole again. It's one of the most effective ways of teaching complex tasks like the consultation. Each part (e.g. initiating the consultation) can be further analysed and deconstructed. Each part is *repeatedly* practised (with *continuous* feedback) until proficiency is reached. It can be done on a 1–1 or small-group basis.

   N.B. Micro-skills teaching is *not* the same as 'see *one*, do *one*, teach *one*'. Micro-skills teaching places heavy emphasis on *repeated* practice and *continuous* feedback.

2 **Contiguity:** Putting together all the individually mastered parts again is called contiguity. It is invariably about teaching your trainee about sequencing, coordination and timing. For a complex task like teaching on the consultation, you may need to teach via a part method – subdividing the consultation into sections and learning one section at a time before putting those back together again.

EXAMPLE OF THE PART METHOD

I tend to teach around the Calgary-Cambridge model of the consultation. I break the model down into its five main parts and concentrate on one part at a time. For example, for 'Initiating the Consultation' we have a *discussion* about what it's all about, why we do it and the micro-skills involved. The trainee will see me *demonstrate* those micro-skills in our joint surgeries. We might do some *role play* to help the trainee get some initial practice. They would then go and *practise* them in their own consultations. There will be surgeries in which I will *observe and monitor* how well they are progressing. Throughout all of this, I will give *feedback* to help them tweak their skills. When they start becoming really good, it's time to move onto the next section. The end is a matter of joining up the various sections.

3 **Practice and feedback:** You need to give trainees sufficient time to *practise* and *reflect* on their skills repeatedly. They also need to be given continuous *feedback* in order to help them refine those skills. This feedback might be intrinsic (comes from within the trainee – for instance, how they feel) or extrinsic (comes from someone else like you). The best type of feedback is intrinsic – because the trainee has already convinced themselves what they need to do and, therefore, are more likely to do it. The good Trainer doesn't simply tell the trainee what they need to do; instead, they help the trainee realise for themselves what they need to do. Helping the trainee develop self-reflection skills in this way also prepares them for their future when you're no longer there to hold their hand. In their book about teaching and learning, Reece and Walker[4] describe a generic pathway for acquiring any skill. We've modified it here for teaching on the consultation.

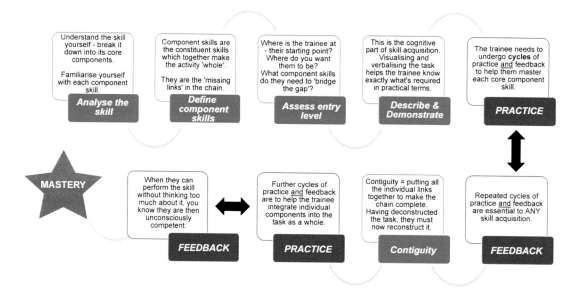

Repeated practice and feedback (the red boxes) are essential to acquiring any skill.

2 Your attributes as a teacher

When you look at someone's video and offer feedback on their consultation skills, what you are really doing is giving advice on the way they interact with other people: an area which is sensitive and personal. You must tread carefully because if you do this badly you risk damaging the trainee as well as irreparably harming your relationship. Adopting the following attributes will result in acceptance and keep you both on the same side.

Attributes of a good teacher

1. A good teacher shows **empathy and sensitivity** towards her learner.
2. A good teacher has **patience** and doesn't lose his rag. He understands that the purpose is to **nurture** the trainee, not to destroy them. Nurturing takes time.
3. A good teacher has a **vision** of where she is ultimately taking the training. To help them with their educational journey, she **asks the right questions** at the right time.
4. A good teacher is **versatile** and **anticipates change**. He is **comfortable with novelty** and is able to use the raw experiential material a trainee offers to help them with their educational journey.
5. A good teacher is **altruistic** – she really wants to help the learner develop and mature without any other vested interest.

---

3 Your teaching style

There are a variety of teaching styles. Let's go through each one.

The authoritarian style

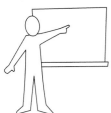

This is often the standard default position that a lot of teachers use where they 'tell and sell': *'I know it, you don't; I'll tell you, then we'll both know.'* The authoritarian style is often frowned upon by educators because if you start 'telling' too much, it goes through one ear and comes out of the other. It also doesn't actively involve the trainee; nor does it get them to reflect. However, the authoritarian style has its place – when balanced with other styles, it gives conciseness and preciseness.

THE AUTHORITARIAN STYLE

Trainee: 'How could I have got the patient to open up and tell me more?'
Trainer: 'To do that, one of the first things you need to do is build rapport.'
Trainee: 'How do I do that?'
Trainer: 'To build rapport, you must allow the patient to talk at the beginning and don't interrupt them. Then explore their ideas, concerns and expectations.'
Trainee: 'Cool. Thanks for that.'

The Socratic style

This is teaching by asking instead of telling – teaching only by asking questions. Socrates used to get his students to reflect and fine-tune their knowledge, skills and attitudes by playing a little naive and asking logically leading questions that would get them to question their own philosophy and core values and thus hopefully change their thinking minds.

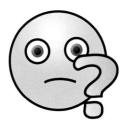

THE SOCRATIC STYLE

Trainee: 'I don't know what more I could have done for that patient.'
Trainer: 'What makes you think you needed to do more?'
Trainee: 'Well, he didn't seem quite pleased at the end, although my clinical management was sound.'
Trainer: 'So, if a clinical plan is good, the patient should always be happy. Is that right?'
Trainee: 'I think so . . . Yeah'
Trainer: 'And in this particular case, your clinical management was sound – yes?'
Trainee: 'Yes.'
Trainer: 'And was the patient happy?'
Trainee: 'I see your point. I suppose there must be more to it than just getting the clinical bit right.'
Trainer: 'What other things are you thinking of?'
Trainee: 'I suppose you've got to find out really why they've come and settle any worries.'
Trainer: 'And did you do that? Did you ask what he had come for and was worried about?'
Trainee: 'Mmmm . . . actually I didn't. If I had, he would have been a lot happier, wouldn't he?'

As you can see, questions (and only questions) are used to arouse curiosity and at the same time serve as a logical, incremental, step-wise guide that enables trainees to understand a complex topic or issue with their own thinking and insights. Some of these questions can be prepared before the teaching session ensues, but some will depend on the dialogue and, therefore, can only be developed as the session unfolds (i.e. extemporaneously). The method necessitates a lot of energy, concentration and thought from the teacher – *but* with practice, *you will get better*. Don't give up on the first round (initial flaws are usually around the sequencing of questions).

The Socratic method helps learners get involved and excited about the material being taught – to think and change things for themselves. Remember: change that originates from the individual is more likely to result in implementation. The method is also stimulating for you (the teacher) – you find out what others think and, sometimes that changes your thinking too!

N.B. Some people **mistake** the Socratic method as a critical process which goes something like *'What am I thinking? . . . No, that's wrong'* and to do it without caring for the learner (akin to trying to change behaviour in patients, but not caring whether they manage it or not).

The heuristic style

This is where you encourage the trainee to find things out for themselves rather than giving them the answer. A heuristic style encourages the learner to adopt learning skills which help them 'seek answers' for themselves rather than relying on others. This helps them cope with new and unexpected situations in the future.

THE HEURISTIC STYLE

Trainee: 'Whenever I ask patients what they think is going on, they invariably look at me in a funny way and say "I don't know. You're the doctor". Everything goes downhill from there.'
Trainer: 'What's the actual phrase you use?'
Trainee: 'Usually, it's something like "What do you think is causing it?"'
Trainer: 'Have you ever thought about using a different phrase?'
Trainee: 'Mmm . . . never thought about it. I suppose I could. Can you give me some of your phrases?'
Trainer: 'The problem is that my phrases work well for me because they fit in with my natural style. They may not work for you, and it's important to use ones that feel natural to you. So, how about collating a bank of phrases from different sources, and then trying some out?'

Trainee: 'Sounds good.'

Trainer: 'So, where do you think you might get some phrases from?'

Trainee: 'Well, that yellow consultation book has a few in there.'

Trainer: 'Great. It's best to get some from a variety of sources. So, where else could you try?'

Trainee: 'I could ask my peers at Half-Day Release.'

Trainer: 'Super, you do that and then next week we'll look at the list and pick a few to try. And then I'll share with you some of mine and see how we compare.'

Trainee: 'Sounds great!'

The counselling style

This style aims to help the trainee *understand* the interactions taking place in the consultation and *make sense* of the material being learned. The teacher must not be authoritarian. SET-GO (see later) works well with this style.

THE COUNSELLING STYLE

Trainee: 'I wish I built better rapport with that patient. Then I think things would have gone better.'

Trainer: 'What makes you think that?'

Trainee: 'From their body language I could sense dissatisfaction with my management plan.'

Trainer: 'Because you hadn't built rapport, was the patient off with you right from the start?

Trainee: 'Mmmm . . . actually, we got on really well. In fact, we even had a giggle about something in the middle of the consultation.'

Trainer: 'From where I'm sitting it sounds like rapport was OK. Are you sure the difficulty was because of rapport?'

Trainee: 'Mmmm, actually most of the consultation was OK. It was just the last bit.'

Trainer: 'So why did the last bit of the consultation go a bit pear shaped?'

Trainee: 'Dunno.'

Trainer: 'Usually, bad endings result from poor explanations or not tackling the patient's agenda.'

Trainee: Oh . . . hang on: he told me right at the beginning that he just wanted reassurance and there's me banging on about medication, investigations and even a referral.'

Trainer: 'And what does that tell you?'

Trainee: 'Well, it tells me that I need to think of what the patient wants and not to be totally self-absorbed in my own agenda. And if there is a variance between the two, to realign things.'

Trainer: 'Sounds good. So, if we could rewind this consultation, what would you have done differently and how? Give me some specific examples.'

Trainee: 'Well, at the point where . . .'

In summary

A good communication skills teacher can flexibly move in and out of these different styles in accordance with what the learning situation demands. It's important that you develop a repertoire of styles. If you are heuristic *all the time*, you will end up with a frustrated trainee who will eventually stop coming to you for anything because they anticipate a woolly answer with nothing concrete in return. Similarly, being authoritarian *all the time* will create a dependent trainee who never becomes autonomous at handling new situations.

Top Tip: Even if you are able to move flexibly between teaching styles, none of that matters if you don't spend time *building rapport*, showing *respect* for your learners and *putting them at ease*. Examining one's consulting style is personal and sensitive territory – and doing these things will encourage learners to engage in an intellectually uninhibited manner in an environment which is apprehension free.

4 The variety of teaching media for the consultation

There are a number of ways of recording, describing and evaluating consultations. The first question you should always ask yourself is: *'What am I trying to achieve?'* Only then try and pick media and facilitation methods which will help you do that.

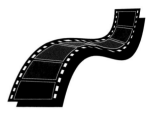

Method	Notes
Verbatim	A verbatim is a written account of a conversation. **Strengths:** Unlike new technology like DVD, verbatims help you to concentrate purely on what is said (i.e. without being infected by non-verbals). The trainee who struggles with how to phrase a question, share their thinking, or how to discover the patient's perspective might find this a powerful tool.
Audiotape	Like verbatims, just because we have newer technology these days does not mean that audiotape has no place in consultation training today. **Strengths:** Listening to a conversation helps us fine-tune what we say and how we say it without it being 'infected' by visual stimuli inherent within videotapes or DVDs. The trainee who struggles with language (e.g. International Medical Graduates) may find this a good way of building their linguistic capital.
Videotape or DVD	Videos and DVDs help us retrospectively observe a real consultation. There are a variety of ways to analyse them too (from highly structured methods to ones that are more 'loose and free'): • using a consultation critique sheet – like the MRCGP COT criteria • using well-known facilitation methods like Pendleton, Gask and ALOBA • watching a video and then letting the discussion run free. **Strengths:** You can see both verbals and non-verbals at the same time. You can rewind and pinpoint areas that demonstrate good skills or need more work.
Trigger tapes	Trigger tapes are video clips that *demonstrate* a particular competency or skill. **Strengths:** Particularly good in terms of showing trainees exactly how to do something (and be clear in their minds) before going out and practising it. Good for consultation skills training where getting consent for recording is difficult, e.g. breaking bad news, a very depressed or psychotic patient.
Sit in Surgeries	An observer sits in on real or simulated consultations and offers advice. **Strengths:** You can directly observe both verbals *and* non-verbals in real time. You can offer advice on things 'hot off the press'.
Sit & Swap Surgeries *(sometimes called Joint Surgeries)*	This is where the trainee and Trainer see alternate patients: giving the learner feedback and praise, then modelling the skills yourself with the next patient. 'Walking the talk' earns you respect. Most Trainers do a 'sit and swap' surgery during induction; but don't stop there! Make it a regular commitment. **Strengths:** You observe verbals and non-verbals in real time. In addition, you can offer advice on things 'hot off the press' and demonstrate the skills. You can choose to focus on – 'beginnings', 'non-verbals', 'giving information' etc.

Joint Visits	A great tool – being off the surgery turf may provide further insights. Just sitting side by side in the car on the way to a visit can create a safe space where the learner can share difficulties, and you can both learn more about each other.
Simulated Consultations	This is where trainees practise consulting with well-briefed actors who play the role of the patient. *See* Chapter 18: The Simulated Patient. **Strengths:** A simulated consultation provides a *safe* educational climate in which a doctor can *practise* consulting skills. The consultation can be rewound and played again, and different techniques tried out without damaging a real patient.

A few years ago, we used to get our new trainees to sit in with different doctors just at induction. The idea was to help them get to know the doctors and see a range of consulting styles. We later found out (from an evaluation) that trainees at this stage are usually more concerned with things like:

- 'How am I ever going to consult in 10-minute slots?'
- 'How does the computer system work?'
- 'How do I deal with stuff I've never seen before?'
- and *not* consultation models and styles!

So now, we get them to sit in with different doctors periodically *throughout their time at the practice* – not just at induction. Trainees love it – especially during the latter half of their attachment where they have a better grasp of consultation frameworks and benefit from seeing a range of versions for specific skills like exploring the patient's perspective, explanations and so on.

Before we move on – the Hawthorne Effect

The biggest problem with any of the recording/evaluation methods listed above is that what you see or hear might not be representative of what really happens when you are not watching them. In other words, whenever someone is being observed (not just trainees), they tend to put on their best performance. Most of the time, this is not intentional; it's just the way it is. You can probably recall doing the same yourself – perhaps in videos of yourself in preparing to become a Trainer or Trainer reapproval. This is called the Hawthorne effect and it is a form of reactivity where the person being observed improves or modifies an aspect of their behaviour that is being measured simply in response to the fact that they are being observed.

The term was coined in 1950 by Henry A Landsberger who analysed experiments from 1924 to 1932 at the Hawthorne Works (an electric factory outside Chicago). Hawthorne Works had

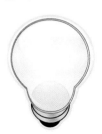

commissioned a study to see if its workers would become more productive in higher or lower levels of light. Landsberger noted that the workers seemed to be more productive in higher levels of light. *However*, productivity seemed to decline after the study was over even though light levels remained high! He suggested that the productivity gain was due to the motivational effect of the interest being shown in them and not the light intervention.[5]

In a similar way, observing and evaluating trainees through video or sit-in surgeries will result in modified behaviour. This can be positive (e.g. they display more empathy than usual) or negative (they get all nervous and mess up the consultation). It's important for Trainers to be aware that the Hawthorne effect may be at play, especially if there is a variance in what you have observed and what others (like staff or patients) say about the trainee. The more trainees are observed and get used to being observed (e.g. videoing), the more it is hoped that the Hawthorne effect will wear off.

5 Different consultation facilitation methods

Whatever resource, educational material or teaching media is used, the educator needs to decide which facilitation method(s) to employ to help bring out the learning points in that material. They won't come out by themselves! Here is a summary of the variety of facilitation methods which lend themselves to a wide variety of teaching media. Most of these are covered in other parts of this book. However, those that aren't – we will cover here.

Facilitation Method	Notes
1 Modified Pendleton's principles[6] 2 The SET-GO method[2] 3 Gibbs's reflective cycle[7] 4 Agenda Led Outcomes Based Analysis (ALOBA)[2]	*All of these are covered in detail in Chapter 7: The Skilful Art of Giving Feedback. Both Pendleton and SET-GO offer a concise and precise method of facilitating feedback.* *Gibbs is good at looking at a particular event that went wrong.* *ALOBA 'cuts to the chase' by working on the difficulty the learner wants help with.*
5 The Gask method[8]	*Covered in more detail this chapter. The Gask method (like ALOBA and Gibbs's cycle) is good for helping the learner resolve some sort of difficulty.*
6 Balint[9]	*Covered in more detail in Chapter 24: Doing Balint. It's good for getting trainees to talk creatively about the doctor–patient relationship with a view to providing new insights.*

The method the authors particularly like is ALOBA, although we often use a combination of approaches to maintain dynamism and variety.

All these facilitation methods involved **evaluating** something and then giving some sort of **feedback**. Most of the time, you try to do the following.

1 Identify what the trainee does well (so that they carry on doing it).
2 Identify what the trainee finds difficult, needs help with or needs to improve on (and how).
3 Feed this back to the trainee in a way that he or she will be positively accepting of.

The Gask method[8]

(Linda Gask is Professor of Primary Care Psychiatry at the University of Manchester.)
In the Gask method, the trainee is asked to bring a tape in which they have had some sort of difficulty (beyond the clinical). You then attempt to resolve that difficulty by first trying to gather more information from three sources:

1 what the *patient said* at the time (the narrative)
2 what the *doctor heard* and *saw* at the time (verbal and non-verbal cues)
3 what the *doctor felt* at the time (emotions).

Ask the learner to select a consultation	Make sure they've not just picked one at random, but that they bring one which they have had difficulty with and would like some help.
Set an agenda with the trainee	Ask the learner to identify areas or difficulties they want to work on. One of the commonest mistakes facilitators make with the Gask method is not teasing out and defining a specific agenda. So, if a trainee says: *'I had difficulty with the end of the consultation'*, **ask** *'What in particular was difficult about the end?'*. **They might say,** *'I got into a right mess when I tried to explain what I thought might be going on'* **to which you might then say** *'Ahhh, right. So would it be helpful if we focus on explaining things to the patient and give you some feedback and suggestions?'*

Set an agenda with the trainee	Keep drilling down until you get specific agenda items which you feel you can work with. Agenda items usually fall into one of two categories: those centred on **problem-detection** skills and those on **problem-management** skills (see table below).
Watch the tape	If you're in a group setting, brief them about what they are meant to be doing. Restate the agenda in simplified and concise terms so that everyone is clear. When watching the tape, ask them to play close attention to: 1 what the *patient says* – the history 2 what the *doctor 'sees' and 'hears'* 3 what the *doctor feels.* The facilitator, the trainee or any other member will need to know that they can stop the tape at points which relate to the agenda. They can stop the tape to draw attention to a skill which was demonstrated *or* to something which could have been done differently.
Stop the tape!	• Remember to focus on specific skills, not generalities. • Focus (in general) on consultation skills, not clinical content.* • If the tape is stopped because something could have been done differently, ask for a specific suggestion for an alternative way of doing it. • Remember to keep feedback constructive. The facilitator should use a hierarchy of prompts before imparting their view. *You can focus on clinical content but if you do, you must overtly structure the teaching session that way: *'I sense that you're not all comfortable with the management of asthma in GP. Shall we take 10 minutes to discuss this? Then we can go back to the communication issues Sofya mentioned.'*
Summarise and close	• Ask the learner what they found most helpful in the discussions. • Ask others for their opinion (if in a group setting). • Summarise key learning points. • Thank the learner for bringing their tape as a gift for others to learn from. • In a group setting where discussions may have become emotive, you may need to take a member or two aside after the session to ensure they are OK.

Problem-detection skills *(These things help identify the problem)*	**Problem-management skills** *(These things help deal with the problem)*
• *Beginning the interview (failures here lead to failures in disclosure from the patient)* • *Picking up/responding to verbal cues (open questions, clarification, examples)* • *Picking up/responding to non-verbal cues* • *Asking about health beliefs and concerns* • *Demonstrating empathy (gets patient to open up)* • *Controlling the interview (to gather the right info)* • *Knowing when and how to end the interview*	*Helping the patient by:* • *ventilating feelings* • *giving information/educating* • *making links with other things they've said* *Working with the patient by:* • *negotiation* • *motivating change* • *problem-solving* • *marital/family interviewing*

The facilitator's role in the Gask method

• When the tape is stopped:
  • Monitor and facilitate discussion – make sure the learner's and group's needs are *both* being attended to.
  • Make sure the group gives constructive criticism: a balance between positive comments and alternative suggestions.

- Label/identify the behaviour of the doctor on the tape and the alternative behaviours suggested by the group.
- Summarise before moving on.
- Stop the tape yourself when the patient clearly exhibits verbal or non-verbal cues. If necessary, prompt group to develop own skills in identifying these by asking a hierarchy of questions like:
    - *'Why do you think I stopped the tape?'*
    - *'Did you notice anything happening at that point?'*
    - *'Did you notice anything about the patient's demeanour?'*
    - *'Did you notice the change in her voice when she talked about her husband?'*
- Ask for feedback at the end from the doctor who brought the tape.
- Give them some praise to go home with!

Using consultation crib sheets

Consultation crib sheets map out the consultation micro-skills that trainees should be trying to master. The one that you're most familiar with is probably the MRCGP COT Criteria. Some educators love consultation crib sheets because they detail specific areas to give feedback on. Feeding this information back still requires careful facilitation and feedback skills. Don't be fooled into thinking that you can simply tick a few boxes, pass it back to the trainee and job done. Other educators despise these tick box assessment sheets because they find them too restrictive for something as complex as the consultation; they say that these crib sheets ruin the narrative thread present in all consultations.

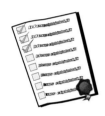

So, what's our view? Earlier on, we talked about variety adding to dynamism. We would encourage you to employ a variety of facilitation methods for looking at the consultation. Yes, use crib sheets by all means but don't fall into the trap of solely relying on them; view them as another tool in your consultation teaching toolbox. They can be particularly helpful:

- if you would like a framework to help guide your consultation teaching session
- if you're not quite sure where the consultation is going wrong; they can help pinpoint the difficulty
- if you'd like to monitor how your trainee is progressing over time.

I hear a lot of Trainers say how much they dislike the MRCGP COT sheet for consultations – saying it is too summative in nature. I actually like it – probably because I've found a way of using it both summatively and formatively. I say to my trainee that we will both mark her consultation video but that we must write down the evidence for a tick. That evidence has to be in the form of something *seen* or *heard* in the consultation. At the end, we compare notes and engage in dialogue. We particularly focus on areas where there was (1) a difference in marks, (2) underperformance and (3) a missed opportunity. This formative process allows us to:

- reach shared understanding through exploring variance
- align our marking grades
- identify future learning needs and how to tackle them.

Structured assessment sheets can be good if you use them in creative ways.

A variety of consultation crib sheets are available on our website (including MRCGP COT, Pendleton, Tate and Calgary-Cambridge).

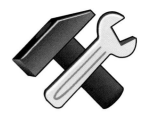

SECTION 2: The practical side of things

In this section, we will look at ST1s, ST2s and ST3s in groups. We will identify some of the contextual challenges they face when teaching them about the consultation. We will then go on to identify some ways in which we can help them on a practical level.

Top Tip: Remember what we said earlier – analysing consultation styles is personal and sensitive territory. Revealing your personal consulting style, especially to a group of others, can be scary stuff and can feel quite threatening. Spend time building rapport, teasing out fears, validating feelings, providing reassurance and putting trainees at ease. Monitor continuously for cues and periodically check how the learners are – particular the one under the spotlight.

Teaching consultation skills to ST1s and ST2s in hospital posts

The challenges

In the first few months trainees are usually more concerned about the ePortfolio and facts relating to specialties than they are about communication skills. They've just joined a new environment (the hospital trust) with new colleagues, and it may be too early for them to talk about their own inadequacies or show consultation videos of themselves to peers.

What makes things even more difficult is that some training rotations only expose the trainee to general practice at the end. Because of a lack of immediate relevancy, it's not surprising to hear about the disengagement of some. Furthermore, hospital service provision often makes it difficult for them to come to Half-Day Release anyway.

Then there is the problem of having little autonomy in junior hospital posts. Trainees are expected to present the patient's history in the time-honoured hospital clerking model of history, examination, diagnosis, investigations and so on. This 'conveyor belt' approach to medicine leaves little space for a more profound understanding of why the patient came and what needs to be achieved within the consultation.

Finally, most senior clinicians, having not been taught consultation skills, usually adopt a doctor-centred approach and germinate negative perceptions about the person-centred approach seen in general practice:

- *'Surely it's all down to your personality and natural ability.'*
- *'You can't teach that stuff; what's there to learn anyway?'*
- *'Being doctor-centred is time efficient and patients don't know what's best for them.'*
- *'You're here as an O&G trainee. You can do GP later.'*

Teaching on the consultation . . .

In general

- Because ST1s and ST2s at this stage are new to one another, it's important to develop some group rules like allowing people to speak and respecting their views. More about group rules in Chapter 13: Teaching and Facilitating Small Groups.
- It's also worth going through the principles of giving and receiving feedback (*see* Chapter 7: The Skilful Art of Giving Feedback). This will enable them to give feedback to others in constructive ways while also being able to receive and accept it from others.
- At the ST1/2 stage, it's important to **tackle attitudes** about the consultation. There is no point practising consultation skills if the learners think it's all about a natural ability, or that it's all over-hyped. For individuals to feel safe enough to reveal their attitudes, you need to create an educational climate which emits honesty, openness, respect and trust.
- It's also important to start introducing them to *some* **knowledge/theory/evidence** about the consultation. How about encouraging them to read a light-hearted consultation book? Perhaps Liz Moulton's *The Naked Consultation*[12], Peter Tate's *The Doctor's Communication Handbook*[13] or Roger Neighbour's *The Inner Consultation*[14] (although some find this last one rather erudite).

At Half-Day Release or consultation skill modules/workshops

Introduce the concept of consultation skills early on in training. Allow trainees to reflect on their strengths and weakness. They are likely to need examples, advice and direction.

- Get trainees to reflect on medical school consultation teaching *and* the consultations they've observed/experienced during their FY years – the good, the bad and the ugly!
- Get them to observe how different doctors approach particular patients and scenarios – the young vs the old, patients vs relatives, breaking bad news and so on. Again, identify the good, the bad and the ugly. Identify positive and negative behaviours.
- How do we communicate with our family and friends? How does this differ from the doctor–patient model? Should it be different? Are there lessons we can learn?
- Get them to consider the pros and cons of the doctor-centred hospital clerking model against the patient-centred model seen in general practice. Some of their perceptions will be wrong. Use the evidence to realign their thinking. The evidence is well documented in Kurtz's green book: *Teaching and Learning Communication Skills in Medicine.*[2]
- Although there is considerable educational merit in using consultation videos, it is difficult for trainees to show videos of themselves for practical, technical and personal reasons. An alternative is to use trigger tapes (see section on 'teaching media') like the one from the RCGP[15] or analysing someone else's video (yours or an agreeable ST3). Showing your mistakes might encourage them to open up and show theirs.
- Do some case discussion – focus on cases where communicating with patients has gone terribly wrong. What was the cause? What could have helped? What have you learned? See some of the scenarios in the box below.
- Encourage role play: hook them in by pointing out that this is an opportunity to practise things in a setting where it is okay to get things wrong. It's better to 'mess up' in role play than in the real thing. Re-enact difficult or confrontational scenarios to help develop consultation skills (*see* box below). Remember to look after the learners' feelings, provide reassurance and occasionally add humour to liven things up. If you feel you aren't particularly well versed in facilitating role play sessions, *see* Chapter 18: The Simulated Patient – your walking, talking, learning tool.

Some concepts worth talking about at the ST1/2 stage:

- verbal and non-verbal cues
- the meaning of empathy ('walking a mile' in the patient's shoes)
- Helman folk model[16] – useful for trying to get inside the patient's head
- McWhinney's disease-illness model[17] – the additional benefits of covering both the doctor's and patient's perspectives in a person-centred consulting model.

Some scenarios to help work on consultation skills at the ST1/2 stage:

- a patient wishing to self-discharge
- a patient refusing to comply with medication
- talking to upset relatives
- talking to demanding relatives
- a difficult ward sister
- breaking bad news.

 Top Tip: Shortly after induction, consider setting up an HDR session where ST3s give role play examples of the main consultation models to ST1s. It can help bond ST1s and ST3s, provide revision for ST3s, provide a non-threatening introduction to consultation models to ST1s and be light-hearted and funny.

Practising consultation skills on the wards

- Summarise benefits of a patient-centred model. Get trainees to review the hospital clerking model – ask what needs to change in order to make it more holistic (e.g. incorporating the patient's ICE, exploring the psychosocial, gathering information from relatives). Is the modified version workable in their busy hospital setting? If not, refine it further until it is.
- Advise them not to shy away from explaining to patients (and their relatives) their clinical suspicions, differential diagnoses and treatment options. Encourage them to explore the expectations of their patients and to manage any variance.
- Encourage them to get involved in complex scenarios like dealing with uncertainty and risk, breaking bad news or complicated discharge planning that involves communicating with patients and their relatives.
- Discuss consultation skill opportunities in specific specialities.
  - Psychiatry – setting boundaries in patients with challenging behaviour, reassuring anxious patients, sensitivity and empathy with depressed patients.
  - Elderly medicine – conversing with the elderly, chunking information, signposting, summarising and checking understanding.
  - Rheumatology – exploring the effect of the illness on the patient's life, sensitively screening for depression.
  - Paediatrics – adapting personal consulting style for communicating with children, talking to parents, identifying their concerns and expectations. The art of appropriate reassurance.
- Get them to ask consultants if there are any specialty-specific consultation techniques or approaches (e.g. Kaye's 10-step approach to Breaking Bad News in Palliative Care). Practise them!

Top Tip: 5 days in general practice – see if hospital-based trainees can take time out or study leave for a 5-day placement in a general practice to enable the GP Trainer to deliver 'a shot' of consultation skills training.

Teaching consultation skills to ST2s in their first general practice post

The challenges

Trainees at this stage may not want to embrace the 'tree-hugging stereotype' of general practice. They will still be preoccupied with the concrete learning of facts for their post and AKT revision rather than the more nebulous but equally important general practice learning areas. However, once trainees reach this stage, they are very receptive to general practice-specific skills.

Teaching on the consultation . . .

In general

- Most ST2s won't be familiar with videoing their consultations. Undoubtedly, they're going to be a bit videophobic – explore feelings, empathise and reassure.
- Start encouraging them to video their consultations and to look at these on their own at first. When they are comfortable with this, they can review them on a 1–1 basis with their Trainer and, later on, as part of a small peer group at Half-Day Release.
- It's also worth going through the principles of giving and receiving feedback again (*see* Chapter 7: The Skilful Art of Giving Feedback).
- When they were ST1s, hopefully Half-Day Release will have provided some knowledge and explored some attitudes around the consultation. At the ST2 stage, while it is still important to **continue with *knowledge* and *attitudes***, it's equally important to **start practising the actual consultation *skills***.

At practice or HDR level

- Revisit some bits of consultation theory – encourage them to read one or two consultation books (see the end of this chapter for a list). Design some tutorials around some of the chapters to consolidate their learning.
- ST2 trainees might still be too reluctant to show their videos or even engage in role play. Consider using trigger tapes or other consultation video resources available from the RCGP.[15] Show one or two of your own – especially ones that aren't particularly great; if you only show trainees your 'star' consultations, they may find it *even* harder to show you their own.
- Design workshops/modules/tutorials which focus on *practising* basic consultation skills – perhaps the micro-skills?

Examples of consultation micro-skills

- Skills for encouraging the patient's contribution (exploring ICE)
- Picking up and responding to signals and cues
- Screening, signposting, summarising
- Agenda setting
- Explaining things
- Making a joint plan with the patient
- Checking understanding
- Safety-netting and following up.

Task sheets for working on these micro-skills are available on our website. There are more on www. bradfordvts.co.uk (click 'online resources' then '02 the general practice consultation'). Silverman's book on *Skills for Communicating with Patients*[3] also offers suggestions as does 'Communication Skills Manual by Chafer' which is available on our website.

Top Tip: Get your trainee to practise a specific micro-skill with every patient in a set surgery. They should continue doing this in subsequent surgeries until they feel competent. When ready, continue the process with a different micro-skill.

- *'Over the next two surgeries, I'd like you to screen for problems other than the presenting complaint with every patient. Try out different ways of doing this. Perhaps jot down some points in your notebook – the pros and cons of various methods. And how about a tutorial next week to see what worked best for you?'*
- *'Over the next two surgeries, I'd like you to pay close attention to how you greet the patient and your opening phrase. Vary the way you do this and what you say. Sometimes, consider saying nothing at all – perhaps just a smile with gestures to encourage them to sit down and talk. Listen carefully to the first couple of things they say. Do these opening gambits add a different dimension to the consultation? What effect do different greetings have? How do patients respond? Are some better than others? Are some best used in a particular circumstance?'*

N.B. A gambit is a remark intended to open a conversation.

Teaching consultation skills to ST3s
The challenges
We know that a lot of teaching on the consultation occurs in GP practices. We know that most Trainers get some form of teaching consultation skills training and a paper by Evans *et al.* says nearly three-quarters of them felt that this training had positively changed their approach to teaching.[18] Trainers value the teaching they have received on the consultation. So, the problem isn't getting Trainers to teach on the consultation. The problem is getting them to use a variety of consultation teaching methods. Different methods offer different teaching and learning perspectives. One needs to be able to vary the method to suit the individual learner and the variable context.

Then there is the problem of the MRCGP's workplace-based assessments. There are so many of them that 'in-house' tutorial time is often hijacked by doing them (mainly COTs and CBDs). This leaves very little time for anything else. Repeatedly doing COTs only looks at the consultation from one angle and blackens out other windows of opportunity.

The final challenge concerns trainees. Once they have successfully undertaken the CSA, many seem to lose interest in doing videos and looking at their consultations further. Prior to this they were dead keen. It is almost as if some trainees see success in the CSA as the end point to their learning! How terribly sad.

Teaching on the consultation . . .
In general

- Remind them that their time with you may be one of the few opportunities where they will get to explore and enhance their consultation skills which in turn will make their working lives easier.
- Your aim is to help them find their own effective, adaptive and personal model.
- The most important aspect of consultation training at the ST3 stage is *practice*. Explore fears and concerns about revealing their inadequacies on video. Empathise and seek to resolve. Remind them that they need to practise and practise until they become unconsciously competent (*see* Chapter 29: Assessment and Competence).
- This will invariably involve 'reflection **on** action' *and* 'reflection **in** action' (*see* Chapter 28: Reflection and Evaluation if you're unfamiliar with these terms).

At practice level

- It's worth going through the principles of giving and receiving feedback again (*see* Chapter 7: The Skilful Art of Giving Feedback). This is a period where they will receive intense feedback from you and others. It's also a period where they will be expected to give feedback to their colleagues! Training is much easier when a trainee accepts, respects and is grateful for the feedback given than when they pull out their defensive barriers. In this chapter, you will have noticed the feedback theme running continuously from ST1 through to ST3; this signifies its importance.
- Encourage the trainee to read an in-depth consultation book like Silverman's *Skills for Communicating with Patients*.[3] Set some tutorials around particular chapters.
- Aim to do more than the minimum requirement for COTs but remember to make time to look at the consultation in other ways too – Gask, ALOBA, other crib sheets etc. Different methods offer different strengths.
- Use COTs as a teaching tool: watch the consultation, teach on appropriate aspects and *then* write it up as a COT.
- Joint surgeries are one of the best ways to see how your trainee is really performing. Consider 'sit and swap' surgeries too (where you can demonstrate some skills).
- Discuss cases and alternative approaches – random and problem cases or during debriefs.
- Role play some CSA scenarios (there are loads of CSA scenario books out there).
- OOH sessions – sit in with your supervisee. A great opportunity to teach!

At HDR level

- Devote some HDR sessions to analysing consultation videos on a small-group basis. The aim, of course, is to collaboratively learn from each other.
- Set up patient simulator sessions to work on particular consultation skills. (There are a whole variety of scenarios available on www.bradfordvts.co.uk – click 'online resources' then '03.7 teaching and learning' then 'OSCE').
- Set up mock practice CSA scenarios.
- Encourage those who have recently passed the CSA to run some CSA sessions.
- Encourage trainees to form CSA small groups to practise scenarios in their own time (many trainees say how they find watching each other's styles helpful).

Specific areas worth looking at during ST3

- Time management – and dealing with 10-minute appointments!
- Consulting with adolescents. Asking parents to leave the room. The GMC guidance 0–18 years[19] gives useful information on consulting with children.
- Three-way consultations (doctor–patient–relative).
- Patients with limited English.
- Dysfunctional consultations – frequent attenders, demanding patients, angry/aggressive patients, dependent patients, self-help rejectors etc.
- Telephone consultation skills.

- Using your body language to talk.
- Framing language in a positive way.
- Exploring the narrative thread.[10]
- Non-violent communication[20] (aka compassionate communication).
- Neurolinguistic programming (NLP).[21]
- Motivational interviewing.[22]
- Transactional analysis.[23]
- Balint's ideas:[9]
1 the flash
2 the drug doctor
3 the doctor's apostolic function
4 the mutual investment fund
5 the collusion of anonymity
6 the courage of one's stupidity.

And don't forget the humanities and creative arts

Use the humanities to introduce and enhance aspects about the consultation. Involve the trainees in the selection process about which resources to use – this enhances enthusiasm and reflection on the process. You can use film clips, TV shows, artwork, novels, poems and even songs! For more ideas *see* Chapter 17: Using the Creative Arts. In addition, we strongly recommend investing in the excellent resource book by Powley and Higson.[24]

Consultation books

Light-hearted – good for new trainees (ST1s/2s)

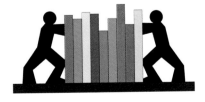

- Liz Moulton's *The Naked Consultation*[12]
  - Full of practical gems and shorter on the theory.
- Peter Tate's *The Doctor's Communication Handbook*[13]
  - A good all-rounder.
- Roger Neighbour's *The Inner Consultation*[14]
  - Some trainees find it light-hearted while others find it heavier.

Heavier going – good for the more experienced (ST2s/ST3s)
- Silverman *et al. Skills for Communicating with Patients*[3] (Calgary-Cambridge)
  - Evidence-based, full of phrases, comprehensive coverage of all micro-skills.

To push the trainee even further
- Salinsky and Sackin's *What are you feeling, doctor?*[25] *(Balint'esque)*
- Donovan and Suckling's *Difficult Consultations with Adolescents*[26]
- John Launer's *Narrative-based Primary Care*[10]
- Lewis Walker's *Consulting with NLP*[21]
- Bub's paper on 'the patient's lament' – overview of how to turn moaning during consultation into a useful therapeutic and diagnostic tool.[11]

How do you know whether a trainee is getting there?

The answer to how you know whether a trainee is making progression lies in Bloom's Taxonomy[27] – *see* Chapter 10: Five Pearls of Educational Theory. He identified three domains of learning: the cognitive (knowledge), the psychomotor (skills) and the affective (attitudes). He also identified the range of learning depths present within each of these learning domains. The spectrum of learning depths, subdivisions and layers is called Bloom's Taxonomy (taxonomy is another word for classification). Each taxonomy is hierarchical – by which we mean that higher levels cannot be reached if lower ones are not attained. The diagram here shows the taxonomy for the psychomotor (skills) domain.

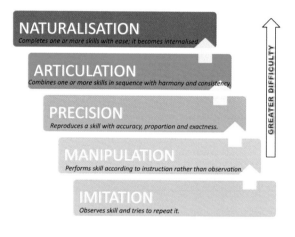

Truth be told, Bloom didn't actually create a taxonomy for the psychomotor domain. This one was formulated by Dave[28] in 1975. This *'skills'* framework should give you some idea of where your trainee is at, whether they're making adequate progress up the ladder towards naturalisation (mastery) and if not, what you need to do to push them up to the next level.

Skill development involves integrating tasks into a coordinated whole. You can tell when a trainee has reached the naturalisation level – their performance becomes habitual or automatic. **Watching a trainee move up this ladder with their consultation skills is one of the most satisfying things you will see as an educator in general practice.**

Closing comments

Our aim is not to produce clones of GPs all reciting the same stock phrases and acting out the same rehearsed consultations. Our aim is to help our trainees achieve a flexible approach to their consultations, allowing them to use a variety of communication skills, draw from different communication models, and tailor their approaches to suit individual patients, while maintaining and developing their personal style.

One might argue that the MRCGP COT crib sheet already defines the clones that we need to produce. However, we would like to highlight one fact – that the COT criteria are outcome-based criteria. What this means is that although the final outcome is predetermined, how you go about achieving that outcome is not. That (most exciting) part of the educational journey is entirely up to you (see example below).

> **COT criterion 1: The doctor is seen to encourage the patient's contribution at appropriate points in the consultation**
>
> *To achieve this you can use active listening skills, open questions, silence, non-verbal encouragement and clarification in whatever combination or sequence you want. As long as it gets you to the end point in a timely way is all that matters.*

A sample of resources on our website
- Various structured consultation assessment sheets – Pendleton, Segue, Cox.
- Discussion, dialogue and Socrates.
- Fundamental concepts in the GP consultation.
- Communication skills manual by Andrew Chafer.
- A survey of GP trainees in the Bath area about the consultation (2011).

Other chapters you may like to read
- Web Chapter: Consultation models
- Chapter 7: The Skilful Art of Giving Feedback
- Chapter 18: The Simulated Patient – your walking, talking, learning tool
- Chapter 24: Doing Balint.

Please give us some feedback on this chapter to help shape it for the next edition.
Go to www.essentialgptrainingbook.com and simply click on the title of this chapter.

References
1 Maguire P, Pitceathly C. Key communication skills and how to acquire them. *BMJ.* 2002; **325**(7366): 697–700. Review.
2 Kurtz SM, Silverman JD, Draper J. *Teaching and Learning Communication Skills in Medicine.* 2nd ed. Oxford: Radcliffe Medical Press; 2004.
3 Silverman JD, Kurtz SM, Draper J. *Skills for Communicating with Patients.* 2nd ed. Oxford: Radcliffe Medical Press; 1996.
4 Reece I, Walker S. *Teaching, Training and Learning: a practical guide.* 6th ed. Sunderland: Business Education Publishers; 2008.
5 Landsberger HA. *Hawthorne Revisited: management and the worker, its critics, and developments in human relations in industry.* Ithaca, New York: Distribution Center, NYS School of Industrial and Labor Relations, Cornell University; 1958.
6 Pendleton D, Schofield T, Tate P, Havelock P, editors. *The New Consultation: developing doctor-patient communication.* Oxford: Oxford University Press; 2003. pp. 75–80.
7 Gibbs G. *Learning by Doing: a guide to teaching and learning methods.* Oxford: Further Education Unit, Oxford Polytechnic; 1988.
8 Gask LL, Goldberg D, Lesser A, Millar T. Improving the psychiatric skills of the general practice trainee: an evaluation of a group training course. *Med Educ.* 1988; **22**(2): 132–8.
9 Balint E, Norell J. *Six Minutes for the Patient: interactions in general practice consultations.* London: Tavistock; 1973.
10 Launer J. *Narrative-based Primary Care: a practical guide.* Oxford: Radcliffe Medical Press; 2002.

11 Bub B. The patient's lament: hidden key to effective communication: how to recognise and transform; *Med Humanit.* 2004; **30**: 63–9.

12 Moulton L. *The Naked Consultation: a practical guide to primary care consultation skills.* Oxford: Radcliffe; 2007.

13 Tate P. *The Doctor's Communication Handbook.* 6th ed. Oxford: Radcliffe; 2009.

14 Neighbour R. *The Inner Consultation.* 2nd ed. Oxford: Radcliffe; 2004.

15 Hull M. *Communication Skills for GPs in Training (2 disc DVD & workbook).* RCGP Midland Faculty; 2005 (available from RCGP bookshop: www.rcgp.org.uk/bookshop).

16 Helman C. Disease versus illness in general practice. *J R Coll Gen Pract.* 1981; **31**: 548–62.

17 Levenstein JH, McCracken EC, McWhinney IR, *et al.* The patient-centred clinical method. *Fam Pract.* 1986; **3**: 24–30.

18 Evans A, Gask L, Singleton C, Bahrami J. Teaching consultation skills: a survey of general practice Trainers. *Med Educ.* 2001; **35**: 222–4.

19 www.gmc-uk.org/guidance/ethical_guidance/children_guidance_index.asp

20 Rosenberg M. *Nonviolent Communication: a language of life.* 2nd ed. Encinitas, California: Puddle Dancer Press; 2003.

21 Walker L. *Consulting with NLP.* Oxford: Radcliffe; 2002.

22 Miller WR, Rollnick S. *Motivational Interviewing: preparing people for change.* 2nd ed. Guildford: Guilford Press; 2002.

23 Berne E. *Games People Play: the psychology of human relationships.* Harmondsworth: Penguin; 1973.

24 Powley E, Higson R. *The Arts in Medical Education: a practical guide.* Oxford: Radcliffe; 2005.

25 Salinsky J, Sackin P. *What Are You Feeling, Doctor?* Oxford: Radcliffe; 2000.

26 Donovan C, Suckling H. *Difficult Consultations with Adolescents.* Oxford: Radcliffe; 2004.

27 Bloom BS, Engelhart MD, Furst EJ, *et al. Taxonomy of Educational Objectives: the classification of educational goals.* New York: Longmans Green; 1956.

28 Dave RH. In: Armstrong RJ, *et al. Developing and Writing Behavioural Objectives.* Tucson, Arizona: Educational Innovators Press; 1975.

24

Doing Balint

PAUL SACKIN – TPD (Cambridge) & lead author   JOHN SALINSKY – TPD (Whittington) & lead author
with helpful advice from
HEATHER SUCKLING – retired GP (London), SHAKE SEIGEL – TPD (West Midlands), LENKA SPEIGHT – GP (London)

Introduction

We hope this chapter will achieve three main objectives:

1 to outline who Michael Balint was and what Balint work is all about
2 to help you decide whether this sort of work is for you and, if so –
3 to give you some ideas as to how you might 'do' Balint as an educator.

Along the way, we will touch on the history of the Balint movement, talk a bit about his wife and collaborator Enid, describe how Balint groups work today (and how you might build it into a GP training programme) and finally consider other contexts where a Balint approach might prove useful.

The history

It all started with a small ad in *The Lancet*

In April 1950 a small advertisement appeared in *The Lancet*, inviting general practitioners to take part in a 'Discussion Group Seminar on Psychological Problems in General Practice' at the Tavistock Clinic in London. The invitation was issued by a dynamic and creative psychiatrist called Michael Balint, who was to become one of the major influences in the revival and rebirth of general practice in the 1950s.

Who was he?

Michael Balint was born in Hungary in 1896. He qualified as a doctor in Budapest and trained as a psychoanalyst. In 1939, he moved to England to escape the Nazi occupation of Europe and, by 1948, he had taken up a consultant post at the Tavistock Clinic in London. He had always been interested in general practice (his father had been a GP) and he had an idea that 'psychologically, much more happens in general practice between patients and doctors than is discussed in the traditional textbooks'.[1]

The unhappy GPs of the 1950s

GPs in the early 1950s were not very happy. The NHS, which had begun in 1948, had detached family doctors from any significant participation in hospital medicine. They felt left out of all the exciting scientific developments going on in secondary care. It seemed that whenever they had 'an interesting case' the patient would be completely taken over by the hospital. Instead, they found themselves having to cope with a flood of miserable people with puzzling symptoms, which could not be made to add up to any of the illnesses they had learned about as students (There was no vocational training in those days and most GPs went straight into practice, often single-handed, after house jobs). Many patients were also depressed and anxious, but referral to a psychiatrist didn't seem to help very much. The patients kept coming back and it was difficult to know what they wanted. Some of the GPs were interested in the psychology of their patients and suspected that some training in this department might help them to make sense of a job that was becoming increasingly frustrating. They were the first to join Michael Balint's Tavistock experiment.

What made Balint think he could help?

- He wanted to find out what general practice was really like by *listening* to the doctors talking about their work.
- He was enthusiastic about group discussion as an educational process. Rather than learning by lecture, he believed that the doctors could only learn by *finding things out for themselves* (an educational principle that still permeates through specialty training programmes today).
- He thought that, as a psychoanalyst, he could help them to be more perceptive about what was going on in the *emotional interactions between doctor and patient*. Much of this goes on at an unconscious level: for instance, a doctor can dislike a patient without ever really knowing why.
- Balint was already taking part in a similar group for marital caseworkers at the Tavistock, where he worked creatively with a social scientist called Enid Eichholz. They devised the 'Balint method' together, although she gets less credit than she deserves. They went on to run GP groups together, and she soon became Mrs Enid Balint.

The Doctor, his Patient and the Illness

In 1957, Michael published a book called *The Doctor, his Patient and the Illness*;[1] it became one of the key texts of modern general practice throughout the world. It describes the work of the early seminars and is often thought to be difficult to read. However, you might want to give it a go – there are lots of case histories similar to the patients we see today. The first story is about a 32-year-old woman with undiagnosable chest and abdominal pains whose attitude to her GP becomes 'aggressively flirtatious'. Okay, perhaps that one's not so typical but no doubt it's caught your eye! As a result of this book the Balints received invitations to talk about their work in Europe and America. By the 1960s Balint groups had begun to appear in many countries including France, Germany, Belgium, Holland, Italy and the USA.

The early groups

By 1952, there was a nucleus of dedicated GPs who wanted to have an ongoing group with the Balints. The group met weekly in academic terms for 90 minutes. Other 'Balint groups' were also started, with Michael's psychoanalyst colleagues at the Tavistock as leaders.

To begin with, the Balints encouraged the GPs to have at least one long consultation of about an hour with any patient they wanted to present at the seminar. This gave the patients the freedom to reveal themselves as *people with difficult lives* as well as patients with difficult symptoms. Follow-up presentations were encouraged and there were often signs of marked improvement. Even if the symptoms persisted, the fact that the doctor and patient were more *emotionally* in touch with each other made consultations much more productive.

Later on the doctors began to feel that their many other patients, who were not receiving long sessions, were being neglected. Michael, who was always open to new ideas, agreed, and the group changed its focus to looking at the doctor–patient relationship in the course of a series of ordinary GP consultations. These were then (in the 1960s) thought to last an average of six minutes. The group published a book called *Six Minutes for the Patient*,[2] a title which led some GPs to think it might contain the answer to their prayers. 'Six minutes' was the beginning of the modern style of Balint work. Group members were now free to present a patient they had only seen once, as well as others they had known for years.

Balint doctors put everything down to sex

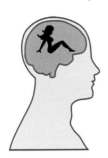

Although Michael's book became well-known and frequently quoted all over the world, its ideas had little appeal for the majority of British GPs, who were not very 'psychologically minded'. There was a general suspicion that doctors in Balint groups spent all their time fantasising about their patients' sex lives. If they weren't doing that, they were pointlessly ruminating about their own personal problems. In fact, the Balints never intended the groups to provide therapy for the doctors and resisted any attempt to swing the discussion in this direction. With the arrival of video recording of actual consultations, the Balint method was regarded by many GP educators as historically important but totally outdated.

How did Balint survive in Britain?

Balint work survived thanks to the enthusiasm and commitment of a small cohort of GPs who had been trained in the early groups. When vocational training started, some of these GPs became Course Organisers (now known as Programme Directors). Naturally, they introduced Balint into their Half-Day Release courses. The next generation of Course Organisers continued this tradition, and gradually it saw itself emerge in areas like the annual conference of the Association of Course Organisers (now called Association of Primary Care Educators – APCE). Other factors that ensured the survival of Balint's work included the following.

1 The continuing presence of Enid Balint, who, after Michael's death in 1970, was active to the end until she died in 1994.

2 The formation of 'research groups' looking at particular topics through the lens of the doctor–patient relationship. Indeed, Balint called the original groups 'research cum training seminars', in that order.

3 The creation of the Balint Society[3] which encouraged new groups to form and started weekend meetings in Oxford in 1978 to offer people 'a taste of Balint'. These have continued annually ever since, and similar meetings now take place in other parts of the country.

The present situation

Today, Balint work is treated more respectfully by GP educators. Its potential role in learning to be a GP is included in the RCGP curriculum.[4] The Balint Society is still active, with groups usually being led by GPs or by a GP and a psychotherapist together. The present and future role of Balint groups in GP education will be discussed later in this chapter.

What's the point of Balint work?

1 **To get a better understanding of the doctor–patient relationship:** Balint compared the doctor to a 'drug', whose 'pharmacology' needed to be understood, including its effects, side-effects and dosage.[1]

2 **To provide training, *not* therapy:** The method Balint used had parallels with group psychotherapy, but he was always keen to point out that the group was *not* therapy but research and training. What Balint's method *did* have in common with psychotherapy was the use of free association. For example, group members were not permitted to use case notes, the principle being that what came into their minds (or didn't) was what mattered. The omission of 'key' facts was seen as a clue to understanding what was happening in the doctor–patient relationship, rather than (as it would have been in traditional medical presentations) a sign of incompetence in the presenting doctor.

3 **To help GPs learn how to listen to and understand what their patients are really saying:** Balint did not aim for group participants to be 'amateur psychiatrists' but instead to help them improve on their listening and understanding skills.

4 **To provide insight into how a patient's feelings could induce similar emotions in the doctor:** Balint was aware that this work was stressful, not easy and difficult to use with doctors whose personalities were 'too rigid' or 'too vulnerable' and looking to the group for therapy.

What characterises a Balint group?

The Balint Society Council considered this in 1994. They came up with a list of 'essential' and 'desirable' characteristics of a Balint group.[5] This should not be seen as the final word on this subject, and they would welcome comments and criticisms. For fear of sending you to sleep, we'll just concentrate on some of the main 'essential' characteristics – some of these we've discussed before.

1 **The clinician should present current cases that are giving him or her a particular cause for thought.** Cases giving rise to distress, puzzlement, difficulty or even just surprise, are likely to lead to a useful discussion.

2 **The discussion focuses on the relationship between the presenting doctor and his or her patient.**

3 **The purpose of the group is to increase understanding of the patient's problems, not to find solutions.** As Balint said, *'If you ask questions, all you get is answers.'* To stop the process from deteriorating into an interrogative Question–Answer session, we suggest that once matters of fact have been quickly cleared up, the presenter should then be asked to move his or her chair slightly out of the circle and not to participate in the discussion that follows. This method allows the group to work creatively together, focus on speculations as to what might be going on rather than on problem-solving and without the worry of the presenting doctor interjecting, correcting and disrupting the flow of the discussion.

4 **Case notes should not be used, as discussed previously.**

5 **The discussion should be in a small group with participants and leader(s) arranged in a *neat* circle.** A group size of between 6 and 12 participants generally works best.

6 **There should be a defined group leader and, ideally, a co-leader as well.** Essentially, leaders should be GPs, psychotherapists or allied professionals (like counsellors) who have had some relevant training in small-group leadership and experience of Balint groups. A GP and a psychotherapist or counsellor would make a good combination.

7 **Remember, the groups are not for personal therapy.** *'Discomfort or distress in the doctor is not ignored but is worked through in the context of the needs and problems of the patient rather than of the doctor.'*[6]

What actually happens? Take me through an example

Okay, let's imagine that we're going to take part in a Balint group for GP trainees. We all sit around in a circle. There are nine of us plus the leader. She's called Claire, and she's also one of the Programme Directors.

So, who's got a case?

'OK,' says Claire. *'Does anyone have a patient they would like to tell us about?'* There is silence for what seems like ages but is probably only 30 seconds, while Claire gazes into space. Some people fidget a bit. Then one of the trainees (Julia) says, *'I have one I could talk about.'* *'Anybody else?'* asks Claire, looking around the group. However, everyone is looking expectantly at Julia. *'OK then,'* says Claire, *'let's start with yours, Julia.'*

Julia presents her patient

So Julia starts her story. *'This patient is a man of 35, and I haven't seen him before. But I did see from the records that he is a drug addict, so that put me off straight away. I don't know what it is about addicts, but I really hate having to deal with them. The way they try to manipulate you and get prescriptions off you.'*

(Murmurs of sympathy from some group members)

'So anyway, [Julia continues] it turns out he's not asking for any narcotics or benzodiazepines. He says he's come about his asthma. He says he has been having numerous attacks and the only thing that helps is a blue inhaler. So can he have three, because he gets through them very quickly! I ask if he is having any other treatment for asthma, and he says he isn't. And, in fact, there's nothing on his prescription list except salbutamol and one of the doctors gave him two of those only a few days ago! He didn't seem breathless, just anxious. He was sweating a lot and kept wiping his face with his sleeve. I listened to his chest which was OK and his peak flow was over 600 so that was OK. I asked him to show me his inhaler technique, and he said when he gets breathless, he holds the inhaler in front of his face and kind of sprays it in his face about 20 times. That's the only thing that makes him feel better. If he didn't do that he feels that he is going to choke to death.'

Asthma or drug abuse?

'So I told him he needed to make an appointment for the asthma clinic and get properly assessed. I showed him how he should use the salbutamol, and he asked if he could have just one more. Then he got sort of desperate, saying, "I don't know what will happen if it runs out and I get another attack. Please give me three or at least two. I beg of you." He actually said I beg of you. He pulled his chair up close to me. I asked if he was taking any drugs, and he said no, he used to but now he's clean. I just wanted to get rid of him. It's a horrible thing to say, but I felt disgusted with him the way he was pleading with me. And the way he made me do something unprofessional. I just wanted him to go. So in the end I gave him a prescription for two inhalers (I know, I know, I shouldn't have) and told him to make an appointment for the asthma clinic. So then he went. I was so upset I was shaking. I really hope I don't have to see him again.'

The group ask questions

'Thanks Julia,' says Claire. *'Does anybody have any questions about factual details?'* The group members are all looking stirred up by Julia's evident distress.

Simon, who is sitting opposite her, says, *'I think you did very well to only give him two and insist that he comes to the clinic. There's something very fishy going on here, I reckon. I wonder if he's getting panic attacks from using cocaine, and he's using the inhaler to bring himself down.'*

There is a general wave of sympathy for Julia. Someone says he may be selling the inhalers on the street. Claire intervenes at this point and says, *'I know we're all a bit disturbed by Julia's experience, but could we just have factual questions for now? And then we'll think about what went on in the consultation.'*

Someone asks what the patient looks like. Was he scruffily dressed? Did he look like an addict? Were his pupils constricted? Was there anything in the notes about his personal life? To which Julia answered that he was neatly dressed, with short hair and looked quite clean. There was nothing about asthma in his record, and she had not been able to ask him about his work or family or anything.

Julia sits back and listens

Questions then seem to naturally die down. Claire suggests that Julia moves her chair back a few inches and stays quiet for about 15 minutes, just listening while the rest of the group discusses the case. *'So no more questions to Julia! She's told us all she can. Now it's our turn to do some work. What do we think was going on between these two, the doctor and the patient?'*

To begin with the group members continue expressing sympathy for Julia and saying that she had done really well in such a difficult situation. Someone thought her Trainer should see the patient next time. Someone else thought he should be screened for drugs or referred to the community substance abuse clinic. A strict limit should be put on his prescriptions, and he must be assessed to see if he really has asthma. If he doesn't comply, he should be removed from the practice list.

The group leader intervenes

Our leader, Claire, gets a bit restless. She says, *'We really don't like this young man very much, do we? We are being quite stern and punitive. But here is somebody who may be in absolute terror of not being able to breathe. We don't know if it's asthma or panic attacks or what, but I guess he must feel really frightened.'*

Then one of the trainees (Alison) says, *'I agree. He probably felt he was going to die or something. It sounds more like panic than asthma. But somehow his manner, all that pleading and sweating! It makes you want to reject him.'* And she makes a gesture with both hands of pushing someone away. Somebody else says it probably is panic disorder, and he ought to be referred for cognitive behavioural therapy. Another trainee says we know he has a history of addiction, and he could be lying about the whole thing. Then Alison comes back and says she doesn't think he was lying, and perhaps we were being hard on him, and perhaps Julia should find out more about his background, next time – if she can bear it! Claire says that some people are very difficult to empathise with because we can't imagine ourselves ever behaving like that. However, what would it feel like to be him, that day? Some people agree that he is probably genuinely frightened. If one got to know him better, he might be helpable. Others continue to be sceptical.

Julia comes back in

Then Claire invites Julia to rejoin the discussion. Julia says it was very interesting listening to everybody, and she was relieved that other people also found him repellent [laughter]. Then she says that when Alison said it might be worth finding out more about his background; she suddenly remembered that he had said he lived with his father who had died suddenly four weeks ago.

Somebody says, *'I feel quite sorry for him now.'* And Simon says, *'If it's true!'*

'Oh, Simon, you're such a cynic,' says Alison.

'Well, no,' says Simon, *'you have to be. I've worked in a drug clinic, and people are just lying all the time.'*

Claire notes that we are somewhat divided in our feelings about the patient. He seems to induce either pity or disgust. She asks Julia whether the discussion was helpful. Julia says, *'Yes it was. I think I do need to find out more about him, and I'm sure he'll be back! I feel I could manage seeing him again, with you all backing me up. I'll let you know what happens.'*

The leader's contribution

Let us summarise the key points of the leader's contribution:

1 She asks the group to stick to factual questions and then asks the presenter to 'sit out'. This encourages the group members to reflect on their own feelings, rather than simply questioning the presenter.

2 She lets the group express their negative feelings about the patient up to a point. She then intervenes, inviting them to try to identify with the patient to get some sense of his feelings. This is partly successful and at least some members become more sympathetic.

3 When the presenter is allowed into the group again she has remembered what the patient said about his father dying. She has become a little more interested in him as a person. The leader observes that the patient has induced mixed feelings in the group.

4 The leader speaks up for the patient, introducing the (possible) perspectives of another person.

Why do Balint in GP training?

Trainees who take part in a regular Balint over a period of a year or more benefit in a number of ways:

At a *basic* level, Balint helps you:

- become a better **listener**
- learn to be more **empathic** and empathise with a wider range of people
- be more interested in **patients' life history**, background and personal relationships
- be more inclined seriously to consider what the patient wants (more **patient-centred**)
- be more **tolerant**
- be able to **find motivation** to help patients who at first seem hopeless or obnoxious.

At a *higher* level, Balint helps you:

- become more aware of **own feelings** about patients
- realise that **patients project emotions on to doctors**: somehow, the patient makes the doctor feel what the patient is experiencing (helplessness, failure, depression, anger, etc.)
- learn how to **recognise these feelings** without letting them get out of control (*'Okay, I'm now feeling a bit irritated but I need to keep this in check in order to maintain the relationship.'*)
- gain **insight** into why some patients frequently arouse negative emotions (*'I can't stand it when he moans. I suppose it can't be easy for him with having xxx and yyy in his life.'*)

In *general*, Balint means you:

- **enjoy work** better
- find **all patients potentially interesting** (even if no major pathology)
- are less likely to suffer 'burnout'
- are less likely to get **complaints**
- and work just seems to be **less stressful**.

You can see that Balint is based on experiential learning – learners self-select the cases that they've come across which they wish to explore further. Learning from Balint is inductive, in contrast to being deductive, in that changes in attitude result from the accumulation of insights from one's own and other colleagues' presentations. As Balint is done in small groups, you also have all the benefits of small-group work thrown in.

- **Providing a safe environment:** to allow members to talk about their feelings without the fear of any backlash.
- **Providing an avenue for cathartic release:** where participants get relief from unburdening themselves about difficult patients to a sympathetic group of peers.
- **Members working in collaboration:** expressing their thoughts and how they would manage a similar patient. Ideas are shared, built upon and assimilated.

- **Being properly facilitated:** the group leader or facilitator helps the small-group process by steering the discussion and giving the group the benefit of his or her knowledge and experience.
- **Providing a supportive environment:** members provide valuable support for each other; this may range from things to do with the trainee's relationship with their GP Trainer, consultant or colleagues to fears about future careers and aspirations.

You're just saying all of that? Where's your evidence?

In the last few years there has been a good deal of research into the effects and effectiveness of Balint group work. This work has demonstrated that Balint-trained doctors:

- show greater evidence of empathy and patient-centeredness[7,8]
- have increased job satisfaction and show greater patient tolerance.[9]

Qualitative accounts have also demonstrated a positive effect on the emotional development of young doctors,[10,11] students[12,13] and mature doctors.[14]

Do trainees like it?

Some take to it straight away. In our experience, trainees with an arts background generally enjoy Balint from the start. Others may need some time to get used it – those with a very medical approach to general practice find it difficult to see the point (and may find it all a bit too 'woolly'). Everyone else is somewhere in between. If the group continues to meet regularly, many in this mid-

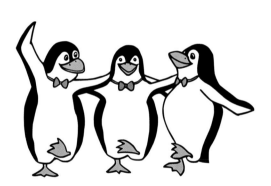

dle group begin to appreciate the Balint sessions more. This may be to do with their development as GPs. They may be discovering that general practice is more about relating to people with difficulties than the diagnosis and treatment of diseases.

If you're new to Balint, don't give up if the participants remain unimpressed after the first session – most of us feel uncomfortable the very first time we try *anything* new. Our own experience in leading trainee groups over many years and in discussion with other leaders at Balint workshops suggests that the benefits accumulate gradually over time. Experiential learning can take place in a hierarchy of levels as the trainees get the hang of what is going on in the group and in the doctor–patient relationships that have come under the microscope. A significant proportion of these will become 'converts' as they discover more about themselves.

Facilitating Balint groups

Let us assume that you are reasonably comfortable leading small-group discussions. If you are not, you need to concentrate on building those skills first (*see* Chapter 13: Teaching and Facilitating Small Groups). We'll start with the Balint process and then look at some of the components in more detail.

<table>
<tr><td>The Balint process</td></tr>
</table>

Setting up

- Neat circle, position of facilitator and co-facilitator, switch off mobiles.

Briefing on Balint

- Find out who is new to Balint. Give an introductory handout?
- (1) Who was Michael Balint, (2) The Balint process, (3) Why we do it (4) Balint rules – dos and don'ts.

'Who's got a case then?'

- Group leader: *'Has anyone got a case they'd like to talk about?'*
- Thank the person who plucks up the courage to do so.
- Remind the group that the case is to be seen as a gift from which we are all going to learn (not as a platform to denigrate one another).

The case is presented

- The presenter presents the case in (1) their own words, (2) at some length and detail, (3) without interruption and (4) without reference to any case notes.

Questions to clarify matters of fact

- Questions from the group only to *clarify matters of fact* – not to elicit the presenter's thoughts or feelings. Don't allow questioning to go on for too long.
- One always useful question is to ask what the patient look liked – their physical characteristics, their clothing and so on.

Presenter asked to sit back

- Presenter moves their chair 6 inches outside the circle.
- No more questions allowed.
- Presenter not to interrupt further group discussion.

Discussion of the doctor–patient relationship ensues

- Remind the group that the session is not about problem-solving but to offer thoughts about the doctor–patient relationship – think about what each one must be feeling and thinking.
- Encourage free association and creative thinking.
- Start off the discussions with something like: *'If I were the doctor, I would feel . . .'* This makes a safe harbour for the presenter and prevents them cutting ideas short by saying things like *'I thought of that, and it didn't help.'*

Group leader intervenes if . . .

Generally, the group leader says very little, but will need to intervene:
- if the group veers away from talking about the doctor–patient relationship
- if the group is not sticking firmly to the individual case being presented (i.e. are becoming anecdotal).

Speak up for the patient

- Protect the patient if you feel they are being unfairly assassinated.
- This degree of empathy may be difficult in the case of a patient who is seen as obnoxious, demanding, or 'untreatable' because of a personality disorder.

Presenter rejoins the group

- As discussions come to a natural close, the presenter is invited to rejoin the group.
- The presenter is given the opportunity to make some comments on what they've heard, although whether they do so is entirely up to them.
- Thank the presenter for offering the case as a gift for us all to learn from.

Additional notes

Setting up

1 Start by making a **neat balanced circle of chairs**. *Balanced* circles are important (it affects individual participation).
2 **Space the leaders** within the group (so that they are neither next to each other nor directly opposite each other).
3 Put a **notice on the door** asking for no interruptions.
4 'Please switch off your **mobile phones**.'

Briefing on Balint

Talk about the following.

1 The Origin of Balint work: Michael Balint, origin of his work and the formation of Balint groups. There is an excellent introductory handout (by Heather Suckling) available from our website.
2 Why we do Balint? In order to 'hook in' your intended participants say something like: *'Balint helps us to explore the **doctor–patient relationship** in order to deepen our understanding of it. This may make you a **better GP** and may help you **avoid burnout** by making the **work more interesting**.'*

The Balint process

1 Briefly go through what happens in a *typical* Balint group session. Don't spend too long on this though.
2 Specifically:
   - That it is *not necessarily to discuss problem cases*, just ones which have intrigued, interested or maybe disturbed.
   - It could be a *continuing* relationship or a *one-off encounter*.
   - This is *not about good or bad* management, or right or wrong answers.
   - Encourage fantasy, lateral, 'right-brain' thinking – this method is more art than science.
   - Work may raise personal issues for presenters or group members and the Balint process might bring those to the fore. The group shouldn't be afraid of that and while Balint is not about therapy, one should respect and acknowledge such difficulties. Give a personal example if appropriate.

Explicit Balint Rules – five dos and don'ts

1 Explain that all material is confidential within the group.
2 Group members should own their statements.
3 Focus on the doctor–patient relationship.
4 Get the group to look at the process rather than seek solutions. The group is not there to solve the presenter's problems.
5 Remember that the case is 'a gift' for the group. We need to *stick with the case*; participants should not venture off and start introducing their own cases or anecdotes.

Notes for the facilitator

1 Enable all members to participate. However, protect them from attacking each other – create a safe environment.
2 Discourage interrogation of the presenting doctor.
3 Maintain focus on the doctor–patient relationship and not on problem-solving. If discussions go off at a tangent, bring them back by saying something like: *'What's going on between this doctor and this patient?' 'What effects are the patient's mood and behaviour having on the presenting doctor and on the rest of us?'*
4 Stay with the presented case only and discourage anecdotes. Intervene if others try to 'infect' the case with their own particular case, i.e. where a member says, *'I had a similar case where the patient was xxx and yyy and what we did was . . .'*
5 Encourage reflection and deflect questions appropriately. Trainee: *'Do you think there's something else causing the patient to be like this?'* Facilitator: *'What did you have in mind Danny?'*
6 Encourage lateral thinking and imagination.
7 Speak up for the patient. More on this below.
8 Watch the time if no one else has been allocated to do this.
9 Don't talk too much! Try to steer the group to come up with insights for themselves, rather than you telling them. If you've got a co-leader, try not to speak straight after them. If in doubt, keep quiet.
10 Ensure the presenter is OK at the end.

Speaking up for the patient

Sometimes, groups can collude with the presenting doctor and 'assassinate' the patient. If you think someone has been unfair and not considered the patient's perspective, encourage them to reflect by saying something like:

● *'I wonder how the patient would feel at this point. I wonder what's going on for them.'*
● *'What do you think the patient might be feeling or going through? I wonder what it's like being in their shoes.'*
● *'How do you think the patient would feel or react to what you've just said? Would anyone care to guess?'*

The aim is to remind group members of the patient's perspective, their vulnerability and the need to protect them. Remember, Balint is all about *understanding* the doctor–patient relationship.

Working with a co-leader or co-facilitator

Having a co-leader is a gift, but also a challenge. Get to know each other before the group starts and share ideas as to how to run it. For instance, you might wish to keep some roles separate, e.g. have one leader as 'chair' to keep an eye on the time, introduce the discussion, etc. while the other leader concentrates on particular interventions. Try not to speak directly after your co-leader has spoken. Listen carefully to what he or she has said, and consider reinforcing it later if the group has not taken up the suggestion. Make sure you debrief afterwards and be prepared to learn from each other in order to modify your approach for the future.

Being creative with Balint – different contexts and application

Inevitably, the Balint method has evolved over the years and taken slightly different directions in different countries and different circumstances. However, the basis of Balint remains the same:

focusing on the fundamentals of human relationships. So far, we've concentrated on Balint as applied to the doctor–patient relationship, but we've seen it providing valuable insights in the following relationships.

1 In a Trainers' workshop to look at a specific Trainer–trainee relationship.
2 In a partnership to look at a doctor–doctor relationship.
3 In the surgery to explore a relationship with a colleague.
4 It's not just for doctors – successful groups have been run for professions such as social workers[15] and the clergy[16] too.

No doubt there are others. In Germany, many leaders are psychotherapists or psychoanalysts and usually only one case is discussed in a 90-minute session.[17] As a result, a greater depth is achieved, and participants probably achieve a better understanding of the unconscious factors involved in their work with patients. The group we described in 'What are you feeling, doctor?'[18] explored, like any Balint group, the doctor–patient relationship but went into more depth about the doctor's end of the spectrum and how difficulties arose because of unconscious factors in the doctor. Educators who are also experienced Balint leaders may want to take up the challenge and offer groups that explore particular aspects of the doctor–patient relationship in more depth.

Training – getting proper Balint experience

For those of you who would like to try giving Balint a go in the presence of experienced others, try 'The APCE annual conference', join a local Balint group or try 'The Balint Society Weekend'.

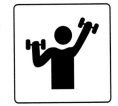

1 **The APCE annual conference:**[19] there is usually a Balint group running in parallel with the normal small groups, led by a couple of experienced Balint leaders who are, or have been, Programme Directors themselves. This group functions as a 'normal' Balint group discussing cases but time is also set aside in each session to discuss the leadership. Participants are encouraged to take a turn at leading or co-leading a session if they wish to.

2 **Joining/forming a local Balint group** – admittedly these are a bit thin on the ground in the UK but the Balint Society might well be able to help you find a group within reach. Alternatively, if you can get some local colleagues interested in forming a new group, the Balint Society might be able to find you a leader.

3 A **Balint Society Weekend** – these are held in various parts of the country, where there will be four or five group sessions helping you to get some concentrated experience. Look on the Balint Society website for details (www.balint.co.uk). Some of the weekends may include workshops for leaders. The Balint Society also runs regular **Group Leaders' Workshops** in London. As you continue with this leadership training, you may be interested in **Balint group leader accreditation**. Details about accreditation can be found in the 2009 issue of the *Journal of the Balint Society*.[20]

Final thoughts

It is now over half a century since Balint's seminal book was published[1] and we believe (because Balint is all about human relationships) that the principles remain perfectly relevant today.

- **It's a learner-centred method in action.** The case 'offered' by the presenter can be seen as a 'gift' for the group. The way the group works increases the presenter's understanding without making them feel 'on the spot'. Guided by the leader(s), the rest of the group supports the presenter while also offering challenge – the basis of a good learning environment. Other group members learn too. They gain insight into their own work with patients by exploring the presented case.

- **It's an alternative to problem-solving.** So much of GP training centres on problem-solving, which is of course extremely important in working with patients, but is a bit uni-dimensional. The Balint experience help trainees to look at their work in a very different and more creative way, thus helping our trainees become more rounded learners and practitioners.

- **It promotes a reflective practice.** The Balint experience is an opportunity for trainees to reflect in a deep way on their work with patients. As well as helping them understand and work with patients better, the experience of reflection should help trainees in all aspects of their work, their continuing professional development and their lives in general.

In these times when 'ticking the boxes' seems a major part of all professional activity, there is a huge need for us to understand and stay with the emotional aspect of our work with patients and colleagues. Balint work offers a highly effective way of doing this – indeed it refreshes the parts that other approaches to medical education don't reach.

A sample of resources on our website

- Balint approach to the consultation.
- Balint facilitator instructions.
- Balint handouts for trainees.
- Troubleshooting Balint.

Other chapters you may like to read

- Chapter 12: How Groups Work – the dynamics
- Chapter 13: Teaching and Facilitating Small Groups.

The Balint Society website

All of the authors and contributors to this chapter are members of the Balint Society. Please come and visit us at www.balint.co.uk

---

Please give us some feedback on this chapter to help shape it for the next edition.
Go to www.essentialgptrainingbook.com and simply click on the title of this chapter.

References

1 Balint M. *The Doctor, his Patient and the Illness.* London: Pitman Medical; 1957 (Millennium edition, Edinburgh: Churchill Livingstone; 2000).
2 Norell J, Balint E, editors. *Six Minutes for the Patient.* London: Tavistock Publications; 1973.
3 www.balint.co.uk (accessed 11 January 2010).
4 www.rcgp-curriculum.org.uk/pdf/curr-2 (accessed 11 January 2010).
5 Balint Society Council. What is a Balint group? *J Balint Soc.* 1994; **22**: 36–7.

6 Campkin M. Is there a place for Balint in vocational training? *J Assoc Course Organisers*. 1986; **1**: 100–4.

7 Kjeldmand D, Holmström I, Rosenquist V. How patient-centred am I? A new method to measure physicians' patient-centredness. *Patient Education and Counselling*. 2006; **82**: 31–7.

8 Nease DE, Margo K, Floyd M. The resident Balint outcomes study: final results of our two-year evaluation. In: *Balint Work and Globalisation. Proceedings of the 16th International Balint Congress*. Brasov: Altus, 2009. pp. 57–62.

9 Kjeldmand D, Homström I. Balint groups as a method of increasing job satisfaction and reducing professional burnout among GPs. *Ann Fam Med*. 2008; **6**: 138–45.

10 Forsell J. Balint groups with young doctors in their foundation year at a county hospital in Sweden. *J Balint Soc*. 2006; **34**: 22–7.

11 Lustig M. A pilot registrar Balint group in Melbourne. *J Balint Soc*. 2004; **32**: 17–19.

12 Shoenberg P, Suckling H. A Balint group for medical students at Royal Free and University College School of Medicine. *J Balint Soc*. 2004; **32**: 20–3.

13 Turner A. Making space for the doctor-patient relationship through Balint training in the first year of medical school. *J Balint Soc*. 2005; **33**: 34–41.

14 Salamon M, Kuntz C. The Ottawa Balint group quantitative research project: how doctors benefit. International Conference on physician health, Ottawa, 2006. Available at: www.cma.ca/imdex.cfm/ci_id (accessed 23 January 2010).

15 Moreau Ricaud M. *Michael Balint: Le renouveau de l'Ecole de Budapest*. Paris: Erès, 2000.

16 Bryant D. A Balint Group is not just for doctors. In: *Medicine, Evidence and Emotions 50 years on. Proceedings of the 15th International Balint Congress*. Lisbon: Cor Expressa, 2007. pp. 45–52.

17 Otten H. Balint-work in Germany. *J Balint Soc*. 1998; **26**: 16–19.

18 Salinsky J, Sackin P. *What are you feeling, doctor?* Oxford: Radcliffe; 2000.

19 www.ukapd.org (accessed 22 January 2010).

20 Balint Society. The Balint Society guidelines for accreditation of Balint group leaders (British). *J Balint Soc*. 2009; **37**: 5.

PART EIGHT

MRCGP, Supervision and Assessment

25

MRCGP in a Nutshell

JIM BARTLETT – TPD (Shropshire) & lead author   NIGEL DE-KARE SILVER – Associate Director (London Deanery)
AMAR RUGHANI – APD (Yorkshire & the Humber Deanery)   BRUNO RUSHFORTH – Clinical Research Fellow (Univ. Leeds)
MARY SELBY – Trainer (East of England Deanery)   RAMESH MEHAY – TPD (Bradford)

> While all the information in this chapter is correct at the time of going to press, please check the RCGP's website for the latest information. To try to ensure most of the things cited in this chapter remain factually correct for as long as possible, we've concentrated on principles and guidance rather than focusing on numbers and tick boxes.

Introduction

The aim of this chapter is to set out an overview of the MRCGP exam with thumbnail descriptions of its components and some suggestions as to how to help guide your GP trainees through the process. We've tried to provide a balance in terms of principles, guidance and information giving because we believe that getting concepts right is more important than getting bogged down by the minutiae.

The very basics

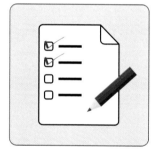

- Since August 2007, the Membership of the Royal College of General Practitioners (MRCGP) is the mandatory **licensing examination** for all General Practice Specialty Training Registrars (GPstRs for short) in the UK – they cannot be let loose on the public without it!
- The MRCGP is an *integrated* assessment programme that has three components:
  1. Applied Knowledge Test (AKT) – an MCQ exam; £400 approx. – max 4 attempts
  2. Clinical Skills Assessment (CSA) – an OSCE style exam; £1500 approx. – max 4 attempts
  3. Workplace-Based Assessment (WPBA) – assessments done *throughout* the entire GP training envelope (currently 3 years); free.
- Each of these components tests different professional competencies (with some overlap), but together they cover the whole spectrum required for specialty training for general practice.
- Evidence for the WPBA is collected in a web-based recording tool called the ePortfolio; each trainee will have their own.
- At the end of their GP training period, if they have satisfactorily completed all the posts and achieved 1, 2 and 3, they can then apply for their Certificate of Completion of Training (CCT). This is the final certificate that allows them to practise as independent GPs. Oh, and they have to pay for that too!

We didn't have to do all of this stuff in my day. Why now?

The MRCGP assessment system has seen a number of different formats in the past. It used to be optional (when Summative Assessment was the compulsory assessment procedure), but now it's mandatory. We believe that the recent changes to GP training are good. Under older GP training models, most GP trainees who were good enough got through successfully. However, because of the lack of any structured and educationally sound assessment procedure, unfortunately some who shouldn't have got through did too. One GP looks after (on average) 1800 patients and one bad egg can affect 1800 lives. It's therefore important to keep the number who get through the net but shouldn't as low as possible.

Summative Assessment was introduced as a way of ensuring this, but in terms of its educational soundness, it was predominantly concerned with *showing* that you *could* do something rather than providing convincing evidence of *doing it* competently on a *regular* basis. The old MRCGP exam suffered the same problem too – showing rather than actually doing!

- For the first time in general practice, the current MRCGP assessment system is based on 12 clearly defined professional competencies. These define what *must* be achieved to be able to function independently as a safe and competent GP.
- The current MRCGP assessment system also consists of a number of components that *assess* at the *'doing'* level (*see* Miller's Pyramid in Chapter 29: Assessment and Competence).

Why the MRCGP is compulsory

- The **'public'** rightly expects GPs to have passed a stringent quality-control procedure.
- The **GMC** would like to prove that all GP trainees have been assessed to the same standard, and that the assessment can be defended and upheld against all challenges (from disgruntled failed GP trainees or patients).

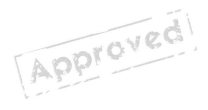

- The **Royal College** would like to uphold and improve standards in general practice. Generally speaking, learners are only interested in learning what they are ultimately going to be tested on. On that basis, the college can 'drive' what GP trainees learn through their assessment system.

What does this changeover mean for established GP Educators?

For established Trainers

Trainers will need to make an adjustment from what may have previously been a cosy mentoring and supporting role to that of an assessor with the potential to derail a career but, nevertheless, protect the public. And switching between the role of being the trainee's teacher, mentor, assessor and even friend is by no means easy. One moment you may be their friendly mentor and on another, their assessor.

Then there are the new assessments. You will have to find protected practice time to do them. Before doing them though, you have to familiarise yourself with them. Ultimately, that means becoming familiar with the 'curriculum statement headings' and the 'professional competency statements' too.

For established Programme Directors

In the old days, you could teach about anything – whatever was relevant at the time, and much of it was about things you cannot get from books. Now, you will be fighting the pressure from our trainees to teach 'to the exam'. If you give in, other equally vital parts of our jobs will be squeezed out. 'MRCGP' will then start to dominate everything, including Half/Full-Day Release. Rather than coaching to the exam, our role could be seen as a much more longitudinal one: improving performance as a GP through **guided reflection over time**. Knowledge and skills will be acquired after reflection: our job being to help steer the process, highlight attitudinal blocks and guide reflective learning.

Curriculum headings and competency statements. What's the difference?

We're glad you asked because it is something to get 'sorted' in your head right from the start. The MRCGP has achieved a first in postgraduate medical exams by setting out from the onset a cross-referenced **curriculum** which is matched against a blueprint of desired **competencies**. But many Trainers still get confused over the terms *curriculum statement headings* and *professional competency statements*.

- The *curriculum headings* tell us *what* GP trainees need to cover and know.
- The *professional competencies* tell us the *level of performance* they need to develop.

The curriculum statement headings (what they need to know)

There are currently 32 curriculum statement headings divided into 15 sections, covering specific clinical, professional and managerial aspects of general practice:

The GP curriculum statement headings as of January 2011	
1 Being a General Practitioner	10 Gender-specific Health Issues
2 The General Practice Consultation	*10.1 Women's health*
3 Personal and Professional Responsibilities	*10.2 Men's health*
3.1 Clinical Governance	11 Sexual Health
3.2 Patient Safety	12 Care of People with Cancer & Palliative Care
3.3 Clinical Ethics and Values-Based Practice	13 Care of People with Mental Health Problems
3.4 Promoting Equality and Valuing Diversity	14 Care of People with Learning Disabilities
3.5 Evidence-Based Practice	15 Clinical Management
3.6 Research and Academic Activity	*15.1 Cardiovascular problems*
3.7 Teaching, Mentoring and Clinical Supervision	*15.2 Digestive problems*
4 Management	*15.3 Drug and alcohol problems*
4.1 Management in Primary Care	*15.4 ENT and facial problems*
4.2 Information Management and Technology	*15.5 Eye problems*
5 Healthy People: promoting health + preventing disease	*15.6 Metabolic problems*
6 Genetics in Primary Care	*15.7 Neurological problems*
7 Care of Acutely Ill People	*15.8 Respiratory problems*
8 Care of Children and Young People	*15.9 Rheumatology, musculoskeletal and trauma*
9 Care of Older Adults	*15.10 Skin problems*

You can see from this that the curriculum is a list of topics that are to be covered in the GP training period. Previously, this used to be 'anything and everything', but it has now been divided and subdivided into chunks to aid study and learning. Most curricula evolve continuously so don't expect this to remain static in the future – it's likely to have things added here and there in response to changes in medical knowledge, priorities and emphasis.

If you go to www.rcgp-curriculum.org. uk/ and click on 'curriculum documents', you will see a link to 'GP curriculum statements'. If you click on this link, you'll be able to click onto any one of the curriculum statement headings to see its 'make up' in more detail – the **intended learning outcomes (ILOs)** and some suggestions of resources. We know it looks a bit daunting but the more you look at it, the more familiar it will become (and there is no need to memorise any of it).

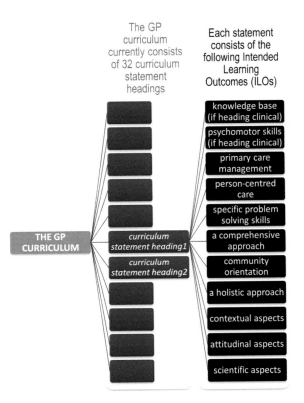

The 12 professional competencies (level of performance they need to develop)

The *core* curriculum statement heading – **'1 Being a General Practitioner'** was written to describe the 'essence' of being a GP, but not to specify what behaviours to look for in someone competent for independent practice. However, a *set of behaviours* has been described to help provide evidence that a trainee has acquired the necessary knowledge, skills and attitudes (KSA). This is known as the **MRCGP competency framework** or as **The 12 Professional Competencies.**

The 12 Professional Competencies for WPBA

1. Communication and consultation skills
   - *Communicating with patients and using recognised consultation techniques.*
2. Practising holistically
   - *Operating in physical, psychological, socioeconomic and cultural dimensions, exploring feelings as well as thoughts.*
3. Data gathering and interpretation
   - *Gathering and using data for clinical judgement, the choice of examination and investigations, and their interpretation.*
4. Making a diagnosis/making decisions
   - *A conscious, structured approach to decision-making.*

5. Clinical management
   - *The recognition and management of common medical conditions in primary care.*
6. Managing medical complexity and promoting health
   - *Aspects of care beyond managing straightforward problems, e.g. comorbidity, uncertainty, risk and the approach to health rather than just illness.*
7. Primary care administration and IMT
   - *The appropriate use of primary care administration systems, effective recordkeeping and information technology for the benefit of patient care.*
8. Working with colleagues and in teams
   - *Working effectively with other professionals to ensure patient care, including the sharing of information with colleagues.*
9. Community orientation
   - *The management of the health and social care of the practice population and local community.*
10. Maintaining performance, learning and teaching
    - *Maintaining the performance and continuing professional development of oneself and others.*
11. Maintaining an ethical approach to practice
    - *Practising ethically with integrity and a respect for diversity.*
12. Fitness to practise
    - *Awareness of when his or her own performance, conduct or health, or that of others, might put patients at risk and the action taken to protect patients.*

Important notes about the 12 professional competencies

- A professional competency is the capability to perform a particular professional task, with skill of an acceptable quality.
- *All* trainees must achieve *all* 12 competencies if they want to get their CCT.
- The different types of work-place based assessments (COTs, CBDs, etc.) will be 'marked' in reference to these professional competencies.
- You can award the trainee one of four grades for each professional competency.

Insufficient Evidence (I)	Needs Further Development (NFD)	Competent (C)	Excellent (E)
From the available evidence, the doctor's performance cannot be placed on a higher point of this developmental scale.	*Rigid adherence to taught rules or plans. Superficial grasp of unconnected facts. Unable to apply knowledge. Little situational perception or discretionary judgement.*	*Accesses and applies coherent and appropriate chunks of knowledge. Able to see actions in terms of longer-term goals. Demonstrates conscious and deliberate planning with an increased level of efficiency. Copes with crowdedness and is able to prioritise.*	*Intuitive and holistic grasp of situations. No longer relies on rules or maxims. Identifies underlying principles and patterns to define and solve problems. Relates recalled information to the goals of the present situation and is aware of the conditions for application of that knowledge.*

- Remember: the standard you are measuring them against is that of someone who is ready to practise independently – *and not the stage they are at.*
  Question: *What grade would you award an ST1 trainee in a GP post who you think is pretty good at practising holistically (way beyond what you would expect for their stage), but not as good as an ST3, who is ready to practise independently?*
  Answer: *Award an NFD (or if available, 'NFD – above expectation') rather than Competent.*
- If you are ever unsure as to what grade to give, refer to the ePortfolio: each assessment will have its own competency guidance framework detailing specific 'competency descriptors' for each of the four grades rather than the generic ones given above.

A little extra on intended learning outcomes

Each curriculum statement heading has a 'set' of intended learning outcomes (usually covering nine domains plus knowledge and psychomotor skills if the heading is clinical). Learners tend to look at the intended learning outcomes in the curriculum statements and assume that by ticking these off, they can become GPs. What they need to do is to look at the ILOs of *each* curriculum statement heading *when the time is right*. Instead of using these in isolation, they need to use them to help build up a picture of what is required of them in different contexts. For example, if a trainee is trying to learn about 'holism':

- An ILO from the ENT statement says: *describe how a holistic mindset would help to improve the patient's management (e.g. understanding why and how earache might affect the child's education).*
- An ILO from cancer care says: *holistic skills should help the doctor to see why and how the family could be involved* and so on.

How it all fits together – curriculum, ILOs, competencies and assessments

There is a clear link between the curriculum, the intended learning outcomes, the professional competencies and the MRCGP assessments. The nine ILO areas have been translated and matched to the 12 professional competency areas – illustrated in the table below. What this table shows is that *all* 12 professional competencies (and ILOs) cannot be observed and measured by any one single assessment. However, all 12 are covered by the whole 'set' of assessments and exams. Individually, they are 'tested' in more than one type of assessment. This table helps you interpret the array of assessments in a trainee's ePortfolio; it tells you what competency areas and ILOs have been covered and where you can triangulate for extra evidence of a competency should it be lacking in one of the assessments. Trainers, Educational Supervisors & ARCP panel members – print this table off and use it!

Intended Learning Outcomes (ILOs) *as per GP curriculum*	The 12 Professional Competencies	Which covers what?								
		Exams					WPBA			
		AKT	CSA	CBDs	COTs	Mini-CEX	MSF	PSQ	CSR	Learning log entries
Primary care management	• Clinical management	☑	☑	☑	☑	☑	☑		☑	☑
	• Working with colleagues & teams			☑			☑		☑	☑
	• Primary care administration & IM&T	☑		☑						☑
Person-centred care	• Communication & consulting skills		☑		☑	☑	☑	☑	☑	☑
Problem-solving skills	• Data gathering and interpretation	☑	☑	☑	☑	☑	☑		☑	☑
	• Making diagnosis and decisions	☑	☑	☑	☑	☑	☑		☑	☑
Comprehensive approach	• Managing medical complexity	☑	☑	☑		☑			☑	☑
Community orientation Contextual aspects	• Community orientation			☑					☑	☑
Holistic approach	• Practising holistically		☑	☑	☑			☑	☑	☑
Attitudinal aspects	• Ethical approach to practice		☑	☑			☑		☑	☑
	• Fitness to practise		☑	☑			☑		☑	☑
Scientific aspects	• Performance, learning and teaching	☑				☑	☑		☑	☑

Triangulation in practice: Let's say that as an Educational Supervisor, you have read a number of the trainee's learning log entries marked by the Trainer as demonstrating an 'ethical approach to practice'. However, you're not so convinced; to you, the link seems tenuous. You can see from this table that one of the other assessments which looks at ethics is CBDs. Therefore, to resolve your dilemma, you could look at a set of CBDs and determine to what extent the ethics competency has been demonstrated there.

So, not reaching a competency in one form of assessment can be searched for in another. Alternatively, you can validate the 'grade' of particular competency from one assessment by comparing results in several assessment methods. The table also helps us spot those areas where we might have to probe a bit harder to see how our trainees are doing. For example, the table tells you that a pass in the AKT, no matter how high the score, will not tell you anything about your trainee's communication skills or ability to *use* ethics.

By specifying the set of behaviours that defines competence *and* the assessments which 'test' for them, both GP trainees and their educators are now in a position where they know:
1 what is expected of them
2 which assessments test what
3 where they might look for evidence to demonstrate particular competencies
4 where they need to focus as training draws to a close.

The three main bits of the MRCGP

The MRCGP is broken up into three readily identifiable chunks, although the GP trainees probably perceive it as 2+1 with the 'exam' sections causing them more worry, even though the ongoing assessment over the three years of training is more time consuming (and more searching). The three components can be broadly thought of as looking at knowledge, skills and attitudes, although there is considerable overlap in what they actually test.

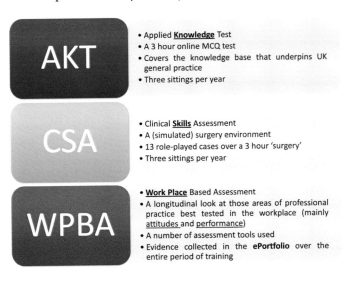

AKT
- Applied **Knowledge** Test
- A 3 hour online MCQ test
- Covers the knowledge base that underpins UK general practice
- Three sittings per year

CSA
- Clinical **Skills** Assessment
- A (simulated) surgery environment
- 13 role-played cases over a 3 hour 'surgery'
- Three sittings per year

WPBA
- **Work Place** Based Assessment
- A longitudinal look at those areas of professional practice best tested in the workplace (mainly attitudes and performance)
- A number of assessment tools used
- Evidence collected in the **ePortfolio** over the entire period of training

Miller's Pyramid and the MRCGP

Miller's Pyramid[1] provides a framework for assessing how good someone's clinical competence is – or their hierarchy of performance. In this pyramid, knowledge-based factual recall (*knows*) sits at the bottom. Applying (*knows how*) or demonstrating (*shows*) that knowledge sits higher. However, the highest order of performance is at the *does* level – where the doctor incorporates the new knowledge (or skill) into everyday actual practice. The

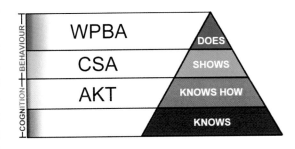

pyramid helps us look at the 'power' of an assessment: if you want to measure how good someone is at something, the best assessment methods would be those that test at the 'shows' and 'does' levels of performance – because they look at the person's behaviour (what they actually do) rather than their cognition (what they know).

You'll be glad to hear that most of the MRCGP assessment tools (other than AKT) are pitched at the 'shows' and 'does' levels of Miller's Pyramid. In other words, they are geared towards examining the trainee's behaviour – what they actually do rather than what they say they know. This in itself should give GP educators faith in the current MRCGP assessment system over previous methods, which tested at the lower levels. The 'spread' of MRCGP assessments not only assures us whether a trainee has the core knowledge and rudiments of clinical skills, but that they can apply these within the complexity of the consultation room to a level which the patient will recognise as being a 'performing' GP. (More on Miller's Pyramid in Chapter 29: Assessment and Competence.)

The Applied Knowledge Test (AKT)
What is it?

RCGP on AKT: The Applied Knowledge Test (AKT) is a summative assessment of the knowledge base that underpins independent general practice in the United Kingdom within the context of the National Health Service. Candidates who pass this assessment will have demonstrated their competence in applying knowledge at a level which is sufficiently high for independent practice. Whilst candidates will be eligible to attempt the AKT at any point during their time in GP specialty training, it is anticipated that the most appropriate point, and that providing the highest chance of success, will be whilst working as a GPStR in the final year of their specialty training programme (ST3).

The AKT is a 3-hour multiple choice exam done online at Pearson Vue centres (centres where people usually do their driving test theory exam).

What does it cover?

The AKT tests topics that are common and/or important in *three* main categories:
1 core clinical medicine and its application to problem-solving in a GP context *80%*
2 critical appraisal and Evidence-based clinical practice *10%*
3 health administration, Informatics and Organisational structures that support UK general practice *10%*.

Reassuringly, in a pilot of experienced Trainers most scored 70+% (well in the pass range), although a few scored scarily more! The questions themselves seem relevant to general practice. The pass mark is somewhere around the 65% mark (it changes with each sitting according to complicated psychometric statistical analysis). The bits that frighten the trainees most (and we suspect Trainers too) are the statistics questions, although there are not too many of those. There are a significant number of questions on informatics and administration issues which are more likely to trip up the unwary (and certainly those less experienced in general practice).

 Top Tip: Key messages: the exam is mostly about applied knowledge in a clinical context, not knowledge per se. The performance of examinees in critical appraisal is generally very poor. A little knowledge in this area can therefore earn valuable marks.

What can you do to help?

> ### General consensus – when to take the AKT
> - You should not take it until you have done at least 6 months in general practice.
> - You should not take it until you've had some exposure to practice management.
> - Do not take it after you have had a period away from work (e.g. pregnancy), as you need to have kept up to date with NICE and SIGN guidelines, etc.
> - Revising with others helps.

- We don't think that the responsibility for preparing for this part of the exam comes into the remit of Programme Directors or Trainers explicitly. Hopefully, all Trainers will be helping their trainees with skills to acquire the knowledge they need to make informed day-to-day decisions.
- Ensure trainees see plenty of patients and get them to reflect on what they are doing with each patient. Such a level of patient exposure and reflective practice should put them in good stead for the AKT.
- Trainers would be wise to point out those areas of practice that trainees may not come across as often as established GPs will; for instance, practice management and administration.
- One way you can help trainees to deal with dilemmas presented in AKT questions is to imagine a consultation scenario and consider which would be the best evidence-based approach to that problem.
- Most GP trainees are grateful for (and need) some teaching on stats and critical appraisal.
- Encourage your trainee to form or join a study group going through questions together.
- Encourage them to use a variety of AKT practice books and websites.
- Perhaps the best advice is to read the AKT Examiners' feedback on the college website which details areas of the exam that candidates do least well.

Clinical Skills Assessment (CSA)
What is it?

> The Clinical Skills Assessment is 'an assessment of a doctor's ability to integrate and apply clinical, professional, communication and practical skills appropriate for general practice'. GPStRs will be eligible to take the CSA when they are in ST3 (the third and final year of their GP specialty training).

The CSA is a mock surgery, held three times a year, at a tailor-made centre in London. The premise is simple – candidates are assessed on their consultation and clinical skills with actors as the patients and an assessor watching. The candidate stays in a mocked-up consultation room while a new 'patient' appears every 10 minutes along with a different assessor until 13 cases have been completed. Candidates are given a brief set of details about each patient and are expected to conduct the consultation (including examination and prescribing) – within the 10 minutes, with a 2-minute gap to read up the notes of the next patient (or, more probably, panic about what they got wrong with the last).

The role player will have been given clear instruction on how to play the patient and clear guidance as to when to reveal additional parts of the history – particularly ideas and concerns if given the appropriate question or opportunity from the candidate. Not all cases require an examination and in those that do the candidate is allowed to continue as he or she would normally. If the examination is not part of the assessment, either the role player will have steered the candidate away (*'Can I come back another time?'*) or the examiner gives the examination findings to the candidate. This is often a slightly awkward moment, as most of us use the time when we examine patients as 'thinking time' and having this suddenly removed can be disconcerting.

Each examiner moves round with the role players marking the same case, so each candidate is assessed by 13 different examiners who each make an independent assessment. A variety of general practice settings will be tested. For example, candidates might be taken off to another room for a 'home visit' or telephone consultation.

What does it cover?
Each CSA case will look at three domains:

	What do these domains mean? **Which ILO areas of the curriculum do they cover? (bold type)**
Data gathering, technical and assessment skills	**Problem-solving skills** – gathering and using data for clinical judgement, choice of examination, investigations and their interpretation. Demonstration of a structured and flexible approach to decision making.
	Technical (Clinical Practical) Skills – demonstrating proficiency in performing physical examinations and using diagnostic and therapeutic instruments.
Clinical management skills	**Primary Care Management** – recognition and management of common medical conditions in primary care.
	Comprehensive approach – demonstrating a structured and flexible approach to decision-making. Demonstrating the ability to deal with multiple complaints, comorbidity and risk. Demonstrating the ability to promote a positive approach to health. Synthesis, diagnosis, appreciation of comorbidity, flexibility and sharing management options with the patient.
Interpersonal skills	**Person-centred approach** – demonstrating the use of recognised communication techniques to understand the patient's illness experience and develop a shared approach to managing problems.
	Attitudinal aspects – practising ethically with respect for equality and diversity, in line with the accepted codes of professional conduct. Communication, respect for others, professionalism and other behavioural indicators.

This is the test that scares the trainees more than anything else – and not surprisingly as it is a very scary beast (and costs a little fortune). The CSA is an 'integrative skills assessment': the candidate is expected to integrate all parts of the consultation into a fluid whole – from the initial 'putting the patient at ease', through history taking (+/– examination), exploring ICE, formulating and to agreeing a management plan. In other words, from greeting to goodbye and all points in between – checking of course that the patient has understood and had their concerns addressed. Phew!

A bit more about the cases

Each case has been written to test some of the intended learning outcomes (ILOs) from a given curriculum statement. The case writers are all active GPs, and the cases reflect the breadth and variety of UK general practice and the sort of problems that you might deal with day to day. Having said that, you wouldn't want to do them all at once and sitting the CSA is a bit like a surgery from Hell – although with the guarantee of no interruptions, late arrivals or QOF templates to fill in.

The starting point for a case might be a clinical scenario encountered that represents:

1 a **diagnostic** challenge: e.g. recognising depression in a man with tiredness or
2 a **management** challenge: e.g. negotiating treatment options where the diagnosis is clear
3 an **interpersonal** skills challenge: e.g. where the patient is upset or angry over something (with the diagnosis and management being straightforward).

In each situation there will be challenges across each of the three areas being tested, although it may be skewed towards one area more than the others by the very nature of the case. The marking schedule is adapted for each case to reflect the key behaviours (which reflect the ILOs) that the case writers would expect to see demonstrated in that situation.

How it is marked

RCGP:

Pass: The candidate demonstrates an adequate level of competence, displaying a clinical approach that may not be fluent but is justifiable and technically proficient. The candidate shows sensitivity and tries to involve the patient.

Fail: The candidate fails to demonstrate adequate competence, with a clinical approach that is at times unsystematic or inconsistent with accepted practice. Technical proficiency may be of concern. The patient is treated with sensitivity and respect, but the doctor does not sufficiently facilitate or respond to the patient's contribution.

For *each* of these domains, the trainee will be given one of four grades: (1) Clear Pass (3 marks), (2) Pass (2 marks), (3) Fail (1 mark), and (4) Clear Fail (0 marks). The marks are added up over all 13 cases to give a possible maximum of 117. The pass mark is determined daily by the 'borderline group method'. This is based on calculating a 'borderline CSA score' for candidates at the border of passing and failing a case. Known as a 'cut score', this is used as the basis for setting a passing standard with a statistical adjustment for measurement error. The standard is set for each day to take account of the differing case palettes (and tends to be in the area 70 to 75). So it would be possible to have a clear fail in one domain in a few cases, but this would have to be balanced by clear passes in others. It is important to note (and to reassure your trainees) that none of the cases hinges on a single issue which might make or break it – so missing a cue or a diagnosis that was not obvious would not be an automatic fail if otherwise the case was handled appropriately (a bit like getting the wrong answer but using the correct method in a Maths paper!)

Reliability

Do the candidates pass who 'should' pass, and the candidates fail who 'should' fail? By and large – yes (in as much as can be possible in any exam). The 'borderline group method' is a way of ensuring reliability and fairness. The passing standard is discussed and approved each time by a panel, including lay members and AITs. It is constantly reviewed and reflected upon as are the cases to ensure they follow changes in prescribing and management with each case checked, prior to the exam, against possible changes in the guidelines.

What can you do to help?

- Remind them that it is not just about consultation skills. They need to be clinically clued up too!
- Keep an eye on your trainee's performance on the Consultation Observation Tool (COT) – this will help guide you as to their 'readiness' to take the CSA.
- Go through some CSA cases with your GP trainee. Ask them to bring one of their CSA books and pick a case and role play it. Don't worry if you feel a bit apprehensive – most CSA books will tell you where the emphasis and focus of the case are.
- Encourage your trainee to form or join a CSA group with others – where they can role play the scenarios themselves.

 Top Tip: Experience in Rotherham suggests that writing cases and role play are valuable ways of helping Trainers *and* trainees to become familiar with the CSA module.

 Red Alert: Some trainees request 'temporary time out' from daily general practice to focus and study for the CSA. Remind them that CSA cases are based on common real presentations in general practice and, therefore, patient exposure is vital to success. The best way to prepare is to see patients and tackle their PUNs and DENs.

Workplace-based Assessment (WPBA)

RCGP: Workplace-based Assessment (WPBA) is defined as the evaluation of a doctor's progress over time in their performance in those areas of professional practice best tested in the workplace. It is a process through which evidence of competence in independent practice is gathered in a structured and systematic framework. Evidence is collected over all three years of training. The evidence is recorded in a web-based portfolio (the ePortfolio) and used to inform six-monthly reviews and, at the end of training, to make a holistic, qualitative judgement about the readiness of the GPStR for independent practice. WPBA is a developmental process. It will therefore provide feedback to the GPStR and drive learning. It will also indicate where a doctor is in difficulty. It is learner led: the GPStR decides which evidence to put forward for review and validation by the Trainer.

What's it all about?

Everything! It's basically a set of assessments that occur repeatedly throughout the training period – testing and providing evidence for the 12 professional competency areas. This is the first time that longitudinal medical assessment has been defined and quantified as part of a professional exam. It is the first time that a GP assessment sits at the top of Miller's Pyramid. And at the end of

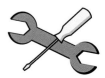

training, when all the evidence has been collected and digested, the Trainer is asked (as the person most likely to know):

- 'In light of the evidence, is this candidate good enough?'
- 'Are they competent to be let loose on the public?'

Is this the 'Jewel in the Crown' for the MRCGP?

Yes – even though it has looked a bit unpolished at times! It is here to stay and like it or not it will consume a considerable amount of your energy, whether as a Clinical Supervisor, Educational Supervisor or as a member of the ARCP panel. Don't let this dishearten you; Wiggins[2] says that you're more likely to see authentic performance in an assessment if:

1 testing is done as close as possible to the situation in which one attacks the problem
2 the assessment procedure is somehow flexible to accommodate the variation inherent in professional practice (otherwise, that variation will always escape capture by a set of rules).

In terms of WPBA, what could be more appropriate than to assess doctors doing what they are meant to be doing rather than saying what they would do, or doing it under artificial circumstances and under the watchful eyes of an examiner? And what a tool for learning and developing skills – with built-in tools for reflective practice and setting up a lifelong habit of learning. Yes, it is a jewel!

Van der Vleuten[3] says: a *useful* assessment instrument has:	How does WPBA compare?
● Cost-effectiveness	*Yes – because you, the Trainers, are doing it all (and for free!).*
● Acceptability	*Yes – we don't see anyone complaining massively.*
● Reliability	*High (i.e. reproducibility) – clear marking descriptors in place.*
● Validity	*High (i.e. measures what it's supposed to measure) – triangulation in place.*
● Educational impact	*High – WPBA connects assessment with learning and the workplace. The assessments consistently feature throughout the trainee's training envelope. These assessments and their mechanism of feedback ultimately drive future learning.*

So it's a jewel without any blemishes?

Not quite. There are three problems with the WPBA.

1 Inter-observer variation: the tendency of one observer to mark consistently higher or lower than another observer.
2 Intra-observer variation: the variation in one observer's marks for no apparent reason (good day/bad day phenomenon).
3 Case specificity: the variation in the candidate's performance from one challenge to another, even when they seem to test the same attribute.

But on the whole, WPBA is good?

Answer – yes.

What are the different assessments in WPBA?

There's quite a number of them and you'll see that someone has gone crazy with the use of mnemonics – don't stress too much about remembering them; in time, they will become second nature. We'll cover the fundamental and important things about each of the WPBA elements here. More detailed guidance is on the college website (www.rcgp.org) and there are additional resources for each on www.bradfordvts.co.uk (click on the MRCGP icon). The only other thing we'd like to mention at this point is that you need to understand and become comfortable with the 12 professional competencies because they form the basis of the grading schedules for most of these assessments (especially COTs and CBDs).

WPBA assessments in a nutshell	
Case-based discussion (CBD)	
Done in hospital and GP posts. 6 in ST1 6 in ST2 12 in ST3	A structured 30-minute oral interview on a clinical encounter. The trainee selects a case which he or she thinks demonstrates particular professional competencies. It is much more than just a conversation about a patient seen a week or so ago. They prepare some written case notes, which are submitted beforehand so that the assessor may formulate specific questions to elicit the evidence for those competencies. Questions like: what the trainee actually did, why they did that and whether they considered anything else at the time. Feedback is given to the trainee at the end. The assessor is the Clinical Supervisor (i.e. the consultant for hospital posts and the Trainer for general practice). **Tip 1:** *Remember, CBD is an official assessment. Do the assessment first and only give feedback and teaching at the end. Do not attempt to dip in and out of teaching when you are meant to be in assessment mode. Otherwise, the whole thing will become an unstructured chaotic mess.* **Tip 2:** *There is a CBD question maker tool available on our website.*
Consultation Observation Tool (COT)	
Only done in GP posts. For each GP post in ST1 or ST2 – only 3 needed. In ST3, 12 needed for the year	An assessment of a **GP** consultation observed either directly (sitting in with the trainee) or retrospectively (by video recording). There is a COT marking crib, which tells the assessor which particular communication skills to look for. An overall judgement is also made before feedback is given to the trainee. There is no rule about consultation length. Ideally, at least one consultation should be assessed by someone other than Trainer. A wide range of contexts is required: at least one child, older person and mental health problem. The assessor is the GP Trainer. In hospital posts, COT is replaced by mini-CEX. **Tip 1:** *Some trainees will have never engaged in video work before and will be very apprehensive. You need to explore their feelings and show sensitivity.* **Tip 2:** *Encourage trainees to submit complex and difficult cases because they're the types of cases likely to yield more evidence.* **Tip 3:** *Try to relate the feedback and the skills you have observed to established consultation theory (well documented in the Silverman, Kurtz and Draper book[4]).*

WPBA assessments in a nutshell

Mini-Clinical Evaluation Exercise (Mini-CEX)

Hospital based equivalent to COTs. 3 per hospital post.	An assessment of a clinical encounter observed in hospital posts focusing on clinical skills, attitudes and behaviours. The assessor is the hospital consultant or a senior grade physician. When the trainee moves to a GP post, they do COTs instead of mini-CEXs.

Direct Observation of Procedural Skills (DOPS)

9 mandatory procedures that can be done at any time in the training period – need witnessing and accrediting by seniors, not peers!	Assessing skills like testing for blood glucose to taking a cervical smear. Assessments can be done in hospital or general practice. There are mandatory DOPS and optional ones. The observations are completed opportunistically. Assessment is made by senior members of the clinical team with appropriate skills (SpRs, Staff Grades, Nurses or Consultants). **Tip 1:** *Fellow trainees are not allowed to assess each other; watch for this.* **Tip 2:** *Try to get trainees to do the essential female DOPs early because they are quite difficult to achieve in the last 3 months (esp. for male doctors).*

Multi-source feedback (MSF)

2 in ST1 (5 clinical) 2 in ST3 (5 clinical + 5 non-clinical)	An online questionnaire completed by clinical and non-clinical team members. Only the clinical members are asked for detailed feedback in certain areas of **clinical performance**. Everyone (clinical + non-clinical) is asked for feedback on **professional behaviour**. Feedback takes the form of a 7-point grading system together with some free text boxes. Once a minimum number of questionnaires have been completed, the ePortfolio will analyse, categorise and display the results – but only when triggered to do so by the Educational Supervisor. The idea behind the ES having to 'release the MSF results' is so that feedback isn't just dumped on the trainee but is imparted in a controlled, structured and developmental sort of way (i.e. accompanied by discussion).

Patient Satisfaction Questionnaire (PSQ)

Only when in GP posts – at least 40 patients. x1 if in GP at ST1/2 x1 in ST3	This questionnaire asks patients for their opinion of the doctor–patient relationship: what was the communication like, did the doctor show respect and empathy, etc. It's only done in GP posts (not hospital). Paper questionnaires are handed out by the receptionists to consecutive patients seeing the trainee until 40 have been returned. The results are transferred to the ePortfolio (in some places the deanery will do this but in others it will be the practice admin team). This will then form the basis for a subsequent feedback discussion with the Trainer.

Clinical Supervisor's Report (CSR)

During every hospital and GP attachment.	The Clinical Supervisor (Trainer in a GP post; Consultant for hospital posts) needs to write a structured report towards the end of each attachment. It needs to be done roughly at month 4 or 5 of each post so that it can be reviewed (and issues explored) in the subsequent Educational Supervision meeting. The report is split into four sections, looking at: **Relationships**, **Decision-Making Skills** (termed Diagnostics – not diagnosis!), **Management** (as in administration and organisation, not clinical management) and **Professionalism**.

WPBA assessments in a nutshell

Educational Supervisor's Report (ESR)

During every hospital and GP attachment.	Towards the end of every post, the trainee and Educational Supervisor need to meet to reflect on the post to: review the evidence for learning, check that the minimum number of WPBA assessments have been completed, identify which competencies have been covered, highlight which ones still need working on and make learning plans for the next post.

Naturally Occurring Evidence (NOE)

Optional, but in some deaneries it is mandatory.	Naturally Occurring Evidence includes things like Significant Event Analyses, which occur 'naturally' during the course of one's work. Other examples include: prescribing, referral analyses, audits and projects. NOE can provide powerful evidence for some of the professional competencies, and they can be used to demonstrate curriculum coverage too. Currently, there is no stipulated minimum requirement for any of these by the RCGP. However, deaneries can enforce their own requirements. Check the position with your local deanery.

Out of hours (OOH)

In hospital, participate in on-call rota. In GP, one 4–6-hour OOH session per month.	In hospital posts, trainees are expected to engage in the normal on-call duty rota (and write up some of the learning that results in their ePortfolio). In general practice, they are expected to do a minimum number of hours with the Out-of-Hours centre. The current benchmark is one session a month lasting 6 hours – this will be checked by ARCP panels! The OOH trainee rota is usually organised by the Training Programme Directors – so if you're a Trainer, you don't need to worry about this. What you do need to do is to make sure that (1) the trainee is engaging, (2) the OOH supervisor is supervising them (i.e. it's not all about service provision), and (3) the trainee is writing some reflective log entries on their OOH experiences.

*This table stipulates the **minimum** number of CBD, COT and mini-CEX requirements: **You should aim to do significantly more!** They also need doing in a timely way (i.e. spread out and not all last minute). The minimum requirement applies to part-time trainees too.*

 Top Tip: Most WPBA assessments have detailed competency descriptors outlined in the ePortfolio to help guide your marking. Refer to these before awarding your grade. It's easy to become 'out of sync' even if you think you're familiar with the marking system.

The ePortfolio

RCGP: The ePortfolio is a web-based tool that records details of achievement, documents all stages of training, and records evidence of WPBA and reviews with Educational Supervisors. A record of personal development and experience is becoming mandatory for all doctors. It provides evidence that training has taken place and allows the GP trainee to reflect on a range of learning opportunities.

MRCGP, Supervision and Assessment

The central premise of the WPBA is that **the trainee has ownership and responsibility** for his or her own learning and collecting the evidence to show that the learning has taken place and the required level of competence reached. The ePortfolio holds together all the *evidence* generated through the WBPA process to show evidence of *competence* – but it is more than just that: it is also a space for the trainee to *record learning*.

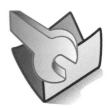

- A trainee is given an ePortfolio when they join a scheme. Ownership and responsibility for the portfolio rests with them, but others have access to it along the way.
- It's where you will find all the WPBA assessment marking tools (e.g. COTs and CBDs). It's also where the Clinical and Educational Supervisor's reports are uploaded. If a trainee has completed formal assessments (AKT/CSA), these too will be automatically uploaded. In a nutshell, the ePortfolio cements everything together.
- Trainees record their own learning, reflection and achievements under a section called 'the learning log'. The Trainer/Educational Supervisor needs to ensure that the learning log is not merely a descriptive account of events or clinical encounters – the trainee needs to reflect, evaluate and learn.
- Learning points do not always need to be developmental. For example, one might choose to describe a case to highlight strengths in (say) management. Learning points that a similar case should be managed the same way is acceptable.
- The ePortfolio will be periodically accessed and assessed by others (e.g. Educational Supervisor and ARCP panels) to ensure that the trainee is making adequate progression and enough evidence is gradually being accumulated for all 12 professional competency areas.

In the ePortfolio, trainees can:

- record educational log entries
- map log entries to curriculum headings
- upload attachments
- formulate a Personal Development Plan
- record CPR and AED certification
- record Out of Hours sessions (and learning)
- self-assess competency progression
- email any ePortfolio user.

In the ePortfolio, educators can:

- record work-place based assessments
- map log entries to professional competencies
- make additional 'Educators' notes'
- file Clinical & Educational Supervisor reports.
- record the ARCP outcome
- advertise meetings/courses to trainees
- rate their competency progression
- email any ePortfolio user.

Knowing the difference: the Clinical vs Educational Supervisor

Before we look at how all of these various MRCGP components fit together, we need to make sure that you're clear about the differences between a Clinical and Educational Supervisor.

- The *Clinical* Supervisor (CS) oversees the trainee's *day-to-day* work and helps the trainee get the most out of the current post they are in. In a hospital, it's the consultant, in general practice it's the Trainer. Hence, the CS changes every time the trainee changes jobs. The CS also signs off Workplace-Based Assessments. He or she needs to hold three formative meetings with their trainee (beginning, middle and end of job) with a final report towards the end (the CSR). The trainee and CS should at all times be aware of their responsibilities for the safety of patients in their care.

- The *Educational* Supervisor (ES) oversees the trainee's progress throughout the entire training programme. He or she does this by periodically meeting up with them every six months. The ES helps the trainee reflect on experience, identify learning needs, look at educational opportunities and formulate a PDP. In summary, the ES makes sure the trainee is on track for training and helps identify trainees in difficulty early. All of this is logged in a report called the ESR. Because the same ES will remain with the trainee throughout their training, the ES-trainee relationship is one of the most crucial relationships to get 'right'.

How does it all come together?

The ePortfolio contains a set of tools to use over time to construct a virtual 3-D demonstration of the trainee's competence in general practice. Consider this analogy:

Imagine a building site for a three-storey building which has a floor plan similar for each floor, each containing 12 rooms. At the start of training the trainee has only the footprint of the building, with the rooms marked out on the concrete foundations. The trainee is met onsite by a site manager in a hard hat marked 'ES' who hands over a toolbox and a list of people who will rotate as site foremen and will wear hard hats marked 'CS'. The tools in the toolbox (ePortfolio) will provide the scaffolding for the project under the supervision of the CS. The building, from foundation to completion, will take 3 years. The site manager (the ES), will visit every six months to check on progress and will generate six-monthly progress reports, which will be passed on to head office (called ARCP) who will decide if the building is progressing at a suitable pace. At the end of the 3 years head office (ARCP) will also check whether all building specifications have been met (the professional competencies), whether each room has been kitted out according to requirements (the curriculum) and whether it is safe in general (patient safety).

We hope this scenario illustrates how the curriculum, the professional competencies, the MRCGP components (AKT, CSA, and WPBA), the ePortfolio, the ES, the CS, and the ARCP panel all fit together.

The Workplace-Based Assessments are not summative, final, career-busting assessments but judgements nevertheless. They help **build a picture**.

1 What the trainee is like now.
2 How they are progressing.
3 Define where they need to get to.
4 Define what they need (i.e. further training) to do to get there.

- Try not see each assessment as a pass/fail thing. Instead, see them as little pixels which together with other 'pixels' will make the bigger 'picture' clearer. On their own they are nowhere near as significant as when they are seen as part of a collective.
- It's okay for a trainee to be scoring lots of NFD (Needs Further Development) grades at the ST1 and 2 level – actually, that is what's expected! It's worthwhile making sure your trainee is clear about this right from the start so that they are not disappointed and don't go off in a huff! (If they were awarded 'Competent' for everything at ST1/2 level, then that would mean they don't need any GP training!)
- Towards the end of each *post*, the Educational Supervisor will make a recommendation whether that stint of training has been satisfactory. At the end of the *ST year*, the ARCP

panel will review the ES reports and the ePortfolio and decide whether the trainee moves on to the next ST year.

What happens to all this evidence? The ARCP

The ARCP panel is a deanery body that performs an *Annual* Review of Competency Progression. In other words, whenever a trainee is due to move up an ST stage, the panel reviews their ePortfolio first and only allows them through if it is satisfactory.

Outcomes the ARCP panel can make	
Outcome 1	**Satisfactory Progress:** *achieving progress and competencies at the expected rate.* *– no action needed*
Outcome 2	**Unsatisfactory progress:** *development of specific competencies required.* *– additional training time not needed*
Outcome 3	**Unsatisfactory progress:** *inadequate progress by the trainee.* *– additional training time required*
Outcome 4	**Unsatisfactory progress:** *released from training programme.* *– i.e. they're kicked out (although there is a right to appeal)*
Outcome 5	**Unsatisfactory progress:** *incomplete evidence presented.* *– additional training time may be required*

 Top Tip: Everything ultimately boils down to the adequacy of 'evidence'. This is why we urge you to spend time 'hooking' your trainee into the ePortfolio at an early stage. Any trainee with a laissez-faire approach is doomed to fail.

A pictorial summary

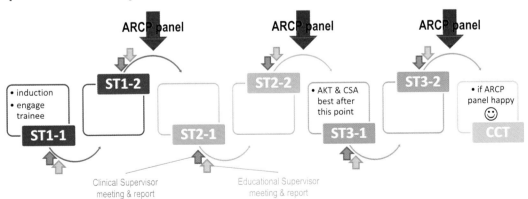

Key: AKT = Applied Knowledge Test; ARCP = Annual Review of Competency Progression; CCT = Certificate of Completion of Training; CSA = Clinical Skills Assessment; CSR = Clinical Supervisor's Report; ES = Educational Supervisor; ST = Specialty Training Year.

Closing comments

We hope the MRCGP nutshell has been cracked open enough to give a flavour of the kernel inside. Our learner has, we hope, now successfully completed his or her training. The virtual building is complete and just requires the topping off ceremony to get the MRCGP.

The completed virtual building will of course grow in other ways; it will need updating and decorating from time to time and perhaps the occasional extension (Appraisal and Revalidation). Perhaps Miller's Pyramid needs an extra level?

If the MRCGP is the jewel in the crown of the College, we (the community of GP educators) hold the cloth to make it sparkle. We feel that the whole MRCGP process lays the foundations for reflective learning, and its continuing development will shape us and the future profession. We urge you to get involved with it at whatever level.

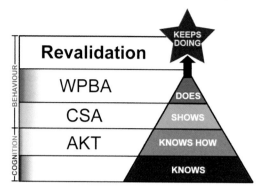

A sample of resources on our website

- WPBA components – which ones at which ST stage? An **excellent** 'at a glance' map.
- A variety of CBD, COT and ePortfolio related material.
- Levels of Reflection; Reflective Writing.

Other chapters you may like to read

- Chapter 26: Effective Clinical Supervision
- Chapter 27: Effective Educational Supervision
- Chapter 28: Reflection and Evaluation
- Chapter 29: Assessment and Competence.

Please give us some feedback on this chapter to help shape it for the next edition.
Go to www.essentialgptrainingbook.com and simply click on the title of this chapter.

References

1 Miller GE. The assessment of clinical skills/performance. *Acad Med.* 1990; **65**(Suppl.): S63–7.
2 Wiggins GP. *Assessing Student Performance: exploring the purpose and limits of testing.* San Francisco: Jossey-Bass; 1993.
3 Van der Vleuten CPM. The assessment of professional competence: developments, research and practical implications, *Adv Health Sci Educ.* 1996: **1**: 46–67.
4 Silverman JD, Kurtz SM, Draper J. *Skills for Communicating with Patients.* Oxford: Radcliffe; 1998.

26

Effective Clinical Supervision

MOHAN KUMAR – Associate Director (North West Deanery)
RODGER CHARLTON – Professor of Medical Education (Univ. Swansea)   RAMESH MEHAY – TPD (Bradford)

Introduction
We all remember the good old-fashioned maxim of **'See one, Do one, Teach one'** of medical learning. This sums up the ethos that was of Clinical Supervision (and may still be in some circles). However, this maxim fails on a number of accounts.

1 It fails to capture vital educational nuances such as learning styles, learner anxiety, supervisor style, supervisor anxiety, reflection and so on.
2 It hints that somehow practising medicine is all about refining a set of 'skills', rather than the triumvirate of *knowledge*, *skills* and *attitudes*.
3 It completely bypasses the art of self-directed learning with support and facilitation.

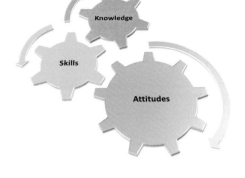

GP training has always had the benefit of the close *'apprenticeship'* model at least in the year we spent attached to a training practice. The role of the Trainer as Clinical Supervisor has always been far more complex and more rewarding than the old maxim seemed to suggest. With the changing face of GP training, the introduction of a more structured three-year GP curriculum[1] and emerging clarity between the role of a 'Clinical Supervisor' and 'Educational Supervisor'[2] it is perhaps time we consider these roles in more detail.

A GP trainee will encounter multiple Clinical Supervisors throughout their training as they rotate through various posts. Therefore, it is vital for the individual Clinical Supervisors (and the Training Programme Directors) to consider what skill sets are required of them. In this chapter, we shall explore Clinical Supervision from five angles:

1 the definitions
2 the elements of good Clinical Supervision
3 models of Clinical Supervision
4 practical Clinical Supervision
5 the training and development of Clinical Supervisors.

Defining clinical supervision
Here are some definitions to help you get started.

> A formal process of professional support and learning which enables individual practitioners to develop knowledge and competence, assume responsibility for their own practice and enhance consumer protection and safety of care in complex clinical situations.
>
> **Department of Health[3]**

Strange though it may seem, there has been very little work in the definition of Clinical Supervision for doctors. Most of the definitions have emerged from the professional development of nurses and counselling therapists. Perhaps this explains the old school mentality among doctors that all consultants are naturally expected to be teachers and supervisors without any formal training. It will also explain our good old *'See one, do one, teach one'* adage! Here's another definition from the world of counselling:

> An intervention provided by a senior member of a profession to a junior member or members of that same profession. This relationship is evaluative, extends over time and has the simultaneous purposes of enhancing the professional functioning of the junior member(s), monitoring the quality of professional services offered to the client that he, she or they see(s), and serving as the gatekeeper of those who are to enter the particular profession.
>
> **Bernard and Goodyear[4]**

The Trainer is not the only Clinical Supervisor during the time a GP trainee is in a GP practice. There are others who have clinical supervisory roles who are not named Trainers within a learning organisation but clearly have the necessary defined skill sets. It also helps if we accept that just being a qualified professional doesn't automatically convey one the necessary clinical supervision skills. An *effective* Clinical Supervisor requires a certain set of knowledge, skills and attitudes (covered later). Finally, here's another definition for you to mull over – perhaps the most concise one yet.

> An exchange between practising professionals which enables development of professional skills.
>
> **Butterworth and Faugier[5]**

Clinical Supervision is a fine balance between developing a self-directed learner and ensuring patient safety.

Elements of good clinical supervision

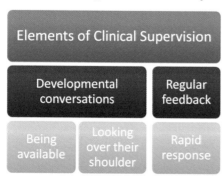

A Reference to Post Graduate Specialty Training in the UK (aka 'The Gold Guide') offers that Clinical Supervision incorporates *'being available, looking over the shoulder of the trainee, teaching on the job with developmental conversations, regular feedback and the provision of a rapid response to issues as they arise'.*[6] This statement actually summarises the components of good Clinical Supervision. Let's tease these out and look at them in more detail.

Being available

There needs to be clear guidance to the learner as to *who* is supervising them and *when*. Although obvious, you will be surprised at how often it doesn't happen. Being clear about this ensures both parties maximise the learning opportunities from a clinical encounter. Often learners entering into general practice may interpret clinical supervision as 'ask only if help is needed'. This approach is fraught with problems as it relies on the trainee to make an assessment of the situation and they may miss many unknown unknowns.

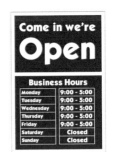

> ## As a Clinical Supervisor, you need to:
> - be clear over what is expected of the learner
> - signpost that you are available, and that you expect to be called upon
> - be available – on an ad hoc as well as a 'protected time' basis*.

This usually means liaising with administrative staff like the Practice Manager to 'make things happen' (e.g. the debriefs).

Rapid response

As a Clinical Supervisor, you need to be able to offer rapid support to the learner. This means looking at your own work commitments to ensure there is sufficient protected time. Slots may need to be taken out of appointment schedules to enable the learner to access help quickly and efficiently.

> ## As a Clinical Supervisor, you need to:
> - have protected time to do the supervision – don't 'squeeze' it in between your daily clinical and administrative chores
> - respond to the trainee in a timely way
> - make sure you don't give off signals indicating that you're in a rush or too busy. Otherwise trainees will refrain from getting in touch with you, which is the opposite of what you want them to do.

Looking over the shoulder

Workplace-Based Assessment is best triangulated by 'looking over the shoulder' of the trainee. You need to make sure your trainee understands that this continuous and regular observation is a mandatory part of your role as Clinical Supervisor. Most learners will not be used to this level of scrutiny from their hospital setting, and may misconstrue this is as a sign of their inadequacy – you need to set things straight.

However, this does not mean all trainees are spoon-fed and advised constantly. New trainees will obviously need close observation at the start. They are relatively inexperienced, and close supervision is necessary to protect patients and help trainees develop competencies. As they progress through training, develop competencies and your confidence in their abilities grows, you may (as Clinical Supervisor) be able to use a lighter touch approach. Those that are clearly able should be allowed to consult freely, develop their own styles of information gathering and be expected to solve problems and fashion management plans.

Regular feedback

The formative aspect of the Clinical Supervisor's role involves regular feed-back loops. This helps trainees develop competencies. However, trainees might not be used to the level of feedback given in general practice training, and some may put up defensive barriers. Therefore, at the start of their post, trainees need to understand the purpose of feedback, that it will feature a major part of their training programme, and that they need to welcome it.

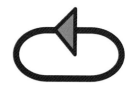

Giving feedback is a skill in itself. As a Clinical Supervisor you may feel you need training in this area – perhaps a workshop on giving feedback and structuring it in a positive way. There are a number of established models you can follow such as 'Pendleton's rules'[7] or 'ALOBA'[8] (Agenda Led Outcome Based Analysis) – *see* Chapter 7: The Skilful Art of Giving Feedback. The use of these is subject to the situation and the time available. Both emphasise the learner-led nature of seeking and receiving feedback. As Clinical Supervisor you also need to be familiar with the GP curriculum and the competency descriptors. The competency descriptors are there to help you offer specific and constructive feedback on areas that are deemed important for general practice and are going to be assessed.

As a Clinical Supervisor, you need to:

- develop your skills in the art of giving feedback (e.g. attend a workshop)
- become familiar with the GP curriculum and the competency descriptors. Otherwise, how do you know what areas to feed back on?

Developmental conversations

The *summative* and *formative* roles of Clinical Supervision (i.e. being their friendly mentor one moment and their assessor the next) can create conflict and tension in the relationship with your trainee. Even so, you need to know what level your learner is at, what their curriculum coverage is, what their competencies are so that you can move them up Miller's Pyramid from *knows*, *knows how*, and *shows*, to *does*. See Chapter 29: Assessment and Competence if you are unfamiliar with Miller's Pyramid.

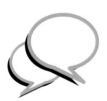

For this to happen, the Clinical Supervisor and trainee need to feel comfortable enough with each other to 'lay their cards on the table'. Both of you need to be open, honest, trusting and respectful of each other right from the start. Both of you need to show a genuine (platonic) interest in each other. You need to remember that difficult feedback is sometimes difficult for your trainee to accept; your trainee needs to remember that difficult feedback may not have been easy for you to give. Developmental conversations (= a proactive dialogue geared towards identifying and tackling needs in a positive and enthusiastic way) can only happen if both the learning environment and the relationship are optimised.

As a Clinical Supervisor, you need to:

- create and nurture a positive learning ethos, culture and environment; *see* Chapter 9: Exploring and Creating a Learning Culture
- spend time building and maintaining the relationship with your trainee. In particular, both of you need to show respect, show trust, be open, and be honest with each other.

Models of Clinical Supervision

You now have some idea of the **key principles** behind good Clinical Supervision. However, there are several ways in which you can actually do the Clinical Supervision at ground level. We describe three models for you below.

Developmental Model[9]

This model classifies learners as beginners, intermediates or advanced based on their behaviour in three areas: Self-awareness, Autonomy and Motivation (SAM).

- **The beginner** may doubt his or her level of skills and abilities (low self-awareness). They will be dependent on the supervisor for advice on nearly everything (low autonomy). They will have little motivation for independent learning and will almost rigidly mimic what the Clinical Supervisor does or tells them to do.
- **The intermediate learner** will be reasonably aware of their strengths and weaknesses. They will be relatively autonomous. They will try to problem-solve and look up things for themselves, only seeking help for the more difficult patients and problems.
- **The advanced learner** is totally aware of his or her limitations. They will be largely self-sufficient and only seek consultation when appropriate.

In this model, the Clinical Supervisor monitors and facilitates a learner's (1) *Self-awareness*, (2) *Autonomy*, and (3) *Motivation*, thereby gradually aiming to move them from beginner to advanced learner in a sequential manner.

Integrated Model

While the intention of Clinical Supervision is to develop a self-directed learner, the integrated model understands that there may be occasions where:

- the supervisor needs to be a **Teacher** – where the *supervisor* is instructive, didactic and informative
- the supervisor needs to be a **Counsellor** – enabling the *supervisee* to identify blind spots and overcome them
- the supervisor needs to be a **Consultant** – where the supervisor and supervisee *work together* and look at particular areas to develop solutions for excellence.

Unlike the previous model where the Clinical Supervisor moves the learner from beginner to advanced in a sequential way, this model says that the Clinical Supervisor needs to be different things (be a teacher, counsellor or consultant) at different times for the same trainee. In other words, not sequentially, but based on what the situation dictates.

Orientation-Specific Model

In this model, the supervisor creates or manipulates 'situations' to 'test' the learner first and then provide debrief and discussion afterwards in order to develop insight. They will help the learner identify areas for learning and appropriate techniques to achieve learning. This may include skills rehearsal (role play), modelling empathy, sensitivity and appropriate communication.

So which one should you go for?

There is no such thing as the best model. We would say that you need to make use of all three – using them at different times. It's difficult to offer you specific advice other than to say that it is context dependent. It's not rocket science either: simply review the situation you are both in and think which model fits best or will achieve the desired outcome.

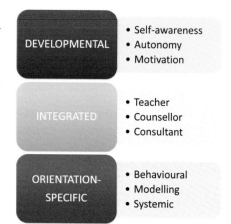

Practical Clinical Supervision

We've just seen three **models** for Clinical Supervision. These can be applied to a number of **teaching tools** that you can use to help you with clinically supervising your trainee.

Teaching tools to help you clinically supervise	
Random Case Analysis (RCAs)	In an RCA the Clinical Supervisor selects a case that the trainee has seen randomly from an appointment list (could be GP Surgery or Outpatients). The trainee is asked questions about the case to identify blind spots. This enables the Clinical Supervisor to teach on those blind spots. It's particularly good for exploring the knowledge domain (although it can be equally good at exploring skills and attitudes in the right assessor's hands). Use it to get some idea of where the learner is at, identify curriculum coverage gaps, and establish safety in the early stages.
Problem Case Analysis (PCAs)	In a PCA, the learner identifies cases from their day-to-day work that are giving them some sort of difficulty. These are then explored. It's particularly good for clinical management. It should be used in balance with other teaching methods. If you do nothing but PCAs, you only ever end up tackling the learner's needs that they're aware of and their blind spots go undetected! It's also very dependent on the learner's ability to identify issues.
Debriefs	A debrief is where the supervisor goes through the learner's clinical encounters for the day. The primary purpose is for patient safety – to ensure they've been clinically handled the right way and have not been put at unnecessary risk. However, debriefs can also be educational – they can signpost curriculum areas covered, competencies demonstrated and other areas still in need of further development.
Joint Clinics	The learner and the supervisor work jointly, perhaps each taking turns in seeing patients. This will work in an OPD setting and in GP surgery. In the case of the latter, it can be with the Trainer, the partners or the practice nurses. There are several advantages to this approach – modelling, assessing, teaching techniques, exploring skills and attitudes, understanding systems and approaches to chronic disease reviews (just to mention a few).
Tutorials	Formal topic-based tutorials are losing their kudos, mainly because knowledge becomes quickly out of date. It's better to teach trainees the lifelong skills of raising self-awareness and educating themselves rather than pouring into their minds knowledge that will no long be useful in 3–5 years' time. Tutorials which work on skills and attitudes are likely to 'last longer' than those that purely focus on knowledge. However, like everything in life, balance is the key – a bit of all three?

Teaching tools to help you clinically supervise	
MRCGP WPBA assessment tools	Don't forget to use some of the WPBA tools to help you clinically supervise the trainee. CBDs, COTs, MSFs, PSQs, ePortfolio learning logs, significant events and other naturally occurring evidence – all lend themselves very well to Clinical Supervision. These are tools you have to learn how to use anyway!

 Top Tip: The Clinical Supervisor needs to assess and facilitate the development of the trainee's knowledge, skills and attitudes (= workplace behaviours). To increase your repertoire of teaching methods see Chapter 5: A Smorgasbord of Educational Methods.

Beginnings are important

Because a trainee's Clinical Supervisor will change as they move through each post in their rotation, it's important that each supervisor (together with the trainee) sets the educational scene right at the beginning and establishes an educational and learning contract. This sounds quite formal and rigid – but it needn't be. All we are saying is to make sure you spend some protected time in which you:

- get to know each other
- discuss what the learning organisation (and supervisor) will provide
- outline other learning opportunities available
- discuss what is expected from the trainee in return
- discuss the assessments – some learners see them only as a 'tick-box' exercise and fail to appreciate them as learning launch pads
- discuss: giving and receiving feedback
- explore other ideas, concerns and expectations (from both parties).

If you get the beginning right, the more likely it will be that the rest falls into place. Problems that emerge at the end of a training post are usually a result of failures at the beginning.

Training and development of Clinical Supervisors

There are clear guidelines set out by the RCGP on the attributes of Clinical Supervisors based on the 'Gold Guide'.[6] It is vital that the training of Clinical Supervisors incorporates these.

Attributes of the Clinical Supervisor[6]		
Knowledge	Skills	Attitudes
• MRCGP and WPBA • GP curriculum • The 12 professional competency descriptors • Principles of adult learning • Basic educational theory • Learning objectives • Assessment tools	• Setting learning objectives • Giving feedback • Teaching skills • Assessment skills • Facilitating reflection • Facilitating self-direction • Involving others in the team	• Approachable • Supportive • Non-judgemental • Valuing diversity • Patient positive • Modelling good behaviour

I don't think I've ever been taught or trained in Clinical Supervision. I suppose I just get on with it. However, our GP training scheme has started up regular Clinical Supervisor meetings – where we all meet regularly to share knowledge and skills. I've found them immensely useful. Although I didn't have any problems with being Clinical Supervisor before, going to them has really made me explore and understand what I am trying to do and to try out other and better ways of doing it rather than sticking to the way I've always done it. Subsequently, the role has become more enjoyable too!

Writing a Clinical Supervisor's Report

Clinical Supervisors need to write a report in order to provide a helpful overview to others of the trainee's performance during that post. To provide an 'all-rounded' view, make comments under the following four headings (often referred to as RDM-p):

Relationship	Diagnostics	Management	Professionalism
• With patients • With staff • With other colleagues (within and outside the practice)	• Assessing patients (and their needs) • Assessing oneself • Assessing staff and colleagues • Decision-making in practice-related activities	• Managing patients • Managing oneself: e.g. performance, health and well-being • Managing staff and colleagues • Managing practice-related activities	• Respect for people • Respect for protocol • Respecting importance of R, D & M • Being aware & carrying out contractual responsibilities

Diagnostics is about decision-making skills in general rather than clinical diagnosis.
Management is about administrative and organisational skills rather than clinical management.

Clinical Supervisor's Report – what makes a good report?		
Not Acceptable (descriptive)	**Acceptable** (analytical)	**Excellent** (in addition to the acceptable column) (evaluative)
Tick box completed inaccurately. Judgements not referenced to evidence from the trainee portfolio. Where the judgements can be evaluated, they do not appear to be justifiable.	Judgements are justifiable and referenced to the evidence.	Comments are more sophisticated/in-depth analysis of strengths and areas for development. Efforts are made to triangulate evidence, with comments based on more than one source.
No comment is made on the current state and the progression of competence. Little or no analysis of the trainee strengths and weaknesses.	The current state and the progression of competence are made clear. The strengths and weaknesses are identified and described.	The supervisor comments on the quality and range of the evidence-set in order to improve trainee insight and future data.
No suggestions for improvements. No PDP formulated and agreed with trainee.	Recommendations for further development are evidential and address the needs identified.	Critically evaluates presented evidence to define recommendations for further development.

Closing statement

It is evident that Clinical Supervision has matured beyond the 'See one, Do one, Teach one' approach. There is a wealth of theory and reflection that underpins the current pragmatic approach to teaching the future GP. The summative and formative nature of the assessments can be a difficult juggling act. However, Clinical Supervision is the foundation of workplace-based learning that is essential in educating the future GP.

> Clinical Supervision helps learners develop by giving meaning to their learning experiences.

A sample of resources on our website

- MRCGP assessments and the 12 professional competencies.
- Random Case Analysis.

Other chapters you may like to read

- Chapter 25: MRCGP in a Nutshell
- Chapter 29: Assessment and Competence
- Chapter 7: The Skilful Art of Giving Feedback
- Chapter 30: Quality – how good are we?

Please give us some feedback on this chapter to help shape it for the next edition.
Go to www.essentialgptrainingbook.com and simply click on the title of this chapter.

References

1 www.rcgp-curriculum.org.uk/ (accessed 2 March 2011).
2 www.mmc.nhs.uk/specialty_training/specialty_training_2011_final/gold_guide.aspx (accessed 2 March 2011).
3 Department of Health. *A Vision for the Future: report of the Chief Nursing Officer.* London: Department of Health; 1993.
4 Bernard JM, Goodyear RK. *Fundamentals of Clinical Supervision.* 2nd ed. Boston: Allyn & Bacon; 1998.
5 Butterworth T, Faugier J. *Clinical Supervision and Mentorship in Nursing.* London: Chapman & Hall; 1994.
6 Department of Health. *A Reference to Post Graduate Specialty Training in the UK.* 4th ed. London: Department of Health; 2010.
7 Pendleton D, Schofield T, Tate P. *The Consultation: an approach to learning and teaching.* Oxford: Oxford University Press; 1984.
8 Kurtz SM, Silverman JD, Draper J. *Teaching and Learning Communication Skills in Medicine.* Oxford: Radcliffe Medical Press; 1998.
9 Stoltenberg CD, Delworth U. *Supervising Counsellors and Therapists.* San Francisco: Jossey-Bass; 1987.

Effective Educational Supervision

GAIL CROWLEY – TPD (Rotherham) & lead author   MEI-LING DENNEY – TPD (Edinburgh) & lead author
RAMESH MEHAY – TPD (Bradford) & lead author   with helpful advice from
AMJAD KHAN – Associate GP Dean (West Midlands Deanery) and CHARLOTTE HART – Course Director (MMedEd, Keele Univ.)

> This chapter is a general guidance, as each deanery can vary in its interpretation and requirements.

Introduction

No doubt you are reading this because you're now an Educational Supervisor. Perhaps you're asking yourself a couple of questions like *'Why am I doing this?'* and *'What am I supposed to do?'* Maybe you're a Clinical Supervisor too and wondering *'What's the difference?'* So let's slow down and start with what Educational Supervision is and take it from there.

What is Educational Supervision?

Educational Supervision (ES) is a forward-looking process which is primarily educational and developmental, and designed to help the individual to progress. Regular ES meetings should provide an atmosphere which highlights strengths and reveals difficulties so that these may be helped to be put right within the framework of the objectives set at the start of the programme.

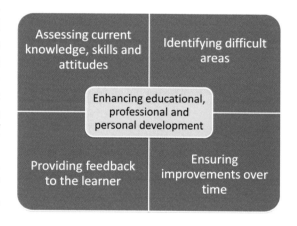

Phew, that was a mouthful, but in essence, ES is about keeping the trainee on track for their training and helping them identify and develop in those areas where there is an identified need. The process involves lots of feedback.

Is it a form of assessment?

Before we answer that, we'd like to remind you of the two types of assessment – formative and summative.

- **Summative assessment** is *evaluative*. It's usually done at the end of a period of time (e.g. the 12-monthly ARCP panels) to assess whether the trainee has made the grade either to move up a stage in their training or attain a certificate of competence.
- **Formative assessment** is *diagnostic*. By that we mean it is periodically carried out during a trainee's time on a training scheme to figure out what needs to be done to improve. It's often called 'educative assessment' because its primary function is to aid learning.

A useful analogy is that given by Stake.[1] He says: *'When the cook tastes the soup, that's formative. When the guests taste the soup, that's summative.'*

So, what kind do you think Educational Supervision is?

Educational purists would say that ES should be formative (i.e. developmental). They argue that in summative assessment (like exams), trainees tend to hide what they are bad at whereas in formative assessment they should be comfortable about displaying it – surely it's the latter that we're after in ES. In addition, ES should be seen as punctuations on a continuous interaction between supervisor and trainee rather than a one-off thing which is so characteristic of summative assessments. But in reality, and especially in the context of GP training, ES tends to be a mixture of formative and summative assessments.

The formative and summative functions of the Educational Supervisor

The Educational Supervisor has three functions.

1 *Formative*: **to support the trainee throughout their training scheme** as a mentor or guide.
2 *Formative*: **to guide the trainee through MRCGP** – especially the Workplace-Based Assessment (WPBA). This will invariably involve giving feedback and helping them develop reflective skills.
3 *Summative*: **to make recommendations to ARCP panels** for ST progression/CCT. This involves assessing evidence for the competencies against the standard that is a global judgement about fitness for independent practice (i.e. using the RCGP's competency descriptors to help define what that 'fitness' means).

Many supervisors have difficulty with the last point because they find it uncomfortable having to mark someone as 'unsatisfactory' or 'refer to panel'. However, others say that in referring someone to the panel you're not actually making a summative judgement – what you're doing is making a referral for a second opinion and that the panel is making the ultimate summative judgement. We're not convinced – it still sounds summative to us!

The knowledge, skills and attitudes required

In order to carry out the formative and summative functions listed above, there are certain requirements of the Educational Supervisor:

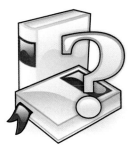

Attributes of the Educational Supervisor		
Knowledge	**Skills**	**Attitudes**
• Knowing what reflection really means – the types and levels of reflection. • The principles of feedback. • Equality and diversity awareness. • Familiarity with the curriculum statement headings. • Familiarity with the 12 professional GP competencies.	• Teaching reflective skills. • Giving feedback effectively. • Assessing the evidence of competency in the ePortfolio.	• Being non-judgemental. • A genuine desire to want to help the trainee develop. • A willingness to get to know the trainee on a personal level in order to develop a mutually respectful, open and honest relationship. • Giving ES the importance it deserves – like making protected time for it. The RCGP refers to ES as the 'glue that holds training together'.

JOB DESCRIPTION (EDUCATIONAL SUPERVISOR)
Responsibilities
An Educational Supervisor (ES) is responsible for overseeing training to:

1 ensure that trainees are making the necessary *clinical* progress
2 ensure that trainees are making the necessary *educational* progress.

Performance is reviewed via the ePortfolio in reference to the GMC's *Good Medical Practice* document. Therefore, they should have knowledge of the ePortfolio and have received training in:
- competence assessment
- appraisal and feedback
- equality and diversity.

Essential qualities of an Educational Supervisor
The relationship will develop throughout the training period and during that time the ES will see the trainee move through a significant change in how they practise medicine. In order to facilitate this change, the ES needs to:
- develop a relationship with the trainee built on mutual trust and respect
- be a good listener
- analyse significant amounts of information
- be skilful in the art of giving constructive feedback.

Accountability
The ES should communicate with the local Programme Directors should a trainee give cause for concern. The normal standards that govern probity and professionalism for GPs are of course expected to apply to Educational Supervisors.

Set-up
It is desirable that the trainee has the same ES throughout the whole of their training. The ES needs to be supported by colleagues, both from their practice and from their local Trainers' group.

So, what's the difference between Clinical and Educational Supervision?

Clinical Supervision is covered in detail in Chapter 26: Effective Clinical Supervision. The main difference is that the role of the Clinical Supervisor (CS) is about the *supervision and development* of a trainee in the work environment for a *particular 4–6–12-month placement*, whereas the ES provides *diagnostic* assessment of performance *throughout the whole 3-year GP training programme*. As a GP Trainer you might find yourself as a Clinical Supervisor to the trainee(s) in your practice and Educational Supervisor to one or more other trainees, who could either be in secondary care or another GP practice (depending on their ST year). So it's worth knowing the difference:

Educational Supervisor	Clinical Supervisor
Looks at the trainee's *overall educational programme* and sees where they are at and where they need to be.	Looks at the trainee's *clinical needs* determined by their performance in the current post.
Highlights educational needs and opportunities to help the trainee get appropriate training and experience in an integrated way throughout training.	Ensures that an individual trainee's timetable allows attendance at formal teaching sessions, is appropriate for his or her learning needs and that there is a correct balance between training and service in the placement.
Reviews assessments (like COTs, CBDs, MSFs etc.) and gives feedback on where to focus next. In doing so, the ES helps the trainee keep on track for MRCGP.	Carries out assessments that will be reviewed in Educational Supervision. Supervises the day-to-day clinical activities, ensuring that the trainee only performs tasks without supervision that they are competent to do so.
Provides an Educational Supervisor's report (in the ePortfolio). Responsible for signing off the trainee at the end of each ST year before progressing to the next level.	Provides a Clinical Supervisor's report (again, in the ePortfolio). Responsible for signing off workplace-based assessments.
The trainee usually has one supervisor throughout the entire scheme. Usually, a Programme Director or Trainer	Clinical Supervisor changes every time there is a change of post. Usually, a consultant if in a hospital or a GP Trainer if in a GP post.
In most deaneries, it is expected that there is a minimum of one meeting per post.	It is expected that there are three meetings per post – at the beginning, middle and end.

Who's the best person to be an Educational Supervisor?

An Educational Supervisor needs to be an experienced GP Educator: often, a GP Trainer or Training Programme Director (TPD). Non-GPs are not well placed to validly assess or guide on what is required to be fit for independent practice. Ideally, the *Educational* Supervisor should not be the same person as the *Clinical* Supervisor: how can you expect a trainee with practice-based difficulties to confide in an Educational Supervisor, who is also their Clinical Supervisor *in the same practice*? There's obviously a conflict of interest and while the two should be separate, in *real life* this is difficult (there's just not the number of Educators in some training schemes to make this feasible). This area is of particular debate. While the trainee is in their first post having a combined Clinical and Educational Supervisor can work well, but it is not best practice for someone at ST3 level; there can be conflict between the roles and judgements may become more subjective. Having an independent Educational Supervisor's opinion to 'back up' the Clinical Supervisor's assessments gives a more solid overview, triangulates better and is more helpful to the ARCP panel: especially when the trainee is not progressing well.

How often should you meet?

Most deaneries expect the ES to meet formally with their trainee at least once every post. Some even suggest two for the first post of the ST1 stage because they say that is where you need to 'get in' and lay some good foundations (like what is expected of the trainee, how to write a good log entry and so on). Others argue and say if anything, the two meetings should be at the ST2 hospital-based stage because that is where we lose contact with trainees, and so we need to put in the extra effort to make sure they're developing an understanding of the competencies and demonstrating this. And

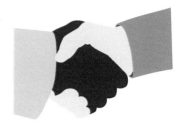

yet others argue that the high level of supervision is more appropriate at the final ST3 year as we need to make sure they're 'on track' for their CCT.

There is truth in all these arguments. Check with your deanery to find out what is locally preferred. We would say that, while there may be variance among deaneries, the number of meetings you have really depends on the trainee – if someone is struggling (e.g. underperformance), you need to review them more. At any time, you may feel it appropriate to have a direct discussion with their Clinical Supervisor, especially if there have been concerns in a previous post or to communicate an unsatisfactory Educational Supervisor's Report and subsequent deanery decisions.

 Top Tip: The Educator's Notes section of the ePortfolio is a useful place for highlighting any concerns or conversations that you may have had with the trainee or CS. It's certainly the best place to document any unofficial ES meetings. It is also worth noting that the ePortfolio's messaging system has a built-in audit trail – useful if a trainee repeatedly ignores the advice you're giving.

Do the reviews need to be done face to face?

As we've said before, it's important to see these meetings as punctuations on a continuous interaction between ES and trainee. Therefore, not all have to be done in person – choosing appropriate media (virtual supervision via phone or email) to do the required formative feedback and communicate the summative assessment judgements could be agreed between the supervisor and trainee.

 Red Alert: TPDs – be careful in trying to 'sell' Educational Supervision to Trainers by saying that they don't need to meet all the time. This might harm the purpose and importance of ES if they become laissez-faire about it as a result.

The Educational Supervisor and the ePortfolio

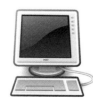

How often you look at their ePortfolio is up to you but this also depends on how well the trainee is progressing. Weekly reading may give you too many snapshots whereas once a month may give you a better feel for how things are going. **Early checking of their PDP after your first meeting is strongly advised** with a follow-up message via email, telephone or the Educator's Notes – really whatever works best for you and your trainee.

You need to look at things which will help you write your Educational Supervisor's Report, like the number of CBDs, mini-CEXs and so on. However, don't forget the ongoing learning log. Someone needs to read these learning log entries because they can provide valuable clues about how the trainee is doing. But the question is who. Some say it should be the Clinical Supervisor, who can do it in a timely way, and as they're overseeing the trainee's day-to-day clinical work, they have a better understanding of the context of each entry. Others say it should it be the Educational Supervisor, because what is needed is an independent person to assess purely on that which is written to see if it provides *evidence* for demonstrating the competencies. There is no consensus, but most schemes encourage the CS to read the log entries because there simply isn't the time to do this in an Educational Supervision meeting. The CS is the Consultant in a hospital post and the Trainer in a GP post. In reality, it's not surprising to hear that getting the CS to read the entries is easier to achieve in GP than in hospital posts.

Even if the Clinical Supervisor reads all the entries, that doesn't mean the Educational Supervisor is off the hook. The ES still needs to 'sample' some of them to see how the trainee is performing. How else can the ES form a view about the quality of reflection, use of PDP, and progression towards competency in the 12 competency areas?

 Top Tip: As an ES, how about reading log entries every 6 weeks or so and making an Educator's Note as appropriate (and even providing a guidance note for the trainee). This makes preparation for the review less demanding.

The Educational Supervisor's Report (ESR)

While a large part of the ESR is summative ('Is progress in xxx satisfactory') it also needs to be formative so that you can guide the trainee along their path towards certification, as well as their future Clinical Supervisors in how best to support their trainee.

● Where is the trainee in their learning and development right now?
● What is missing?
● What do they need to do now?
● How can this be achieved?

Doing Educational Supervision – the bit that's really important!

In order to be able to make informed evidence-based judgements about the trainee, they will need a reasonable amount of evidence within their ePortfolio. The more assessments you look at, the better the picture you get of the trainee and the more accurate your *holistic* judgement is going to be at the end of it. Because it is anticipated that a trainee's demonstrated competence will increase as they progress through their year, the later assessments should show more evidence of competence than the earlier ones. The same thing applies to the Learning Log and PDP. If there are few entries, it's worth 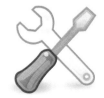 looking at the majority of them, but if you have an enthusiastic trainee who has a large number of entries, you may need to use judicious sampling.

This is what the ePortfolio's left navigation menu looks like and a summary of what to do:

Trainee's Name	Here's what you need to do (in 10 easy steps):
Summary	
Learning Log	←❶ Click here first, read the entries and map to competency areas.
PDP	←❷ Review the PDP – is it alive and kicking?
Evidence	←❸ Review the regular WPBA assessments (CBDs, COTs, Mini-CEXs)
Posts	←❹ Then review the infrequent WPBA assessments (MSF, PSQ, CSR).
Educator's Notes	←❺ What do the Educator(s) have to say? What themes emerge?
Curriculum Coverage	←❻ What areas of the curriculum are low and need more work?
Skills Log	←❼ Are the DOPS being achieved in a timely way?
Competence Areas	←❽ Which competence areas lack evidence and need further work?
Reviews	
Create Review	← Finally, click here to create a review and fill in the online ESR but also:
Continue/Edit Review	❾ Review Trainee's Self Rating of the 12 Competency areas
	❿ Rate them on the 12 competency areas yourself (**objectively**).

Let's look at each of these 10 areas in turn. There's a document on our website called *A Proforma for Doing Educational Supervision*, which covers the same material outlined below but *with extra technical advice*.

❶ The Learning Log (including NOE)

The Learning Log: Read as many entries as is necessary for you to get an accurate idea of how the trainee is using the log and performing. Look at the quality of the entry – determine whether it's reflective (see ISCE criteria below). Are there *enough* entries of a *variety* of types being recorded? Try to educate the trainee how they could improve on their log entries so that they can be better the next time around.

A good log entry will:

- show a good depth of **reflection** (more on reflection below)
- clearly highlight the **learning outcome**
- demonstrate coverage of one or more **curriculum areas**
- provide evidence for one or more **professional competencies**.

Time out – let's talk a bit about reflection

To be able to judge whether a log entry shows good reflection, you need to understand what reflection is. It is a **skill** which we all do to varying depths; being a skill means it can be strengthened through practice.

Why do we go on and on about reflection?

Reflecting on or during some experience in light of known theoretical concepts or previous learning should lead to new insights into different aspects of that situation. Therefore, effective learning won't happen unless you reflect. The outcome of reflection *is* learning (Mezirow,[2] 1981).

The proper definition

- Kemmis[3] (1985) – the process of reflection is more than a process that focuses 'on the head'. It is a positive active process that reviews, analyses and evaluates experiences, draws on theoretical concepts or previous learning and so provides an action plan for future experiences.
- Johns[4] (1995) adds that reflection is a personal process that enables the practitioner to assess, understand and learn through their experiences. This results in some change for the individual in their perspective of a situation or creates new learning for the individual.

Judging the depth of reflection in a log entry – the ISCE criteria

We've decided to call them the ISCE criteria (adapted from Richardson and Maltby[5]).

The ISCE criteria for reflection

- **Information:** How well does the trainee *describe* what happened or was *observed*? Is it in enough detail?
- **Self-Awareness:** Is the trainee *open* and *honest* about performance (usually through writing about own *feelings* and/or that of others)?
- **Critical Thinking:** Does the log entry show evidence of *analysing* the bigger and smaller pictures, *problem-solving* and describing own *thought processes*?
- **Evaluation:** Does the trainee pull together the above three things (*synthesis*) before going on to describe *what* needs to be learned, *why* and *how*?

Levels of reflection – what's acceptable and what's not		
Not Acceptable (descriptive)	**Acceptable** (analytical)	**Excellent** (in addition to the acceptable column) (evaluative)
Information Provided		
Entirely descriptive, e.g. lists of learning events/certificates of attendance with no evidence of reflection.	Limited use of other sources of information to put the event in context.	Uses a range of sources to clarify thoughts and feelings.
Self-Awareness		
No self-awareness.	Some self-awareness demonstrating openness and honesty about performance and some consideration of feelings generated.	Shows insight, seeing performance in relation to what might be expected of doctors. Considers thoughts and feelings of others as well as himself or herself.
Critical Analysis		
No evidence of analysis, i.e. an attempt to make sense of thoughts, perceptions and emotions.	Some evidence of critical thinking and analysis, describing own thought processes.	Demonstrates well-developed analysis and critical thinking, e.g. using evidence base to justify or change behaviour.
Evidence of Learning		
No evidence of learning, i.e. clarification of what needs to be learned and why.	Some evidence of learning, appropriately describing what needs to be learned, why and how.	Good evidence of learning, with critical assessment, prioritisation and planning of learning.

Have you ever read a trainee's log entry and thought it was a bit dire (and that was putting it politely)? Did you struggle to pinpoint where it fell down? Then use the ISCE criteria to help you figure this out. It's often because the trainee has written endless descriptive notes without further analysis or evaluation.

 Top Tip: The descriptors under the 'excellent' column in the table above summarise the key features of a really good reflective log entry. Why not print off this table and keep it with you while reading log entries? Share it with the trainee and get them to lead you through their own log entries. They're more likely to enhance their reflective skills in this way.

Another way you can get them to learn is to pick a poor log entry and get them to apply Kolb's[6] experiential learning cycle to it. Kolb's learning cycle is covered in greater depth in Chapter 10: Five Pearls of Educational Theory, but we've outlined it briefly for you here.

Kolb's Learning Cycle

- **Concrete Experience** – something that has happened to you or you have done.
- **Reflection** – reviewing the event or experience and exploring what you did and how you and others felt about it.
- **Abstract Conceptualisation** – developing an understanding of what happened by seeking more information or bringing in theoretical concepts or previous learning to form new ideas about ways of doing things in the future.
- **Active Experimentation** – trying out these newly formed ideas.

The more you can coach your trainee to do reflection properly, the more you move them from ignorance to understanding. That should help them progress and develop more swiftly, requiring less and less input from you, and ultimately making your work as Educational (or Clinical) Supervisor easier. Bliss!

My trainee doesn't like writing it all down. He says he does all this reflective stuff in his head anyway and all this ePortfolio stuff is unnecessary!

It's not uncommon to hear this but, remember, reflection is an active process rather than a passive thinking one. The problem with thinking 'in your head' is that people often rush through the stages of the reflective process. Writing it down encourages them to slow their pace, leading to a better description, better critical analysis, better self-awareness and better evaluation (and hence better learning): Richardson and Maltby[5] 1995, Zubizarreta[7] 1999 and Tryssenaar[8] 1995. Is that enough evidence for you?

Back to log entries – validating them
When a trainee adds a log entry, it needs to be 'mapped' to two things:

1) The GP curriculum statement headings	2) The 12 professional competencies
Examples:	Examples:
• *The General Practice Consultation*	• *Practising holistically*
• *ENT problems*	• *Data gathering and interpretation*
• *Sexual Health*	• *Making diagnosis/decision*
The GP Trainee needs to do this mapping.	Only the supervisor can do this mapping.
The supervisor needs to validate them.	

- The trainee maps their log entries to one or more curriculum statement headings.
- The CS or ES needs to validate them, i.e. checking to make sure the trainee's linkages are appropriate (and that they are not over-linking).
- So, when you are validating a log entry against a curriculum statement heading like *Care of Older Adults*, all you are saying is: '*Yes, this log entry is something about the Care of Older Adults.*' You are *not* making a judgement call as to whether the trainee is competent in this area or not.
- However, the story is different when it comes to mapping to professional competencies. Only map to a professional competency if:
    - the written log entry is **clearly about that competency and**
    - the trainee has made a clear **reflection and analysis** in terms of that competency.
- This mapping process is important because all the mapped entries can then be displayed in a structured way in reference to the GP curriculum and the 12 professional competencies. This is useful information for your ES meeting.

❷ The PDP

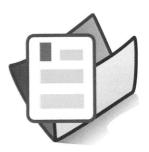

The PDP should show a number of entries that relate to the personal learning needs of that particular trainee. Mandatory requirements should not be entered on the PDP, and most entries should fulfil SMART criteria (Specific, Measurable, Achievable, Realistic, Time-bound). Alarm bells should ring when there is nothing planned, no thought about what to get out of the job, and when nothing is signed off.

WHAT'S A PDP AND HOW SHOULD YOU ASSESS IT? A PERSONAL VIEWPOINT

A useful analogy would be to view the PDP like a shopping list. We might go shopping with a list of items we know we need to buy, but we may find we need to change the items when in the shop because of lack of availability, etc. We may also spot things we didn't know we needed until we saw them on the shelves. Therefore, I think the PDP is great for planning learning (and particularly useful at the beginning of each post and at review points), but in my view, day-to-day small items of learning can be addressed perfectly adequately through the learning log. The PDP is a tool to aid reflection and learning, and is not an end in itself.

Comparing sophisticated PDPs to more rudimentary plans is like comparing a Rolls-Royce to a Mini. The Rolls is considerably more expensive and sophisticated, but may be no more effective in getting from A to B, and in certain circumstances (e.g. climbing a snowy hill) the mini may be the better vehicle. The difference between an elaborate and basic PDP may be more about preferred learning style than effectiveness of learning strategies. The key question is whether the trainee has shown understanding of the process, and has planned and completed learning journeys.

In terms of assessment, we need an approach that is more qualitative than quantitative when looking at PDPs, and I think the PDP has to be seen as just one element of the bigger portfolio, rather than something to be judged in isolation. I am looking for evidence in the ePortfolio that the trainee can identify and address learning needs, and demonstrate the application of learning to practice. If the PDP is scantily populated, but the learning logs demonstrate reflective practice and completion of learning cycles, then I think this is acceptable. A PDP where nothing is signed off does of course raise concerns.

I think one also needs to be careful about labouring the importance of 'SMART' objectives (although I know it borders on heresy to say so!). It's a great concept in theory, and it is useful to ask a trainee 'What exactly do you need to know when you say you want to learn more about diabetes?' but tidying up objectives to make them SMARTer doesn't necessarily add value to the learning in my experience. I think the discussions about 'SMARTness' are important, and it is of course helpful to clarify the nature of the need and how it will be addressed and completion demonstrated. However, specificity, in particular, can sometimes be difficult to define in advance of learning, and sometimes useful outcomes may be achieved that bear little resemblance to initial objectives. I don't think this necessarily matters, although it is great if trainees include some reflection on this.

Going back to the qualitative vs quantitative argument, as experienced educators we are in a position to make credible judgements about PDPs, even if our judgements may differ about the same PDP. I suspect that criteria that give best inter-rater reliability may be the least useful, and maybe we shouldn't get too hung up about this.

Nick Field (APD Sheffield)

❸ Reviewing the regular WPBA assessments (CBDs, COTs, Mini-CEXs)
Explore your confidence in the Clinical Supervisor
As you look at each set of assessments, try to get a feel for the accuracy of the grades given under the various competency or other headings.

⚠ Red Alert: Alarm bells should ring if you see:
- the same grade being given under every heading
- an excessive number of 'Excellent' grades
- grades awarded under headings that are unlikely to have been tested in a hospital post (e.g. *'Primary Care admin and IMT'*).

CBD, COT and mini-CEX mapping
After sampling enough CBDs, COTs and mini-CEXs for confidence in the rating, it's then important to step back and get an overall view. To do this, get the trainee to map out the competency 'marks' for each assessment so that you can see if any patterns emerge. For example, you may notice that out of the eight CBDs done so far that there's a competency that has never been assessed, or has always been graded as needing further development – thus helping you to advise the trainee. There are competency mapping sheets on the Bradford VTS website (www.bradfordvts.co.uk, then click 'Ed Supervision'). We urge you to encourage your trainee to fill them out; your life as ES will be easier if you get the trainee to do some preparatory work for *their* own ePortfolio. The mapping sheets also help you get an overview of the *context*, *complexity* and *level of difficulty* of the cases seen. This may have a bearing on the ratings given by the assessor, and you will need to take this into consideration. If they are of low challenge, making it difficult to judge your trainee's competency, it is worth noting this in your comments in the ESR.

❹ Reviewing the infrequent WPBA assessments (MSF, PSQ, CSR)
Multi Source Feedback (MSF)
In a general practice post, trainees need five clinicians and five non-clinicians to complete an MSF report, but in a hospital post they need only five clinicians, whatever their ST year. When you click on 'MSF', you will be offered a bar chart and spyglass icon 🔍. Click on the bar chart icon to see the collated evidence. This will be split under the two headings of (1) professional behaviour and (2) clinical performance. The free text comments in the MSF are especially useful, giving insights that would not be gained from other assessments.

- Pick out **themes** (positive and negative) from the free text entries for both professional behaviour and clinical performance.
- Formulate **suggestions** *with* the trainee to help them perform better.
- Incorporate these into the final **ES report**.

Patient Satisfaction Questionnaire (PSQ)

A PSQ is only ever done when the trainee is in a primary care placement. In simple terms, **compare the trainee's median to that of the peer median**.

- If the same: trainee performed similarly to the average GP trainee population.
- If trainee > peer: trainee performed better.
- If trainee < peer: trainee performed less than the average (a concern!).

As with the MSF, make some comments in the ESR: pick out positive and negative *themes* and *suggestions* (having discussed these with the trainee first).

Clinical Supervisor's Report (CSR)

There needs to be a Clinical Supervisor's Report for each post a trainee has been in. This should be done *before* the Educational Supervision meeting. The report is there to provide a helpful overview of the trainee's performance during that post. The CS is asked to provide comment under the following four headings:

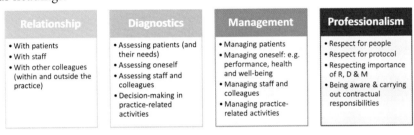

Relationship	Diagnostics	Management	Professionalism
• With patients • With staff • With other colleagues (within and outside the practice)	• Assessing patients (and their needs) • Assessing oneself • Assessing staff and colleagues • Decision-making in practice-related activities	• Managing patients • Managing oneself: e.g. performance, health and well-being • Managing staff and colleagues • Managing practice-related activities	• Respect for people • Respect for protocol • Respecting importance of R, D & M • Being aware & carrying out contractual responsibilities

Diagnostics is about decision-making skills in general rather than clinical diagnosis.
Management is about organising and managing oneself or others rather than clinical management.

- Review each of the R, D, M and P categories and pick out positive and negative *themes*.
- Consider looking over previous CSRs to see whether current themes were noticed then, whether there were additional themes and whether progress has been made.
- Engage in dialogue with the trainee – explore and problem-solve together.
- Summarise all of this in the ESR.

The college has produced some guidance on how to write a CSR. It might be worth sharing this with the Clinical Supervisor before they do the report:

Clinical Supervisor's Report		
Not Acceptable *(descriptive)*	**Acceptable** *(analytical)*	**Excellent** (in addition to the acceptable column) *(evaluative)*
Tick box completed inaccurately. Judgements not referenced to evidence from the trainee portfolio.	Judgements are justifiable and referenced to the evidence.	Comments are more sophisticated/in-depth analysis of strengths and areas for development.

Clinical Supervisor's Report		
Not Acceptable *(descriptive)*	**Acceptable** *(analytical)*	**Excellent** (in addition to the acceptable column) *(evaluative)*
Where the judgements can be evaluated, they do not appear to be justifiable.		Efforts are made to triangulate evidence, with comments based on more than one source.
No comment is made on the current state and the progression of competence.	The current state and the progression of competence are made clear.	The supervisor comments on the quality and range of the evidence-set in order to improve trainee insight and future data.
Little or no analysis of the trainee strengths and weaknesses.	The strengths and weaknesses are identified and described.	
No suggestions for improvements.	Recommendations for further development are evidential and address the needs identified.	Critically evaluates presented evidence to define recommendations for further development.
No PDP formulated and agreed with trainee.		

❺ The Educator's Notes

How you use the Educator's Notes is not set in stone. Although only Educators (Trainers, Clinical and Educational Supervisors) can write stuff in it, the section is viewable by all stakeholders (trainees, ARCP, etc.). ARCP panels find them particularly helpful.

Top Tip: Use the Educator's Notes to:
- document *performance concerns* discussed with the trainee (including performance that is at odds with the evidence from the learning log)
- document *exceptional circumstances* like family problems and sickness
- *communicate something* to you or others – reminding the trainee to follow up on something, reminding yourself about things to note in the ESR, tutorial planning and agreed preparation, providing additional information to ARCP panels and so on.

- Read through the Educator's Notes to get an overall picture of how training is going.
- Pick out any obvious positive and negative themes (and discuss with the trainee).
- Add to it *if* you feel what you have to say will help the trainee or others.

❻ Curriculum Coverage

- Decide whether the coverage pattern is broadly appropriate for the level of the trainee and the posts they have done so far. For example, if they're in Paeds, there should be a number of entries in the curriculum heading *8 Care of Children and Young People.*
- Click on a heading and sample some of the evidence to make sure entries have been appropriately tagged. You can unlink items that are not.
- Are there any obvious lacunae in the curriculum, taking account of the posts they have already covered?
- Even at ST3 stage there may be low numbers for certain headings like Learning Disabilities and Genetics. But remember: the GP curriculum was designed for a lifetime career in general practice; it's too much to be covered adequately in a GP training programme. Dip into the sparse areas: the few log entries might be comprehensive and reflective enough to be considered as acceptable. So, while numbers may be low for some areas, what you're assessing is whether there are adequate 'learning cycles' happening.

❼ The DOPS

These only need to be completed *by* the final review in ST3, but may be done throughout their three-year training. Only the DOPS that have actually been observed and independently assessed can be counted.

 Red Alert: Make sure the trainee is gradually working on their DOPS and not leaving everything until the end of their training. Furthermore, make sure that they're not getting other trainees to assess them – be clear that this is unacceptable.

❽ Competence Areas

This section provides the available evidence for the 12 competence headings. The two columns to the right will give you the number of linked entries from their learning log, and the number from their assessment forms respectively.

● First note which areas are sparse with evidence and need working on.

● In a similar way to the 'Curriculum Coverage', click on each competence heading and sample the learning log entries or WPBA forms that have contributed to the evidence.

● Make a note of some specific pieces of evidence to quote when you come to do your rating of the trainee (point 10 below).

❾ The Trainee's Self-rating (of competence areas)

Before the Educational Supervision meeting, the trainee has to rate themselves on the 12 Professional Competency areas. It is quite interesting because it provides information on the trainee's reflective skills and their level of insight, which may warrant further discussion if there is a large variance in their ratings from yours. The spy glass Q on the right of each competency enables you to compare current comments and ratings to past ones. Look at each competency and see if what they've written in the 'evidence' box marries with the rating they have awarded themselves. If not – educate! Then compare their ratings with your scores – discuss any variance. Are there weak areas where they lack insight?

 Top Tip: Before an Educational Supervision meeting, remind the trainee to rate themselves. Ask them specifically to do the following.

1 Pretend to be someone who doesn't know them and make a judgement according to the evidence within their ePortfolio (like COTs, CBDs and log entries). Refrain from personal subjective comments.

2 Record the analysis and judgement in the 'Evidence' box – be specific.

3 What do they feel they need to do in the future to better the evidence for that competence? Write this up in the 'Actions' box.

❿ The Educational Supervisor's ratings (of competence areas)

This is where *you* have to assess the trainee's ePortfolio and rate them under the 12 professional competence headings. If you do not feel that the evidence is there, or that the evidence displayed is not sufficiently robust for you to be able to make a judgement, give the rating of 'NFD – Below Expectations'. The expected grade by the end of ST3 is 'Competent for Licensing'. The 'Excellent' grade is reserved for exceptional trainees and should not be not be awarded in a willy-nilly way.

● In the **'Evidence' box**, specify the evidence that justifies your rating.

  ● For example: '*5 COTs & 4 CBDs show competence in practising holistically*'.

- Sometimes it can be helpful to signpost even more specific evidence: *'The last CBD case was about xxx and the trainee did yyy which indicates practising holistically'*.
  - There is a fabulous document on our website called *Finding the evidence for the rating scales*.
- In the **'Actions' box**, specify what the trainee need to do (in terms of evidence) to better their score.
- If you haven't already done so, **compare your ratings with the trainee's self-rating. Discuss any variance** and summarise it in the ESR.

Filling out the online ESR form (the 'Finish Review' section)

As you read through the evidence, it's a good idea to make notes at the same time (either on a piece of paper or open up a second ePortfolio browser). There's a lot to read, and it is difficult to keep it all in your head by the time you come to do the ESR (especially the bit where you have to rate the trainee according to the evidence).

Quality of evidence presented

Make a comment on the quality of:

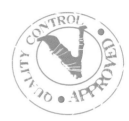

- log entries – level of reflection, types of learning activities
- CBDs – complexity of cases and a range of cases
- COTs – complexity of cases and their context (e.g. palliative care, children, etc.).

Make a recommendation

1 Satisfactory	All of the evidence is complete, and there are no concerns.
2 Unsatisfactory	The trainee's portfolio is severely lacking, *or* there is evidence to suggest that their progress is unsatisfactory, *or* there is some other cause for concern. Let the Training Programme Directors know early on.
3 Panel Opinion Requested	The portfolio is incomplete in some way, *or* you may be in doubt as to whether you can pass it as satisfactory for some other reason. With this option you are *not* failing the trainee – you're merely asking for a second opinion. Again, let the Training Programme Directors know early on.
4 Out Of Post	The trainee has taken a break from specialty training, for example Maternity Leave or 'Out of Programme Experience'.

The Agreed Learning Plan

Give feedback on the following areas of development and try to be specific.

- What is lacking in the trainee's ePortfolio?
- What should they be doing to improve their ePortfolio (content and process)?
- How they can maximise their learning opportunities?
- How they can address any other concerns or deficiencies?

Food for thought

We'd like to close by leaving you with this to ponder over:

Making judgements (and having to justify them in a concrete way) about competencies (even if their nature is understood) on the basis of what trainees have written demands both an in-depth assessment of the log entries and a new skill of assessing that material. The majority of Trainers are much more used to making judgements based on regular close personal contact rather than remotely via an e-record. For instance, most of us have no problem with the Clinical Supervisor's Report.

The fundamental question of narrative truth is also raised. How much is lost in translation from the clinical event to the written word? How many people 'subconsciously adjust' the notes written about a patient following consultation to fit with their interpretation and direction of diagnostic travel? I recently had to challenge a trainee when their description of what actually happened in a significant event was at variance with what they had recorded in their ePortfolio log.

Roger Higson (TPD, Northallerton)

 A Final Top Tip: Please look at Bradford VTS's website. There are a whole host of downloadable resources to make your life easier: www.bradfordvts.co.uk

A sample of resources on our website

- A year in the life of an Educational Supervisor.
- How many assessments and when.
- Evidence for the rating scales.

Other chapters you may like to read

- Chapter 25: MRCGP in a Nutshell
- Chapter 26: Effective Clinical Supervision.

Please give us some feedback on this chapter to help shape it for the next edition.
Go to www.essentialgptrainingbook.com and simply click on the title of this chapter.

References

1 Scriven M. *Evaluation Thesaurus*. 4th ed. Newbury Park, CA: Sage Publications; 1991.
2 Mezirow J. A critical theory of adult learning and education. *Adult Educ.* 1981; **32**(1): 3–24.
3 Kemmis S. Action research and the politics of reflection. In: Boud D, Keogh R, Walker D, editors. *Reflection: Turning Experience into Learning*. London: Kogan Page; 1985. pp. 139–63.
4 Johns C. Framing learning through reflection within Carper's fundamental ways of knowing in nursing. *J Adv Nurs.* 1995; **22**(2): 226–34.
5 Richardson G, Maltby H. Reflection on practice: enhancing student learning. *J Adv Nurs.* 1995; **22**(2): 235–42.
6 Kolb DA. *Experiential Learning*. Englewood Cliffs, New Jersey: Prentice-Hall; 1984.
7 Zubizarreta J. Teaching portfolios: an effective strategy for faculty development in occupational therapy. *Am J Occup Ther.* 1999; **53**(1): 51–5.
8 Tryssenaar J. Interactive journals: an educational strategy to promote reflection. *Am J Occup Ther.* 1995; **49**(7): 695–702.

28

Reflection and Evaluation

JOHN HART – TPD (Kettering, East Midlands) & lead author   MARK WATERS – GP Educator (West Midlands)
AMAR RUGHANI – APD (Sheffield)   RAMESH MEHAY – TPD (Bradford)

Reflection and evaluation are skills most of us perform to varying degrees in different aspects of our lives. These feature prominently in GP training, especially in our role as Clinical and Educational Supervisors – to help the trainee develop or enhance the skills they already have (and, of course, ourselves too).

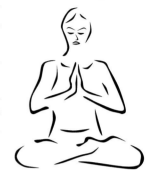

The very nature of being labelled as *skills* means that most of us can improve or enhance them. And that is what this chapter is all about – helping you to improve your skills of reflection and evaluation through better understanding. Some will find this as natural and self-evident as a duck to water; others will feel adrift and exposed, but we will help you, nevertheless.

Now you mention it, what exactly is reflection?

As you will see in the table below, many eminent people have defined this.

Defining Reflection	
Dewey[1]	**Active, persistent and careful consideration of any belief** or supposed form of knowledge in the light of the grounds that support it and the further conclusions to which it tends.
Boud et al.[2]	Reflection in the context of learning is a generic term for those **intellectual and affective activities** in which individuals engage to **explore their experiences** in order to lead to **new understandings and appreciations**.
Kremmis[3]	The process of reflection is more than a process that focuses 'on the head'. It is a **positive active process** that **reviews, analyses and evaluates experiences**, draws on **theoretical concepts or previous learning** and so provides an **action plan for future** experiences.
Johns[4]	Reflection is a **personal process** which enables the practitioner to **assess, understand and learn through their experiences**. This results in some **change for the individual** in their perspective of a situation or creates **new learning** for the individual.

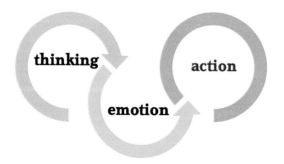

We particularly like the definitions given by Kremmis and Johns; they are specific, comprehensive, and make the explicit link between thinking, emotion and action in the reflective process. Reflection is this whole process – thinking, which leads to some sort of emotion, which together lead to some sort of action.

Hey, what about Schön? Where does he come into all of this?

We're glad you've brought up Schön – who is often regarded as the godfather of reflection. The two books published by Schön[5,6] in the 1980s have had enormous influence on our ideas about adult and professional learning. The key to appreciating Schön is to understand that he is talking about knowledge. He challenged the idea that knowledge can be written down, established, and agreed on in an objective way. For him, it is the job of the professional to be able to *create* his or her own knowledge. And the crucial tool that professionals use to create this personal, subjective knowledge is reflection. He described several kinds of reflection, including 'reflection-in-action' – which is the ability of professionals to 'think what they are doing while they are doing it'. He regards this as a key skill. There is a lovely section near the beginning of his book[5] where he describes the crisis he perceives in professional knowledge:

> In the varied topography of professional practice, there is a high, hard ground overlooking a swamp. On the high ground, manageable problems lend themselves to solution through the application of research-based theory and technique. In the swampy lowland, messy, confusing problems defy technical solutions. The irony of this situation is that the problems of the high ground tend to be relatively unimportant to individuals or society at large, however great their technical interest may be, while in the swamp lie the problems of greatest human concern. The practitioner must choose. Shall he remain on the high ground where he can solve relatively unimportant problems according to prevailing standards of rigor, or shall he descend to the swamp of important problems and non-rigorous enquiry?
>
> Schön[5]

He asserts that the only way to manage the 'indeterminate zones of practice' is through the ability to think on your feet, and apply previous experience to new situations. But for Schön it wasn't just about creating knowledge. Professionals also have to use their knowledge, and look back critically on their actions. He had particular terms for these things which we will cover below in the section 'Types of reflection'.

Why do we go on and on about reflection?

Effective learning won't happen unless you reflect. Reflecting on or during some experience in light of known theoretical concepts or previous learning should lead to **new insights** into different aspects of that situation.

Ultimately, the outcome of reflection is learning (Mezirow)[7]

1 It widens our perspective on a problem (broadens **knowledge**).
2 It helps us develop strategies for dealing with it (develops **skills**).
3 It helps us acquire new insights into our behaviour (changes **attitudes**).

Types of reflection

Don't confuse *types* of reflection with *levels* of reflection. *Levels* of reflection (covered later on) refers to how *deeply* one reflects and *types* of reflection to the *different ways* in which you can do it. Schön[5] in his work identifies two **types** of reflection; these are 'reflection *on* action' and 'reflection *in* action'. He suggests that reflection is used by practitioners when they encounter situations that are unique, and when individuals may not be able to apply known theories or techniques previously learnt through formal education.

Reflection-*on*-action (retrospective thinking)

We start with this one first because it is the one that is most familiar to us and that many of us do quite often. This is **reflection after the event**. In other words, you allow the event to happen, and then you consciously decide to reflect on it afterwards (and some of you will even go a step further to document it). For those of you familiar with Honey and

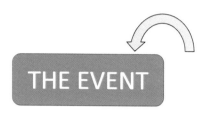

Mumford,[8] it is this activity that their 'Reflector' learning style is referring to (more in Chapter 11: Learning and Personality Styles in Practice).

Reflection-*in*-action (thinking on your feet)

This is the kind of reflection which occurs while a problem is being addressed, in what Schön calls the 'action-present'. It is a response to a surprise that occurs during the event; something which throws you off from your usual way of doing things – where the expected outcome is outside of our 'knowing-in-action' (see below for more on 'knowing-in-action'). The

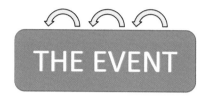

reflective process is at least to some degree conscious, involves 'thinking on your feet' but may not be verbalised. Reflection-*in*-action is about thinking again, in a new way, about a something we have encountered – challenging our usual assumptions.

Knowing-in-action

Knowing-in-action is another way of talking about 'tacit' or unspoken knowledge. When someone does a task expertly in 'automatic mode' they must have some unspoken yet internalised knowledge necessary for that task in the first place. The **knowing** is **in** the **action**. It is revealed by the skilful execution of the performance. That 'unspoken' knowledge is derived from the *evidence*, from the individual's *experiences* and from their *reflections*.

> #### KNOWING IN ACTION: AN EXAMPLE
>
> Jaya is a GP trainee sitting in with Ed, her Trainer. The next patient is a 54-year-old woman who comes in with a shopping list of five problems. Jaya thinks to herself, 'Gosh, I'm glad I'm not in Ed's shoes. How's he going to manage this in 10 minutes?' However, when she comes back from her own world to the present, she's realised that Ed has already managed to sort out one of the problems. He's now onto the second problem which is about some tummy problem. He takes a history and examines her and thinks she might have had a bit of a tummy bug. The usual advice is given and the patient (who is satisfied) then goes on to say, 'So, I'll come and see you next week about the other three things?' to which Edward nods with a warm smile. Jaya is taken back thinking how on earth did he manage to do this so efficiently and effortlessly? Jaya asks him about it afterwards, but Ed says he can't really say because he wasn't paying that much attention to what he was doing. However, one thing is for sure – he must have internalised some powerful knowledge and skills about negotiation – perhaps from what he has read, experienced or reflected on in the past – because this is clearly evident in his actions.

So what? What's the big deal about these two types of reflection?

As we have said before, most of us are familiar with reflection-*on*-action. And this is the bit that we often capture in our appraisal folders. It's also the type of reflection that GP trainees write about in their ePortfolios. All we are saying is to use *both types* of reflection – don't ignore 'reflection-*in*-action'. Quite a lot of us do 'reflection-in-action' on automatic pilot yet we fail to capture that in our appraisal-revalidation-ePortfolio worlds. Is it possible to write up our 'reflection-in-action' as well as think about it afterwards in a more conscious way? That would help us to 'reflect-*in*' and 'reflect-*on*' the same learning event. If we've managed to confuse you in this last sentence, try reading it just one more time (and slowly).

The ISCE levels (depths) of reflection

Study this table for a few minutes.

Levels of reflection – what's acceptable and what's not		
Not Acceptable (descriptive)	**Acceptable** (analytical)	**Excellent** (in addition to the acceptable column) (evaluative)
Information Provided		
Entirely descriptive, e.g. lists of learning events/certificates of attendance with no evidence of reflection.	Limited use of other sources of information to put the event in context.	Uses a range of sources to clarify thoughts and feelings.
Self-Awareness		
No self-awareness.	Some self-awareness demonstrating openness and honesty about performance and some consideration of feelings generated.	Shows insight, seeing performance in relation to what might be expected of doctors. Considers thoughts and feelings of others as well as him or herself.
Critical Analysis		
No evidence of analysis, i.e. an attempt to make sense of thoughts, perceptions and emotions.	Some evidence of critical thinking and analysis, describing own thought processes.	Demonstrates well-developed analysis and critical thinking, e.g. using evidence base to justify or change behaviour.
Evidence of Learning		
No evidence of learning, i.e. clarification of what needs to be learned and why.	Some evidence of learning, appropriately describing what needs to be learned, why and how.	Good evidence of learning, with critical assessment, prioritisation and planning of learning.

This table has been derived from original work done by Atkins and Murphy[9] in 1993. Good reflection will encompass all four ISCE areas, and to the level described in either the acceptable or excellent columns. Let's talk about each of the components in turn.

- **Information Provided:** Describing what happened or what was observed in enough detail. It should be honest and unbiased. This should be sufficient to give the feeling to an independent person that they were actually there. Care is needed to include information that is assumed to be known or self-evident.
- **Self-Awareness:** Being open and honest about performance but also writing about own feelings and/or those of others.
- **Critical Analysis:** Breaking the bigger picture into smaller parts and analysing the bigger and

smaller pictures. It involves identifying and challenging assumptions, problem-solving, describing own thought processes, and developing alternatives.

- **Evidence of Learning** = [SYNTHESIS + JUDGEMENT + EVALUATION][9]
  - Synthesis – pulling together the above three things (I, S and C) and integrating new information with the old (while also considering feelings).
  - Judgement – considering the possibilities, weighing them up and describing what needs to be learned, why and how.
  - Evaluation – looking back to see what difference it made.

EXERCISE: HOW GOOD A REFLECTOR ARE YOU?

Pick a reflective entry from your own appraisal or revalidation file. If this is too painful, take a peek at one of your trainee's reflective entries in the learning log section of their ePortfolio.

Q1:   In terms of this table, how reflective is that entry?
   a Were all four components covered?
   b To what level was each component described? (Which column?)
Q2:   What advice would you give yourself (or the trainee) to make the entry more reflective?
   a Which of the four components were missed?
   b For those components that were anything but 'Excellent', how could you move them into the 'Excellent' grade?

 Top Tip: Use the ISCE table to evaluate your trainee's learning log entries. Refer to this table if you feel a trainee's log entry is poor but cannot figure out why.

Other ways of reflecting – Kolb

Going through the ISCE components in order is not the only way you can encourage someone to reflect widely and deeply. The two other ways we will talk about are Kolb and Gibbs. Both are learning cycles, which means that they are reflective cycles too (at the beginning of this chapter, we said that the outcome of all reflection is learning). Here is a diagram illustrating Kolb's learning cycle.[10] So, to reflect deeply and widely on an experience, just start at 1 (the experiencing stage) and work your way through to stage 4 (experimenting).

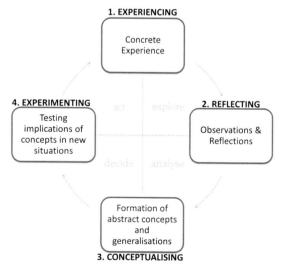

1 **Concrete experience** is the something that has happened to you, or that you have done.
2 **Reflection** is concerned with reviewing the event or experience and exploring what you did and how you and others felt about it.
3 **Abstract conceptualisation** is about developing an understanding of what happened by seeking more information or bringing in theoretical concepts or previous learning to form new ideas about ways of doing things.
4 **Active experimentation** is about trying these newly formed ideas.

Other ways of reflecting – Gibbs[11]

Using your experiential event, start at 'description' and work all the way around the cycle to the 'action plan' stage.

Gibbs's reflective cycle is particularly useful in helping trainees reflect on their consultations (especially the difficult ones).

So far, we've looked at three reflective frameworks – can you remember them?

[Ans: 1. ISCE, 2. Kolb, 3. Gibbs.]

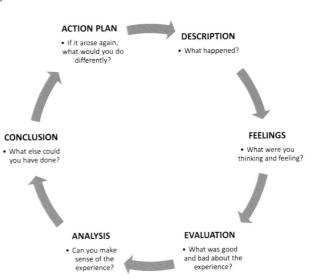

ACTION PLAN
• If it arose again, what would you do differently?

DESCRIPTION
• What happened?

FEELINGS
• What were you thinking and feeling?

EVALUATION
• What was good and bad about the experience?

ANALYSIS
• Can you make sense of the experience?

CONCLUSION
• What else could you have done?

Reflective Writing and Learning Journals

Reflective writing and learning journals – you having a laugh?
No – Moon[12] and Bolton[13] say that *Reflective Writing* and *Learning Journals* have additional power compared to other more traditional forms of learning as outlined below.

Educational benefits
● Reflective writing slows down the learning process, making sure we fully take account of the situation and, therefore, learn deeply and widely from it.
● Re-reading and rewriting is an educative process that deepens the quality of learning. It enables the learner to understand their own learning processes. It facilitates learning from one's own experience. It raises self-awareness skills – helping you explore 'the self' and one's own views of the world. It can help you make connections you didn't expect and understand things in new ways.
● Re-reading and rewriting develops a questioning attitude that helps one to get closer to what one wants. It aids progressive thought, which can be worked on later. This enhances problem-solving, reflection and creativity skills as well as promoting intuitive understanding.
● Re-reading and rewriting is a therapeutic process which supports behaviour change by questioning our own beliefs and attitudes. Writing is private: one can share it if they so choose. It is also safer (i.e. you cannot unsay verbal comments). There is personal ownership of the learning and because we become teachers and learners in our own lives, it enhances personal worth and self-empowerment.

Other benefits
● Reflective writing provides an alternative voice for those not good at expressing themselves verbally.

- Use of metaphors is easier in writing.
- Fiction is appropriate in writing (not so acceptable verbally and can be seen as lying). Recounted as through the writer's own experiences.
- Speech can be forgotten or changed. Writing leaves clear record.
- Writing can be torn up.

Okay, I'll give this reflective writing thing a shot. Got any guidance?

We'll do better than that. Here's an exercise for you to try either by yourself or with others (a group of GPs/trainees would be good). It's an exercise developed by Maggie Eisner, one of the Programme Directors for the Bradford GP Training Scheme. She uses it at induction with new trainees to expand their thinking and make them more open to creative ways of learning.

REFLECTIVE WRITING EXERCISE

This session requires 90 minutes. Everyone needs a pencil and paper in front of them. Split into balanced groups of 6–7. By balanced, I mean in terms of gender, experience, culture, talkativeness, reflectiveness, etc. – as far as you can judge it! In this exercise, the facilitator should write too.

Introduction
- The purpose of this exercise is to show you one way you can reflect on your experience – this is an essential phase of the learning cycle.
- It can help you make connections you didn't expect and understand things in new ways.
- Some people will take to it easily because they enjoy writing, others don't – it may remind you of school – try not to dwell on that but just get into it.
- It isn't anything to do with how well you write, although it may have the side-effect of improving your writing style.
- Later, we'll be talking about the experience, and if you want to we may share some of the writing, but if you don't want to share it, that's OK.

Warm-up
- This is a warm-up exercise like warming up for physical exercise. It's to get your creative writing juices flowing.
- We're going to spend 6 minutes on it.
- Write whatever is in your head – like a stream of consciousness.
- It's important to keep writing. Don't stop to think. If you feel you're drying up, keep writing the same word until something else comes into your head.
- This is only for you. You won't be asked to share it with anyone else.
- Facilitator – set your mobile alarm for 6 minutes.
- Facilitator – after the exercise, you can have a brief chat about how that felt but not for long.

Main exercise
Try this title. Write it on a flip chart. *'An important learning experience I had . . .'*
- We will have 20 minutes for this exercise.
- The theme is 'an important learning experience I had'.
- It can be something from your medical education, but it doesn't have to be – could be from any part of your life.
- Afterwards, I hope some of you will be willing to read out what you've written.

- If you do, it will of course be confidential in the group.
- If you don't want to, no one will force you to.
- Let's write – we'll have 20 minutes.
- Facilitator – set your mobile alarm for 20 minutes.

Facilitator's Notes
The repeated instruction re: 20 minutes is intentional as some always think it's 6 minutes again.

Group discussions – which will eat up the remaining time (about an hour).
- Start by asking about the process and discussing it a little – 'how did that feel?'
- Strongly encourage them to *read out* their stuff rather than them just telling the group what they've written about.
- In the discussion, try to make sure that both the process and content get discussed.
- Don't forget about all the usual stuff about keeping it safe for participants, etc. – reflective writing can be powerful and make people feel *unexpectedly* vulnerable.

 Red Alert: Although frameworks like ISCE, Kolb's and Gibbs's can be useful for helping someone develop reflective skills, be careful in using them for reflective writing. You don't want them to dampen the freedom, creativity and spontaneity offered by free thinking (and after a while, many of you will find them constraining too).

Other writing activities to try
These activities are taken from Kathleen Adams' wonderful book *Journal to the Self*.[14] Some will take your fancy, and others won't – that's okay! Try some of these things with someone else – a good way of building rapport.

Daring to be even more creative . . .

- **List 100 things** *off the top of your head. Group them into themes and write about reality next to them.*
- **Stepping stones:** *When you look back on something, try to split it into 12–15 significant points. You can do this for different areas of work, interests, etc. Write down a comment on each memory in time from the earliest to the present.*
- **Writing from a different perspective:** *e.g. how the (neutral) pot plant might see the consultation. Roads chosen and not taken. 'Never judge a man until you have walked in his shoes.'*
- **Write unsent letters** *so that you can express emotion without the risk of the fallout. For catharsis, completion and/or clarity.*
- **Character sketch:** *everyone we know is our teacher – we can see things in others that we love or hate in ourselves. Pick someone. Ask yourself: 'What is it about that person that always annoys me and am I avoiding seeing that in myself?'*
- **Write in an extended metaphor:** *e.g. what sort of house or car would you or others be?*
- **Topics du jour:** *write down one area of life to monitor for each day and review different process each day.*
- **SWOT:** *Strengths, Weaknesses, Opportunities and Threats in a situation.*
- **Captured moments, dreams and imagery:** *keep a notebook. Write these down immediately as they appear.*

Reflecting and evaluating as a GP Educator

Adapted from *Becoming a Critically Reflective Teacher* by Stephen Brookfield.[15]

Ways of reflecting and evaluating yourself
Seeing ourselves through our students' eyes *Use formal and informal evaluation forms to get feedback directly from the audience.* *'4 fundamental questions to evaluate a GP training post' – document available on our website.* *'Tynedale questionnaire' – document on our website.*
Getting feedback from others *'360 degree feedback form for GP educators' – available on our website.*
Using self-evaluation questionnaires *'Trainer's Needs Questionnaire' – available on our website; good for your Trainer's Appraisal.*
Videotaping your teaching sessions *Peer observation usually needs someone who has a wide variety of experience as a teacher and who can verbalise their thoughts and suggestions. Brief the observer on what sort of information you need.*
Keep reflective logs *Of stressful events, surprisingly pleasurable events, times of puzzlement, moments when the audience were least or most engaged, situations of greatest anxiety and other events which took you by surprise. Reflect on them. Discuss with a colleague. There's a 'Critical Teaching Incident Questionnaire' on our website, but you may want to use something less structured and restrictive.*
Ideology critique *Dominant ideologies are uncritically accepted and embedded in everyday situations. When things go wrong, re-examine the basic principles and assumptions to see if they still hold true. Turn logic on its head. Who benefits from the dominant view? Who loses by it? Do we need a new dominant view? What would that new structure look like? (Look up 'double-loop learning' on the net.)*
Teacher learning audits/appraisal *Get into the habit of seeing yourself as a learner. Reflect and be aware of how much you've learnt over the last year. What knowledge and skills have you acquired? What attitudinal shifts have occurred? What triggered these changes? How did it all happen?*
Role model profiles *Pick some role models/heroes – people who embody talents and characteristics absent from us. Define those missing qualities. How might you emulate them?*
Survival advice memos *Write a guide on the best advice to survive the job. What you need to know to survive. What you need to be able to do to stay afloat. What you wish others had told you. What your successor needs to avoid doing, thinking, assuming. Now write about what has happened to give you evidence for your advice (thus highlighting how you have developed).*

 Top Tip: *'Critical Conversations about Teaching'* groups'.[6] Reflective groups in which you can discuss evaluative data about you as an educator with experienced others. Remember: ground rules to stop aggressive attacks. Perhaps prefacing any criticism by a meritorious comment? The group needs to keep a healthy bank balance – of credits (positive comments) and withdrawals (negative comments). Everyone needs to respect differences, be willing to listen, and have a certain degree of tolerance and patience.

Reflection for Appraisal and Revalidation

With Revalidation, we will all have to demonstrate what we learn, why we learn it, how we learn it and what impact this has on our practice. What better way of doing this than using the reflective thinking and writing tools we've discussed so far? Most experiences (significant events, patient feedback, courses attended) lend themselves well to these reflective tools. Appraisal templates now include many of the prompts we've seen in the reflective frameworks, and it is useful to encourage GP trainees to think and record issues in this way too (they're ultimately going to have to for appraisal/revalidation anyway).

What sorts of things can I reflect on?

Lots of things! The obvious one is reflecting on a clinical event that was interesting, difficult, or dysfunctional. But you can also reflect on:

- **Good clinical care:** reflecting on *systems* that allow effective care and what can be done to improve them.
- **Maintaining good medical practice:** reflecting on your level of knowledge and skills around clinical topics. PUNs and DENs.[16]
- **Relationships with patients:** reflecting on the doctor–patient relationship and your communication skills. Did the patient have sufficient opportunity to tell their story? Did they feel respected? Did the patient feel a partner to the outcome of the consultation? You may need to carry out a Patient Satisfaction Questionnaire or do some video consultations to provide a source of data.
- **Relationships with colleagues.** Carrying out a multi-source feedback questionnaire (a 360-degree type thing) is clearly one way of gathering data.
- **Teaching and training:** using feedback sheets after teaching sessions, peer observations or video of teaching sessions.

My trainee isn't particularly reflective. Help!

I've looked at a few of the log entries in my trainee's ePortfolio and they aren't reflective!

You cannot make a global judgement of the trainee just based on a few log entries. You need to read as many as it takes to help you get to that point of certainty where you can safely say, *'I now think I have a clearer picture of what this trainee is generally like.'* Here's a list of characteristics of superficial and deep reflectors (Entwistle[17]) which may help you further.

Superficial reflectors

- Tell their story from one point of view – theirs!
- The account is sequential.
- No reference is made to their emotional reaction and how this subsequently impacted on them.
- Little attempt to focus on particular issues.
- Most points are made with similar weight.
- Often give merely a descriptive account of the experience.

I've had another look and, actually, 80% or so aren't particularly reflective. What now?
It really depends on why your trainee isn't particularly reflective.

1 Is it because your trainee's attitudes need to change? In other words, is it because they can't see the point of reflection or aren't particularly hooked in? *Or*
2 Is it because they lack the skill to do it? In other words, their attitude is OK (i.e. they value reflection) but simply don't know how to go about it. This one is easier to tackle than the first.

My trainee values reflection but is simply finding it difficult to do or write down
All you need to do is to introduce them to one of the reflective frameworks – ISCE, Kolb or Gibbs. Pick a reflective log entry to assess from their ePortfolio. Work through it using one of the frameworks (we suggest the ISCE one – easiest to do). Show them how they could have made the entry more reflective *and* highlight the *new insights* that result.

Other things to remember:

- When reflecting-*on*-action, encourage trainees to record details of incidents that have either troubled or surprisingly pleased them soon after the event as possible (as memory cannot be relied on).
- Encourage the *non*-reflective trainee to sum up each day with a reflective comment in his or her diary, spending only a few minutes doing it. You may also set them an example by keeping a reflective diary of your own professional practice or, indeed, your experiences as an Educational or Clinical Supervisor, thus demonstrating that learning is always ongoing!
- The more you can coach your trainee to do reflection properly, the more you move them from ignorance to understanding. As they get the hang of it and require less and less input from you, the more autonomous they become. And your work as Educational or Clinical Supervisor becomes easier.

 Top Tip: Print the ISCE table and keep it with you when reading log entries. Encourage your trainee to do the same when writing them up. Revisit log entries *together* and get the trainee to gradually start *leading you* through the reflective process with their entries.

My trainee thinks reflection is a load of rubbish
What's needed here is for you to somehow trigger an attitudinal shift in the trainee and that's not going to happen overnight! How you do this depends on your trainee – who you will know better than we do. Therefore, we cannot give you specific advice, but we can offer some general guidance.

First, do it in a sensitive way: **acknowledging, validating and empathising** with their feelings – just like you would do with patients. Secondly, help the trainee to recognise and embrace the need for an attitudinal change themselves. People are more likely to adopt **behaviour change that they realise for themselves** than when others tell them. The types of attitudinal things we are talking about are listed in the rounded box below.

> ### The key qualities (attitudes) individuals need to do proper reflection
> 1 Open-mindedness
> 2 Commitment to self-enquiry
> 3 Motivation and
> 4 Readiness to change practice.
>
> Richardson and Maltby,[18] Gillings[19]

Naturally, good reflectors are all of these four things. Which of these is your problem trainee lacking? It's probably more than one! What can you do to strengthen them?

He says that he particularly hates writing it down and does it more quickly and efficiently in his head anyway. What do you say to that?

Loads of trainees say that they do it in their head but, remember, reflection is an **active process** not a passive thinking one. The problem with thinking 'in your head' is that people often rush through the reflective process. Writing encourages them to slow down and think through things properly. Slowing it down promotes a better description, better critical analysis, better self-awareness, better evaluation and, therefore, better learning (Richardson and Maltby[18], Zubizarreta[20] and Tryssenaar[21]). That should be enough evidence to convince them.

A 2-minute guide to Evaluation

Until now, we've not said much about evaluation. The reason is that if you were to draw a Venn diagram with one circle representing reflection and the other evaluation, you would realise that there's a big overlap between the two. To reflect on something is to evaluate! What more is there to say? However, what follows is specific to evaluation. We've adapted it from a '2 minute guide to Evaluation' (part of a series of '2 minute guides' in relation to Revalidation) which was written by GP Tutors from the former Yorkshire Deanery.[22]

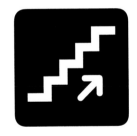

What is Evaluation?

Evaluation allows us to examine the *value* of a task which we've just completed to ourselves and others (**value** is at the heart of this word). This is not just about saying the task has ended, or we have achieved a goal but what *effect* this work has had on us. We can evaluate two things: the **outcomes** (what we achieved) and the **process** (how we did it).

What outcomes can be evaluated?

Outcomes can take many forms.
- You may gain new **knowledge** (facts about a disease, developments in therapy).
- You may have learnt a new **skill** (an ability to do something, e.g. inject a joint).

- Your **attitude** to the subject may have changed (e.g. you have decided that you now wish to offer a service you were previously unsure about).
- There may be a change in **performance** in you or in the practice because of working in new or different ways.

How can outcomes be evaluated?

Kirkpatrick[23] developed a hierarchy of evaluation (see table below for an adapted version). In this table, you can evaluate any task at one of four levels. The further down the table you decide to evaluate, **the more impact and effect** your task will have had (providing you get positive feedback indicators). The *ultimate* purpose of GP training, Appraisal and Revalidation is to provide high-quality patient care. Therefore, it's not surprising that Kirkpatrick puts anything that measures patient care at the highest rank at level 4.

Kirkpatrick's Levels of Evaluation	Outcome measured by	+ve = achieved	-ve = failed to achieve
1 **REACTION** Own sense of achievement	Surveying your feelings and thoughts after the activity.	Satisfaction with having undertaken the activity.	No satisfaction with undertaking the activity.
2 **LEARNING** You actually learned something!	Testing knowledge, surveying attitudes, demonstrating new skills.	New knowledge, skills or attitudes acquired.	No new knowledge, skills or change in attitude.
3 **BEHAVIOUR** Your behaviour changed and you use the learning	New protocols and practice guidelines, change in performance (e.g. captured through video or looking through individual patient records).	Applying new knowledge and skills to work. Approaching a problem differently because of a change in attitude. In summary, a change in performance.	New knowledge, skills or attitudes are not put to use, i.e. not being used to improve patient care.
4 **RESULTS** Your patients have benefited from your learning	Audits, surveys, significant events and quality indicators show improved patient care.	Patients have benefited – their management or care has improved.	No benefits seen for patients. No change in patient management or care.

- GP appraisers can now start looking at PDPs in this manner. Has a PDP item been achieved? If so, how? At what level did the GP evaluate? Changes at level 4 may take many years to achieve, and it may be your wish to review the activity in a couple of years (e.g. changes as a result of a new protocol for managing patients with high cholesterol may only be visible in cholesterol levels via an audit in 1–2 years).
- Programme Directors can use Kirkpatrick's table to decide at what level they want to evaluate a teaching course they've just run. Sometimes, it is not practically appropriate to evaluate at level 4 – you may have to settle for level 3 or 2 – as long as you know what that level represents.
- Trainers can evaluate the effectiveness of their consultation teaching in this way. Reviewing the trainee's video consultations – that would be level 3. However, a positive change in a trainee's Patient Satisfaction Questionnaire score (the start vs the end of post) is surely going to be the best measure – level 4.

Don't forget to evaluate the process too

It is also helpful to think about how you did the work – the **process**. What worked and what didn't and why? What would you do differently next time? Are there any learning needs that you have identified?

Closing remarks – role modelling reflection

We know from research that years after GP trainees have qualified, they continue to display attributes picked up during training from their GP Trainers. Therefore, as GP Educators, we are powerful role models. This means we need to role model reflection too – to 'walk the talk', to 'practise what you preach' and so on. Make time during day-to-day practice to do this and encourage the trainee to take 'time out' with you to reflect together. Don't rush it; give it the time it deserves. Avoid saying *'Let's reflect on that later . . .'* – do it when it's 'hot off the press'. Make it become an integral part of both of your working lives.

A sample of resources on our website

- Creating a culture of reflection.
- Exercises to help build skills in reflection.
- Trainer Needs Questionnaire.
- 4 fundamental questions to evaluate any GP post.

Other chapters you may like to read

- Chapter 4: Powerful Hooks – aims, objectives and ILOs (especially Constructive Alignment)
- Chapter 30: Quality – how good are we?

Please give us some feedback on this chapter to help shape it for the next edition.
Go to www.essentialgptrainingbook.com and simply click on the title of this chapter.

References

1 Dewey J. *How We Think: a restatement of the relation of reflective thinking to the educative process*. Massachusetts: DC Heath; 1933.
2 Boud D, Keogh R, Walker D. *Turning Learning into Experience*. London: Kogan Page; 1985.
3 Kremmis S. Action research and the politics of reflection. In: Boud D, Keogh R, Walker D. *Turning Learning into Experience*. London: Kogan Page; 1985.
4 Johns C. The value of reflective practice for nursing. *J Clin Nurs*. 1995; **4**: 23–60.
5 Schön D. *The Reflective Practitioner*. Aldershot: Ashgate Publishing Limited; 1991.
6 Schön D. *Educating the Reflective Practitioner*. San Francisco: Jossey-Bass; 1987.
7 Mezirow J. A critical theory of adult learning and education. *Adult Educ*. 1981; **32**(1): 3–24.
8 Honey P, Mumford A. *The Manual of Learning Styles*. Maidenhead, UK: Peter Honey; 1986.
9 Atkins S, Murphy C. Reflection: a review of the literature. *J Adv Nurs*. 1993; **18**(8): 1188–92.
10 Kolb D. *Experiential Learning*. New Jersey: Prentice-Hall; 1984.
11 Gibbs G. *Learning by Doing: a guide to teaching and learning methods*. Oxford: Further Education Unit, Oxford Polytechnic; 1988.
12 Moon J. *The Use of Learning Journals: reflection in learning and professional development*. London: Kogan Page; 1999.
13 Bolton G. *Reflective Practice: writing and professional development*. London: Paul Chapman Publishing; 2001.
14 Adams K. *Journal to the Self*. New York: Warner Books; 1990.
15 Brookfield SD. *Becoming a Critically Reflective Teacher*. San Francisco: John Wiley & Sons; 1995.

16 Eve R. *PUNs and DENs: discovering learning needs in general practice.* Oxford: Radcliffe Medical Press; 2003.

17 Entwistle N. *Styles of Learning and Teaching: an integrated outline of educational psychology for students, teachers and lecturers.* London: David Fulton Publishers; 1998.

18 Richardson G, Maltby H. Reflection on practice: enhancing student learning. *J Adv Nurs.* 1995; **22**(2): 235–42.

19 Gillings B. In: Burns S, Bulman C (eds). *Reflective Practice in Nursing: the growth of the professional practitioner.* Oxford: Blackwell Science; 2000. pp. 106–21.

20 Zubizarreta J. Teaching portfolios: an effective strategy for faculty development in occupational therapy. *Am J Occup Ther.* 1999; **53**(1): 51–5.

21 Tryssenaar J. Interactive journals: an educational strategy to promote reflection. *Am J Occup Ther.* 1999; **49**(7): 695–702.

22 Kapur S, Parkin A. A two minute guide for GPs on Evaluation. In: *Revalidation Without Tears – a series of 2 minute guides.* Developed by GP Tutors in the former Yorkshire Deanery; 2004.

23 Kirkpatrick DL. The Four Levels of Evaluation. In: Brown SM, Seidner CJ. *Evaluating Corporate Training Models and Issues.* Boston: Kluwer Academic Publishers; 1998.

29

Assessment and Competence

NIGEL DE KARE-SILVER – Associate Director (London Deanery) & lead author
RAMESH MEHAY – TPD (Bradford)

Becoming comfortable with *assessment*

Assessment is something most of us as doctors have considerable experience with. Assessments may still create those hair-raising, spine-tingling, nauseous, cold and sweaty moments but most of us, as doctors, have been subjected to assessment so often that we have an innate confidence about being able to get through.

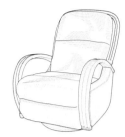

As qualified GPs, we know with every challenge there are hoops to get through and walls to climb – and **we have done it!** We have worked our way through these successfully. We have intellectual and organisational abilities that have brought us to this point in our careers.

- We *can* assimilate, reproduce and apply knowledge to everyday situations.
- We *can* analyse and communicate our thoughts to others.
- We *can* organise ourselves to remain on top of our work loads.

We have these precious gifts, and that makes us qualified enough to undertake specialty teaching and training (and the assessments therein).

Becoming comfortable with *competence*

Competence is something new to many of us. Competence may seem like the latest buzzword, but if you think about it, it is the most important parameter of the suitability to perform any job. Competency is widely used across many industries as a core recruitment tool. It can also be used as an instrument at various career stages to help an individual develop by defining strong and weak areas of competence.

To help assess whether a training doctor is competent to perform as a GP, the RCGP has defined 12 areas which they must be competent in if they are to satisfactorily complete training. Competence is important at many levels – for patients, for you, for other doctors and so on. Therefore, competence is something you must be able to demonstrate to others (and thus assessors too). Assessors themselves should similarly be assessed on their ability to demonstrate their competence to carry out the task of assessing others. Gone are the days where one was deemed a competent assessor just through the very nature of being a hospital consultant or a doctor with an immense number of experiential years under his or her belt. Sure, experience gives you the foundation to become an assessor, but it is no substitute for being trained up for the role.

Why assessment? Aren't we clever enough?

Yes, medics are very clever people (actually, it depends how you define cleverness). If we take the intelligence quotient (IQ), the lowest IQ of qualified doctors is around 120. Many are higher than this! It's competitive to get into medical school in the first place. Intelligence wise, doctors in general are in the top 2% of the population.

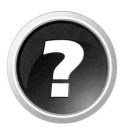

If doctors are clever and organised people and have passed the very stiff examination-based assessments to get into and through medical school, why do they need to go through yet more assessments during their specialty training? Why not let them progress through their training, enjoy the richness of their experiences, and allow their naturally clever minds to transfer their knowledge into applied skills? Can't assessments dominate and interfere with learning to such an extent that they become disadvantageous? Don't trainees end up worrying more about the assessment than the learning?

Yes, learning is indeed often dictated by assessments and this can mean that learners adopt an immature attitude to learning. They only bother picking up books when they have an exam to pass. Those taking exams work hard to make sure they understand what is needed in order to get through an exam, and the standard needed to pass. They often familiarise themselves with the techniques and subtleties expected in the language of their presentations, and work hard to talk the language expected by their examiners. Assessments, therefore, can hijack and drive the learning.

This means that if assessments aren't reliably measuring something of value (i.e. something which makes a difference in the real world), then the learning that results (the outcome) will be valueless too. And the worrying thing is – that happens! What's more worrying is that despite this misalignment, trainees will continue to work hard to be successful, with the mark of success being their exam achievement and *not* their clinical performance. In fact, this group of highly intelligent competitive people would work so hard for the success of an exam pass, that if they were commanded to jump through hoops of raging fire in step to a specified piece of music in order to succeed, they would learn to do so and would learn to do it well.

> Question: Is the candidate's purpose of undergoing assessment to pass or to learn?

So, back to the original question: aren't we clever enough? Yes, we are clever enough *but* competency assessment is not an assessment of intelligence but an assessment on the ability to apply that intelligence within the expectations of one's role in work – the ability to work with other people (colleagues and patients), cope with pressures, be professional and so on. Competency is more interested in our *performance than our intelligence* – and that's what makes a difference to patient care. Competency-based testing thus assesses our ability to perform, not our ability to pass the test! And we need to continually revisit the assessment processes we have, tweak them to make them as robust as possible and be prepared to redesign them in the light of changes to the expectations of practising GPs and changes to best practice thinking in assessment design.

Mark Twain was scathing of doctors: 'I was once a sharp shooter but I now practice a far more deadly profession.' In his day, the acquisition of title of 'doctor' was lost in a mist of nepotism, wealth and personal networks, as was the process of getting into medical training in the first place. Medical degrees were in place and had been since the 9th century. However, their relevance to the job the doctor was expected to perform was questionable. Doctors were a variable set of individuals with questionable backgrounds and abilities yet possessed a self-imposed divine right to command respect and obedience. They were thus dangerous.

Defining *and* assessing competence

Let's look at some models of competence. You can use any of these models to:
1 define the different levels of competence and therefore:
2 gauge how competent someone is becoming and therefore:
3 develop an assessment (or marking) grid to match.

And they're quite easy to understand too. So let's work our way through them.

The Conscious Competence Model

Nobody really knows the origins of this model. Some say Confucius, others say Socrates! Some even say it comes from Johari's Window (*see* Chapter 4: Powerful Hooks – aims, objectives and ILOs), but actually the two are completely different (one looks at self-awareness, the other is about skill acquisition). Actually, who cares! Let's just get on with the model.

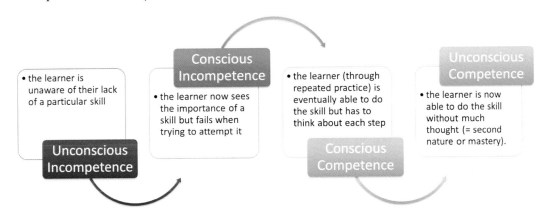

This model outlines how we acquire a skill. It tells us how much of a novice or master someone is at something (i.e. how competent they are). The model is pretty self-explanatory – think back to when you started to tie your own shoe laces and read the model again in relation to that. Someone has suggested yet another level – the **'conscious competence of unconscious competence'**. What a mouthful! This level describes a person's ability to recognise and develop unconscious incompetence in others – teaching your own kids how to tie shoe laces, for instance.

Learners can feel uncomfortable (frustration and despair) during the conscious incompetence and conscious competence stages. It's useful to remind learners that these uncomfortable feelings are good because they mean one is no longer in their comfort zone but on the journey to their desired state. Unconscious competence (i.e. mastery) can only be achieved through practice, practice and practice – and it is here where those uncomfortable feelings fade away.

- If you've got a trainee who is struggling with a particular skill, use the model and figure out where they are in the learning process. This should then help you determine what needs doing to move them to the next level.
- You can also use the model to define individual descriptors for an assessment or evaluation grid (see table below).
- If you decide to share this grid with the trainees, it will tell them exactly what is expected of them.

For example, let's consider 'doing a neurological examination'.

Performing a neurological examination – Conscious Competence model			
Unacceptable *(Unconsciously Incompetent)*	**Needs Further Development** *(Consciously Incompetent)*	**Competent** *(Consciously Competent)*	**Excellent** *(Unconsciously Competent)*
The learner *knows* little and/or *demonstrates* very little. He or she *might* be able to demonstrate a *few* of the micro-skills – but the operative word is few.	The learner's knowledge is good. There is mixed performance in demonstrating the skills – some are done well, others need work.	The learner's knowledge is good. The performance for all of the micro-skills is acceptable, although they clearly have to think about some of them and might not do them with flair.	The learner's knowledge is good. They perform all micro-skills effortlessly and with elegance. It is second nature to them.

I decided to learn how to sail – don't ask me why, but I did. Okay, my life is sad, and I needed a hobby! I didn't see the need to read anything about it beforehand – after all it's a physical task and what's there to read anyway? One just needs to 'do', don't they? And I'm pretty good with my hands, and I thought that after a lesson or two, I'd probably be ready to go.

[This is Unconscious Incompetence]

At my first lesson, I became aware that there were right and wrong ways of doing things – lots of rules for dealing with ropes, wind, health and safety and reading maps. My knowledge was definitely low and, clearly, you needed all of this first to be able to sail properly and safely.

[This is Conscious Incompetence]

After a while, my ability to handle the boat developed. Sure I made mistakes, but one does need to get a feel for what needs to be learned. I could now do things pretty much okay, although I was acutely conscious of every move and every error and never certain or confident that anything was done right. One may be deemed sufficiently proficient at this stage to be allowed to sail alone, albeit on a restricted basis. At this stage, I could see how many of my fellow learners were really pleased with themselves, but nevertheless, we were all aware we had little confidence.

[This is Conscious Competence]

On reflection, when mistakes are common [*usually the period between Conscious Incompetence and Conscious Competence*], progress can be slow and enjoyment can be so fragile that some of my fellow learners decided it was not for them, and they dropped out! I was disappointed that our teacher didn't pick this up and failed to protect them.

Anyway, finally came the day when I could sail and handle the boat with familiarity and ease. One's mind can then concentrate on the route and weather reports or on the radio rather than thinking about each of the component sailing skills. And at this stage, if something is not quite right, you pick up on it and deal with it. But also at this stage, you can really start enjoying the journey.

[*This is Unconscious Competence*]

The Dreyfus model[1] – Novice to Expert
This is simply another model that describes something similar to the Conscious Competency model we've just looked at.

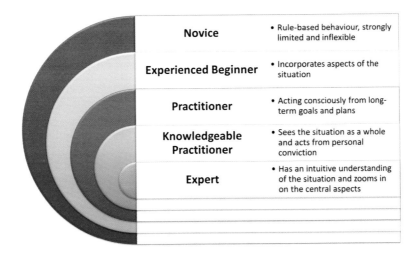

Novice	• Rule-based behaviour, strongly limited and inflexible
Experienced Beginner	• Incorporates aspects of the situation
Practitioner	• Acting consciously from long-term goals and plans
Knowledgeable Practitioner	• Sees the situation as a whole and acts from personal conviction
Expert	• Has an intuitive understanding of the situation and zooms in on the central aspects

Introducing competency progression
The more a trainee practises a set of skills, the more likely it is those skills will become internalised. Once internalised, the trainee can then start to practise the next order of skills and so on. During this process, as more and more competencies are developed, the trainee moves from Novice to Practitioner to Expert (although in some areas the latter may take several years after training). This progress is called 'competency progression'.

Patients aspire to be seen and treated by doctors who are competent, safe and in whom they can be confident. While they recognise and appreciate the need to train, they will often prefer to be seen by the 'Expert' than the 'Novice' or even the 'Practitioner'.

● The expert can look at the situation in front of him, managing it correctly and safely. *But* he also has the spare capacity within his consciousness to have insight and know when to look at the bigger picture – the wider issues that may not be obvious to the Novice or Practitioner.
● The expert will have experience behind her; she will have developed nuances in understanding, analysis and communication, which are not expressed in textbooks or standard training materials.

- He will have abilities, which reach beyond the classroom – abilities which have only emerged as a result of a wider understanding and knowledge.

When trainees start a training programme, it's important to determine where they are at in terms of competence. Clearly, they're not going to be experts but the important thing is for the Educational or Clinical Supervisor to review this regularly to ensure they are gradually developing competencies as they move through their training programme. In general practice, deaneries formally review this competency progression through ARCP panels (short for **Annual** Review of Competency Progression). And if a trainee fails to show adequate competency progression, they can stop them from moving onto the next training year.

Which assessment method do I use?
The Conscious Competence or Dreyfus **models** help you:
1 define what is competent
2 develop an assessment grid against which you can benchmark your trainee.

What these *models* don't tell us is which assessment *method* to use. We may well have developed an assessment or marking grid for say 'Practising Ethically' – but how do we test it? Do we set an MCQ, a viva, and OSCE, a combination or what? Luckily, Miller's Pyramid helps us to choose an appropriate method.

Miller's Pyramid[2]
The psychologist George Miller proposed a framework in the 1990s which helps you answer the question:
1 *What level of clinical competence are we aiming for?*
2 *Which assessment method would adequately measure that?*

Miller's Prism of Clinical Competence (a.k.a. Miller's Pyramid)

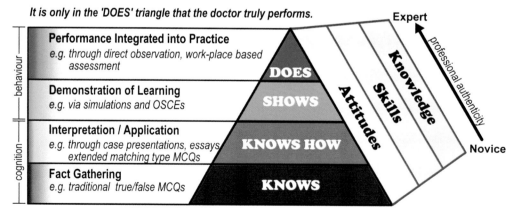

Based on work by Miller GE. The Assessment of Clinical Skills/Competence/Performance. *Acad Med.* 1990; **65**(9): 63-7. Adapted by Drs. Ramesh Mehay and Roger Burns (January 2009).

Originally, Miller represented his framework as a two-dimensional pyramid. In our diagram above, we've adapted it to include the knowledge, skills and attitudes domains of learning and thus called it **'Miller's Prism'***. Dent and Harden[3] have added a fifth level called* **'Mastery'** *that sits above 'Does' to* *make the distinction between one who can perform a skill with competence to one who can perform it in an expert or masterful way.*

In this pyramid, the lower two levels only test *cognition* (or knowledge), and this is where inexperienced trainees usually sit: they either 'know' or 'know how' to do something. The upper two levels test *behaviour*, that is, whether they can apply ('show' or 'do') what they know in practice? Ultimately, the best zone is the 'Does' level because it is at that level a doctor truly performs. For instance, if you were planning on installing a conservatory, would you get someone who 'knows' something about building conservatories or someone who actually builds conservatories for a living (the 'does' zone)?

The problem with assessment methods aimed at the cognition zones is that trainees can get away with 'brushing up' their knowledge a few weeks before. This knowledge then fades shortly after, making any learning temporary. This is less likely with assessment systems aimed at the 'behavioural zones', and that makes them more valid and better preparation methods for professional life. But that is not to say assessing at the lower levels is valueless – they may be appropriate for someone who is in the early stages of learning a new skill.

So, if we apply Miller's Pyramid to 'practising ethically':

● At the **Knows** level, the learner **has some knowledge** about ethics. *It may be appropriate to test at this level in (say) a first-year medical student who is just starting to learn about ethics for the first time. At the end of the year, you might assess knowledge around ethical theories and concepts using factual recall tests like MCQs.*

● At the **Knows How** level, the learner **knows how to** practise ethically. *A fifth-year medical student has moved on from acquiring knowledge and might be learning about ways in which you can apply that knowledge to patients and real situations. At the end of the year, you might assess them by setting an essay on the application of ethical principles or perhaps a case presentation.*

● At the **Shows** level, the learner **can show you** that they can practise ethically. *An ST1 trainee in a GP post may have a 'flash' moment on the importance of an ethical approach to practice. They've refreshed their knowledge and now wish to try some ethical frameworks out on real patients. Towards the end of the post, you might assess them through a case-based discussion – focusing specifically on what the doctor actually did that proves that they practised ethically. At a scheme level, the Programme Directors might assess them via a patient simulation exercise or an OSCE – and see whether they can reproduce the skills.*

● At the **Does** level, the learner **routinely practises** ethically in their daily work. *An ST3 trainee should be practising ethically regularly in consultations. You can assess whether they are doing this by directly observing their day-to-day work or some sort of workplace-based assessment – perhaps analysing random videos, random cases or sitting in with them periodically.*

We hope we have not confused you. At the very least, we hope you can see how doing an 'MCQ' to test a trainee's ability to examine a knee just doesn't cut the mustard (but a skills station does). Here's a little test for you: can you use Miller's Pyramid to explain this:

I struggled to get through medical school – I failed my first, third and final years but always managed to pass the retakes. Luckily, in the end, I caught up with my peers (many of whom were also my mates) and I continued my house-officer year with them.

There was one particular colleague who I want to talk about. She always got exam distinctions at medical school. After exams, I would look at the list bottom-up to see where I was; she would look top-down. She actually graduated with honours! But what I found amazing was that she struggled as a house officer. She was abysmal at putting in Venflons, doing ECGs and always seemed anxious about managing newly admitted patients. If the ward staff had any queries, they tended to approach me instead!

So how is it that I struggled in medical school but was pretty good on the wards? And how is it that she was a grade A student who seemed to have lost her halo on the wards? Life is weird!

ANSWER: Her learning was always at the 'Knows' and 'Know How' levels (cognitive competence)and unfortunately that was the level the medical school examinations tested (through MCQs, short answers, essays and vivas). Working on the wards requires behavioural competence.

Formative and summative assessment

How should assessments be used? What is their purpose?
- Is it to enhance or drive learning?
- Or is it to check whether a candidate has reached a certain level?
- Can these two purposes be combined?

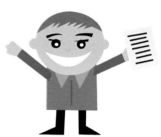

Some assessments are about checking to see whether a trainee has reached a certain level or grade so that they can be given a 'ticket' to go on to the next stage. This is termed **summative assessment**. However, other assessments are done just to determine strong and weak areas so that the learner knows what they need to carry on doing and what they need to work on in a developmental sort of way. This is termed **formative assessment**. Formative assessment is a reflective process that intends to promote student attainment.[4]

If the primary purpose of assessment is to support high-quality learning, then formative assessment ought to be understood as the most important assessment practice.

In summative assessment, an assessor always makes the judgement. In formative assessment, the judgement of good and weak areas can be made by the assessor, teacher or the learner themselves.

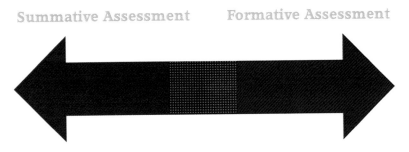

Summative Assessment

- It's all about the end point.
- It's often numerical.
- The stakes are usually high.
- Ensuring high reliability is therefore essential.
- *Example: end of term written exams.*

Formative Assessment

- It's all about words and feedback.
- It's about truly wanting to help learners learn.
- Particularly good for helping learners acquire generic skills.
- *Example: the day-to-day clinical supervision on wards or in a GP post.*

 Top Tip: In formative assessment, ask your learner:
- how near or how far he or she feels from the required standard
- where he or she feels his or her training needs to be targeted.

Summative assessment	Formative assessment
Is *usually* a single process like an exam.	Is a continuous process that occurs throughout the training period.
Is about giving the learner a 'ticket' or certificate to proceed.	Is about helping the learner develop.
Results in a grade of competence.	Identifies strengths and weaknesses.
Results in a certificate or grade of competence.	Results in developmental feedback.
Often quite cold, remote and detached from teaching.	Results in a Personal Development Plan.
Is often seen as a negative process, e.g. *'Thank goodness the AKT is over.'*	Is seen as a positive process because it's all about *helping* the trainee, not telling them off.
Examples in GP training:	Examples in GP training
• *AKT*	• *Clinical Supervisor meetings*
• *CSA*	• *Educational Supervisor meetings*
• *The Workplace-Based Assessments like COTs, mini-CEXs, CBDs and so on.*	• *Tools that are not formally part of MRCGP like: Problem Case Analysis, Random Case Analysis, appraisal and so on.*

> ## Summative assessment is an assessment *of* learning
> Formative assessment is an assessment *for* learning.
> In summative assessment, the trainee tries to hide what they are bad at.
> In formative assessment, they should be comfortable about displaying it.

The problem is that trainees get so anxious about the summative type of assessments, which then end up driving the learning. Therefore, educators need to make sure right from the start that the summative elements are truly testing the things we want our learners to learn.

Can you combine formative and summative assessments?
Yes. Take the Consultation Observation Tool. You might start by doing it in a summative way – observing your trainee's video, marking and writing comments along the way. You might even ask the trainee to do the same. Once the video is over, you could then feed back the summative bits in a formative way – for instance, by asking the trainee about their views first before engaging in dialogue. Alternatively, you may even decide to compare grades followed by dialogue focused at areas of large variance. The important thing in both cases is the dialogue. In these two examples, the data is gathered in a summative way but the results are fed back in a formative developmental way in order to direct the learning. Clearly, the assessor needs to be good in the art of giving feedback in order to do this process justice (*see* Chapter 7: The Skilful Art of Giving Feedback).

Why does everyone bang on about reliability and validity?
Why? It's simple – because they're important. After reading this section you'll agree: they are pretty much the keystones of assessment planning. It's important that tests or assessments have a high degree of reliability *and* validity – but this is often difficult to achieve.

Reliability
Reliability is about reproducibility. In other words, if you took a test twice, would it give you the same result? Because if it didn't, how can you *rely* on the result? Reliable assessments are repeatable and reproducible. For example, the reliability of an MCQ test is going to be much higher than that of an assessor-based test (like a viva) because of examiner bias. This doesn't necessarily mean we opt for MCQs over assessor-based tests. The question might be how to make assessor-based tests more reliable (answer – assessor training and calibration).

Validity

Validity is about relevance: does the assessment measure what you are trying to measure? For instance, you will remember from Miller's Pyramid that an MCQ has high validity if all we are simply trying to assess is a candidate's level of knowledge. However, it has low validity if you're going to use it to test how good they are at *doing* a knee examination. For a knee examination, you would have to *see* them *doing* it!

The inverse relationship between reliability and validity

Assessments with high reliability, like MCQs, often have low validity. For instance, MCQs are good at assessing knowledge but what most of us really want to test are more complex things like a learner's analytical skills, ability to deal with complexity, perform a task and so on. MCQs are poor at assessing these. In addition, MCQs often succumb to testing rare things that have little relevance to the daily practice of medicine.

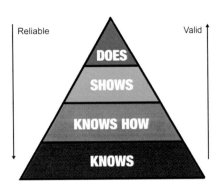

This is not to say all MCQs are rubbish. Some variants (like Extended Matching Questions) are better at testing the *application* of knowledge. This must not be underestimated, as doctors need to have a lot of knowledge and general practitioners, generalists, need to have a very wide field of knowledge. But knowledge alone is not sufficient – doctors need to be able to practise by the application of knowledge in conjunction with other skills like communication, awareness and team working. These skills cannot be tested by traditional knowledge-based assessments because they have low validity in this regard.

To test these more complex skills the trainee needs to be tested in their workplace to see what they actually do there. Workplace-based assessments have high validity, but the inverse relationship exists here too – they often have high validity at the expense of reliability (reproducibility). So, assessing a video consultation using the COT criteria has high validity – you are measuring specific consultation micro-skills that matter. But the fact that different assessors might score the same video differently means the assessment might not be so reliable.

Validity and transference

Having been taught, a medical student can undergo an examination. This may be based on many aspects of the taught course and include expectations on their wider reading and wider research. But despite having undergone extensive teaching and assessment can the trainee, now a newly qualified doctor, perform the task on a real patient? Can they transfer their learning into the real situation and apply their knowledge to the patient, the real person?

Invariably, the answer is no – in order to transfer learnt knowledge and learnt skills there needs to be direct experience of working in the real environment. If this experience only occurs *after* training is completed and *after* assessments on suitability to practise have been concluded, there is nothing in the system, nothing in place, to check that the trainee can actually perform the work they are supposed to be able to do – to serve their patients well.

Therefore, for an assessment process to be valid, it must include assessments on those features of a normal doctor's working practice/working day to be able to judge whether a trainee completing their programme can now perform as a doctor in the real-life environment.

The reliability and validity of various MRCGP WPBA assessments

This table shows you how reliability and validity are applied and used in the real world. Reliability and validity are not just theoretical concepts. They add a new dimension of meaning. They tell you how much respect a particular assessment tool deserves.

Assessment	Reliability	Validity
MRCGP WPBA assessments:		
CBDs *Case Based Discussion* *Trainee presents a patient they have seen which they are questioned over in a focused way.*	Low because of assessor variability. You might have thought the reliability was around a 'medium' for CBDs because of having precise assessment sheets with grading descriptors. We've ranked it low because Trainer calibration is currently poor and the CBD criteria are not universally understood (unlike COT criteria).	High for • Knowledge • Application of knowledge • Consultation skills • Problem-solving skills • Decision-making skills • Attitudes • Analytical skills But if trainees can select which CBDs to present, are they showing their best behaviour rather than their usual?
COTs *(either sitting in and directly observing or via video)*	Medium because of assessor variability. We've decided to go higher with COTs than for CBDs. Although there are precise assessment sheets with grading descriptors for both, we feel Trainer calibration is better. Most Trainers have a good understanding of the COT criteria (because they've been built on previous consultation video criteria and because they do these themselves in daily practice).	High for • Knowledge • Application of knowledge • Consultation skills • Problem-solving skills • Decision-making skills • Attitudes But if trainees can select which videos to present, are they showing their best behaviour rather than their usual? And what about the Hawthorne effect? (*See* Chapter 23: Road Maps for Teaching on the Consultation)

Assessment	Reliability	Validity
MSF *Multi-Source Feedback from Clinical and Non-clinical Colleagues*	High The questionnaire consists of highly focused questions. There aren't that many questions to fill in either – therefore you don't lose the concentration of the person filling in the form. Both of these things mean that a person who had to fill in a duplicate MSF would hopefully write almost as exactly as he or she did in the first.	High for ● Knowledge ● Ability to apply knowledge ● Consultation skills ● Problem-solving skills ● Decision-making skills ● Team working ● Organisational skills ● Attitudes But validity becomes low if trainees select which people to give the questionnaires out to because you are less likely to get a true representation of how others see them (therefore not measuring what it is supposed to measure).
PSQ *Patient Satisfaction Questionnaire*	High The questionnaire consists of highly focused questions. There aren't that many questions to fill in either – therefore you don't lose the concentration of the patient. Both of these things mean that a patient who had to fill in a duplicate PSQ would hopefully write almost as exactly as he or she did in the first.	Moderate for ● Consultation skills ● Attitudes Validity is lowered if the trainee chooses which period to hand out the questionnaires. He or she might behave 'exceptionally well' that day! There is also a risk that those who do fill out and return the questionnaires are a select group of people – those who are prepared to spend time filling out forms. Those people may be polarised on their attitude to the doctor who has seen them between those who think he or she was great and those who think he or she was terrible.

A fuller analysis of the MRCGP components in terms of reliability and validity can be found on our website. Look for the document 'The reliability & validity of different MRCGP assessments'.

MRCGP in terms of assessment and competence
What standard is used for the assessment of competence in MRCGP?
The standard against which the GP trainee is judged is always the level of competence expected of a doctor who is certified to practise independently as a GP. This is the standard that is used *throughout* the years of training. That means an ST1 trainee is judged against a doctor who is certified to practise independently and *not* in relation to their peers at the same stage. You might think this is unfair, but it's not – surely the most important question is where the trainee is in relation to a fully qualified GP?

In the early stages of training that means it is unlikely that a trainee will be able to provide the evidence for the readiness to practise. And that's quite OK (and is the expected norm). What's more important is competency progression (which we talked about earlier). It is hoped that as training progresses the trainee will be able to collect more evidence of competence and be able to build a richer picture of readiness for practice as they come towards the end of training.

My trainees react badly when I grade them NFD. Do you have any advice?

Consider the life journey of the trainee who has just started their first year of GP training with you. They were high flyers at school – passing exams with grade As. They then went to medical school and passed more stringent exams. After that, it was their foundation years – receiving 'competent' or 'excellent' grades for their Workplace-Based Assessments. Then they come to general practice and start getting 'Needs Further Development' (NFD). Having never tasted failure, are you surprised that they react badly to being awarded NFD? Most will react negatively *unless* you prepare them for it. You need to tell them that NFD is the expected norm and get them to see how they wouldn't need to be on a training programme if they were excellent in all 12 professional competencies – do all of this as early as possible. And when you do award an NFD, explain your rationale behind awarding it so that you're both on the same wavelength. So, reassure them that NFD is okay and start talking to them about competency progression instead.

General rules for doing any sort of assessment

Be sensitive

A trainee will be anxious before, during and after an assessment. Be sensitive – assessment is all about what they can or cannot do, and you need to give them a level platform to be able to demonstrate that. Assessment is not about getting them to crack under pressure – if it was what would be the point?

Beef up your feedback skills

Feedback is central to any process of assessment. The purpose of feedback is to give a clear message to the trainee where they should direct future activity. A broad mark, a vague breakdown that cardiology was good and diabetes bad does not give the required detail of feedback that identifies the areas where the trainee needs to focus their learning. Feedback needs to be given clearly and in a balanced way, even where the overarching message is that the trainee is underperforming. Feedback that leaves the trainee distraught and humiliated may give the supervisor some perverse sense of superiority but does nothing to foster learning and development. Give feedback in a way which will make the receiver look towards working on it in a positive way.

> I carry out my assessments by asking my trainees how they think they should be rated. The trainees are often nervous and dislike being put into this position – especially the first few times they are asked to work in this way – but it soon fades. The trainee can work down the list of criteria as easily as I can. At first their ratings might be at variance with mine, which would then lead to some sort of discourse. It often provides a good measure of how much insight the trainee has into their abilities. If a trainee has little insight, it's important to start working on that otherwise they will continue to see and focus on the wrong things. The more you both start grading together, the more likely it is your grades will eventually converge. When that happens you are both on the same wavelength – and your assessment job becomes easier!

Keep assessments alive and dynamic

If you find 'hot spots' during your assessment, stay there and explore. Capture the moment as opposed to the tedium of carrying out exercises line by line.

During a CBD, if I ask a specific question and the trainee gives a woolly reply, my alarm bells start ringing. I will stay there and ask deeper questions that direct the trainee to be more specific. In that way, I only move on when I am satisfied in my own mind as to whether the trainee has demonstrated that competence or not.

Closing comments

As with anything, the future of assessments and the ePortfolio is uncertain. However, we hope you now understand the differences between formative and summative assessments. We also hope you've realised that the MRCGP Workplace-Based Assessments have been carefully thought out and chosen. The chosen ones *generally* tend to tackle the top two rungs of Miller's Pyramid *and* have high validity (although reliability is still variable). One can be confident that now the system is embedded into medical education every effort will be made to improve and build on it continuously. Try not to get frustrated or flustered with any future changes and bear in mind that the new version is probably more reliable *and/or* valid than the old.

A sample of resources on our website
- The reliability & validity of different MRCGP assessments.

Other chapters you may like to read
- Chapter 7: The Skilful Art of Giving Feedback
- Chapter 25: MRCGP in a Nutshell
- Chapter 26: Effective Clinical Supervision
- Chapter 27: Effective Educational Supervision.

Please give us some feedback on this chapter to help shape it for the next edition.
Go to www.essentialgptrainingbook.com and simply click on the title of this chapter.

References

1 Dreyfus SE, Dreyfus HL. *A Five-Stage Model of the Mental Activities Involved in Directed Skill Acquisition*. Washington, DC: Storming Media; 1980.

2 Miller GE. The assessment of clinical skills/competence/performance. *Acad Med.* 1990; **65**: 63–7.

3 Dent J, Harden R. *A Practical Guide for Medical Teachers*. Edinburgh: Churchill Livingstone; 2001.

4 Crooks T. The validity of formative assessments. Paper presented to the British Educational Research Association Annual Conference, University of Leeds, 13–15 September 2001. Available at: www.leeds.ac.uk/educol/documents/00001862.htm

Quality – how good are we?

MARK PURVIS – GP Director (Yorkshire & the Humber Deanery)   IAIN LAMB – Associate Advisor (SE Scotland)
SARAH LAYZELL – TPD (Nottingham)   RAMESH MEHAY – TPD (Bradford)

> 'The place to improve the world is first in one's own heart and head and hands.'
>
> Robert M Pirsig[1]

People don't set out to do a bad job. A bus driver doesn't get up in the morning and think *'How shall I drive my bus today? . . . I know, badly!'* A teenager aspiring to a career in teaching, when asked what sort of teacher they wish to become, does not answer *'a bad one'* or *'one who puts young people off learning'*.

- People . . . educators . . . medical educators, *want* to do a good job.
- We *want* to see learners meet their full potential.
- We *want* to inspire, recapture and share the excitement and enthusiasm that we have for the practice of medicine.

There is something very powerful about 'catching people doing something right'.[2] Frankly, if your approach to quality assurance is to 'catch people out', then you are probably getting in the way of quality improvement.

Concepts such as 'quality control' are limited. Quality should not just be controlled; in many circumstances, quality should be liberated!

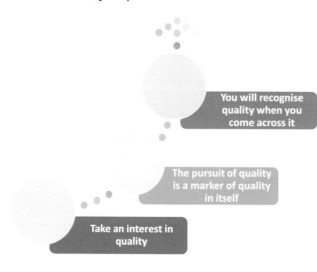

You will recognise quality when you come across it

The pursuit of quality is a marker of quality in itself

Take an interest in quality

- **And that's it!** That is all you *need* to know about quality. The rest is detail.
- You have our **permission** to **skip the rest of this chapter** and move on.
- **But before you do**, take a moment to **contemplate this . . .**

Think of a picture – something like a sky or sunset. Then ask yourself two questions.

1 When do I/we get in the way of quality?
2 How do I/we **liberate** quality in my/our work?

A brief history of quality

If you are still reading, it is because you want to know more . . . are you sitting comfortably? Then we shall begin. Let's start at the beginning, with a brief history of quality. If you are a 'theorist', you will really like this.

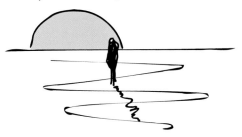

Period	Notes
13th century onwards Crafts and Guilds	Entry to guilds was controlled, with a system made up of apprentices, journeymen and masters. Apprentices served time, assisting other guildsmen. They learnt their basic skills through practice and repetition, progressing in time to become journeymen. Journeymen had to produce 'masterpieces' (probably not summative assessment videos or five-point audits) in order to become a master in the guild. In the 21st century, medical education retains many aspects of the apprenticeship system. The work of the craftsmen was individual, every piece of work unique, but the quality of the work was assured by the mark of the guild.
1770 to early 1800s Industrial	The industrial revolution was characterised by rapid changes in the organisation of the workforce and the introduction of mechanised tooling. The emphasis shifted from the assurance of craftsmen (a skills-based approach) to output-based methods of quality assurance. For example, product inspection and benchmarking. Was this the early, non-medical world's version of QOF?
1910 to 1960s Scientific	A major driver was two world wars – Allied armies using equipment produced by different suppliers on different continents required reliable interoperability. The underlying philosophy was that of modernism: the belief that traditional approaches to quality 'held back' progress and that science and technology can drive progress, leading to improvement. This was the era of mass production and production-line techniques. A scientific approach to quality in the GP world is characterised by: selection, planning, observation, measurement, analysis, improvement and incentives.
1930 to 1970s Human Relations	Between 1924 and 1932, a series of experiments were carried out on Western Electric factory workers in the Hawthorne Works, Cicero, Illinois. The rationale for the experiment was scientific, but the findings heralded a new understanding of the importance of human factors on quality. The Hawthorne Effect[3] (coined by Henry Landsberger) demonstrated that subjects improved their behaviours simply because they were being observed. Key thinkers in the Human Relations era of quality assurance were: 1 Henry Murray (1938):[4] four 'needs' – inclusion, power, autonomy, achievement. 2 Douglas McGregor (1960):[5] Theory X and Theory Y. 3 Frederick Herzberg (1959):[6] complex motivational theory – hygiene factors and motivators. 4 Abraham Maslow (1943):[7] hierarchy of needs.

Period	Notes
1950s onward Total Quality	This era represents an amalgamation of the Scientific and Human Relations approaches, where the sum is greater than the parts. A major driver of this movement was the need to reconstruct the Japanese economy following World War II. A Total Quality Management approach embraces all aspects of the organisation, including processes and people. Key thinkers were: 1 William Edwards Deming[8] (profound knowledge and transformation), who with Walter Shewhart introduced the Plan, Do, Check (Study), Act cycle and placed a greater importance on management in the pursuit of quality. 2 Joseph Juran[9] who focused on planning, improvement and control, using tools such as the Pareto analysis to determine where the greatest effect of quality improvement would be made. The Pareto Effect states that 80% of effects originate from 20% of causes. 3 Kaoru Ishikawa[10] who described seven basic tools of quality, emphasised the human side of quality within a total quality ethos and company-wide control. The Ishikawa diagram (aka fishbone diagram) describes quality as an outcome with materials, processes, equipment and measurement as the causes of quality. 4 Shigeo Shingo,[11,12] who distinguished human error (which is inevitable) from defects (which are preventable) when the error causes effect. Shingo championed immediate feedback, analysis of the root cause of problems and checklists to help prevent lapses.

We can recognise elements of this history in medical education today.

- Our *apprenticeship* model of training that has its roots in the crafts and guilds era.
- *Assessments* that reflect the output-based methods of quality assurance stem from the industrial era.
- A focus on *competencies* and *selection* for training grows from a scientific approach to quality.

Different ways of looking at the truth

In the history section above, you might be wondering:

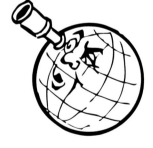

- How can we mention scientific approaches to quality without writing about John Henry Ford and his motor car production line?
- How can the history of a human relations approach to quality fail to mention the work of Charles Handy on motivation, Meredith Belbin and his understanding of how roles within a team impact on performance, John Adair on leadership, or Bruce Tuckman on group processes?
- How can Total Quality Management fail to mention Rosabeth Moss-Kanter, Kaizen or Six Sigma?

It's beyond the scope of this chapter to cover all of these in detail. Yes, we would urge you to delve into some of these because all of them provide a different window for looking at quality – and ultimately different aspects of 'the truth'. You can find more about each of these on our website and even more on Wikipedia and www.businessballs.com – treat them as your friends.

Beware: every way of seeing is also a way of not seeing

At this stage, you may be wondering which theoretical frameworks you should concentrate on. Do you look at Robert Pirsig's stuff or Charles Handy's? Later, you will realise that there are different ways of measuring quality. Again, which do you choose?

KUNG-FU

Remember the 1970s American TV series 'Kung-Fu'? Kwai Chang Caine (David Carradine) is the orphaned son of an American man and a Chinese woman in mid-19th century China. After his maternal grand-father's death, he is accepted for training at a Shaolin monastery, where he grows up to become a Shaolin priest and martial arts expert. The series follows his journey to 'enlightenment' guided by blind Master Po (who gives the young learner Caine the nickname *'Grasshopper'*). Here's a conversation that many of you will remember and which we feel demonstrates the point that although we may have eyes, many of us will fail to see.

After blind Master Po easily defeats young Caine in combat . . .

Master Po: Ha, ha, never assume because a man has no eyes he cannot see. Close your eyes. What do you hear?

Young Caine: I hear the water, I hear the birds.

Master Po: Do you hear your own heartbeat?

Young Caine: No.

Master Po: Do you hear the grasshopper that is at your feet?

Young Caine: [looking down and seeing the insect] Old man, how is it that you hear these things?

Master Po: Young man, how is it that you do not?

Whatever you choose, remember this and keep it at the back of your mind: every way of seeing is also a way of not seeing. Each shows you a different perspective of 'the object' but not one of them will show you all angles.

The metaphysics of quality

There is one thinker on quality whose contribution is important and whom it is difficult to place in a particular movement. Indeed, a central tenet of **Robert Pirsig's** postmodern text[1] is that quality cannot be classified or pigeonholed. Quality is indefinable. Like good music, we all know quality when we experience it, but as soon as we analyse quality, we change it. Quality precedes any intellectual construction. In order to understand quality better, Pirsig presents a dialectic: static and dynamic quality. (*A dialectic is single idea/truth, which can be better understood by examining the argument, usually presented as a contrast/tension between two extremes.*)

Robert M Pirsig: the metaphysics of quality

Static quality: As soon as quality is 'defined' it becomes static. Static quality can be conceptualised and put into patterns. Pirsig defines four patterns: inorganic, biological, social and intellectual.

Dynamic quality: At this extreme of the dialectic, quality is a universal force and is ever changing. In striving for dynamic quality, we know that we will never get there, but we also know that this is unimportant. The striving and the journey become the destination. In climbing to the unseen, unattainable and ever-changing quality summit, the richness is found on the sides of the mountain!

So, what matters to you: is it the journey or the destination? In fact, what's the ethos of the organisation to which you belong and is that at variance with yours? Do you need to realign yourselves before you move on? At this point, you may find it helpful to sit cross-legged on the floor, close your eyes, raise your palms heavenwards and gently hum

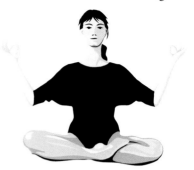

'Ommmmmmmmm'

Those readers who have not achieved a state of oneness with the universe may be forgiven for screaming aloud: *'Enough of the history!'* Indeed, *Grasshopper*, we must move on and look at how these ideas shape the principles of quality assurance in medical education.

Defining quality

Different people see quality as meaning different things, and it's not surprising that there are a number of different definitions flying around in the healthcare sector. Actually, the next time you see a fellow medic, your Practice Manager, and a suitable patient, ask them what they think quality is. A colleague might say something about clinical acumen, a Practice Manager about access and a patient about communication skills. And what's even more interesting is that different people within the same subgroup will have different opinions: some patients (especially those with chronic diseases) might stress good communication skills or continuity of care while others focus on clinical diagnosis and management.

So, back to the question – how do we define quality? The definition of quality is always context dependent; the definition of quality in healthcare is constantly changing because the NHS is forever changing. You need to determine first what the different stakeholders' perspectives on quality are. If you then incorporate a *balance* of these different dimensions you will end up with a definition of quality that is context driven and tailored to your needs.

Some of you will be disappointed by our suggestion at developing your own definition of quality. Perhaps you were hoping for a 'universal answer'. But we hope you can see that the truth (quality in this case) has to be socially negotiated. For those of you still disappointed, perhaps the following generic way of looking at quality might make you happier.

In simple terms, quality is

- Doing the right *thing*, at the right *time* and in the right *way*.
- About best performance within the available resources.

The right thing, the right time and the right way have to be socially negotiated among the different stakeholders.

What's your ethos towards quality?

Before looking at quality ask yourself what it is you are trying to do.

1 **Driving quality improvement:** are you interested in quality because you want to see how you are doing, and because you genuinely want to do things better?

or

2 **Simply measuring quality in itself:** are you more interested in assessing quality for regulation and performance management?

 Top Tip: In the current climate, there is too much focus on measuring quality in itself: productivity targets, waiting times and so on. These measurements are usually politically driven and often used to highlight things to the public (public accountability). However, when people engage in quality with their own hearts and minds (i.e. their own desire to drive quality improvement), that's when quality is truly liberated – that's when it becomes alive, dynamic and automatic.

Quality in a sea of jargon

Management gurus like to use jargon – perhaps to make themselves look better or make you feel 'they know what they're talking about'. We've listed some here for the sake of completeness. However, we'd like to stress that fine tuning your ethos and understanding of quality is more important than any of these terms.

Quality improvement (QI)

- Answers the question: how can we provide a better service?
- Quality improvement is about individuals or organisations wanting to *drive* improvement (preferably from within rather than external pressure) – because they're engaged with its true meaning.
- It offers people the opportunity to excel and therefore leads to an increase in motivation and job satisfaction.

Quality assessment

- Answers the question: how good are we?
- It's a systematic approach to assessing performance compared with selected performance standards; measuring quality in a particular setting using various tools.
- It usually helps people develop a clear understanding of what is expected of them or the organisation.
- The 'results' tell you how well (or badly) you might be driving but not the responsible causal factors (which could be something external to the organisation like deprivation, the recession and so on).

Quality assurance (QA)

- Answers the question: can you help us assure others that we're good enough?
- The focus is on accountability to the stakeholders: in higher education, assurance is a process of establishing stakeholder confidence that the provision (input, process and outcomes) fulfils expectation or measures up to threshold minimum requirements (often called data quality objectives). The aim is to reduce the uncertainty about how good a quality of service someone or an organisation provides.

- UNESCO says it's not just about assuring stakeholders about the quality. It's bigger than that and that QA should embrace all of assessing, monitoring, *guaranteeing*, maintaining and improving quality.[12]
- The Council for Higher Education Accreditation's (CHEA) definition in respect of education is: a planned and systemic review process of an institution or programme to determine that acceptable standards of education, scholarship and infrastructure are being maintained and enhanced.[13]
- Quality assurance versus quality improvement: quality assurance is about problem *detection*; quality improvement is about problem *prevention*. Therefore, quality assurance is *reactive* whereas quality improvement is *proactive*. Quality assurance is usually driven by a *few* high-level managers, but quality improvement is the responsibility of *everybody*.
- And don't confuse quality assurance with accreditation. The former is only a prerequisite for the latter.

Total quality management (TQM)
- A management philosophy that emphasises a commitment to excellence throughout all levels of an organisation (people and processes).

Continuous quality improvement (CQI)
- A term used to denote the constant striving for and pursuit of *excellence*.
- That's all we'd like to say about CQI!

Enough terminology and jargon – we're even falling asleep ourselves here. Let's move on to something more meaty, like developing a quality assurance programme.

The four tenets of quality assurance[14]
Think about these four things whenever you need to develop a quality assurance programme:
1 QA should be oriented towards meeting the **needs and expectations of the different stakeholders** (especially patients and the community; in education, think about educators and trainees).
2 QA doesn't just focus on outcomes. It focuses on **structure** and **processes** and **outcomes**. This allows a deeper understanding of what's going on.
3 QA must use **data** to analyse service delivery processes. Effective problem-solving should be based on facts and **what is real** – not assumptions and perceptions.
4 QA should encourage a **team approach** to problem-solving and quality improvement. Collaborative participation in quality improvement builds consensus and reduces resistance to change.

Developing a QA programme from scratch

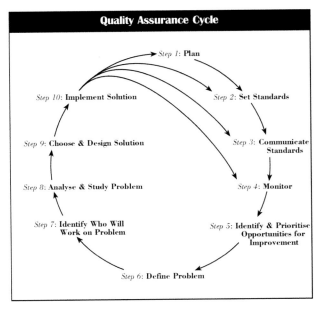

QA cycle by DiPrete Brown et al.[14]

Most of what follows in this section has been adapted from a wonderful document called *Quality Assurance of Health Care in Developing Countries* by DiPrete Brown et al.[14] If you've been set the task of developing a new QA process from scratch, we strongly urge you to get a copy.

Most organisations already engage in activities related to QA without realising it. This means that you already have a foundation upon which you can build a more comprehensive QA programme. QA should be a cyclical and iterative process; the more rounds of the cycle an organisation experiences, the more comfortable they will become with it; it is impossible to improve the quality in all areas at once on the first round. So, take it easy!

Selecting indicators
- The quality indicators that are selected must represent activity that is **important to measure** (and hence be 'fit for purpose'). Otherwise, clinicians and trainees start neglecting areas that are never measured.
- In addition, think about the **practicalities** of measuring that indicator. Sometimes an indicator has good evidence behind it (i.e. it is important) but is impractical to implement. It's all a balancing act.
- As time goes on, some of the quality activities and indicators will need **renegotiating in light of change** – which, in the NHS and GP training, is inevitable.

Setting standards
Standards provide some sort of yardstick against which to benchmark performance. Most people go for statistical measurements (a quantitative approach) – like 80% of your diabetics having a HbA1C below whatever or 95% of a scheme's trainees passing the CSA on the first attempt. Even so, this needn't be all about numbers; think about using qualitative approaches for those things that are harder to measure. Qualitative approaches (e.g. patient satisfaction questionnaires) often reflect reality (and, therefore, quality) more closely and facilitate a deeper understanding of what's really going on. There's an excellent document on our website called *Probophilia* which explores the tension between the quantitative and the qualitative – we urge you to read it and later in this chapter we will check if you have! ☺

When setting thresholds of performance:

- You *must* set **minimum** levels of acceptable performance.
- You *should* set a **range** of acceptable levels of performance.
- You *could* define what makes an **excellent** level of performance.

Identifying and defining problems to work on

- Meaningful and sustainable quality improvement effort depends on identifying problems, understanding them (e.g. root causes) and then working on them.
- Therefore, problems need to be defined precisely. If they're too general (e.g. *'We don't get on as a team'*), it becomes difficult to provide specific/concrete solutions. So take the time to develop clarity about the problem.
- Problem definition is an iterative process: as a team tries to define a problem, they will challenge and change each other's thought processes. They may decide to address one aspect of a multifaceted problem but whatever is chosen, **team consensus is essential**.
- Once you've identified and clarified your problems, refer to your team and get some sort of consensus about how important each one is. Only tackle those that are within your remit.
- Beware of problem statements that blame rather than define the problem (*e.g. 'The doctors are arrogant and horrible to patients'*). Problems should refer to specific processes or activities so that the improvement effort is well focused and measurable. So, in this example, the problem might be that *'patients don't feel welcomed, respected and valued'*. The improvement effort might be *'to deliver communication skills training – specifically helping doctors to build rapport and develop a shared management plan'*.

Problem-solving

- One must build up an accurate and detailed picture of a problem (and its root causes) before one can think about problem-solving it. And we are going to say it again: numbers do not tell you the whole story. Therefore, try to use a combination of qualitative (e.g. surveying people) and quantitative (e.g. statistical analyses) approaches to deepen your understanding of the problem.
- Make sure you and your team prioritise and pick the right problems to work on. Prioritise the small number of problems with the greatest potential impact (see Pareto principle later) and concentrate on problems that are amenable to change. Working on the manageable problems will pay more dividends than the chunky complex ones – and 'early wins' improve team confidence as the team experience the progress being made.
- Finally, when the team is engaged in problem-solving encourage them to think creatively. Think about a pilot project if the solution requires substantial resources or if there is considerable uncertainty about its effectiveness.

The QA process

- If you're the QA champion, you don't have to do all of this on your own. Use the workforce around you for every step of the QA cycle: from setting the standards to problem-solving and generating solutions. They often understand local conditions better than the managers and as a result the standards or solutions developed are more likely to be appropriate, real and effective. They are also more likely to accept and engage in QA activities more readily if they're involved with it right from the start.

- Don't be directive: as the QA champion your role should simply be to facilitate, coordinate, coach and advise.

- And an ideal QA programme is one where the data collection, quality assessment and improvement activities are either part of or incorporated into the organisation's routine management functions. In other words, that it doesn't intrude too heavily on the day-to-day activities. You will make enemies if you increase the burden on training practices or other organisations by getting them to do lots of data generation. And service delivery (which is ultimately what matters) becomes affected as the effort is hijacked by the QA process.

  Ask yourself:

  1 *'What is just enough and won't involve too much extra work?' 'Can some of the indicators go?'*
  2 *'Is there data that is routinely available that we can use – like prescribing or referral data?'*
  3 *Am I using qualitative data that is simply too much hard work to collect? Is there an easier way?*

- There is a continuing debate whether quality assurance is best done internally or externally. Askling *et al.* suggest a compromise: 'A national quality assurance system might offer conceptual tools and basic facts for internal debate about the nature and purpose of higher education'.[16]

- Oh, and don't forget to **re-evaluate** your new QA process – did it work, lessons learned, tweaks for the future and so on.

 Top Tip: Refine your QA process by sharing your experiences with others – get some ideas from those within the organisation and outside. How you present this data depends on who you're talking to: clinical teams might want outcome and statistical measures, commissioners perhaps value for money and for patients – something that's easy to understand.

Your approach to QA in medical education

1 Ambition

Some of you may be uncomfortable with the notion of being ambitious. Personally, any mention of a 'world class service' has us reaching for the prochlorperazine and the barf bag. Harry Potter aficionados will remind us that ambition is the quality most valued by Salazar Slytherin. **Suspend such negative associations with the word ambition.** Perhaps ambition is the wrong word? President Barack Obama used the word 'audacity' in his book about reclaiming the American dream: *The Audacity of Hope.* Yes, audacity. We *ought* to allow ourselves to dream the impossible dream, to dare to be excellent. Quality *is* a bold, dynamic and exciting prospect. We should encourage one another to set ourselves developmental, aspirational and continuously rising standards. We don't get out of bed in the morning to be average.

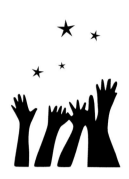

2 Inclusivity, integration, cooperation and collaboration

Quality is everyone's concern. Before it merged with the GMC, the Postgraduate Medical Education and Training Board (PMETB)[17] stated that **'Quality Assurance'** is undertaken by the regulator, **'Quality Management'** is undertaken by deaneries, while **'Quality Control'** is undertaken by Local Education Providers. It may, or may not, be helpful to subdivide and delineate responsibilities in this way; but *everyone* involved should be empowered to deliver quality in medical education. We should recognise the need for collaboration and cooperation. We should acknowledge that some of the important factors that impact on quality for our learners cross organisational boundaries. Those who manage integrated systems should be concerned about quality in the systems that they manage. Those who provide education should be concerned about the quality of that provision.

3 Proportionality

> A Medical Director of one of our medium-sized trusts told me that in the last 12 months his trust has had 51 days of on-site visits by regulators and agencies involved in external quality control.

You might wonder how any organisation can function and focus on quality when the organisation is subject to that degree of external inspection? Perhaps this was an extreme case? Could any of those visits have been coordinated to reduce the impact on the trust? Could the regulators have used processes other than on-site visits? Did the visiting regulatory bodies even realise that there had been so many other regulatory visits? Our efforts to assure quality should be proportionate. We should target quality assurance processes based on probability and risk. We should remember the Pareto principle[18] (that 80% of the effects come from 20% of the causes) and target our efforts at the areas that generate most opportunity for improvement. We should assess the impact of any quality assurance process and align our processes with other parallel processes where there are synergies.

Proportionality is dependent on context. Many systems work on a principle of 'earned autonomy' where parts of the system with a proven track record of delivery of quality may be subject to 'light touch' external monitoring. The wider environmental context (political, economic, technological and socio-demographic factors) will also shape our approaches to assuring quality. For example, during economic downturn, approaches may be more focused on best value and cost reduction, rather than added value.

4 Clarity, transparency and accountability

The purpose of quality initiatives should be clear. Processes and standards should be simple, joined up, consistent, fair and clearly understood by all stakeholders. Aspirational standards should be differentiated from minimum acceptable standards. Lines of accountability should be stated, particularly with respect to regulation. Where processes are designed to be independent there should be no conflicts of interest. There should be appropriate scrutiny of quality, including scrutiny by stakeholders who are external to the organisation or system. For example, the inclusion of lay members in quality processes.

5 Measurement and triangulation

- If I measure something, that gives me data . . . but data is *not* quality.
- If I collate the data, give it some context, then I have information . . . but information is not quality.
- If I comprehend and understand the information (what it tells me and what it fails to tell me), then I have knowledge . . . but knowledge is not quality.
- If I use this knowledge to create choice, have impact and to change things for the better . . . **then I might have quality** (and not all change is improvement!).

These days we live in an age of regulation and measurement. Even so, let's put that down to one side for a moment and rediscover the true spirit of measurement. When we set out on an ambitious task, we need to know how we are doing. We measure ourselves to find out whether we are making progress. We don't measure ourselves to create a carrot or a stick! We need to be able to see how close we are getting to our desired destination – and that won't happen if there aren't any measurable milestones along the way. For that purpose, we need 'SMART' objectives, which are **S**pecific, **M**easurable, **A**chievable, **R**ealistic and **T**ime-bound.

And all measurement is subject to error. We may have blind spots, we may not measure the right thing, we may measure it in the wrong way, or we may measure without accuracy. Therefore, it's important to triangulate. **Triangulation** is a process where something is measured in different ways or from different sources/perspectives to build up a more accurate picture of where we are.

6 Judgement

If measurement is prone to error, then judgement is even more challenging. Judgement requires the evaluation of measurements (qualitative and quantitative – see below), including consideration of corroborating and conflicting evidence, in order to come to a synthesis and a decision with respect to quality. Some judgements, for example, whether a training placement is fit for purpose, are 'high-stake' judgements.

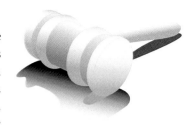

Measurement – what's more important: quality or quantity?

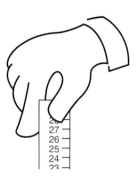

Quantitative measurement tends to focus on numbers and frequencies rather than on meaning, description or experience. Quantitative data invites statistical analysis. It is worth remembering that *'the numbers are not the story'*, and it is worth asking: *'What's the story behind the numbers?'*

Qualitative measurement tends to collect data that describes meaning. Qualitative measurement can tell the story and can aid a focus on understanding. **It tends to measure the more hard-to-measure aspects of quality.** Examples of qualitative instruments include multi-source feedback, patient satisfaction questionnaires, review meetings, interviews, reviewing case notes and analysing significant events.

So, if you want to assess the quality of the therapeutic relationship between doctor and patient, you would want to use qualitative methods (like patient satisfaction questionnaires) rather than quantitative ones. Some of the following vignettes will hopefully add further clarity about which to use and when.

SCENARIO 1: QUANTITATIVE VS QUALITATIVE

A *quantitative* analysis of Clinical Skills Assessment (CSA) results for the May 2010 diet shows that, compared to national pass/fail rates, one training programme has 10% higher than expected numbers of trainees who have failed.

   Question 1: Does that mean that this particular training programme is a poor performer?

   Question 2: Does that mean that this programme offers poorer training compared to the rest?

   Question 3: Does that mean that this particular training programme needs to buck up its ideas and do some better consultation skills teaching (which is a strong component of the CSA)?

   What if we now told you that a *qualitative* analysis showed excellent consultation skills teaching and feedback? And that this particular training programme was particularly good at identifying and putting on extra training for trainees who needed additional help with CSA.

Answers:

Q1 – This training programme was a poor performer this time around, but you cannot make a global judgement about it being a poor performer in general without comparing today's figures with those of the past. Perhaps they just had a higher cluster of below average trainees this year? The numbers *do not* tell you the story.

   Q2 – This training programme does not necessarily offer poor training compared to other programmes. You simply cannot make this inference; you need to talk to them and find out what they actually do. Again, they may be providing good training but just have more than their fair share of underperformers. The numbers *do not* tell you the story.

Q3 – No, this training programme does not necessarily need to buck up its ideas and consultation skills teaching. In fact, you can see from the qualitative survey that they went the extra mile.

The only thing the numbers do is to make you want to make other comparisons – longitudinal comparison against the previous pass/fail rates in the same programme and comparison to other training programmes in the deanery.

SCENARIO 2: QUANTITATIVE VS QUALITATIVE

A small voluntary medical team visits a village of 1500 inhabitants where 300 people are identified as having TB. The medical team manages to give *all* those with TB (and close contacts) either treatment or prophylaxis. The numbers sound great, don't they? The team deserves a pat on the back for its *100%* success rate (quantitative).

But what if we told you that a year later 25 people from the village died of TB. Now you're asking, 'How can that be?' Answer – the numbers don't tell you the whole story! Talking to some of the members of the community (a qualitative approach) highlighted that while people were given medication, they were not counselled on taking it. Many were so frightened of the red urine (a known harmless side-effect of TB treatment) that they stopped medication prematurely. In the future, we now know what needs to be done to reduce wastage (in both effort and cost) and, more importantly, to save lives (the ultimate measure of quality).

What should we measure?

'It is not possible to learn without measuring, but it is possible – and very wasteful – to measure without learning.'

Donald Berwick, Administrator for Medicare and Medicaid Services

'Not everything that counts can be counted; not everything that can be counted counts.'

Albert Einstein

'The most important things cannot be measured.'

William Edwards Denning, American Statistician (1900–93)

 Top Tip: Did you read that document on our website called *Probophilia*? If you haven't, we suggest you take a moment to do that now. It won't take long, and it explores the tension between the quantitative and the qualitative.

Quality is a comprehensive and multifaceted concept. In terms of the quality of GP training, there's so much rich information that tells a story that we probably **don't need more measurement**; we may **need better measurement** and **better ways of understanding and learning**.

One approach is to introduce some structure to our data; a skeleton on which to hang our observations, qualitative and quantitative. Avedis Donabedian,[19,20] a public health pioneer, described three distinct aspects of quality in healthcare: *outcome*, *process* and *structure*: **the Donabedian triad**.

Although he had misgivings about using outcomes *alone* as a measure of quality, he still believed that outcomes remained the ultimate validation of the effectiveness and quality of medical care.[19] However, others (including us) argue that good outcomes are impossible unless you have good structures and processes, and it's the process and structure levels that will make a real difference at a practice level.

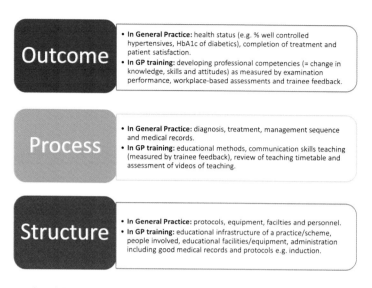

Examples of the Donabedian triad as applied to general practice and GP training

The Donabedian triad is one way of grouping observations. Remember that every way of seeing is also a way of not seeing. The Donabedian triad does not encompass the assessment, measurement or evaluation of culture or values, for example.

Observations can also be grouped into themes or domains. In the Department of Health publication: *The Next Stage Review*, Lord Darzi[21] describes three elements of quality:

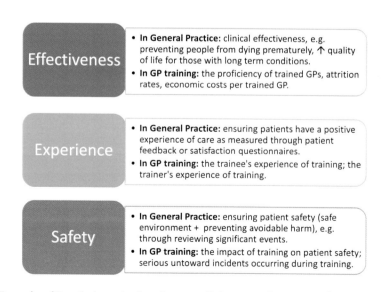

Examples of Darzi's elements of quality as applied to general practice and GP training.

Quality domains in education

In the UK, the current set of quality domains in education are in a state of flux. Therefore, anything we write here will become out of date by the time of publication. We've decided to put something together in a document called *Quality Domains in Education* on our website, which will be updated in line with future changes. This practical document illustrates exactly how to select and define indicators for the current dimensions of quality in education that are in place.

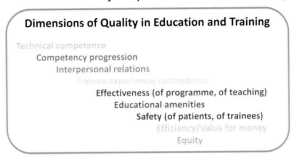

Dimensions of Quality in Education and Training

Technical competence
Competency progression
Interpersonal relations
Trainee experience/centredness
Effectiveness (of programme, of teaching)
Educational amenities
Safety (of patients, of trainees)
Efficiency/Value for money
Equity

Triangulation in education

Over-reliance on one method of assuring quality is a source of error. *'If your only tool is a hammer, then all your problems will be nails.'* There is often an overlap in data and obtaining data from different sources can improve reliability and tell a more accurate story. Try to develop different ways of looking at the same thing to see if they match (and whether that version of 'the truth' is real).

> As an Educational Supervisor, I noticed that one of my trainees seemed to have 'Needs Further Development' grades for the competency 'Working with Colleagues and in Teams' in a number of his Case Based Discussions. That was pretty odd because I got on well with him and thought he was of quite a personable nature. Was I getting a skewed picture from his CBDs or was my own face-to-face interpretation of his personable nature a wrong picture? I decided to triangulate by looking at his recent Multi-Source Feedback and his Clinical Supervisor's Report – both assessments have specific elements about working with colleagues and in teams. I was relieved to see a glowing MSF and CSR which I felt were stronger (i.e. more valid) indicators of this competency because they measure what the trainee *does* rather than what they *say* they do.

This vignette demonstrates the importance of triangulation in terms of checking out competencies. Something similar needs to be done when checking out the data you have on quality; is it representative of the truth? Consider triangulating with data from the overlapping metrics in this Venn diagram.

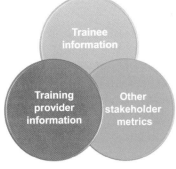

- **Trainee data:** feedback, significant events (triggers), surveys (internal and external), attendance, assessments, ARCP, CSA, AKT, completion rates.
- **Training provider data:** facilities, staffing, policies (e.g. induction), teaching syllabus, Trainer appraisal, feedback from other educators and peer review, trigger events, visits and inspections (triggered visits, routine visits, themed visits), attendance, Trainer qualifications, assessment of teaching skills, clinical quality markers (QOF, patient safety data etc.).

- **Wider metrics:** training outcome data, examination data, completion/attrition rates, equality and diversity data, economic data, annual reports.

Perhaps the most important triangulation is between **education governance** and **clinical governance**. If we place our trainees in environments where clinical governance (clinical processes and clinical outcomes) are poor, our trainees are likely to emulate poor practice. It is possible to have good service and poor training (i.e. good clinical governance and poor education governance), but it is almost impossible to have poor service and good training (i.e. poor clinical governance and good education governance). Poor service is almost invariably linked with poor training. Perhaps the most dramatic example of this is the report of the Care Quality Commission into the Mid Staffordshire Hospitals NHS Trust,[23] where poor education and training (which was identified) ought to have raised concerns about the standards of clinical care.

Quality assurance or triangulating through visits

One of the most popular quality assurance tools is the visit. We have already stated the danger of over-reliance on one tool for quality assurance. If you are thinking of employing 'the practice visit', make sure it doesn't become a bureaucratic, complex, high-stake, mini-accreditation tool in itself. Instead, use the practice visit to:

1 **understand** the context
2 **see** *actual* practice at a ground level, and to
3 **feel** the quality culture of an organisation.

Comprehensive visits where the visiting team 'turns over every stone' are characteristic of low trust highly regulated systems. In contrast, the 'leadership walk around'[24] is a good tool for improving patient safety; more can be found at www.patientsafetyfirst.nhs.uk

Synthesis and judgement

How often should you quality assure? A typical approach is to review quality data periodically. The period can be annual (e.g. for the purposes of providing an annual report on the quality of training), or the period can be for longer time scales (e.g. limited approval for x years). A 'periodic' approach to quality is a pragmatic way of making sure that progress is reviewed. However, it also runs *contrary* to our earlier assertion that quality improvement is a comprehensive and *continuous* process. There are, however, other approaches.

- Triggers – sentinel events to trigger more detailed review of the quality of training.
- Review precipitated by external regulatory review.
- Continuous monitoring: using 'Dashboard', 'Scorecards' and 'RAG ratings'.

Dashboards and Scorecards are ways of grouping and presenting important data from a variety of sources 'at a glance'. Dashboards and scorecards enable organisations to measure how well they are doing and compare themselves with others. They also allow other stakeholders to do the same. NHS Hertfordshire has produced a Scorecard which you can see on our website. Perhaps you can tweak it to develop something for your own purpose (benchmarking GP practices, GP training practices, GP training schemes or dare we say GP consortia!)? Even simpler are RAG ratings – RAG stands for Red, Amber, Green and is a visual way of indicating progress or level of risk – sometimes called the Traffic Light Rating System.[25]

Summary

We started this chapter with three top tips.

1 Take an interest in quality.
2 The pursuit of quality is a marker of quality in itself.
3 You will recognise quality when you come across it.

We can now add some additional advice.

- Be bold in your quality goals.
- Be 'SMART' when setting quality objectives and think in terms of structure *and* process *and* outcome *or* effectiveness *and* safety *and* experience.
- Develop a set of indicators that truly measure what you truly regard as quality. Indicators must be 'fit for purpose'. Try to use data that is routinely available to reduce the burden of data gathering.
- Avoid over-reliance on a single indicator or single source – triangulate!
- Improving quality should not be seen as an isolated activity – it should be continuous.
- Improving quality is the remit of everybody. It should percolate through *all* levels of an organisation. Individuals needn't resist or be scared of it. Instead, they should embrace it and see it as a friend, not a foe. To achieve this: involve others, be transparent, and adopt cooperative approaches to quality. Spend time creating a positive, open and honest culture. Get them to help you with selecting indicators, setting standards – in fact, involve them in all parts of the QA cycle.
- Your role (as quality champion or lead) should be to facilitate others in their quest for quality improvement and not to dictate it. Of course, this also means providing the necessary resources and tools to do this.
- And, remember, it's not all about number crunching – be creative and think about the qualitative angle for the hard-to-measure domains.

Improving quality doesn't cost anything – often it pays instead! Even so, remember that too much measuring can be overkill. The following quote may resonate with many of you. It serves as a warning to those in the pursuit of quality – **and that is all of us**.

> Imposing national standards and continuously monitoring performance jeopardises the essence of the welfare state, which is autonomous professional judgement. Imposing yet more insensitive monitoring and national standards can only be catastrophic – wasting more money, further exasperating staff and driving out common sense.
>
> Simon Jenkins writes for *The Guardian* and received a knighthood for journalism

Finally, we leave you with a couple of quotes from the report commissioned by The King's Fund[26] on quality in general practice (a document really worth reading).

Quality is complex and multidimensional, and no single basket of indicators is likely to capture all perspectives or cover all dimensions of quality in general practice. Nonetheless, we have no doubt that important dimensions of quality of care in general practice can be measured, and routine data sets used, to assess the comparative performance of practice.

The King's Fund: 'Improving the Quality of Care in General Practice' (2011)[26]

The King's Fund went on to review the different ways in which quality was being assessed in general practice and this is what they found:

We found a crowded landscape of quality measurement and reporting initiatives. We conclude that there is a strong case for simplifying and rationalising these activities in order to reduce wasteful duplication of effort and avoid confusion. This would potentially reduce the growing burden on commissioners and general practices and create a more accessible, transparent and coherent picture of quality – one that is more easily understood both by professionals and the public.

The King's Fund: 'Improving the Quality of Care in General Practice' (2011)[26]

We believe the same applies to GP training and education.

A sample of resources on our website
- Probophilia.
- The Dark Side of Quality Measurement.
- Quality Domains in Education.

Please give us some feedback on this chapter to help shape it for the next edition.
Go to www.essentialgptrainingbook.com and simply click on the title of this chapter.

References

1 Pirsig R. *Zen and the Art of Motorcycle Maintenance: an inquiry into values.* London: Corgi; 1974.
2 Blanchard K, Johnson S. *The One Minute Manager: the quickest way to increase your own prosperity.* New York: William Morrow & Co; 1982.
3 Landsberger HA. *Hawthorne Revisited.* Ithaca, New York: Cornell University Press; 1961.
4 Murray HA. *Explorations in Personality.* New York: Oxford University Press; 1938.
5 McGregor D. *The Human Side of Enterprise.* New York: McGraw Hill Higher Education; 1960.
6 Herzberg F. *The Motivation to Work.* New York: John Wiley & Sons; 1959.
7 Maslow A. *Motivation and Personality.* New York: Harper; 1954. p. 236.
8 More on William Edwards Deming at: http://deming.org (also covered very well in Wikipedia).
9 Juran J. *Quality Control Handbook.* New York: McGraw-Hill; 1951.
10 Ishikawa K. *Introduction to Quality Control.* JH Loftus (trans.). Tokyo: 3A Corporation; 1990.
11 Shingo S. *A Study of the Toyota Production System.* Portland, Oregon: Productivity Press; 1989.
12 Vlăsceanu L, Grünberg L, Pârlea D. *Quality Assurance and Accreditation: a glossary of basic terms and definitions.* Bucharest: UNESCO-CEPES; 2007. Available at: www.cepes.ro/publications/pdf/Glossary_2nd.pdf (accessed 29 January 2011).
13 Council for Higher Education Accreditation (CHEA). *Glossary of Key Terms in Quality Assurance and Accreditation.* 2001. Available at: www.chea.org/international/inter_glossary01.html (accessed 4 February 2011).
14 DiPrete Brown L, Miller Franco L, Rafeh N, Hatzell T. *Quality Assurance of Health Care in Developing Countries.* Available at: http://pdf.usaid.gov/pdf_docs/PNABQ044.pdf

15 Shingo S, McLoughlin C, Epley T. *Kaizen and the Art of Creative Thinking: the scientific thinking mechanism.* PCS Inc. and Enna Products Corporation; 2007.

16 Askling B, Hofgaard Lycke K, Stave O. Institutional leadership and leeway – important elements in a national system of quality assurance and accreditation: experiences from a pilot study. *Tertiary Education and Management*; 2004: **10**: 107–20.

17 PMETB, *The Quality Framework for Postgraduate Medical Education and Training in the UK.* 2007. Available at: www.pmetb.org.uk/index.php?id=qualityframework&tktest=72

18 http://en.wikipedia.org/wiki/Pareto_principle

19 Donabedian A. Evaluating the quality of medical care. *Milbank Memorial Fund Quarterly.* 1966; **44**: 166–206.

20 Donabedian A. *The Definition of Quality and Approaches to its Assessment.* Ann Arbor, Michigan: Health Administration Press; 1980.

21 Department of Health. *High Quality Care For All – NHS Next Stage Review Final Report.* Department of Health; 2008. Available at: www.dh.gov.uk/en/publicationsandstatistics/publications/publicationspolicyandguidance/DH_085825

22 General Medical Council. *Quality Improvement Framework for Undergraduate and Postgraduate Medical Education and Training in the UK.* GMC; 2011. Available at: www.gmc-uk.org/education/9038.asp

23 www.cqc.org.uk/_db/_documents/Investigation_into_Mid_Staffordshire_NHS_Foundation_Trust.pdf

24 www.institute.nhs.uk/safer_care/general/leadership_walkaround.html

25 http://en.wikipedia.org/wiki/Traffic_light_rating_system

26 The King's Fund. *Improving the Quality of Care in General Practice.* 2011. Available at: www.kingsfund.org.uk/publications/gp_inquiry_report.html

PART NINE

The Trainee in Difficulty

The Trainee Experiencing Difficulty

JULIE ECCLES – GP Trainer (Gateshead) & lead author
JULIE DRAPER – Retired GP (Cambridge); Freelance Consultant (Communication Skills)
GRAHAM RUTT – Head of School (Northern Deanery)   RAMESH MEHAY – TPD (Bradford)

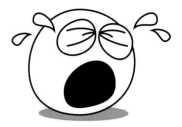

Many trainees experience hard times during their training, but the majority will deal with these instances themselves. A minority may experience difficulties which impact on their training in some way. This is distressing for the trainee and may present challenges for the Trainer or Training Programme Director, particularly where there are real concerns about performance.

This chapter sets out to explore the background and context of the trainee who is experiencing difficulty, and will consider: the size of the problem, some bare essentials you should know, and a framework for assessment and management.

The size of the problem

It is difficult to quantify the number of trainees who experience difficulty, because the majority of problems are successfully managed within the normal training period, either by the learner themselves, or with help from the training programme. However, the National Clinical Assessment Service (NCAS)[1] says that even in the most serious cases, two-thirds of doctors are back at work after remediation.

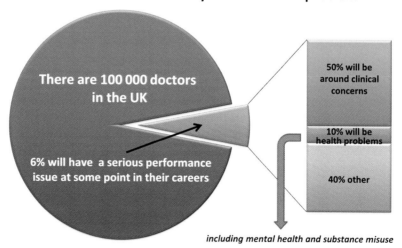

Doctors in difficulty: the size of the problem

There are 100 000 doctors in the UK

6% will have a serious performance issue at some point in their careers

50% will be around clinical concerns

10% will be health problems

40% other

including mental health and substance misuse

*Figures quoted in Donaldson IJ (1994) Doctors with problems in an NHS workforce. BMJ. **308**: 1277–82.[2]*

Does that mean 6 out of every 100 trainees will have serious performance difficulties? Probably, but the important thing to remember is that **with support and remediation, *the majority* of these trainees will complete their training.**

The trajectory of a 'normal' trainee

In your medical student days, do you recall the old adage that 'you have to feel a hundred **normal** abdomens before you can recognise the abnormal one'? The same is true with trainees in difficulty: you need to be clear about what is normal so that you can spot deviations from it.

With a normal trainee, over time you can expect to see:

- a gradual diminution of the number of questions per surgery and a change in the nature of the questions
- a gradual reduction in the consultation length
- an increased ability of the trainee to deal with complex cases independently
- an increasing ability to discover the patient's agenda and address their concerns
- a move from only considering the presenting complaint to addressing other areas such as modifying health seeking behaviour, health promotion and QOF targets
- a move from considering just the needs of the individual patient to enquiring about those of the practice population as a whole, for example, showing awareness of gaps in service (= community orientation).

What are the signs and symptoms of a trainee in difficulty?

Sometimes it can be difficult to spot the trainee in difficulty: many will cope superficially, and some will be very good at hiding the problem (especially if nothing serious has resulted). Hopefully, the following symptoms and signs will help.[3,4]

- **Asking superficial (rather than deep) learning questions:** Over time, the nature and number of questions for a 'normal' trainee alters as they move from requiring information to actively learning about general practice. Different learners spend different lengths of time in each stage but reverting to an earlier stage may be an indication of things getting difficult. Of course normal gradual progression involves occasional backward steps too, but the challenge for the Trainer is to recognise when the trainee is becoming stuck and not moving forward.
- **Never progressing from a low work rate:** The trainee arrives early, stays late but still seems to run behind. They may have little insight into this and complain that they are overworked.
- **Having overt clinical problems:** Strong trainees make the occasional minor error. Average trainees make mostly minor errors. Weak trainees (although they may do well in quite a number of cases) have a pattern of cases with a cluster of errors, some of which are major. The most frequent clinically related performance issues are:
  - poor note keeping
  - inappropriate prescription writing
  - inappropriate investigations
  - failure to follow protocols
  - problems with practical procedures
  - failure to recognise or respond to clinical urgency.

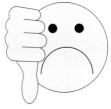

In general, when a catastrophic event happens, it's not usually the result of a major error but rather a succession of minor errors, which together deliver a powerful punch. The problem for the Trainer is to decide at what point this pattern of errors goes beyond reflecting the learning needs of the trainee to constituting a serious cause for concern.

- **Doing the disappearing act:** Not answering their bleep, staff not being able to find them (they go missing), frequent unexpected absence such as Monday and Friday sick leave.
- **Bypass syndrome:** When other members of the team approach anyone except a particular trainee (even if that trainee is the duty doctor), there is a problem!
- **Expelling bursts of anger or tears:** Some trainees who are struggling may become frustrated and irritable but others will show the opposite – withdrawing, not gelling with the team, and becoming insular.
- **Coming across as rigid or inflexible:** Where the trainee appears unwilling to compromise, rejects criticism and is defensive (tending to blame others).

    The MRCGP provides additional pointers:

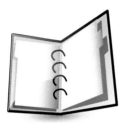

- **Not demonstrating a progression of competence over time:** Mapping out the COT and CBD competency domains over time will help you see a lack of progression and the areas in which it is most marked. (Mapping sheets available at www.bradfordvts.co.uk – click MRCGP > COT, CBD or MiniCEX.)
- **A pretty poor ePortfolio:** Look at their ePortfolio and you'll see: insufficient entries, high numbers of poor-quality entries, little evidence of reflection, and learning needs not being addressed.

 Top Tip: When defining a trainee's performance concern, start from the evidence you have about their performance or behaviour, rather than ticking things off from the anecdotal list above.

A framework for assessment and management: RDM-p[5]

The RDM-p approach is a diagnostic framework to help *guide* your support for *any* trainee, but *especially* when you have one in *difficulty*. It was developed in 2006 by Tim Norfolk, an independent occupational psychologist with extensive experience of working with doctors in difficulty.

 Top Tip: We will attempt to describe a condensed but functional version of the RDM-p approach here, but there is a comprehensive version available on our website (called *The RDM-p Manual*).

---

1 Why RDM-p?

The RDM-p approach stops us from rushing through things and drawing premature conclusions when we've only got a hunch about some of the things going on. Poor performance is often a symptom of things which are usually complex and multifactorial. The RDM-p approach slows us right down. It makes us think about things sequentially, and that starts with carefully defining the actual *performance* concern first. It does this by encouraging us to go back to the *behavioural evidence* we have and re-examine it for themes. Only then are we allowed to explore causal factors. In doing this, it also keeps the performance problem ('symptoms') and the cause ('aetiology') separate. Many other models blur the boundary between these two things, resulting in faulty inferences and hence plans that fail to 'hit the mark'.

> GPs tend to assess patients initially on 'intuitive' pattern recognition. This is fine in principle, provided a GP has the knowledge, training and experience. The key is getting the balance right between this initial recognition (the 'gut feeling') and confirmation through evidence (i.e. being alert for contradictory symptoms and signs). The same should apply when dealing with GP trainees in difficulty. The problem is that most GPs don't have sufficient training or experience in the day-to-day assessment of doctors to risk relying on 'hunches'. Hence, one sometimes hears loose and faintly prejudicial talk, based on questionable assumptions drawn from limited but weary experience. If you think about it, compare the number of trainees a GP might have trained with the number of patients seen – more patients in a day than trainees in a lifetime! And assessment often based on a few days' specific preparation to be a GP Trainer in contrast to 8+ years of medical training. This is why I encourage Trainers to be very deliberate in their approach to analysing performance, and why I've encouraged them to view assessment of their trainees in much the same holistic way as they would their patients. But to bring an additional rigour and care to the process, because of their relative lack of experience in handling such assessment, and the associated risks of making early assumptions. Without that rigour, any complex analytical process is put at unjustifiable risk.
>
> Tim Norfolk[6]

2 The logic underpinning RDM-p

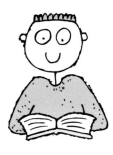

1 *Performance concerns begin with performance*, not personality or health or work relationships – though the latter may be the *cause* of the performance concern.

2 *Therefore, ensuring an accurate **diagnosis** of the problem first through the RDM-p framework* (covered below) is the central part of the process. Start with the *evidence* about the trainee's performance rather than making subjective judgements on what a few people have said. Comments *based on observed events* are more likely to point you in the right direction than the stab in the dark approach which results from analysing subjective comments.

3 *Only then do you start a step-by-step search for causes via the SKIPE framework* (also covered below), which explores whether there are deficiencies in Skills and/or Knowledge or whether there are Internal, Past or External factors contributing to the problem.

4 *The RDM-p approach (via SKIPE) explores how several causal factors may be interacting with each other to cause the problem.* Most other models are deeply flawed because they only get you to look at each individual causal factor in isolation (i.e. as separate entities). In real life, under-performance is a result of several causal factors interacting and influencing each other.

5 *In summary, you use RDM-p then SKIPE to fully diagnose 'the what and the why' of underper-formance.* Only then can appropriate development plans be created to target the specific needs or issues emerging from the 'diagnosis'.

3 Diagnosing the *problem* (through RDM-p)

When you're concerned about a trainee's performance, those concerns usually stem from some sort of evidence about their behaviour – things you, others or the trainees themselves have noticed. For the RDM-p model to work, it's important you collect as much of these *specific* bits of 'evidence' (both negative *and* **positive**) as you can, because the quality of the outcome depends on the quality of the input.

RDM-p

Generally speaking, a trainee's performance concern or difficulty will fall into one or more of the following four categories.

1 Problems with building **relationships**.
2 Problems with **diagnostics** or decision-making *(and not just clinical, but in making decisions for other parts of their lives too*).*
3 Problems with **management** *(management in this sense relating to organisational management rather than in the clinical sense; managing our personal routines and systems).*
4 Problems with **professionalism**, thus honesty, integrity, trust and respect *(a problem here means that there is an attitudinal problem to be addressed by the trainee).*

---

*For example, a trainee who fails to seek medical treatment or advice for their own deteriorating health indicates a problem in the diagnostic domain because of a lack of insight. Accurate self-assessment (i.e. turning the diagnostic eye onto oneself) is a vital part of day-to-day practice.

Let's step aside and look at these in more detail:

Relationship	Diagnostics	Management	Professionalism
• With patients • With staff • With other colleagues (within and outside the practice)	• Assessing patients (and their needs) • Assessing oneself • Assessing staff and colleagues • Decision-making in practice-related activities	• Managing patients • Managing oneself: e.g. performance, health and well-being • Managing staff and colleagues • Managing practice-related activities	• Respect for people • Respect for protocol • Respecting importance of R, D & M • Being aware & carrying out contractual responsibilities

In essence, general practice involves a subtle interaction between three core activities: relationship, diagnostics and management. They could perhaps be visualised as three interlocking 'cogs in the wheel', for which professionalism then provides the essential oil. Within the dynamic interaction between these three areas lies every component of the job, though most attention centres on relationship and diagnostics.

Norfolk and Siriwardena[5]

Signs and symptoms of difficulty in R, D, M or p	
Signs & symptoms of a concern in **RELATIONSHIP**	• Communication and consulting skills – like a lack of empathy, not adapting language and style to the circumstance, not picking up and responding to verbal and non-verbal cues, poor negotiating skills. • Working with colleagues and in teams – not working in a team could be due to poor communication skills, poor delegation or poor leadership skills (not being able to encourage or persuade people/patients to respond willingly or positively to one's decisions or suggestions).
Signs & symptoms of a concern in **DIAGNOSTICS**	• Data gathering and interpretation – not doing enough of this for optimal decision-making (whether for patients, colleagues, other staff or oneself). • Analytical skills – once the data has been gathered, difficulty in prioritising it or offering alternative options, suggestions or explanations. • Decision-making skills – where the trainee has a difficulty in reaching that pivotal point (imagine the peak of a triangle) where a decision has to be made: e.g. when to treat, refer or wait and see. • Examination and technical skills (i.e. practical diagnostic skills) – not doing these in an appropriate manner.
Signs & symptoms of a concern in **MANAGEMENT**	• Managing particular events – a lack of structure to the consultation, not managing their referral letters or pacing a meeting badly. • Managing ongoing events – not maintaining adequate records after home visits, not keeping on top of one's other roles within the practice. • Managing performance – falling behind with ePortfolio entries. • Managing relationships – not providing continuity of care or not routinely *monitoring/ maintaining* one's relationship with colleagues. • Managing oneself – displaying stress-related behaviour, not establishing an effective work-life balance (e.g. no longer playing sport because you're 'too busy', or 'too stressed to relax').
Signs & symptoms of a concern in **PROFESSIONALISM**	• Respect for others – not showing equal respect for patients, colleagues, staff and others; being judgemental. • Respect for one's position – not acting within one's professional roles/boundaries, not appreciating the effect of one's behaviour/actions on others (e.g. running late and showing no regard for the poor patients who have been kept waiting), not minimising risk (e.g. where one's own health might compromise someone else's safety). • Respect for protocol – not adhering to established clinical *and* professional codes of practice. When someone doesn't do referral letters in a timely way, it is clearly a management issue. However, it might also indicate a lack of respect for its *importance*; this lack of respect for process or protocol is a professionalism issue. **This won't necessarily be true in all cases** – some individuals respect the idea of doing letters on time but simply can't quite deliver (i.e. are simply disorganised = a management issue).

Coming back to the evidence . . . after collecting behavioural data about a trainee's underperformance from various sources, (including the trainee, whose perspective is obviously crucial), rather than jumping to conclusions at this point the RDM-p approach gets you to map the evidence to the four RDM-p performance domains. Mapping the evidence in this way helps you to step back, generalise away from those specific bits of evidence, and move towards building a clearer picture of where the performance difficulty lies. The true nature of the difficulty will emerge when you review all four RDM-p areas and see where negative evidence is the most dense (Please note: some pieces of evidence may need to be mapped to more than one domain.)

4 Diagnosing the *causes* (through SKIPE)

Once you've identified which of the four performance domains are problematic, you then need to explore the *causal* factors that lie behind them **and** the *influential* factors that may be maintaining them. This exploration may *start* by exploring the views of relevant others, but should always be *concluded* through discussion with the trainee, where their ideas can be tested against those of others, and a truly holistic understanding can then be reached.

The RDM-p approach again provides a structured and comprehensive way to connect and facilitate discussion around the causal factors – through the 'SKIPE' framework. SKIPE stands for **S**kills, **K**nowledge, **I**nternal factors, **P**ast factors and **E**xternal factors. SKIPE defines the full set of causal and influential factors, which can affect an individual's development in any of the three performance domains (Relationship, Diagnostics, Management), and can also affect the professionalism that underpins them. The SKIPE framework is intentionally kept separate from RDM-p to emphasise the fact that Trainers need to draw on the same principles that should guide clinical practice: searching first to diagnose the **nature** of the problem (via RDM-p) and *only then* searching for possible causes (via SKIPE).

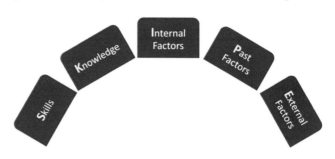

SKIPE in a nutshell	
Skills & Knowledge (the initial 'SK' check)	**When exploring causation, always start with an initial SK check:** *'Is there a skill and/or knowledge issue here?'* Visible behaviour (performance) is a direct glimpse at someone's *skills* and you cannot perform a skill without having some *knowledge* underpinning it.
	So, once you've identified a performance concern, first assess how well the trainee is actually demonstrating the relevant Relationship, Diagnostic and Management **skills**. If there's a problem, then check whether the trainee **knows enough** about those skills; things like how well they understand what the specific skills are in the first place, and how, when and where to use them!
Internal Factors	These are factors currently *acting within* the individual like attitudes/values, personality traits/styles and health/capacity. The trainee's attitudes will largely determine their *professionalism*.
Past Factors	These are the foundations on which individuals build their professional life; they include both early influences (such as upbringing, cultural and educational roots) and more recent influences (such as their experiences in training practices and hospitals). Any of these could be having a dominant or lingering effect on an individual's thinking and behaviour, e.g. a trainee who shows a chronic lack of confidence or strong values based on an upbringing which stressed 'right and wrong'. Tread carefully: it is sensitive territory.
External Factors	These are factors currently *interacting with* the individual – either at home or at work (like relationships, resources and expectations). For example, a single mum trying to cope with two little ones and yet trying to stay on top of being a full-time GP trainee. Or an overworked Trainer becoming frustrated with his 'slow-to-learn' trainee, which leads to a breakdown in their relationship and low self-confidence in the trainee.

All of this is summarised in the diagram below. Study it for a few moments.

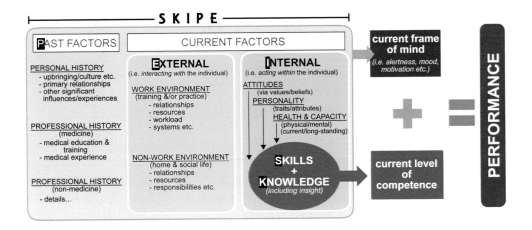

Read the following in reference to the diagram above

Competence is primarily defined in terms of a trainee's knowledge and skills (i.e. what we can actually hear and see as they perform). If these are poor, a trainee is unlikely to have basic competence and, therefore, cannot *perform* well. So when a trainee underperforms, we naturally tend to focus on strengthening their knowledge and skills, hoping that this will redefine and raise competence and hence ultimately improve performance. There's nothing wrong with that; if a trainee lacks knowledge or skills, we clearly need to strengthen them. But the problem is that is all we tend to do – and much of the underlying story may lie elsewhere. The other part of the story is embedded in Internal, Past and External factors, as illustrated in the SKIPE diagram above. These interact with each other to help determine a trainee's current state of mind, as well as potentially influencing the development of *knowledge* and *skills*.

For example, if your colleagues tell you that your trainee's clinical knowledge isn't up to scratch – yes, it may be that his clinical knowledge is indeed poor. However, the fact that he is having relationship difficulties at home and is moonlighting to support a heavy mortgage and three kids is probably leaving him little time for his own personal study. Giving him a bit of extra tutorial time (to improve knowledge) isn't going to have much impact on the situation. Some things in his personal life have to change.

'SKIPE' simply suggests the natural route through these various factors.

- *First* consider the level of **Skill** being demonstrated and the **Knowledge** underpinning it.
- Then step back and think about current **Internal factors** that might be having an impact.
- Then whether any **Past factors** might be having a lingering effect on the individual.
- Finally check whether any **External factors** (i.e. 'outside the individual') are at play.

In summary: Sometimes the 'SK' bit is enough to account for the problem – as we have suggested, not knowing something or not being able to articulate or activate a particular skill has led to problems. So all that is needed might be a straightforward, practical, self-contained entry in the PDP. But often, it is more than just that and for a comprehensive approach, we need to check the 'IPE' bit too. Taking this approach, **SKIPE** gets us to look at potentially influencing factors from within the individual (whether current internal or in their past), and from without (i.e. external factors), and importantly invites us to consider them *together*. From here, appropriate development plans can then be created.

5 The discussion with the trainee

The individual trainee *must* be interviewed at the heart of this process, and in a non-judgemental way that allows *apparent* evidence about a problem, and its causes, to be qualified after weighing the trainee's perspective against the views expressed by others. The discussion has two purposes:

1 For you and the trainee to build an accurate picture *together* (data gathering).
2 To generate *workable* solutions likely to have a greater impact (planning).

The RDM-p approach should parallel the principles of 'good consulting' – in essence, it's a similar journey, and the skills involved are similar: showing respect, building rapport, data gathering, defining the problem, formulating a joint agenda, shared decision-making, joint future planning and so on. In summary, it should be:

1 **Person-centred** – this encourages self-evaluation. Involve them as much as possible right from the start. Give them time and space to digest and reflect on the situation.
2 **Systematic and thorough** – spend time gathering information properly and exploring it to the appropriate level (remember: quality of the input = quality of the output).
3 **Fair and respectful** – listen to what the trainee has to say. Don't prejudge them based on what others have said. Step into their shoes and see their perspective.

In Transactional Analysis[7] terms, try and aim for an adult–adult relationship (where you treat the trainee like an adult and not as a child who needs a telling off). An adult–adult relationship is more likely to result in behaviour change than a parent–child one. This is because an adult–adult relationship encourages trainees to think and determine action for themselves. We are more likely to adopt changes we suggest for ourselves than when they are imposed upon us. No doubt you can relate to that!

How to achieve an adult–adult relationship with your trainee

1 Establish a **safe climate**: comfortable, open and honest.
2 **'Start *low*, then go *slow*'**: By *low* we mean initiating the discussion with items that are not likely to evoke a strong *negative* emotional bite-back response (see Top Tip below). Go *slow*: don't rush from one theme to the next.
3 **Build an accurate picture *together***: Collecting and discussing evidence from all sides.
4 **Don't dive in** and suggest a trainee's perception is wrong. **Validate feelings** and **explore the specifics** first.
5 Encourage as much **reflection and self-evaluation** as possible.
6 Find an appropriate and **specific route to change (collaboratively)**: using the SKIPE framework, get the trainee to come up with specific suggestions. Plan together and follow the patient-centred model you are familiar with.

 Top Tip: Judgements about professionalism are likely to evoke a strong emotional response. How would you feel if someone questioned the level of respect, importance or value you place on things? Wouldn't you bite back? Instead, start with an issue centred within one of the R-D-M domains, where poor professionalism may have influenced outcomes. Only start tackling the professionalism aspect when you feel you have developed enough rapport, the trainee is positively engaged and the focus is already on identifiable RDM evidence.

To prevent conflict

Firstly, make sure you have good feedback skills. If you haven't, build on them by going on a course or something. Then, do the following.

- Establish the purpose of the session: something along the lines of trying to help them and not to punish them.
- Never start discussions by talking about a negative issue first. Instead, concentrate on building rapport. Then accentuate the positive: this will add balance to the discussion so that it doesn't come across as all negative.
- When you're ready to move onto a more tricky area, always gather more information first and explore the other person's perspective. No immediate judgement – just an invitation to explore. Engage in a true two-way dialogue. Don't use judgement words like 'lazy' or 'rude'. Don't dictate; instead use something like Socratic questioning[8] (see brown text below) to help them gain insight about inconsistencies in their current beliefs, so that they automatically search for an alternative point of view.
- Maintain an eye on their verbals and non-verbals and appropriately explore what you hear and see. Tread carefully, be sensitive and validate feelings.
- You may need to revisit and remind each other about the purpose of the session: especially at sticky moments.

Socrates used to get his students to examine their own value and belief statements by asking simple questions, which would gently draw out inconsistencies or contradiction in them. This, in itself, often provided proof for an alternative point of view (the antithesis). Socrates wasn't out there to prove he was right and others were wrong but instead to 'improve the soul of his learners' by freeing them from unrecognised errors.

(There is a document called 'Discussion, Dialogue and Socrates', which tells you more. It can be found on our website as a resource for Chapter 10: Five Pearls of Educational Theory.)

6 To summarise

- Three broad domains define the work of a GP (Relationship, Diagnostics and Management), all underpinned by professionalism. Professionalism is looked at separately because it is clearly not a 'skill', but a reflection of the *approach* taken to one's work (the R-D-M areas). Actually, these four components together map the essence of *any* service profession: **relate** to someone, **diagnose** their needs, **manage** the process, and at all times ensure you act **professionally**. The difference between general practice and many other services is that to be a 'competent' GP, all four elements need to be demonstrated at consistently high levels. The RDM-p model helps you determine which of these are problematic for a trainee in difficulty.
- Each of these domains demands a particular knowledge and skill set (the 'SK' of SKIPE), but their development may also be helped or hindered by wider factors (the 'IPE' of SKIPE).
- The key to using the model with struggling trainees is to first define what's going wrong (using RDM-p). Only then try to determine what's *causing* or *influencing* the problem (by searching the 'SKIPE' framework for clues). In this way, the SKIPE framework helps you to determine causal factors with greater precision, leaving both of you in a position that will generate 'remedies' more likely to succeed.

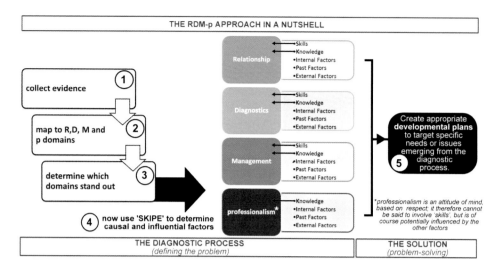

THE DIAGNOSTIC PROCESS
(defining the problem)

THE SOLUTION
(problem-solving)

1 **Collect evidence** from a number of different people (including the trainee) – verbal comments, written statements, things you've noticed, things the trainee has noticed. Don't do anything with this evidence just yet – simply collect it.

2 **Map each piece of evidence** (or statement) – write out each piece of evidence on a separate line and then figure out which of the four RDM-p domains it *possibly* relates to. Some items can be mapped to more than one of the four areas. Mark the statement with one or more of the letters R, D, M or p. Put a '+' sign next to it if it is a positive indicator of that domain and a '–' if it's a negative one (i.e. a criticism). Put a domain in brackets if you think the evidence may be a *weak* (positive or negative) indicator of it. Examples below:

The evidence	RDM-p category	Reasons for the categorisation and areas we might want to explore
Unenthusiastic trainee	(M-) p-	*If a doctor has a poor attitude in terms of their approach to work, this is a **professionalism** issue. If the doctor is unenthusiastic because there's so much else going on in their life, then it becomes a **management** issue (failure to manage one's own life).*
Doctor-centred consultations	R- p-	*A doctor-centred consultation says something about the doctor–patient **relationship** and possibly about the attitude of the doctor. Attitudinal problems always relate to **professionalism**.*
Poor patient feedback and complaints	R- D- p-	*Poor patient feedback usually signals a **relationship** problem, but can also suggest a **diagnostic** problem (perceived errors of judgement, missed cues, etc.). The attitude of the doc may also need looking at (**professionalism**).*
Is *always* punctual, hardly ever late	M+ p+	*A punctual doctor is someone who obviously **manages** their time well. A strong positive word (i.e. '**always** punctual') also suggests clear **respect** for time-keeping and not keeping others waiting (**professionalism**). However, **routine** efficiency is not tagged as professionalism because that is simply doing one's job.*

3 Step back and **review the collated evidence** as a whole and the RDM-p areas you have linked them to. Which RDM-p domain(s) have the most evidence?

4 **Meet with your trainee and discuss.** Let them digest what people have written, then invite them to comment. This is vital – to ensure there is agreement about exactly what has happened. If the trainee challenges the supposed evidence, this needs exploring sensitively, otherwise your chances of later agreeing causes and finally reaching a shared plan of action will be greatly reduced. Once agreed, use the **SKIPE framework** to explore *with* the trainee what might be causing, influencing or maintaining the performance problems identified in the R, D, M domains, and any related professionalism issues.

5 Finally, discuss ways of making things better and incorporate these into a **development plan**. Guide the trainee by 'pulling together' and summarising discussion highlights *from each of the RDM-p domains* and their relevant SKIPE areas. Get the trainee to problem-solve and generate solutions – each of which should be SMART (Specific, Measurable, Achievable, Realistic and Time-bound).

Additional notes on *internal* factors

Reminder: internal factors are about a trainee's **core attitudes**, **personal traits** and **health/capacity**. We've mentioned the role of **attitudes** earlier and there's a document on our website called *Changing Attitudes* which we would encourage you to read. So let's now consider the other factors briefly.

Personal traits

A recent powerful meta-analysis (Morgeson *et al.*, 2007[9,10]) suggests that **personality tests have very low validity** for predicating job performance. Do not use personality measures to *predict* performance – it is dangerous territory, and you'll get your fingers burnt! Look at traits *only if they emerge* as possible causal factors from the evidence of performance and the discussion that follows. In other words, do not blindly start with personality measures. Only go there if the evidence and discussion suggests you need to go there. Unfortunately, those promoting personality measures keep pumping out these 'sexy' lists, based on flimsy evidence, and inviting a passive acceptance of traits as factors. Rather than using personality questionnaires, perhaps this simpler approach might help:

---

1 **How self-critical is your trainee?** Self-criticism is a trait that shows a U-shaped relation to performance; with too much or too little being problematic. High levels of self-criticism are related to depression in doctors but a lack of the ability to be self-critical may also be a problem.

2 **How much of a perfectionist is your trainee?** Perfectionism can lead to difficulties such as over-checking or difficulty making decisions for fear they are not right. Perfectionism also correlates well with other mental health disorders like depression, anxiety and eating disorders. The converse, taking responsibility for one's actions but not blaming yourself for everything that goes wrong, is clearly a healthy approach.

3 **How much self-esteem or confidence does your trainee have?** Self-esteem, like self-criticism, also shows a U-shaped relation to performance; with too much or too little being problematic. Most trainers are wary of the new trainee who thinks they know everything and never asks for help. You need to be the same for the trainee who needs reassurance about all that they do.

Learning styles

Something worth doing is a learning style questionnaire like that of Honey and Mumford[11] (*see* Chapter 11: Learning and Personality Styles in Practice). This questionnaire describes four learning styles (activist, reflector, theorist and pragmatist), and it would be interesting to see how much of these your trainee is.

1 Activists like to learn from experience.
2 Reflectors like time to think and reflect before assimilating new learning.
3 Theorists like to learn from theories, models and concepts.
4 Pragmatists like to learn from practical situations.

> A Trainer was struggling with a trainee, wondering if his knowledge was adequate. He seemed very slow to respond when asked for questions or opinions in the tutorial setting, but his clinical management was satisfactory. A learning styles questionnaire revealed that he was a highly reflective learner, whereas the Trainer was not, and the problem was that the trainee simply needed time to reflect on the question or issue before responding.

Sometimes a trainee is struggling because the learning/teaching methods you are using are at odds with their preferred learning style. Do *you* adapt *your* teaching style to the learning style of *your* trainee?

Health

Raising the matter of illness is challenging for both Trainer and trainee. The Trainer may feel that enquiries might be seen as prying into an area that should remain confidential for the trainee. However, if the trainee is not aware of the effects of illness, making the suggestion might be very useful. Evidence suggests:

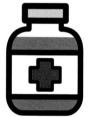

- doctors have similar levels of physical illnesses to the general population
- but they take less than the average sick leave
- they adopt maladaptive behaviours such as working when ill, self-prescribing and informal self-referral rather than using their GP.

In their study, Baldwin, Dodd and Wrate[12] noted that a third of young doctors were not registered with a GP. And the more hours worked the more likely the doctors were to complain of somatic symptoms. While emergency admissions and long hours may not be an issue in GP posts, they do affect GP trainees in hospital posts, and so educators need to be mindful of this.

Physical illness does not commonly affect performance, other than interrupting the training period (but the disruption to the trainee's rotation can be considerable).

> An ST1 trainee was unwell with hyperemesis gravidarum and had several weeks' sickness absence during a four-month hospital post. Even though her performance when well was good, she had missed sufficient training to require an extension and did not complete the minimum three-month full-time equivalent experience in that post for it to count for her CCT. Her rotations had to be reorganised to take into account the sickness absence and her maternity leave, and also to allow her to make up the missing clinical experience in that specialty.

Mental health problems, *including* stress and substance misuse, are a different matter and affect performance significantly. Did you know that they are more common in doctors than in the general public?[13,14]

Alcohol and drugs: A survey of house officers revealed that drinking in excess of safe limits was common and 10% admitted to using illegal drugs.[15] This may affect performance either because of the direct effect of the drug (hangover, drowsiness) or indirectly through social withdrawal, financial problems, driving offences and so on. In industry, absences on Monday mornings and Friday afternoons are recognised as pointers towards a drug or alcohol problem.

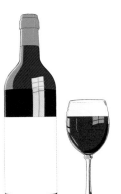

Stress and depression: Surveys suggest that stress is a larger problem than depression, and doctors have lots of it![16]

Trainees may be reluctant to admit to physical or mental health problems, either because they might see it as a sign of weakness, for fear of the consequences or because of lack of insight into the problem. This is made worse if they come from a cultural background where there is little recognition of psychological or mental health problems. Therefore, **tread gently, read verbal and non-verbal cues, show compassion and show empathy**.

It is important to **refer the doctor to their own GP and/or to a consultant Occupational Health Physician** as per the GMC requirements;[17] the trainee may need to be reminded of these. Referral will help clarify whether the trainee is fit to work, unfit, or whether adjustments to the working environment are necessary (such as going part-time). **Do not rely on your own assessment of the risk to patients and never try to fix their health problem by becoming their temporary GP.**

Possible markers of an underlying health problem

- In general, if a trainee (or even a work colleague) shows a recent deterioration of performance, think physical or mental health problems (including alcohol/drugs). If they are suddenly experiencing difficulty in decision-making or attention loss, explore whether they are stressed, depressed or have bad sleeping hygiene.
- If patients keep complaining about your trainee who has 'bad attitude', maybe their anger with patients stems from being stressed. Don't assume it's part of their persona.
- If there are a series of short absences from work, think physical or mental health problems. Absences on Monday mornings and Friday afternoons may be a pointer to drug or alcohol problems.

Additional notes on *past* factors

Reminder: our distinctive personality traits affect our behaviour. Those personality traits will derive from particular influences in our upbringing such as our cultural and educational roots. So if you notice, for example, that your trainee displays characteristics such as perfectionism, or a chronic lack of confidence, or strong values based on 'right and wrong', these will often have their roots in deeply established patterns of thinking or living instilled by others. It can be very useful to touch on this with your trainee, because a reflective dialogue in this area can lead to important 'light-bulb' moments for both of you. This often allows the trainee to temper the influence of particular traits once they realise their roots and impact.

Wider culture and language: Trainees from different cultural backgrounds may have difficulty understanding and adapting to the culture of the community they are working in. Think about it. They have to:

1 adjust to working in a second language
2 work in a system with which they are unfamiliar
3 work with cultural norms that they are not accustomed to.

> 'I was simple enough to think that the British people were all the same, all speaking the same sort of language, the language which I learnt at English school in India. I was surprised I couldn't understand the English nurse and was even more surprised because she did not understand English – my English!'
>
> Indian man (Ahmed and Watt, 1986)[18]

So, what can you do?

- The first thing is to get into a positive frame of mind. We should not forget the positives of having trainees who speak other languages, e.g. what these trainees can teach you about other languages and culture.
- Your job as a Trainer is to help your trainee work effectively in the UK. You need to help them with all the skills that are needed for this – not just the medical ones. Don't bury your head in the sand and don't assume that it will just happen.
- Start by exploring the learner's cultural background, values, beliefs and previous style of medical practice. There are particular areas that a trainee may not be familiar with which you may want to explore later, such as the following.
  1 A patient-centred model of care (ICE, joint management planning, etc.)
  2 Recognising the psychosocial aspects of a problem.
  3 Holistic care.
  4 A non-hierarchical approach to working with colleagues.
  5 Self-directed learning.
- Encourage them to improve on their linguistic capital.
  1 Perhaps join night school conversational classes in English.
  2 Encourage them to go out and socialise with British-born trainees.
  3 The local university will probably have an 'international students' club'.
  4 Encourage them to watch and follow a TV soap opera and maybe discuss a few episodes now and then. Coronation Street (if you're in Manchester), *East Enders* (London), *Brookside* (Liverpool), *Emmerdale* (Yorkshire) or *River City* (Glasgow).

Top Tip: For further advice, read Chapter 20: Understanding and Teaching about Diversity and Chapter 21: Supporting GP Trainees Who Graduated Outside the UK. There are two additional resources on our website that you will find interesting – one is called *Trainees in difficulty – culture and language* and the other *Cultural and Linguistic issues in relation to the CSA*.

Additional notes on *external* factors

Reminder: these are factors currently interacting with the individual, either at home or at work (like relationship, financial and employment issues). Let's look at a few of these.

Employment issues: Workload issues seem to be particularly prevalent in hospital settings, where the work intensity can be high and long hours are the norm, European Working Time Directive not withstanding.

> A Clinical Supervisor for a hospital post had recently raised a number of 'professional' concerns over a couple of trainees, mentioning things like 'not pulling their weight', 'not being team players' and 'being distant with staff'. The trainees too expressed great dissatisfaction with the job. They felt that there were 'not enough people on the shop floor'. The department confirmed understaffing in terms of nursing. The trainees were therefore doing a lot of nursing tasks on top of their own workload. When these trainees moved to a different post (one to A&E and another to General Medicine), they both seemed to get glowing reports – even in the competency areas ear-marked as a cause for concern!

When you receive a complaint about a trainee (for example, from a Clinical Supervisor), don't automatically assume that the trainee is the one with the problem. Likewise, when a trainee complains of difficulties in a post, don't automatically assume the post is the problem. What you need to do is to hear both sides of the story before making any sort of judgement. Speak to the trainee, speak to the department and speak to others on the shop floor. Get as much information as you can from a variety of sources in order to formulate a more rounded picture of what's really going on.

Family, financial and even criminal problems

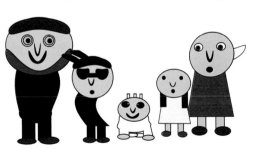

Trainees are, by and large, young adults and are in a transitional phase of their lives. Here are some of the things they may be going through:

- They are often embarking on long-term relationships.
- Maybe they're already partnered but now thinking of having a baby.
- Some already have a young family: juggling training and young children is challenging.
- Some will have relocated to take a training place and may therefore have lost their local network of family and friends to act as informal support.
- Others may still be living in the same place but commuting long distances: this can be fatiguing and may damage relationships.
- Some are separated from their partners or young family, because the partner's job is elsewhere and far away (in the UK or abroad). The NHS still imports doctors from overseas into training schemes – for them, difficulty around the geographical separation from their family is compounded by the cultural and linguistic difficulties of living and working in a different country and healthcare system.

- Trainees of overseas origins increasingly encounter problems with their visas, which will cause anxiety and may interrupt their training programme.
- Some trainees will have fallen foul of the law (driving offences, for instance) and this will disrupt training because of repeated problems with CRB checking.
- It's also not uncommon to hear about trainees having to deal with illness or death of a close family member, or occasionally in their partners or children.

An ST3 trainee in the last six months of training was felt to be progressing more slowly than expected by her Trainer. There had been no previous reported concerns with this trainee. She was on a two-year shortened scheme and, consequently, only had 12 months of general practice, rather than the usual 18 months. In discussion with the trainee, it became apparent that she had a three-year-old child and was effectively functioning as a single parent (her husband had moved with his work and was only coming home at weekends). This was clearly having an adverse effect on her ability to maximise the learning opportunities available to her. The educational plan had to take this context into account and push for an inter-deanery transfer to enable them to live as a family unit again.

i-SID principles

The RDM-p approach provides a framework for assessing and managing the trainee experiencing difficulty. iSID, however, is simply a mnemonic to help you remember some overarching principles that need to be adhered to throughout the entire process.

i is for Identifying Problems Early

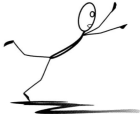

- Use the RDM-p approach to explore these as early as possible – define the problem and identify the cause(s). Prompt identification and action at an early stage offers by far the best chance of avoiding damage to patients and the colleague in difficulty, and of putting things right. It is the kindest and most responsible thing to do'.[4]
- If there is evidence of real risk to patient or person safety, the practice should invoke their own employment procedures, and remove the trainee from clinical work pending consultation. Fortunately, such situations are rare.

S is for Share Your Concerns with Others

- It is important to share your concerns with others and share them *early*. Do not try to deal with complex scenarios on your own.[3] By sharing, we mean *concisely* sharing all the data gathered at the 'Identify' stage above.
- Always talk to your Programme Director(s). Don't be scared about contacting them over something that might turn out to be trivial – that's what they are there for. They have greater experience of trainees in difficulty, and they will tell you whether or not what you say is a poor performance indicator and guide you on what to do next.
- Some schemes have Trainers' workshops where part of it may be devoted to discussing trainees with whom there are difficulties. These can also help you decide whether there is a cause for concern and help you find a way through it. They're also a great source of support in general.
- Talk to the deanery – there will be an Associate Postgraduate Dean for your region who should be able to advise further.

I is for Involve the Trainee

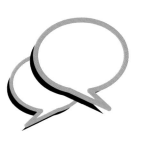

- Involve the trainee in the identified problem as early as possible: create a dialogue and explore the issues with them. There is nothing worse than being the last one to be told about a problem, especially when you're the focal point of discussion. Explain what has been observed (describing actual events) and why this causes concern. It's important not to use judgement words like 'lazy' or 'rude'.
- You need to show you want to understand their perspective, and that you've not simply rushed into 'passing judgement'. However, for this to happen, you have to have created an open, honest and trusting relationship with the trainee. If you set the right *supportive* atmosphere, it's less likely that they'll reject the problem, be defensive or counterclaim.
- The discussion should be in an appropriate protected environment (not in the corridor or in front of others). Show genuine interest and concern. Help the trainee to self-challenge.
- Don't doubt your ability to handle this. Yes, you do have to tread carefully but the skills needed are the same you use in your day-to-day consultations – listen, clarify, summarise, joint planning and so on. You have all the skills to do it; believe in yourself!

D is for Document Facts and Discussions

- Document facts, subsequent discussions and plans. Share this with the trainee.[3]
- The purpose of documenting is to make sure everyone is clear about the difficulties and the collective approach being taken. It's also to protect you should the situation spiral out of control and the trainee appeals for a tribunal.
- Each performance area of concern should be documented along with action points to tackle it. The information you record should be: accurate, factual, objective (i.e. non-judgemental), justifiable, relevant and contemporaneous.

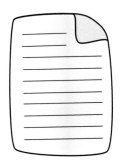

EXAMPLE OF A WRITE-UP

The performance concern: *Management*
Several GP colleagues have concerns over Tim's clinical abilities. Tim says he is unfamiliar with many of the clinical guidelines and isn't clinically up-to-date because he hasn't any time to do this. He finds it difficult to *manage* his time.

We have agreed the following:
1 Tim is currently doing a lot of A&E locum work in order to support his family. He has agreed to drop this so that he has free evening space to do more study.
2 In terms of home finances, he will talk to his wife (a) to see if she can get a part-time job, (b) to identify extravagances that have to go, and (c) to see whether the in-laws can help (and thus release the child-minder).
3 We talked about developing a list of PUNs and DENs after each surgery which Tim will work on during surgery hours, and which will provide a focus for his evening learning.
4 We will schedule regular educational time for Random Case Analyses to identify and tackle other gaps in clinical knowledge.

5   We will review the situation in 6 weeks.

Key points to take home
- **Early identification and intervention** may help resolve problems before they become entrenched, with benefits for the Trainer, trainee and patients. Do not hope the problem will go away.
- **Do not try to deal with the problem alone**, particularly if it is complex or potentially serious. *Patient and personal safety takes precedence over all other considerations.*
- **A detailed 'diagnosis' can lead to effective remediation.** Remember that the presenting problem is a 'symptom', and it is essential to establish the facts and circumstances first. Get information from a variety of sources in order to define the real nature of the problem. Only then explore the underlying causal and contributory factors, to which subsequent intervention must be tailored (the RDM-p approach).
- **Keep clear and contemporaneous documentation.** The trainee must be informed that you are keeping records and has a right to see what is said about them. Don't hide things – be open, honest and involve them as much as you can. After all, it is about them.

 Red Alert: The Data Protection Act[19] governs how personal information is collected and stored. Any data on a learner's performance will be classed as personal data and be subject to the Act. Justify what you have recorded and be prepared for it to be shown to others. It's good practice to share things with the trainee anyway. Avoid subjective judgemental comments. Back things up with evidence. **You must not keep a secret set of records.**

A final word

Don't assume that a trainee who *performs* badly is a bad trainee. They may be good but have unfortunately been unable to demonstrate this through the impact of other factors – like a divorce, depression and so on. And their Trainer needs to be humble enough to ask themselves the difficult question about their own potential role in this.

A sample of resources on our website
- The RDM-p manual.
- Training Programme Directors & Doctors in Difficulty.
- Discussion, Dialogue and Socrates (under web resources for Chapter 10).
- Changing attitudes.
- Cultural and Linguistic issues.

Other chapters you may like to read
- Chapter 33: First Aid for the Remedial Trainee
- Chapter 32: The Top Five Educational Difficulties
- Chapter 7: The Skilful Art of Giving Feedback
- Chapter 29: Assessment and Competence
- Chapter 28: Reflection and Evaluation.

Please give us some feedback on this chapter to help shape it for the next edition.
Go to www.essentialgptrainingbook.com and simply click on the title of this chapter.

References

1 The National Clinical Assessment Service (NCAS). Available at: www.ncas.npsa.nhs.uk

2 Donaldson IJ. Doctors with problems in an NHS workforce. *BMJ.* 1994; **308**: 1277–82.

3 Young A. *Managing Trainees in Difficulty: practical advice for educational and clinical supervisors.* National Association Clinical Tutors; 2008. Available at: www.nact.org.uk/parsedownload?docid=2381

4 Paice E, Orton V. Early signs of the trainee in difficulty. *Hosp Med.* 2004; **65**(4): 238–40.

5 Norfolk T, Siriwardena AN. A unifying theory of clinical practice: Relationship, Diagnostics, Management and professionalism (RDM-p). *Qual Prim Care.* 2009; **17**(1): 37–47.

6 Tim Norfolk, 24 May 2011 (personal communication).

7 Berne E. *Games People Play: the psychology of human relationships.* London: Penguin; 1973.

8 Gaarder J. *Sophie's World: a novel about the history of philosophy.* London: Phoenix Publishers; 1996. pp. 59–63.

9 Morgeson FP, Campion MA, Dipboye RL, Hollenbeck JR. Reconsidering the use of personality tests in personnel selection contexts. *Pers Psychol.* 2007; **60**: 683–729.

10 Morgeson FP, Campion MA, Dipboye RL, *et al.* Are we getting fooled again? Coming to terms with limitations in the use of personality tests in personnel selection. *Pers Psychol.* 2007; **60**: 1029–49.

11 Honey P, Mumford A. *The Manual of Learning Styles.* Maidenhead, UK: Peter Honey Publications; 1982.

12 Baldwin PJ, Dodd M, Wrate RW. Young doctors' health: how do working conditions affect attitudes, health and performance? *Soc Sci Med.* 1997; **45**(1): 35–40.

13 Wall TD, Bolden RI, Borrill CS, *et al.* Minor psychiatric disorder in NHS trust staff: occupational and gender differences. *Br J Psychiatry.* 1997; **171**: 5919–23.

14 Cox J, King J, Hutchinson A, Mcavoy P, editors. *Understanding Doctors' Performance.* Oxford: Radcliffe Publishing Ltd; 2005.

15 Brooks A. Many junior doctors abuse drugs and drink excessively. *BMJ.* 1998; **317**(7160): 700.

16 Firth-Cozens J, Greenhalgh J. Doctors' perceptions of the links between stress and lowered clinical care. *Soc Sci Med.* 1997; **44**(7): 1017–22.

17 GMC Thresholds (Fitness to Practise). Available at: www.gmc-uk.org/concerns/employers_information.asp

18 Ahmed G, Watt S. Understanding Asian women in pregnancy and confinement. *Midwives Chron.* 1986; **99**: 98–101.

19 Data Protection Act: Available at: www.ico.gov.uk/for_the_public/personal_information.aspx

The Top Five Educational Difficulties

IAIN LAMB – Associate Advisor (SE Scotland) & lead author
JULIET DRAPER – Retired GP (Cambridge), Freelance consultant (Communication Skills)
GRAHAM RUTT – Head of School (Northern Deanery)   RAMESH MEHAY – TPD (Bradford)

Introduction

All trainees will have difficulties but, for the majority, they are relatively minor and a skilled Trainer will be able to help. But what are those skills? Sometimes trainees will have, and cause, significant difficulty, creating huge anxiety and a lot of work for Trainers.

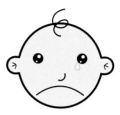

What doesn't work

- Ignore and it will go away – it doesn't, and they don't.
- Challenge without evidence – you get challenged with evidence.
- Tell them what to do – well my dad told me, and I didn't learn.
- Assume what the problem is – and get it wrong just like assumptions with patients.
- Try to deal with it on your own – afraid of being seen to be stupid leads to being discovered to be really stupid.
- Feel it's your entire fault and make excuses for them – it usually is their issue and making excuses leads to passing those who should fail. Sometime failing someone is your success!

Chapter 31: The Trainee Experiencing Difficulty and Chapter 33: First Aid for the Remedial Trainee provide a general approach for dealing with trainees in difficulty. In this chapter, we're going to cover the following five *specific* **educational** difficulties.
1 The trainee with poor knowledge.
2 The trainee with poor motivation.
3 The trainee who is constantly uncertain and unable to make decisions.
4 The trainee who always wants their hand held and be told what to do.
5 The trainee who is a muddly consulter.

But before we do, don't forget about SID

SID was covered in detail in Chapter 31: The Trainee Experiencing Difficulty. SID talks about three overarching principles that you should stick to when dealing with any difficulty a trainee might be experiencing.

The SID Framework

SHARE
- Share your concerns with others. Don't get stuck with trying to solve things by yourself.
- Some issues will simply benefit from discussion with colleagues but others will need discussion or referral to professional bodies like the deanery.

INVOLVE
- Involve the learner in those concerns and discussions (despite the level of difficulty).
- It is important to speak to the learner because there are always two sides to a story and they may reveal the ROOT of the difficulty in the process.

DOCUMENT
- Keep detailed specific documentation of the facts of what has happened and any other relevant issues.
- What you record should be **factual, accurate, relevant, objective,** and **justifiable.** Use **descriptive, specific** and **non-judgemental** language.

 Red Alert: Always keep in the back of your mind that any educational difficulty might just be the symptom. The root cause may lie elsewhere, such as:
- a competence or conduct problem
- an underlying health problem
- an issue in or out of work.

 Top Tip: For a comprehensive approach to diagnosing and managing trainees in difficulty, read about the RDM-p approach in Chapter 31: The Trainee Experiencing Difficulty.

---

1 The trainee with poor knowledge

A GP trainee is usually on the scheme for at least 3 years. That gives us enough time to help them improve their knowledge base (Remember there is now a clear curriculum to guide us.)

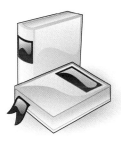

Define the real problem

A trainee with what appears to be poor knowledge might have a bigger problem. Try to figure out which of these four matches the trainee.

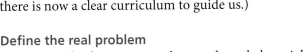

1 **General poor knowledge**

   Knowledge of the areas covered in the AKT is poor across many areas compared to peers at the same stage of GP training.

2 **Specific areas of poor knowledge**

   There is reasonable knowledge of certain areas but gaps are identified that need to be addressed.

3 **Problem with application**

   There is good knowledge but an inability to put it into action.

4 **Lacks insight and is dangerous**

   The trainee lacks insight into the limits to their knowledge, leading to possible overconfidence and a risk to patient safety.

In this section, we're only going to provide guidance for the top two. As for the bottom two, you need to seek advice from your local Training Programme Director(s) – it's more complicated and the trainee will need properly 'diagnosing' (e.g. dyslexia) by others more qualified to do so.

Practical points for (1) and (2)

Things you can do

Try to identify knowledge gaps as *early* in their training programme as possible.

- Look at their **AKT results** and feedback – it often gives you a good breakdown of which areas need work. Look at this in conjunction with the **'curriculum coverage'** page in their ePortfolio (which may or may not be reliable).
- Get the trainee to evaluate their own knowledge. You can use something like the **Curriculum Self-Assessment Rating Scale** (preferred) or the Trainee Initial Self-Assessment (TISA tool) – both available from our website.
- Do lots of **Random Case Analyses** – to tackle knowledge blind spots (*see* Chapter 5: A Smorgasbord of Educational Methods, which tells you more about Random Cases and how to do them).
- **Practice Nurses** are better at following **guidelines** than doctors are – get the trainee to help run nurse-led chronic disease clinics.
- Look at *AKT resources by Mike Tompson* – available on our website.

Things they can do

- Get them on an **AKT course** – perhaps your local deanery runs one?
- Suggest trainees work together in **small study groups** – sharing the workload in terms of up-to-date guidelines, evidence-based medicine and critical reading.
- **Examiners' comments** on past AKT examinations are available from the college website (www. rcgp.org). They provide invaluable information about questions answered badly!

Web resources

- www.e-GP.org – free e-learning resource specifically designed to support trainees learning the curriculum for general practice.
- www.nPEP.org.uk – for questions.
- www.rcgp-innovAiT.oxfordjournals.org – a journal with some AKT questions.
- The RCGP's Essential Knowledge Challenge, available at http://elearning.rcgp.org.uk. Updated every 6 months. Free.
- 50 mock AKT questions are available from www.rcgp.org.uk (click on the MRCGP section).

The first time my trainee failed the AKT, I thought that there was nothing much I could do for him: you either know or you don't, and if you don't only *you* can brush up on that. Then he failed again. On both occasions, his scores were abysmal and that made me think, 'I've got to do something'. What surprised me was that I didn't think he was all that bad when sitting in with him in consultations. And when I asked him directly for knowledge, he could often answer me. He told me that he was reading at least 2–3 hours a day, practising online mock AKTs, and I had no reason to doubt him.

I still felt clueless in terms of helping him, so we both agreed to do a few mock online AKT tests together. The set-up went something like this: he would sit in the corner of our large meeting room, answering questions on a PC. That PC would be linked to a projector which would display things to me. I would be sitting at the back of the room so as not to interfere with him. I would then read and answer each question at the same time as him but I would also note how much extra time he spent on each question. At the end, there were a quite a number of questions where he spent significantly more time than me. We looked into these to explore the difficulty.

We found that he was having to translate the questions into his mother tongue (Punjabi) and then translate the answer back into English! And this is what he had to do when he communicated with patients (no wonder he was consulting at 20 minutes at ST3). This finding was instrumental as to what we did from there on. And if it wasn't for 'hitching a ride' on his mock AKT journey, I would never have realised this finding in a zillion years. Did he pass in the end? Unfortunately not, but I can honestly say that I gave him my best shot.

Finally, there comes a stage for Trainers when all the trainees seem to know more than them. Well do they know how to put it into action? Perhaps not, and that's what keeps us in a job.

I didn't know whether to laugh or cry when a fifth-year medical student, after observing my surgery, said, 'You don't seem to know much medicine, but you seem to get it right every time!'

IL

2 The trainee with poor motivation
Poor motivation can suck the enthusiasm out of Trainers. Here are four things that might help you.

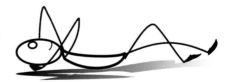

a) Goals: Stephen Covey's *The Seven Habits of Highly Effective People*[1] (Habit 2)
'Begin with the End in Mind': find out what the trainee really sees themselves doing and being in the future.

Your personal image

Your personal image of the long-term end is what matters to you and provides an image of the end of your life as a frame of reference to which everything is examined. Consider:
1   What **roles** do you play in your life?
2   What **goals** do you have for them?
3   Write a personal **mission statement** that is based on your principles and values.

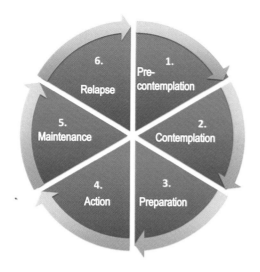

Does this sound like a bit over-the-top psychobabble? Well, it may be but at least take the kernel of the idea and make sure you understand your trainee's motivations for the future. Use awareness-raising questions like What, Where, When, How and Who to raise awareness in the trainee. Awareness is the first fundamental step in DiClemente and Prochaska's Cycle of Change[2] that many of us are familiar with.

Exploring some of my ex-trainees' goals (when they were with me) was one of the most effective things I think I did for them. I have had many trainees who initially seemed to lack motivation but after understanding what they want out of life – what drives them – I could get them to open up, talk about obstacles, help *them* resolve issues and generally move them in a direction that was right for them. Some of them now do a bit of medicine but their main vocation is something else (one's a Baptist minister and another is a politician!). And I still keep in touch with most of them.

b) Core values and the wheel of life (NLP)

Another way we can motivate the learner is to start understanding their true core values. There's an exercise resource on our website, which will help you define a person's 'core value set'. This set is made up of the very things which *drive* (and motivate) them. The resource is called *NLP – The Wheel of Life and Core Values*, and before you try it with your trainee, consider trying it out on yourself first.

c) Motivational Interviewing[3]

When getting people to change, Rollnick and Miller[3] discovered that there are two axes that you need to explore. One is the person's *motivation* to change, and the other is their *confidence* in being able to carry out that change. To help you understand this better, think of the patient who comes to see you wanting to lose weight. Before doing anything, Motivational Interviewing dictates that you figure out how truly *motivated* they are about losing weight and how much *confidence* (belief in themselves) they have that they can do it. If one is high but the other low, exploring methods to make the weak one stronger will help that person with their ultimate goal (in this case – to lose weight).

Likewise, with the trainee who seems laissez-faire:

1 Explore their disinterest – what's behind it? Is something kicking off elsewhere (like at home)?
2 Is a particular change truly worthwhile? Explore the pros and cons.
3 Use the 'motivation and confidence to change' rating scales to determine whether there is a difficulty in motivation, confidence or both.
4 Explore methods to work on motivation and/or confidence to help them get to their destination.

	PROS	CONS
Change		
No Change		

MOTIVATION RATING SCALE
How strong is your motivation (or desire) to change right this very moment?
Motivation to change 0---**10 (v. strong)**

CONFIDENCE RATING SCALE
How strongly do you believe in yourself that you can do it? How confident do you feel?
Confidence to change 0---**10 (v. confident)**

 Top Tip: Exams have a powerful influence in motivating people to learn – use that as a positive lever in your training.

d) How motivating are you and your practice?

Read the article: Role modelling: making the most of a powerful teaching strategy. *BMJ.* 2008; **336**: 718–21 by Sylvia R Cruess *et al.*[4] Then ask the following questions.

● Am I good role model for my trainee?
● Do I share with them how I deal with my own difficulties?
● Is the practice providing the right explicit and implicit environment for trainees?

If yes, then you are providing the right environment to motivate trainees.

 Top Tip: As a role model there's another way you can influence a trainee's motivation. If you show lots of energy and enthusiasm, some of that will rub off on to them too. If you look demotivated, so will your trainee.

3 The trainee who is constantly uncertain and unable to make decisions

In the bad old days of being a junior hospital doctor we worked twice the number of hours now allowed by European law. Much of this was poorly supervised so in some ways it became the good old days of experiencing loads of decision-making. Reducing working hours has made it more difficult for trainees to experience decision-making. And more decisions are informed by rigid and inflexible protocols or referral to a senior colleague for advice.

Trainees who have just started GP training will require help with decision-making. This does not mean there is a problem! However, if that difficulty with decision-making does not lessen with time, there may well be a problem. Before we discuss specific ways of remedying this, let's turn our attention to complexity theory.[5] Complexity theory can help us discuss with trainees the issues that create uncertainty and how we become capable of dealing with complex situations.

There are five elements you should cover when talking about complexity theory: Competence, Capability, Complexity, Certainty and Chaos (the 5 Cs).

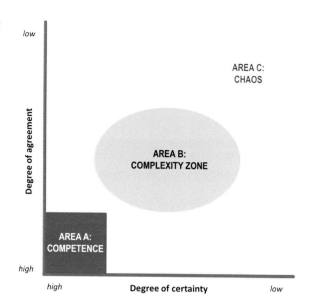

It is easy to measure competence in area A

Competence is something that individuals know or can do in terms of knowledge, skills or attitudes. In Area A, everybody agrees what should be done and there is a high level of *agreement* for the trainee to follow. Commonly, this high level of agreement is based on protocols which in themselves should be underpinned by good evidence. If a trainee has a protocol to follow, they become more confident *and certain* that they are doing the right thing. In discussion with trainees, the majority *think* their Trainers are good GPs because they know lots and are usually very certain what to do. In other words, GP trainees *think* GP Trainers work with a very large Area A.

The marshy swamplands of area B

However, GP Trainers know that most of the work we do is in Area B (often called the Marshy Swampland) – much of what we deal with does not have a good evidence base to support clear agreement. Nevertheless, GPs have the *capability* to manage complex situations. Capability is the ability to adapt to change, to generate new knowledge and continue to improve on performance. For instance, we reduce uncertainty through:

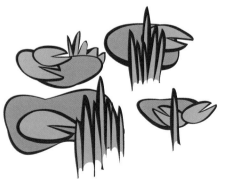

1 discussion and discovery with patients
2 developing shared agreement with patients.

And we're usually comfortable about it being OK for an individual patient to be managed outside the usual norms. We also know that chaos is sometimes the lot of certain patients (Area C). We know that many things influence how we manage individual patients and most protocols don't allow for this. So in Area B there will be some things moving us to certainty and others towards chaos. Complexity Theory dictates that these different pull factors will eventually reach equilibrium in a *non-linear* way. Experienced GPs are used to non-linear thinking but GP trainees are not – and that's not surprising taking into account the fact that most of their teaching, until now, has been linear (based on structure and knowledge).

Practical points – helping your trainee with uncertainty and decision-making

Discuss complexity theory with the trainee to help them realise how most of us operate in Area B (the complexity zone) and not Area A. Therefore, we need to start getting comfortable with being in Area B. Instead of getting all flustered about not knowing what to do, we need to find ways of moving us closer to Area A (i.e. towards certainty and/or agreement). Some of the things below may help.

1 New discoveries are made as trainees engage in deeper dialogue with the patient and, in particular, their **ideas, concerns, expectations and beliefs**. Some of these new discoveries will help reduce their volume of uncertainty.
2 Discussing dilemmas with patients and developing a **shared understanding and agreement with patients** will also help lessen their uncertainty.
3 **Facilitate decision-making rather than giving the answers.** If a trainee comes to you saying they've got a lady who is pregnant and has been in contact with a person with chicken pox, and they don't know what to do, rather than giving the answer you might ask, *'Where else could you look to resolve your problem?'*
4 Where the opportunity arises (for example, during joint surgeries), explicitly **explore your own difficulties with decision-making with them**. Share your PUNs and DENs. This should help them open up the 'façade box' of their personal Johari Window (if you're unfamiliar with Johari, *see* Chapter 4: Powerful Hooks – aims, objectives and ILOs).
5 Finally, encourage trainees to start **learning in a non-linear way**. Get them to share their learning journey with others and watch how the uncertainties change over time. Things like: self-directed experiential learning by keeping a discomfort log; situational learning through shadowing others; small-group learning like role play, problem-solving and for general peer support; problem-based learning through working in teams.

4 The trainee who always wants their hand held and be told what to do

Hang on a minute, isn't this just the same as the uncertain trainee but said in a different way?

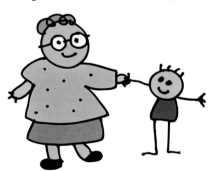

Well, perhaps, but *'It ain't necessarily so'* as the song goes. And since this is something I'm currently trying to learn, in my quest to conquer jazz piano, I note that sometimes I'm totally uncertain about what I'm trying to do *though at other times I'm pretty certain but just need a bit of reassurance* that I'm on the right lines and to be offered a bit of add-on help (IL). Yes, this is indeed about *uncertainty* and a lot of what has been said earlier in the chapter is relevant but there is also something about *confidence*. We need to explore how to lessen the hand-holding by the time the trainee is ready to go it alone.

To understand what might be going on, let's look at a simplified version of what is called 'The Transition Curve'.[6] It is a useful tool for understanding the sorts of issues people might be facing during a change. It maps out their journey from Unconscious Incompetence to Unconscious Competence (*see* Chapter 29: Assessment and Competence, for more on the Conscious Competency Model).

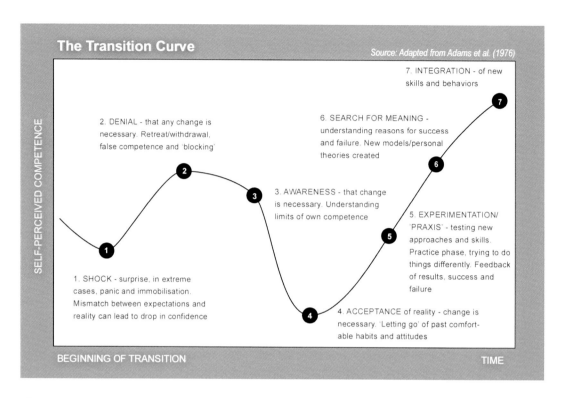

In business, it is estimated that when someone changes a job, they expect it will take 18 months for them to integrate fully into a full-time post. The change from hospital to general practice is a huge transition and when this change happens, you can usually follow a trainee's journey along this curve. They will be fragile during stages 1–5 and, therefore, will need hand-holding to help them through new beginnings while maintaining the level of activity or service. **Realising where the trainee is on the curve will help you initiate appropriate actions and respond effectively.**

- **Stage 1:** the flood of information, new people and new systems threatens to overwhelm. *Hold their hand and provide a good induction.*
- **Stage 2:** the person may resort to previous successful behaviour. For example, the trainee who was an efficient consulter in outpatients persists with a hospital disease model – forcing it to work even though it's not right for general practice. There is a level of unconscious incompetence here. *Help them see the limits of their own competence and help them gain insight into change being necessary.*
- **Stage 3:** the individual shows awareness of difficulties but also has a level of conscious incompetence that frustrates and their confidence can become low. For instance, they might say: 'In hospital, patients didn't come back to see me, and I thought they were fine. Now in spite of trying my best some patients are coming back no better.' *Get them to let go of past comfortable habits and attitudes and get them to embrace the diverse ways of doing things in general practice.*
- **Stages 4 and 5:** moving them on sounds easy but there is often a roller-coaster of success and failure during this conscious competence phase. Watching a trainee's video where they have tried to think about all the COT competencies can look very clunky, and it takes a lot of practice with good feedback to move onto stages 6 and 7. *Help them understand their successes and failures so that they can develop new personal theories or models. Help them search for meaning.*

Practical points – helping the trainee who wants their hand holding

If the hand-holding is a reflection of being uncomfortable with uncertainty, follow the above section on uncertainty. Otherwise, it signals that the trainee is either at stage 1 (where hand-holding is entirely appropriate) or stuck at stage 5. For the latter, try some of the suggestions below.

- Show them the Transition Curve and ask them where they think they're at. Tell them where you think they're at. If you're at variance with each other, engage in dialogue. If you both agree that they're at stage 5, explore what is needed to get them to stages 6 and 7. Put a plan into place. *Help them search for meaning.*
- We need to help the trainee move from Conscious Competence (stage 5) to Unconscious Competence (stage 6/7). Someone at stage 5 still operates in a chunky-clunky sort of way – the competencies are there, but they're not performed with fluidity or fluency. Why is this? Have they had enough patient exposure? Are they reflecting enough? Is there enough formative feedback?
- Hand-holding is, in part, a reflection of how trainees are used to being told what to do rather than developing their own autonomous method of practising and learning. Continue facilitating the process of helping trainees resolve difficulties for themselves rather than directly giving them the 'answers'.
- Encourage them to discuss their anxieties with their peers – hopefully this will lead to shared relief, which might help them to move on.

Top Tip: Look at the document *How a trainee develops – Maslow* on our website. It provides an alternative map of the trainee's journey adapted from Maslow's Hierarchy of Needs (covered in Chapter 10: Five Pearls of Educational Theory).

5: The trainee who is a muddly consulter

The trainee who is a muddly consulter often has deeper problems at several levels.

1 A lack of structure (or order) to the history and management plan.
2 A deficiency in clinical reasoning and problem-solving skills (not uncommon).
3 Poor time-keeping.

It's not uncommon to see these trainees fail the CSA because of disorganised data gathering and failing to reach shared management plans within the time that is allocated. To help the trainee one needs to tackle the above three things.

Adding structure to the history and management plan

- This is usually because of a failure to *signpost* and *summarise* periodically. There are skills worth practising with your trainee.
- Sometimes, a consultation looks unstructured because the doctor fails to take appropriate *control*. Instead, the patient 'runs the show' and takes it in all sorts of directions.
- Encourage the trainee to tease out an agenda (presenting complaint + screening) and take appropriate control.

Clinical reasoning and problem-solving skills

There is now a considerable body of theoretical knowledge about how doctors diagnose and problem-solve.[7,8,9,10] The cognitive processes used by an experienced doctor when an ill-looking patient walks into the consulting room are complex and initially unconscious. Discussing how we develop clinical and analytical reasoning can be extremely useful both to the Trainer and trainee alike – we need to understand before we advise.

How We Develop Clinical Reasoning

Hypothetico-Deductive
- Guess and test as you go
- Go and then think

Schema Driven
- Akin to a flow chart

Pattern Recognition
- Unconsciously pegged to individual patients

increasing knowledge and experience

After Silverman JD[11]

- **Hypothetico-deductive:** This is the least sophisticated approach to reaching a differential diagnosis; it is cognitive, used by inexperienced doctors and entails the practitioner taking a reasonably comprehensive history and then thinking of the diagnostic possibilities later. A variation on this theme is generating various hypotheses as the consultation proceeds, and then confirming/refuting them through using specific questioning techniques, examining the patient and the use of subsequent investigations.
- **Schema driven:** When the doctor is in less familiar territory, for example, a GP consulting a patient with jaundice, he or she will revert to some sort of template or protocol. Here, the doctor may consciously work out whether the jaundice is pre or post-hepatic in order to reach an accurate diagnosis and appropriate management.
- **Pattern recognition:** Recognising familiar patterns of presentation is mostly unconscious and enables the experienced practitioner to take short cuts to assessment and diagnosis. The experienced doctor will then follow this by testing for an accurate 'fit'. In general practice, the doctor uses this method with familiar presentations, for instance, sore throat or a urinary infection, while at the same time being mindful of a symptom or sign which *'just doesn't feel right'*.

Practical points for developing clinical reasoning and problem-solving skills

Faulty clinical reasoning and problem-solving skills are most easily assessed or 'diagnosed' by the Trainer observing the trainee consult – using a *combination* of video and direct observation (sitting in). In these sessions, encourage a formal re-examination of the way the trainee formulates the diagnosis and/or management plan.

- *Consultation videos* – stop at 2-minute intervals and ask the trainee:
  1 What was going on in your head at this point?
  2 What potential diagnosis were you considering at this point? Why?
  3 Was there anything else you had you already considered but rejected?
  4 How were you planning to proceed next?
- *Direct observation* – **consider being explicit with the patient that you may stop and start the consultation to help the trainee learn and develop** (and make sure the trainee is happy with this too). Explore *with* the trainee their reasoning process. Perhaps the patient could be used to give some feedback as well – patients love being involved and contributing. In these sessions, you must monitor the educational climate continuously to ensure that your desire to genuinely help the trainee develop comes through (and not one of superiority).
- Pause at the *data-gathering stage* and explore. There is a stage in data-gathering where the trainee needs to focus and work out a list of discriminatory questions for common and serious presentations (e.g. does the patient cough at night?). Does the trainee need to work on this?
- Pause at the *explanation* and *management planning* stage. Bad decisions might not be because of poor data gathering but the result of premature closure (i.e. proceeding down one line of 'hypothesis testing' too early). Involving the patient in the management planning stage helps formulate a plan they're more likely to stick with (a better decision = hopefully, a better outcome).
- *Model good clinical reasoning* by sharing your own clinical thinking out loud. The good teacher needs to step back from their own unconscious competence to the stage of learning their trainee is at so that they can share how that competence was achieved.

Many years ago I had a student who said at the end of the surgery, 'Gosh that was full of surprises. I didn't know what was going on most of the time and wished you had information bubbles coming out of your head.' That made me start to talk out loud to students and trainees and explore the things that were in my head that were reflective and how they helped me think of choices and the next step.

 Top Tip: The National Prescribing Centre (NPC) has produced a fabulous set of videos exploring *How to make better decisions*. The best one, in our view, is the one called *Individual decision-making*. Available at: www.npc.nhs.uk/evidence/eidm3_individuals/less_than_sixty.php

Time keeping

Muddly consulters take twice as long to consult and muddly ST3s will still be consulting at 20 minutes. With our pastoral/caring hat on, we might be reluctant to shorten the consultation time in case it makes things worse. But the truth of the matter is that by leaving it alone, you are allowing the trainee to continue in their comfort zone – consulting slowly. Why should they consult more efficiently if nothing has changed? Moving them to 10/15-minute consultations creates the necessary (mild) discomfort to encourage them to think of more effective questions, think about their consulting behaviour, and think about more effective ways of handling the consultation in general.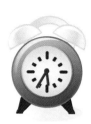

Conclusion

The early stages of a new post can be overwhelming. I remember when I started as a trainee in a practice based on two sites. Mostly, things seemed OK but there were times when I knew I wasn't getting it right. I watched my Trainer closely and, for example, how he left the notes on his desk at the end of the surgery. So I did the same. It seemed fine but there were some mutterings about the new trainee. No one explained until I asked and was told it was fine for the 'old yin' to leave his notes, but I was young, fit, and I should be competent enough to lift some notes and bring them to reception. The next glare was when I apologised and thanked Jenny for the advice. I then discovered that it was only first names in one end of the practice, and I should have thanked Mrs Black.

This little reflective piece demonstrates two key points that we'd like to finish off with. Firstly, how a good induction programme could have prevented a lot of the things mentioned. And, secondly, that not all 'perceived' problems are 'real' problems.

A sample of resources on our website
- The way a trainee develops – Maslow.
- NLP – The Wheel of Life and Core Values.
- The Time Management Matrix.

Other chapters you may like to read
- Chapter 31: The Trainee Experiencing Difficulty
- Chapter 33: First Aid for the Remedial Trainee.

Please give us some feedback on this chapter to help shape it for the next edition. Go to www.essentialgptrainingbook.com and simply click on the title of this chapter.

References

1 Covey S. *The Seven Habits of Highly Effective People.* New York: Simon and Schuster Ltd; 2004.

2 Prochaska JO, DiClemente CC. Transtheoretical therapy: toward a more integrative model of change. *Psychotherapy: Theory, Research, and Practice.* 1982; **19**(3): 276–88.

3 Rollnick S, Miller WR, Butler C. *Motivational Interviewing in Health Care: helping patients change behavior.* New York: Guilford Press; 2008.

4 Cruess SR, *et al.* Role modelling: making the most of a powerful teaching strategy. *BMJ.* 2008; **336**: 718–21.

5 http://tamarackcommunity.ca/ssi8.html provides a good précis of the work of Professor Brenda Zimmerman on complexity theory and GP relevant papers are: Greenhalgh T. Coping with complexity. *BMJ.* 2001; **323**: 799–803 and Innes AD, Campion PD, Griffiths FE. Complex consultations and the edge of chaos. *BJGP.* 2005; **55**: 510.

6 The Lewis-Parker 'Transition Curve' model is a seven-stage graph, based on original work by Adams JD, Hayes J, Hopkins B, in their 1976 book *Transition* (Baltimore: Johns Hopkins University Press). Ralph Lewis and Chris Parker described their ideas in a paper: Beyond the Peter Principle: managing successful transitions, published in the *Journal of European Industrial Training.* 1981; **5**(6): 17–21.

7 Norman G, Barraclough K, Dolovitch L, Price D. Iterative diagnosis. *BMJ.* 2009; **339**: 747–8.

8 Bowen JL. Educational strategies to promote clinical and diagnostic reasoning. *N Engl J Med.* 2006; **355**: 2217–25.

9 Scott I. Errors in clinical reasoning; causes and remedial strategies. *BMJ.* 2009; **339**: 22–5.

10 Falk G, Fahey T. Clinical prediction rules. *BMJ.* 2009; **339**: 402–3.

11 Silverman JD. *The New History Taking/Clinical Reasoning Course 2009.* Unpublished. Cambridge: University of Cambridge Clinical School.

First Aid for the Remedial Trainee

GRAHAM RUTT – Head of School (Northern Deanery) & lead author
JULIE ECCLES – GP Trainer (Gateshead)   **ALISON McDONALD** – TPD (Northumbria)

- Have you been approached with a view to helping a trainee who has had severe and repeated difficulties?
- Have you been asked to help a trainee with some specific targeted training?
- Maybe you've been allocated a trainee who has been given an extension to their training?

Then this chapter is for you. Although a lot of what is written below is mainly about repeated CSA failures, the concepts hold true whatever their reason for repeatedly failing.

Why you?

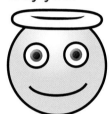

You should have been selected because you have some special skills to give to the situation, rather than just because you are available. Make no mistake: you have agreed to a really challenging, but potentially extremely rewarding, experience. With help and support, most of these trainees can successfully address their learning needs and progress to CCT (their final certificate saying they've completed training).

The five commandments for taking on a 'remedial' trainee

The five commandments

1 Do not think of them as remedial.
2 Keep an open mind about why they are having difficulties.
3 Use a different strategy (don't use lots more of the same).
4 Make patient safety your first concern.
5 Be open to surprise.

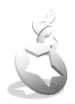

---

1 Do not think of them as remedial
Here are two definitions of the word remedial.
- Intended to improve deficient skills in a specific subject.
- Concerned with the correction, removal, or abatement of an evil, defect or disease.

We hope you can see that neither mindset is particularly helpful for our purposes – the first is too simplistic, the second is simply wrong!

2 Keep an open mind about why they are having difficulties
However much you respect the opinion of those who have assessed the trainee, you must remember that no one reaches this stage without having enough intelligence to pass finals, get through

an increasingly rigorous recruitment and selection process and know quite a lot of medicine. Although the problem will be complex, multifactorial in origin and not easily identified, *the strategies you can use to help are often simple*. It may be that these doctors feel the hard work they have put in to get this far is not appreciated or valued by their Trainers. Time spent understanding and showing respect for positive achievements in the past may help generate a mutually respectful relationship. But at the same time, **do not let your understanding and compassion blind you**. It's a fine balancing act. To be in this situation, they must have a serious impediment to their natural progress – it's highly improbable that they have never been given a chance because all their previous teachers were poor or had personal vendettas against them. It's better to take the view: *'whatever the mitigating circumstances, we are where we are now and we have to help you get out of it'*.

3 Use a different strategy; do not use lots more of the same

There is one thing that you can be certain of: whatever strategies have been used so far have not been successful. They do not need more of the same – but rather something different.

4 Make patient safety your first concern

Even when the teaching is not specifically related to medical knowledge, if any evidence of unsafe behaviour becomes apparent, then you have a duty to raise the matter with the trainee, their Educational Supervisor and the Training Programme Director.

 Top Tip: If a trainee really does have a poor knowledge base and patients are therefore unsafe, remove them from clinical practice and call for help (your Programme Director and the deanery).

---

5 Be open to surprise

For instance, be open to the idea that the previous training practice might not have been quite as good as everyone thought. Or perhaps the problem is that the remedial trainee is unable to recognise their skills. Yes, a remedial trainee has skills! For instance, many trainees, attempting to consult to the formula they believe the RCGP demands (such as trying to identify the patient's ideas, concerns and expectation), are simply unaware that they often demonstrate these skills intuitively during the history taking stage. Their attempt to demonstrate them overtly later in the CSA leads to the feedback about 'disorganised history taking' or 'muddled thinking'.

The essential groundwork

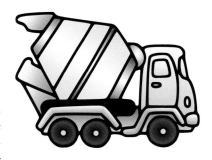

Let's now concentrate on some of the practical steps you will need to take. Hopefully, the trainee will arrive with (or be preceded by) paperwork documenting the evidence that underpins their status as 'remedial' together with what strategies have been used so far to help them.[1] If they have failed the CSA element of the MRCGP exam, they will also come with feedback suggesting why[2] (see the web resource *CSA – how are trainees performing?*). If they have struggled for other reasons, hopefully it should be clear which aspects of what regulation the evidence suggests they are contravening. The regulations being: (1) *GMC Duties of a Doctor*,[3] (2) GP curriculum,[4] (3) MRCGP competence areas.[5]

Top Tip: If you don't get any documentation, ask your deanery for it. You need to clarify where the difficulty lies so that you have a better idea on where to concentrate the training and what strategies you might take. If it is not clear in the documentation, you may need to do some diagnostic work yourself. For instance, you could define which areas of the *GMC Duties of a Doctor*, MRCGP competence areas and the GP curriculum need working on. Alternatively, you may wish to use the *RDM-p approach* covered in Chapter 31: The Trainee Experiencing Difficulty.

The first practical steps

1 Get your practice team on board

Your partners and Practice Manager: Be clear about the challenges the incoming trainee has faced and your plans to help them. This is not the time for trainee confidentiality taking precedence over their learning needs, and the whole practice has to work as a team to help them. We would suggest you share the *general need* (for example, '*we need to help the trainee with time management and consulting skills*'), but not the personal details about how they came to struggle. You will also need to be open with the trainee about what you have shared. Oh, and make sure your partners don't say something like: '*Hello, I'm Dr X. You must be the new trainee with some difficulties that Dr Y talked about the other day at our practice meeting.*' It's unlikely to put the trainee at ease, will embarrass them and may obstruct the relationship-building process that is so crucial at the beginning. Your practice colleagues must all be geared up to helping this

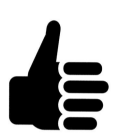

trainee get through; that means getting involved and being comfortable with being interrupted. Practices that have a shared ethos towards training do it better than those where everything is just left to the Trainer. You can learn more about creating an effective learning environment and enhancing a practice's ethos towards training in Chapter 9: Exploring and Creating a Learning Culture.

Rest of the practice team: Your practice team needs to take the approach outlined above too. Again, be careful of sharing the personal details around how they came to struggle and concentrate more on what their needs are, and how they might help.

2 The beginnings

Induction: Decide how to structure the all important 'introduction and induction' in advance. Please sit down and think about it. Tailor it to the needs of your trainee. Don't just hope it will all sort itself out. Involve your Practice Manager. *See* our Web Chapter: Induction for more details.

The educational contract: An educational contract is a negotiated agreement between a teacher and a learner which addresses four elements: needs, expectations, roles, and content. Essentially, it spells out what is expected of them and what they can expect in return. Being clear about this right from the beginning means that you both start off on the same wavelength with a common vision or goal in mind. Educational contracts are also helpful when one side 'breaks the rules' of engagement – they can be used to help re-establish 'connection'. Again, our Web Chapter: Induction tells you more about educational contracts; our website has one for you to download and use.

Patient safety: Work out how you are going to monitor patient safety while allowing them to consult without fear of being watched by 'big brother' all the time. This is a difficult balancing act with all trainees – and especially with those who clearly have problems. Trainees in this position have often been on the receiving end of 'over-vigilance' and nitpicking all their mistakes in the past. *Talk to them* about it and get them to see why it's important for you to do this and the risks you will be putting your practice and patients under if you don't: *'As with all trainees, I need to make sure patients are safe, so initially I will . . . How does that make you feel? Is that okay?'* Get them to agree with what you are ultimately going to do.

> **Top Tip:** Trainees will not object to a strategy that appears restrictive, providing they can see the logic for its need.

Debriefs: We would suggest:

- review every case to start with
- however, ensure that you only criticise *important* issues, not ones where the trainee is simply following a different protocol.

Make sure the debriefs actually happen – review timetables and ensure regularly scheduled protected debriefing slots are in place. Get your Practice Manager involved – they'll be able to do most of the organisational legwork. Debriefing is covered in more detailed in Chapter 26: Effective Clinical Supervision and in our Web Chapter: Induction.

Validate feelings and set a positive climate: Be upfront about you knowing that they have struggled so far. Acknowledge and validate their difficulties and feelings and then go on to explain that you are there to help them overcome their problems: *'From what you've said, I sense that you felt demotivated in your last practice by being watched all the time. And you mentioned that some of the doctors said one thing to your face and something completely the opposite in your ePortfolio. I can understand why you dreaded going into work. I hope you will be happier here. All of us in this practice are here to help you. I'm sure you will like it here, and I hope that if there is anything that upsets you, you'd feel comfortable enough to come and talk to me about it. How does that sound? Is that fair?'*

3 Supervision and support

Make sure you have mapped out all the channels of support in your practice and that the trainee is aware of them too. There should be a Clinical Supervisor nominated for every surgery they do, and it doesn't always need to be you; get your colleagues involved. Your Practice Manager will prove invaluable in the planning process. The more you share the training workload, the more enjoyable you will find the whole experience.

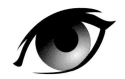

Top Tip: Half of you needs to be task-focused to get all the organisational bits sorted. The other half of you needs to be a soft, gentle and less task-orientated supporter to help the trainee through this difficult time.

What do I do then?

Do what you normally do. Paradoxically, although the presentation may be complex, and the underlying cause multifactorial, the solution is often very simple. The basic building blocks will not surprise you as they represent some old values:

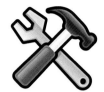

Creating the right educational climate

- Create an atmosphere of **trust and welcome**.
- **Respect and praise** what they *are* good at – perhaps over-egging it a little on occasions: it helps build a really good Trainer–trainee relationship and motivates them to learn.
- Set realistic **achievable goals** while keeping the bigger picture in mind.
- Be prepared to **share your learning needs** with them. This will help them realise that we all have learning needs as well as getting them to open up: *'Mmmm . . . I'm not quite sure what the features of Diddlysquat syndrome are either. Shall we try to find out together? Where shall we start?'*

Some specific things to consider

- Assess their knowledge early using the RCGP's **curriculum checklist tool** or equivalent.
- Do **joint surgeries** where they see some patients but so do you (to enable you to demonstrate skills and model desired behaviour).
- Do lots of **video work** (helps you see what they actually do in practice).
- Do lots of **random case analyses** (especially if knowledge is a particular concern – focusing, in particular, on the clinical aspects of the case).
- Do lots of **problem case analyses**: structure it with a clear separation of:
  - what do you know about the case? (data-gathering)
  - what might be going on? (hypothesis formation)
  - how do you tell? (hypothesis testing)
  - how do you choose what to do? (management plan).[6]
- Engage in **role play** where possible (helps you get an idea of how they would actually behave in practice rather than what they say they would do).
- Do lots more than the minimum number of **CBDs and COTs** (although these are assessment tools, they're also good educational tools that will help you keep an eye on progress and determine where more work is needed).
- Set **learning tasks** appropriate to learning needs as they are identified.

Skills you need to develop and use
- **Listen** attentively.
- Be alert for **cues**.
- Explore **feelings**.
- Help them **reflect** – link the learning to their experience.
- **Summarise and signpost** often.
- **Explain.**
- Give **feedback** often; encourage immediate feedback from the patient where possible.
- **Reframe negative feedback as positive things to do.** Saying: *'Unfortunately, **you did not tackle her concerns** about what she read in her magazine'* would be better phrased *'Would you agree that the patient might have been happier **if you had tackled her concerns** over what she read in her magazine?'* Other examples of positive reframing can be found in a document on our website (called *'Positively reframing the MRCGP feedback'*).

Everything you've said so far is similar to what I already do with all trainees. So what should I do that is different?

- **Be lavish in your praise of what they do well.** It is not uncommon to hear remedial trainees say how previously they have been told (directly and indirectly) how 'rubbish', 'no good' or 'incompetent' they are. Their confidence that they are right and the exam process is wrong will at best be a defensive response of a *frightened* individual. We need to lavishly praise them when they do things well in order to (1) build their confidence, (2) shift the balance of feedback from always being negative and (3) help strengthen the Trainer–trainee relationship.
- **Work on observed or documented behaviour.** This may be from:
  - observations forwarded by Clinical Supervisors or other colleagues
  - discussions with your local Training Programme Director – maybe what they've observed at Half/Full-Day Release
  - behaviour seen in 1–1 role play or videos
  - case notes brought by the learner.

  Formulate and agree learning tasks jointly with the trainee, and review at the next session.
- **Be *very* task-focused, work on specific areas of need and use those around you.** Is there someone who can deliver on a particular deficiency or learning need? Perhaps Dr Hart (a GPwSI in Cardiology) can help fill knowledge gaps in curriculum domain *15.1: Cardiovascular Problems*. How about using Dr Listener to help build on communication skills. You might even involve organisations outside your practice, for example, the diabetic satellite clinic or the local drugs and alcohol misuse service.

- **Stick to your guns if you are clear that the evidence demonstrates something.** Trainees may well be in denial of the truth. For example, whatever trainees say, they fail the CSA if either their consulting skills are not good enough or their exam technique is poor – and they only get negative feedback if the same problem has been noted by two assessors. If necessary demand that the learner continues to work on a point even if they feel they have nothing more to learn about it. The trainee may say: *'I mean no disrespect for you as a teacher, but I think this is a waste of time'*, but if you are certain the evidence suggests they still need to learn a particular point, you should follow on with a clear instruction that nonetheless this is what they are going to do. Of course, you should try to use negotiating techniques to get them on board but, as a last resort, you may just need to be decisively directive!

A trainee was sent for remedial training because he was having difficulty problem-solving during consultations and in discussion would never suggest more than one possible explanation for any given set of symptoms, let alone a changing list of possibilities as the consultation evolved. Not a problem in simple consultations, where they were usually right, but a real problem in complex consultations because they were unable to develop hypotheses let alone evaluate them. They were asked to sit in, watch the Trainer consult, given a pen and paper and asked to write all the possible causes for the patients' presentation that occurred to them as the consultations developed. The list was discussed after every consultation. The lesson was repeated and repeated until the trainee could generate satisfactory lists. Only when feedback from colleagues suggested an improvement in problem-solving in the clinical setting were they congratulated on their new, wider-thinking hypothesis-formation skills.

- **Where necessary, challenge their educational paradigm, and teach them a new one.** A paradigm is a framework, pattern or set of practices that define a particular discipline. In this

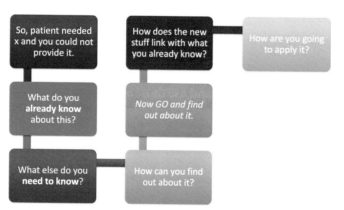

instance, an educational paradigm is another name for a learning framework or mindset. Changing their learning mindset is particularly necessary if, for example, their response to any given situation is simply to read a book. In this instance, you may wish to extend their educational paradigm by encouraging them to engage with PUNs and DENs (see diagram right).

Often, trainees who have been deemed as remedial arrive with entrenched beliefs that they are right and those assessing them are wrong. These will need challenging – but *sensitively*. For instance, they may cling onto learning strategies to help them pass exams, which have clearly not worked in the past. And then there are those who say *'but my friend who has passed said that they did x, y and z'*. Many remedial doctors are members of self-formed study groups consisting of other trainees who are struggling too. These other members (especially if they've finally managed to get through) will often impart bad advice. This ends up providing a recipe for maintaining and reinforcing counterproductive failing behaviours.

- **Do lots of video work.** Why so much video? Videos capture behaviour which helps identify the true nature of the performance problem. This 'evidence' is difficult to argue against and is more likely to be accepted by the trainee. If they continue to be in denial – simply rewind the tape to prove your point! A common problem among remedial trainees is following 'scripts' or rehearsed phrases without them being contextually modified to the patient. The consultation then lacks fluency and appears clunky. You will need to *sensitively* challenge their mindset about 'following the script' and persuade them to 'follow the patient' instead.

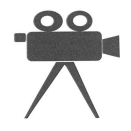

- **Encourage self-evaluation and self-reflection first.** Trainees often yearn for 'answers' or to be told what to do, but we need to help them find strategies to help themselves. After all, what will they do when you're no longer around to hold their hand? Encourage them to self-evaluate and reflect before dishing out any advice yourself. Use a feedback framework like ALOBA or SET-GO, which starts with the learner's perspective and self-evaluation first (more about them in Chapter 7: The Skilful Art of Giving Feedback). These frameworks make the trainee come up with a range of non-scripted interventions, which can then (hopefully) be put into practice through repeated rehearsal. Generating their own solutions means they are more likely to remember them too.

'So in that consultation video, you felt the patient wasn't too pleased with the management you offered him. And you want to know what to do next? . . . Okay, let's look at this in a slightly different way. Let's replay that part of the video where you felt there was difficulty, and I'd like you to note down and tell me afterwards what you actually saw going on. And then we'll take it from there. Is that okay?' . . . Trainer then goes onto use the SET-GO framework.

- **Constantly review progress.** It might be worthwhile time-tabling regular periods to ensure review happens. If the trainee is not making progress, first ask yourself the question *'Have I got things right?'* If the evidence says 'yes' stay with the lesson in hand and go over and over it again. If there are clear signs of progress reward lavishly – build their confidence and their desire to do well.

What have other Trainers said?

A recent meeting of Trainers who had taught trainees in a remedial position concluded that progress is greatest in the following situations.

- It is understood by both parties that the role of the remedial teacher is *primarily* educational and not supportive (although the latter is important too).
- The Trainer keeps sufficient distance between the teacher and learner to enable that *educational* role to be kept in focus while also communicating that they value and believe in them.
- The teacher provides the right balance of positive feedback and challenge.
- The teacher is prepared to be very directive and didactic when necessary.
- The teacher resists the trainee's attempts to persuade them that things are really satisfactory. If they were we would not be where we are now!
- Work is focused, time-limited and based on known facts and demonstrable (i.e. witnessed, video-taped or documented) behaviours so that there is no room for excuses/avoidance of issues.
- Suggestions for change are specific, rehearsed at the time and discussed immediately afterwards.

- There is a consistent approach by all the teaching team, both on task and method. Other people within the organisation make it clear that they value the trainee as a person, believe in their ability to succeed and provide the necessary support they need.

The most difficult issues for the Trainer seem to be:
- coming to terms with not always treating the trainee as an adult learner
- maintaining an emotional distance from the trainee when necessary
- not entering into general discussions not directly related to the task in hand
- developing a workable relationship within these parameters.

 Top Tip: If there are several remedial trainees in your locality, chat with the Programme Directors – see if they can occasionally run a small group specifically for them at Half-Day Release. It can work really well: once the facilitator starts to challenge the trainees, they often see the learning point in each other before they see it in themselves.[7]

All this sounds exhausting. How can I keep my energy levels going?

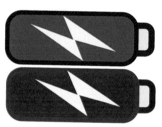 It is exhausting if you don't get the rest of your team members involved. Just because you're the nominated Trainer doesn't mean you have to do all the clinical, educational and organisational stuff. **Share out the workload!** Another thing that will protect your energy from being sapped by targeted training is to arrange reflective **debriefing sessions** with another senior educationalist. Ask your local Programme Director to see whether this is possible – perhaps one of them might volunteer.

 Top Tip: How about developing a separate Trainers' group for those who have remedial or difficult trainees. You could meet periodically to discuss issues, share ideas and generally provide support for each other. Your local Programme Directors can help you set one up.

A little note about the previous training practice

The TPD should try to keep the previous Trainer informed on the progress of the trainee. They should also explore and help them get rid of any crooked thinking they may have developed about themselves. For instance, the Trainer in the original practice can feel bruised at not being able to help the trainee succeed. They can feel like a failure – questioning themselves about what they did wrong. Sometimes, this is appropriate because there is a training need that needs tackling in that practice. However, the majority will have done a good job as far as was possible for that particular trainee.

Are overseas (international medical) graduates different?

We cannot ignore the fact that overseas (particularly male) graduates struggle more with CSA than UK-trained graduates, and much research is currently going on to understand why.[8] Experience suggests that there are strong cultural influences at play. If you want to read more, *see* Chapter 21: Supporting GP Trainees Who Graduated Outside the UK. The following points are worth keeping in the back of your mind.

- **Not all cultures value patient or learner-centredness** to the extent that Western European culture does.
- There is a significant subgroup of doctors whose learning needs are not met because they are **not able to adjust easily to a UK style of teaching/training** rather than any innate lack of skill.
- In trying to adjust, **many follow the 'script'** they perceive the examiner wants to hear rather than the dynamic of the consultation.
- Many overseas doctors **learn by rote** (the same educational paradigm taught in their medical school), and they may therefore have problems with reflective practice.[9]
- **Language difficulties are common.** Again, this may result in 'scripting'.

 Red Alert: Please be careful with this list. It does not hold true for *all* doctors educated overseas – so no assumptions please.

An overseas graduate trainee who was naturally person-centred had problems with language. He said that in all of his consultations, he would have to translate what the patient said into his mother tongue Punjabi in order to digest and understand it. Although he knew how to respond empathically in Punjabi, he would have to spend time thinking how to do it in English. As a result, his consultations were lengthy with uncomfortable pauses, which made him come across as hesitant, uncertain and emotionally detached.

Closing statement

You may have noticed that the remedial approaches described in this chapter use a more teacher-centred, directive style, more akin to some of the learner's original style, which may explain why they were beneficial. It may be that some of these doctors are failing because the *adult* teaching methods that we normally use (which are less restrictive and more creative than the pedagogic directive teaching methods) are inaccessible to them. Some trainees are simply not ready for the freedom they have never experienced before and thus cannot cope with it, and some will even resent it. It's interesting that a group of Trainers with remedial trainees said they felt they were treating these trainees very much as recalcitrant children, at least to start with and not as adult learners – but that it was *very effective* in effecting change.

A large proportion of remedial trainees trained outside the UK. Many of them will be unfamiliar with the healthcare system in the UK. They may just simply need inducting into the NHS and its ways![10] But doctors who have come to the UK often have additional problems. Some have had to work extremely hard just so that they could apply for specialist training. Others (refugee doctors) will have come from very traumatic backgrounds and in such circumstances, in order to maintain that sense of self, many adopt the firm conviction that they are right and everybody else is wrong. These defences, once established, may be difficult to break down, leading to significant unconscious blocks to learning from experience. Such doctors may perceive constructive feedback, even if well founded and well intentioned, as an attack on their sense of selves, thus failing to take it on board and responding in an undesirable way. This may in turn lead to a breakdown in the Trainer–trainee relationship.[11] This group often ends up being labelled 'remedial' when actually they are far from it – just locked into it.

A sample of resources on our website
- Educational contract.
- CSA – how are trainees performing?
- Positively reframing MRCGP feedback.

Other chapters you may like to read
- Web Chapter: Induction
- Chapter 31: The Trainee Experiencing Difficulty
- Chapter 32: The Top Five Educational Difficulties.

Please give us some feedback on this chapter to help shape it for the next edition.
Go to www.essentialgptrainingbook.com and simply click on the title of this chapter.

References
1 Rutt GA, Bedi A, Chalmers H, Eccles J. Supporting struggling registrars. *Educ Prim Care*. 2006; **17**: 260–4.

2 Rendel S. *Feedback from the May 2009 Clinical Skills Assessment*. RCGP Circular to Deanery assessment leads. 2009. Personal communication.

3 GMC. *Duties of a Doctor*. Available at: www.gmc-uk.org/guidance/good_medical_practice/index.asp#Good%20clinical%20care (accessed May 2011).

4 RCGP. *GP Curriculum Statements*. Available at: www.rcgp-curriculum.org.uk/rcgp_-_gp_curriculum_documents/gp_curriculum_statements.aspx (accessed May 2011).

5 RCGP. *The Competence Framework*. Available at: www.rcgp-curriculum.org.uk/nmrcgp/wpba/competence_framework.aspx (accessed May 2011).

6 Rutt GA, Bedi A. A tool to help structure, process and outcome of problem case analysis. *Educ Prim Care*. 2006; **17**: 162–5.

7 Rutt GA, Eccles J. The role of group-work in teaching general practice specialty registrars. *Educ Prim Care*. 2008; **18**: 506–13.

8 Knight C. Diversity: what is behind the CSA failure rates? *Educ Prim Care*. 2009; **20**: 397–401.

9 Chalmers D, Volet S. Common misconceptions about students from South East Asia studying in Australia. *Higher Educ Res Dev*. 1997; **16**: 87–98.

10 Eccles J, Dodd M. *What if I have a doctor new to the NHS?* Available at: www.nvts.co.uk/train_nvts.asp?cont=doctor (accessed May 2009).

11 Youll B. *The Learning Relationship; Psychoanalytical Thinking in Education*. London: Karnac Books. 2006.

PART TEN

Management
and I.T.

The Virtual World of E-learning

DANIEL WEAVER – GP trainee (Pembrokeshire) & lead author   RAMESH MEHAY – TPD (Bradford)
VERONICA WILKIE – Senior Clinical Teaching Fellow (Univ. Warwick)
JOHN LORD – Professor of Primary Medical Care (Univ. Huddersfield)
BRAD CHEEK – TPD (East Cumbria)   IAIN LAMB – Associate Advisor (SE Scotland)

Introduction

E-learning – like it or loathe it, but patients are doing it, their families are doing it as are their friends. So, how can we busy doctors possibly keep up? There is a huge unfiltered world of information and misinformation online. This can be empowering for both doctors and patients but is also a potential Pandora's box if not approached sensibly.

'Hello there, what would you like to talk about today?' I said with a broad smile to Peggy, an octogenarian patient who shuffled into the room and made a beeline for my swivel chair, before being gently ushered away and into the non-swivelling one by her 50-something daughter. As she settled into the seat, I noticed Peggy seemed to be brandishing a large wad of A4 printout with a degree of menace.

'Well doctor, it's like this . . .' she muttered, accidentally dropping some of the sheets onto the floor. As I gathered them up for her, I noticed at least one the papers said PubMED and the others appeared to be printouts from online forums. 'I've been doing some reading, and I think I've got Ankysomethingorother . . . Have a look at the sheets; I got my grandson to print them out on my new printer. It's a marvellous thing really.'

'Mum's wrong!' said the daughter abruptly, 'You've got this fibrosomyalgica thing that they were talking about on the TV the other day . . . Hold on!' Out of her handbag came a half a dozen more printouts. 'Here! And I think she needs to be referred to these people.' Out came a flyer for an expensive medical company in Ohio.

Yes, we all use the Internet daily – it is undoubtedly an efficient way to stay in touch with friends, keep track of current affairs and information. It has also become a part of our careers, with the

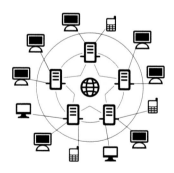

delights of the ePortfolio, online CPD and useful references such as Map Of Medicine,[1] GP Notebook[2] and Web Mentor[3] if uncertain about management. However, despite dipping our toes into the digital world, all in all, medicine and doctors remain quite traditional. This is especially true for medical education, where there is a reliance on text books, handouts and lectures delivered in the main via PowerPoint (with copies of the slides passed to keen trainees, usually on brightly coloured USB drives emblazoned with the name of an expensive medication). We still raise an eyebrow when we see a new flashy whiteboard in a postgraduate department, without knowing how to use it fully, and presentations with bells and whistles often produce grumpy mutterings about how 'less is more'.

Did you know that schools no longer operate in this way; children no longer learn this way. Schools have begun to embrace virtual learning environments. Young people spend huge amounts of time on the Internet. The use of websites such as YouTube[4] and social networks, like Facebook,[5] have taken the place of more traditional hobbies. It is difficult to engage this digital generation with books and didactic teaching. Schools are aware of this trend, and they are taking it seriously.

One teacher told me that her school had recently spent £40 000 on the construction of an e-learning system via a private company. The result was a super slick online environment that resembled a social-networking site such as MySpace[6] or Facebook,[5] but with learning materials, web links, forums and lessons built in. The lessons and resources can now be used in or out of the classroom, and the computer will often be the hub around which the teacher runs the lesson.

The superficial reasons for schools investing in this technology are obvious:
1 making lessons available online if children miss a class
2 to make learning seem more engaging or fun and
3 to reduce paperwork (many of the online tools will record who has completed the lesson and can even mark answers based on tick boxes or key word recognition).

The reality is that the generation in school at present interact, communicate and learn in the electronic world. This is their default, and they have never grown up in a time without computers. Touch screens and spell-checkers are the norm; these are not people who have developed an interest in computing and the Internet like the 'geeks' of the past. It is this same generation of children who will become the medical students and doctors of tomorrow. Surely, the way we teach and communicate needs to evolve too? Therefore, in this chapter, we will consider some of the useful aspects of e-learning and virtual learning environments that can be applied to GP training, as well as some useful websites and services.

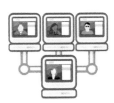

Golden rules of using new technologies
Here are a few principles when you're thinking of using a new form of teaching media.

1 Don't use it just because it's the latest craze
Figure out the purpose of the new gizmo. Then go back to your own purpose and see if it marries with that.

> I once had a person ask me if I could help him develop some teaching podcasts simply because he'd heard about podcasts, although he still didn't really know what they were!

2 Old things might lose a bit of flavour, but they don't lose their function
Just because there is a 'new kid on the block' doesn't mean you should dump the old. Older things, like PowerPoint and paper handouts, still serve a function.

> At a Trainers' workshop, we discussed how we (the Trainers) could communicate and collaborate with each other better. The conclusion was for a subgroup to look at setting up some sort of e-group. We couldn't decide whether to use the new-style social-networking sites like Facebook or the older more traditional Google/Yahoo newsgroups.
>   One of the members helped us resolve this dilemma (the new vs the old). He said our discussions reminded him of the situation where a pharmaceutical drug becomes generic, only shortly to be followed by the birth of a newer version. We've all come across the enthusiastic drug rep who starts extolling the virtues of a new isomer – an exciting looking box, works a tiddly bit better, but we know it costs more. He reminded us that we usually stick with the old because we know it will achieve the outcome we want

anyway. Furthermore, the limitations and side-effects of the old one are well known, so better the devil you know . . .

So we stuck with the old-style discussion groups – they have been around for so long, they have been thoroughly debugged, are very stable and unlikely to run into technical hitches. They're run by well established firms with less likelihood of disappearing in the medium and long term. However, because they do not create significant revenue for the firms, they do not receive new investment. This group of technology has not evolved much recently and has poor compatibility with smartphones. Nevertheless, we still opted for a Yahoo e-group.

3 Check things out with the intended audience before rolling anything out

One of the Training Programme Directors thought it would be good if our scheme had a Facebook page, linking all of us (TPDs, trainees and admin) together. But the rest of us (also TPDs) suggested we ask the trainees first. When we did, it was clear that it was a no-go area – unanimously (and understandably) they wanted to keep life and work separate. The same TPD then asked the audience whether they would like to receive RSS feeds or Twitter messages about news, events and announcements. One of them asked why this would be any better than the email notification system currently in place.

4 Don't dismiss the experts – at least consider them

For example, you might want to have a go at web design, and although you may be able to *deliver* your ideas, it's the professionals who can help you *build* on them and use tricks to make them come *alive*.

We decided to build a surgery website. One of the partners had dabbled in web design, and it was better than forking out £5000 to a professional company. But for some reason, things just didn't work out. After a year, the website still had not gotten off the ground. Fortuitously, someone (a web developer that one of us knew) got in touch with us and asked if we would like him to do us one for a reasonable £1500. Discussions with him helped us realise that there was so much more that websites could offer than our previous conception of simply displaying information. For instance, he incorporated a system where patients could register to receive e-updates and e-announcements. How cool is that?

5 One model does not fit all

Just because you fall in love with a new form of media doesn't mean others will. Different people have different learning styles and, therefore, prefer to communicate or receive information in different ways. To 'capture' the majority, use a variety of media.

In recruiting authors for this book, the Editor used several forms of media to hook in GP Educators up and down the country. The first was a video slide show with accompanying 'feel good' music – working on the visual, auditory and kinaesthetic domains. The second was a colourful A4 pdf flyer (visual domain). These were sent to the masses via email. Some areas received a paper copy of the A4 flyer too. He went to conferences and talked to people (auditory) and finally encouraged others to 'spread the news' by word of mouth (also auditory). The response rate was remarkable. Over 120 GP Educators wanted to get involved – giving up their personal time for free.

The e-landscape – trends and technologies
Smartphones, iPads, and other PDAs

I remember vividly as a teenager being jealous of my dad's Personal Digital Assistant (PDA) – it was a very primitive Palm which he enjoyed prodding with a stylus. It had a calendar and looked very futuristic but had few functions beyond this. The lack of processing power meant that the majority of these early PDA machines could not run useful software. Those that could were extremely slow and expensive. Synchronising them with a computer was often a soul-destroying battle with cables, docks and error messages. Higher-end PDAs could run applications such as Excel and word processing, but their price put them out of reach of the masses, not to mention their geek stigma. How things have changed with iPhones, iPads and so on.

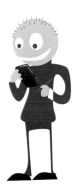

The emergence of companies such as Blackberry, the growth of Wi-Fi (wireless networking), and 3G-capable phones have ushered in a new era. The idea of a phone on which the user can check emails, access the Internet, send text messages and talk to people has gained popularity. In recent years, the smartphone market has exploded. Products such as Apple's iPhone, and phones using Google's Android operating system, have captured the public imagination. These phones have flourished due to the innovation and range of the applications or 'apps' that can be downloaded onto them. Wi-Fi and 3G/4G services allow large amounts of fast data transfer which previously has not been possible. One is never more than 20 yards away from a smartphone user!

The great benefit (or curse) of smartphones is that you can potentially access your emails and even the Internet from anywhere that has a mobile phone signal – making winning pub quizzes infinitely easier for early adopters. You no longer have to boot up a computer to access the Internet, and the easy portability is undeniably useful. You can even chuck your heavy medical reference books out of the window as there are now a variety of useful apps and e-books for the busy clinician. Many trainees without broadband Internet access will depend on their smartphone as their link to the Internet. This alternative method of Internet access is particularly useful because of the poor Internet access in many hospitals, and the extreme measures taken by them to block as many websites as possible in an attempt to improve productivity and reduce computer virus exposure.

In one hospital I worked at, the only available websites appeared to be citation indexes, university pages and the cricket website cricinfo.com (possibly unblocked due to a threatened revolt by locum doctors). This made Internet research almost impossible, and keeping track of emails and the world in general was hard when working a string of long days or nights.

Pros
- Companies such as **Skyscape**[8] offer a download of entire medical textbooks (like the Oxford Clinical Handbook range and the BNF) onto a smartphone.
- There are free apps for things like BMI calculations, paediatric drug dosages, etc.
- Most smartphones have GPS – allowing satellite navigation for house calls.

Cons
- A difficulty with smartphones is that their screens are small and conventional web pages do not always work well.

Websites

Simple websites (often from novice web designers) at a basic-level offer information for the user to read. In this process, there is little interactivity between the user and the website – the user simply reads the web pages. Web design has evolved dramatically in recent years primarily in ways to make the user experience of a website more interactive, dynamic and alive (e.g. through things like flash animations,[9] video clips and customised ways in which web pages can be displayed).

In the early days, you could only create a website if you understood the language of the web – called html code. Then came software that enabled one to simply drag and drop items onto a web page. However, that was only good for simple web pages. The latest craze is something called WordPress.[10] They say that if you spend a couple of weeks studying and playing around with WordPress, you'll be able to create some amazing web pages to which you can add various apps to liven them up: www.wordpress.org

A few of the things you can do with websites include the following.
- Display information – knowledge, timetables, events and courses.
- Upload resources like pre-course material, handouts, pictures (e.g. dermatology images) and video clips (e.g. of communication skills).
- Create links to other useful websites and resources.
- Enable users to communicate with each other (email, posts and forums).
- In general provide a 'one stop' centre.

> **Top Tip:** Be creative: how about creating a chat area on your website? This would provide real-time communication for individuals who are geographically miles apart.

RSS feeds

RSS feeds[11] are news streams that are often embedded in websites. An RSS feed basically provides a periodic summary of the changes or additions to a website. This is then sent out to all the subscribers. For example, part of the RSS feed from say the RCGP website might say *'We have now uploaded new guidelines around Consent and Confidentiality'*. Clicking on that item will navigate to the full story. RSS feeds are a good way of:
- telling you what's new or different about a website without you having to laboriously go through every single page since your last visit
- receiving a concise summary of news streams at a time where there is information overload all around us
- putting you in control – letting you decide which items you want to explore deeper.

Wikis[12,13]

The Hawaiian word for 'fast' is wiki, which is apt because these are websites that allow users to work collaboratively in order to quickly create, edit, update and expand web pages using their usual web browser (like Internet Explorer or Mozilla Firefox). In this way, **a wiki is a living, evolving resource** and can remain current in a way that traditional encyclopaedias cannot. They are also incredibly easy to set up, access and use. The content can be open to all or for an invited few only.

The wiki most familiar to us, our trainees and our Internet-using patients is wikipedia.org.

Wikipedia[14] can be a fantastic free resource but be careful – it can also be a bit misleading if a mischief maker has been at work. Administrators try to moderate any misinformation placed on the website. Articles will contain links to references and sources of information, and many words are hyperlinked – clicking on them will transport you to their own page. www.ganfyd.org[15] is a medical wiki and has the benefit of being edited only by registered medical professionals and invited experts, although its content is open to all. It has a small but growing range of information, which is aimed at multiple specialities. Articles are often linked to relevant guidelines and peer-reviewed sites.

 Top Tip: In the GP setting, a potential application for use of a wiki could be:
- to share course notes or recent reading
- to collate and update information about local services or referral pathways.

Pros
- They encourage people to work collaboratively.
- In so doing, web pages can be created and updated in a jiffy.
- They are basically a living and evolving web resource.

Cons
- Its content might not be 100% reliable, especially if a rogue user has signed up.

E-groups – private or public groups
Yahoo[16] and Google[17] both offer free e-groups – web space where subscribed members can create and reply to conversation threads as well as upload files to share. They're often free because they are paid for by advertising banners. The success of an e-group depends on its members. It is not sufficient for users to simply access the site; they must also participate and contribute ideas.

Our local VTS scheme has used a Yahoo e-group since 2005. Although technology and services have moved on since then, it still serves a useful purpose as a means of discussion and storing files.

Pros
- They are an easy way for a group of people to hold discussions about a hot topic or issue.
- They enable members to work collaboratively and share files.
- They can be set as private to prevent outsiders accessing data and discussions.
- Easy to set up.

Cons
- Each time a post is made every user receives a notification email. It can fatten up your email inbox if the group is too active!
- Only rich text format (RTF) might be supported. That means it will strip messages of colour, formatting or other embedded styles.

e-Forums
Forums (or 'fora' for those who prefer a little Latin) are traditionally the most frequently used form of topic discussion on the Internet. They have been for many years and still continue to remain

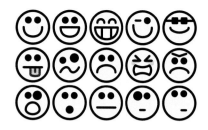

strong (despite new things like Twitter). Conversation threads are searchable – useful for quickly finding a particular topic debated or discussed in the past. Any responses or replies to original posts will be elegantly contained within them. Doctors.net.uk[18] has a good example of a well-constructed forum with broad categories (Clinical, Non-Clinical, Politics, Training) and subcategories (GP Trainers, GP trainees). The beauty of this system is that the user can target their audience.

If you want to have a general discussion, then post to a general forum, otherwise select a specific subgroup.

Social networks

Facebook[5] is the most widely used social-networking site worldwide where you can choose who to connect with. It works best for fire-and-forget type posts or quick feedback on brief statements.

I love Facebook. I can quickly build up a list of my family and friends just by using Facebook's search box. This contact list will gradually grow and grow as Facebook shows you friends of friends who you might also know. And you can keep in touch with your mates in several ways. You can private message or 'PM' them, post something on their front page or 'wall' (which can then be viewed and commented by others), or even 'poke' them. There's a whole host of other things that you can do too – like share pictures, video and web links.

Pros
- Use them to advertise events, as a forum for debates or sharing of materials.
- Most have a downloadable phone app – they're designed to be easily accessible.

Cons
- Like Marmite, social networking has an extraordinary ability to polarise people.
- Every member needs to set up their own profile with the site.
- There are privacy concerns (Facebook's settings sometimes have a mind of their own). The GMC isn't keen on docs posting work-related messages in public domains.

Blogs and Twitters

The term 'blog'[19,20] comes from an abbreviation of the word 'weblog' which usually refers to a website maintained by an individual and used either as a public diary or a means to commentate on various issues. There is no limit on the amount you wish to write about in your blog. Twitter[21] is a micro-blogging website – by micro-blogging, we mean that it's similar to a blog except that each post has a limit of 140 characters.

Advantages of Twitter over blogs
- It encourages authors to make their point concisely. It gets rid of the waffle.
- Shorter posts are easier to browse through and take less time to make.
- Shorter posts mean you obtain information more quickly.

Disadvantages of Twitter over blogs

- Character limits can reduce the potential depth of discussion.
- Hard to make complex points.
- All members need to be familiar with the system (e.g. # and @ tags to link posts).

Online e-learning modules

There are loads of online CPD modules covering a wealth of medical knowledge with embedded video and quizzes. Most take 1–2 hours to complete, and you usually get an electronic certificate of completion at the end. **Doctors.net.uk**[18] hosts many modules as does the **BMJ Learning** website[22] and **e-GP**[23] (an RCGP curriculum based e-learning service). In the context of teaching a relevant module could be a useful and novel form of pre-reading for a tutorial or half-day teaching, and the certificate is a good way of checking that this has been done.

 Top Tip: Why not have a go at creating your own e-learning modules from scratch. Do a Google search on 'creating e-learning modules' and take it from there. Alternatively, if you just want to focus on writing while leaving the technical stuff to someone else, contact Doctors.net,[18] BMJ[24] or RCGP.[25] Some even reward you with payment for each time a module is completed, and it looks good on your CV too.

Podcasts

Podcasts have become a popular feature of iTunes[26] (iTunes being Apple's multimedia player and online shop for varied content from music, to TV and films to books). They are virtually always free and can be downloaded and listened to either on a computer or on a portable media player – such as an iPod or smartphone. Some academic institutions will record lectures and publish them as podcasts. iTunes U[27] (accessed through iTunes) has been expanding this form of e-learning, allowing people to download audio of an academic nature free from places such as Oxford University, etc. The major drawback with this avenue is that creating an account to be able to actually publish content in iTunes U, for GP trainees for example, is arduous, difficult and potentially expensive.

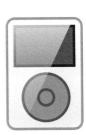

Screencasts

This is a video version of podcasting and is growing in popularity as Internet speeds increase. This is useful for recording and archiving interesting lectures or skills but video can take up a lot of space and be expensive to save remotely. Screencasts aren't particularly difficult to make and may be hosted on video-sharing websites such as YouTube,[4] Vimeo[28] or directly embedded within websites. We (the authors) prefer Vimeo over YouTube.

Teleconferences

A teleconference is a real-time, video meeting experience over the net between participants in two or more locations. It's particularly good for people who need to meet but where other logistical factors (like geography) make it difficult. The quality of the video depends on your connection speed. Most hospitals and some practices have the hardware for this. However, you don't need expensive hardware to teleconference:

- **Skype**[29] provides a free low-frills package for those with webcams and microphones.

- **dimdim.com**[30] also provides free web-conferencing for up to 20 users, with the option of paying for extra users or facilities.

Virtual learning environments (VLEs)
aka Course Management Systems (CMS) and Learning Management Systems (LMS)
The popularity of the Internet with younger generations and the growth of distance learning have led to the creation of VLEs. A VLE helps a teacher construct a lesson or tutorial which learners can then work through either collaboratively or in isolation. However, there are other things VLEs can do:
- VLEs can turn a smartphone into a portable nanny: telling students what time lectures, events or meetings are happening. Telling them where they need to go. And if they still don't know, the app can display a virtual map and slap a virtual pin on the exact location).
- VLEs can provide updates and disseminate other data in general.
- Students can 'quick link' to pod and screencasts made within the organisation.
- Diligent students can check the availability of a book in the library.
- VLEs provide a place to publish contact details for staff and services.

However, the app cannot (yet) iron clothes, cook for them or ensure that they call their mum every week.

Pros (over traditional didactic lectures)
- The interactive nature of the environment helps sustain learner interest.
- Experience indicates that learners are more likely to express their views on a VLE than through small-group discussion.
- It reduces the need for handouts or paper summaries – a significant cost saving.
- The software is usually free as it is open source and under an educational licence.

Cons
- You need to set up a username and password for *every* user.
- VLEs don't work particularly well on smartphone devices.
- You need to get to grips with the software (and the process of creating a lesson).

Some of the commercial VLE services like **Blackboard**[31] offer a bespoke service for organisations such as universities but for an eye-watering price! However, **Stanford University VLE app**[32] is free as is **Moodle**.[33] Moodle tutorials can be incorporated into other websites. **Udutu**[34] is another free tool for web presentations, although it requires hosting. **Edu2.0**,[35] one of the easier ones to use, is mainly for schools but can be adapted to medical teaching. Finally, take a look at **LAMS**.[36] Commercial VLEs are at the moment expensive. Perhaps this is the sort of technology GP training schemes are more likely to consider in the future when they become more affordable.

Cloud computing
Cloud computing is the latest of all the crazes. It helps you access your data from anywhere! Previously, one's pocket or key ring might have accommodated a USB stick, but with cloud computing you don't have to do any of that! In cloud computing your data is uploaded and stored securely, via third-party computer

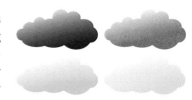

servers, on the World Wide Web (or the Internet cloud). The data can then be accessed from any computer (or smartphone) with an Internet connection. Some cloud services, like **Dropbox**,[37] enables you to make a copy of the files and folders on your PC/laptop too. This enables you to work on them offline if you need to with the reassurance that they'll be synchronised once you're back online again. There's also the added peace of mind from knowing your data is stored safely online (should your PC or lappy get pinched).

 Top Tip: Please check out Dropbox[37] – it's a free cloud service that helps simplify your life. Never email yourself a file again! No more confusion with different versions of the same document. And best of all, other people can be *invited* to work collaboratively on one particular file. Did you know that Chapter 5: A Smorgasbord of Educational Methods was created in this way?

I'm not particularly techno-savvy. Who can I turn to for help?

- Your local hospital – nearly all hospitals have an IT department. Go and visit them face to face. Most will be delighted and honoured that you thought of them.
- Universities – contact the university's IT department.
- Someone always knows someone else who's an IT geek – another Trainer or trainee?
- Search the Internet – just plug your query into Google.

Our GP training scheme (Bradford) runs 'Weds Tutorials' – 1½ hour weekly group tutorials (in addition to Half-Day Release) delivered by Trainers, mainly to cover clinical knowledge. Organising this was always a logistical nightmare with different Trainers picking the same dates and topics. I wondered if we could develop an online booking system – listing topics and dates available on a first-come first-served basis. I tried looking up stuff on the net, but it was all a bit above my head. So I contacted Bradford Hospital's IT department, met with them and posed my problem. They were extremely delighted I'd thought of them, and within a couple of weeks had developed exactly what I was looking for. It's been over five years since the booking system was developed – and it is still online and running. All it cost me was two boxes of chocolates – for the two developers who helped me.

A final note . . .

The Internet and *new* technology seems to be the cultural centrepiece for our new young learners – and we must keep up with them. How else can we 'hook' them in? That doesn't mean we need to make use of every new piece of software or technology out there! Whether you decide to use something or not still depends on those two *old* questions about purpose: *'What is it that you're trying to achieve?'* and *'Will this help you to get there?'* And don't worry if you're not particularly great with technology. Most software developers for the masses know that their product has to be easy to use (i.e. intuitive) and pleasing on the eye. Step out of your PowerPoint comfort zone and start playing with something new and exciting . . . you might just like it! We hope that this chapter has whetted your appetite.

A sample of resources on our website

- Behaviour in e-groups: lurkers, blue mooners and the virtuosos.
- The 5-stage model of e-learning (Gilly Salmon's work).
- How to write a virtual lesson for a VLE.
- Some Dos and Don'ts of Internet Technology.

● Working Creatively with Technology and Hidden Internet Gems.

Please give us some feedback on this chapter to help shape it for the next edition.
Go to www.essentialgptrainingbook.com and simply click on the title of this chapter.

References

1. Map of Medicine: www.mapofmedicine.com
2. GP Notebook: www.gpnotebook.co.uk
3. Web Mentor: www.webmentorlibrary.com
4. YouTube: www.youtube.com
5. Facebook: www.facebook.com
6. MySpace: www.myspace.com
7. Twitter: http://twitter.com
8. Skyscape: www.skyscape.com
9. Flash: http://en.wikipedia.org/wiki/Adobe_Flash
10. WordPress: http://wordpress.org
11. RSS: http://en.wikipedia.org/wiki/RSS
12. Wikis: http://wiki.org
13. Wikis: www.wikispaces.com
14. Wikipedia: www.wikipedia.org
15. Medical wiki: www.ganfyd.org
16. Yahoo groups: http://uk.groups.yahoo.com
17. Google groups: https://groups.google.com
18. Doctors.net.uk: www.doctors.net.uk
19. www.blogger.com
20. www.webblog.com
21. http://twitter.com
22. BMJ Learning: http://learning.bmj.com
23. e-GP: www.e-lfh.org.uk/projects/egp/index.html
24. BMJ: www.bmj.com
25. RCGP: www.rcgp.org.uk
26. iTunes: www.apple.com/itunes
27. iTunes U: www.apple.com/education/itunes-u
28. Vimeo: http://vimeo.com
29. Skype: www.skype.com
30. Dimdim: www.dimdim.com
31. Blackboard: www.blackboard.com
32. Stanford University VLE app: http://itunes.apple.com/us/app/istanford/id292922029?mt=8#
33. Moodle: http://moodle.org
34. Udutu: www.udutu.com
35. Edu2.0: www.edu20.org
36. LAMS: http://wiki.lamsfoundation.org/display/lamsdocs/LAMS+Tutorials
37. Dropbox: www.dropbox.com
38. The Times Online: www.thetimes.co.uk/tto/news/?CMP=KNGvccp1-times%2520website

Growing Tomorrow's Leaders Today – leadership skills

VERONICA WILKIE – Senior Clinical Teaching Fellow (Warwick Medical School) & lead author
MARION LYNCH – Associate GP Dean (Oxford Deanery)
MARK WATERS – GP Trainer (Hereford)   RAMESH MEHAY – TPD (Bradford)

Clinicians are expected to offer leadership, and, where they have appropriate skills, take senior leadership and management posts.[1]

Clinicians and doctors are frequently being asked to show 'more' or 'better' leadership on a range of issues. There are frequent high-level documents asking for better leadership in response to a wide range of ills in the health service, both in terms of training and service delivery.

- But what is meant by leadership?
- Is it really needed?
- Is it necessary for GPs in training to know anything about it or is it solely the preserve of those doctors who go on to various positions outside their practice?

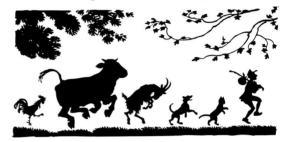

What leadership is and what it isn't

> Management is about tasks, systems and processes but leadership is about people. You lead a team but manage a bank account. Leadership is about identifying and delivering a vision.[2]

Leadership has a long and detailed history. Airport lounges are full of books written by leadership gurus, telling all and sundry that if only we followed their path, we too could lead a major North American corporation. History texts describe the attributes of war leaders. And, finally, the UK's monarch showers honour on those who are thought to have led the way to a better system for us all in Great Britain. But does any of this have an immediate effect for today's hard-working GPs?

The need for medical leadership arose from a multiplicity of sources. In 2005, a report of the National Confidential Enquiry into Patient Outcome and Death (NCEPOD) found that leadership and teamwork by consultants was wanting.[3] Poor communication on the wards was observed frequently between doctors and other clinical staff.[4] This tells us that leadership affects patient care and safety.[5] The need for clinical leadership has also been emphasised in the 'Darzi report'[1] (*Every clinician should be a partner, practitioner and leader . . .*') and in the context of training doctors in the 'Tooke report'[6] (on Modernising Medical Careers).

A very brief history of leadership studies

Early 20th-century description of leaders came from the 'Great Man Theory' (and yes, they were generally descriptions of 'great' men!). This theory tried to identify leadership traits that natural leaders were believed to have been born with.

During the 1940s '*Style* Theory' was written about, with certain styles advocated as being favourable to successful leadership. Many favourable styles were thought to be inclusive of a participative culture, more humanistic, with little attention to the situations and tasks the leaders were faced with. The theory behind style theory was that different styles fitted different situations and thus matching the leadership style to a task produced better effectiveness.

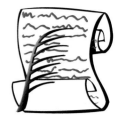

⚠ **Red Alert:** The wish to identify traits is still popular today – often done in recruiting executives of leaders through various personality or 'psychologistic' tests. Listing these traits as 'desirable' in job descriptions can be at risk of then recruiting 'clones'.[7]

Blanchard, Hersey and Johnson delivered a model of '*Situational* Leadership'[8], recognising that no one style fitted every situation. Effective leadership has a democratic and less scientific nature to it.[9] Charles Handy[10] took this one step further in his 'best-fit' approach in which he says that different situations require different types of leaders.

Effective leadership performance depends on:	
1 the power or position of the leader 2 the relationship with his or her group 3 the organisational norms	4 the structure and technology 5 the variety of tasks 6 the variety of subordinate. <div align="right">Charles Handy</div>

It goes without saying that a leader is nothing without followers, and when discussing leadership within the context of general practice it is as useful to discuss when a member of a primary health-care team should lead and when they should follow (a central part of '*Shared* Leadership' theory[11]).

Modern day leadership theory has a whole raft of definitions and it's outside the scope of this chapter to go into all of them in detail, but two descriptors help when thinking of what leadership means to GPs and GPs in training – transformational and transactional leadership.

Transformational and transactional leadership

In the late 1980s and 90s Bass's work[12] on transformational leadership became popular (built on further by the work by Burns[13]).

Transformational leadership is where one or more persons engage with each other in such a way that leaders and followers raise one another to higher levels of motivation and morality.[13] Transformational leaders are able to inspire, motivate, provide intellectual stimulation, while taking into account the considerations of those around them.[12]

Transactional leaders work in the more traditionally described managerial sense – making order, planning and describing what means to be done. Transactional leaders emphasise rewards of immediate value whereas transformational leaders place a higher value on symbolic engagement or commitment. One is not necessarily better than the other – a transformational style is needed to promote change and a transactional style to promote order.

One is not better than the other and in healthcare both are needed, either through one individual who can adapt between the two states or more usefully as collaboration in a team. Junior doctors tend to identify with transactional leadership traits, as their role is mainly to make order of the potential chaos in hospital wards, or 'manage' complex healthcare needs of individual patients in primary care. Transactional leadership is necessary for the hospital wards to function, but transformational leadership traits can still be facilitated. For instance, you might encourage a small team of *interested* people (docs, nurses, admin) to engage in a little project – where they're left to decide how to do it. They would clearly need to engage with each other in order to develop a shared vision, shared direction and shared enthusiasm.

TRANSFORMATIONAL AND TRANSACTIONAL PARTNERSHIP

An ST3 GP trainee in his final three months in general practice noticed how two leadership traits were used to the benefit of the practice. Several months ago the reception manager had been asked to look at a new way of organising the appointments – the practice had less than good access, and was suffering financially. She had written some documents on the status quo and where she thought the practice needed to go, but was not making any headway in getting other staff members to change. At a practice meeting one of the partners offered to help. His position in the practice enabled him to arrange an afternoon for all to be involved. The office manager, *in collaboration* with the reception team, was then able to work out the pros and cons of two main plans as well as the pros and cons of the status quo [*transformational leadership*]. The practice used this information to make a decision, and both the doctor and the office manager were then able to work out a plan to introduce the changes [*transactional leadership*].

Positional and shared leadership

> Organisations, of course, are not objects. They are micro-societies. Those who lead them need to understand the needs and motivations of people in them.[14]

Martin[14] studied 350 middle to upper level managers across many countries to ascertain how leadership has changed. He felt that leaders now need to achieve results through **collaboration, teamwork and innovation**. There was a clear shift towards skills tied to relationships and collaboration, and that leaders needed to become 'organisational architects', to allow an organisational shift to one that allows collaboration and spread of individual skills more widely. He writes: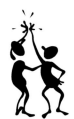

> It is no longer the time of the heroic leader. Instead the job of today's leader is to create space for people to generate new and different ideas, to encourage meaningful conversation between people and to assist people in becoming more effective, agile and to respond to complex challenges.[14]

Shared leadership:
- is about knowing when to step forward to take the lead, and when to follow or encourage another to take the lead. It's not about having too many chiefs and not enough Indians

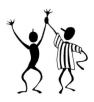

- is more likely to allow individuals within a multidisciplinary team to work to their full potential for patient care.

Positional leaders are still needed (within shared leadership the term 'Super Leader' was coined). These might be modelled by partners in a practice, PCT clinical leaders or those that take on leadership roles within education.

The Medical Leadership Competency Framework (MLCF)

Acknowledgements: we are grateful to the NHS Institute for Innovation & Improvement for providing the illustrations in this section in relation to the MLCF. © NHS Institute for Innovation and Improvement and Academy of Medical Royal Colleges 2010. All rights reserved.

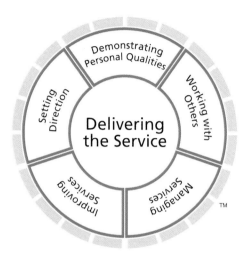

The Competencies

In 2007, the NHS and the Academy of Medical Royal Colleges (a body representing all the medical royal colleges) commissioned a piece of work to see what leadership training was required for all doctors in the UK. A steering group of individuals representing the GMC, BMA, the Academy of Medical Royal Colleges, and Undergraduate and Postgraduate Medical Deans was formed. They worked with three big reference groups (which included doctors, medical students and educators at every level) to develop a competency framework in medical leadership.[15] This also defines the curriculum for medical leadership.[16]

The MLCF is now embedded in every specialty curriculum and forms part of the RCGP's Core Curriculum on being a GP. The competencies will need to be introduced to all doctors in training, but as part of a continuum, rather than just at ST3 level or being the sole responsibility of a hard-pressed GP Trainer. Undergraduate and Foundation Year curricula will need to incorporate these competencies and embrace leadership training in a way that:

- promotes the principles of *shared* leadership
- is taught as an *integrated* part of training, not as a separate course
- is *developmental* – allowing doctors to develop at a pace that is both appropriate and within the context of the job they do.

General practice offers a great experience for many of these competencies to be identified because of the one-to-one nature of the relationship between GP trainee and Trainer/Educational Supervisor, the teamwork within the GP training schemes and because each practice will need to institute some changes at some point. So let's now look at each competency section of the MLCF with examples of how these competencies can be developed in real practice.

Personal qualities

Most of these competencies are difficult to teach but easier to show and reflect upon. For instance, they can be integral to a **case-based discussion** or reflection on a **significant event**; in both cases, reflecting on a trainee's actions or reactions to events. When we teach medical students we often use the term **personal leadership** when looking at personal qualities and working with others.

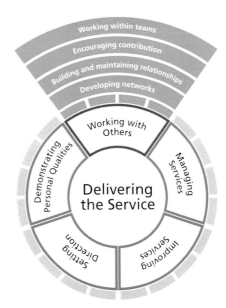

PERSONAL QUALITIES

Dr L came in to help with a swine flu clinic at her training practice. To her horror, she noticed that she had got 17 doses out of the first vial. When she inspected it, she found that she'd been withdrawing to the first mark, which was 0.25 mL, half the dose for adults. She immediately told one of the other GPs. They identified the 17 incorrectly dosed adults, and she drafted a letter which was sent out apologising and asking them to contact her or the practice nurse to be fitted into another clinic to have a second dose at the correct volume.

During a tutorial she discussed what led up to her error and how she'd handled it with her Trainer. They identified that she'd rushed the demonstration video, and not looked clearly at the syringe. Her Trainer felt that by noticing the mistake and acting to apologise and rectify the problem she had demonstrated that she had acted with integrity, and shown awareness about rushing through the training video. As a result of her mistake she had read up on all the aspects of the vaccination programme she could find, and felt confident enough to join the practice flu subgroup.

Competencies demonstrated: acting with integrity, CPD and developing self-awareness.

Working with others

This component is relatively easy to discuss – most junior doctors can identify with certain elements of this. All of them will have ideas based on experiences in other jobs, and show a variety of abilities to reflect on their own role. These competencies are already assessed through some workplace-based assessments like **case-based discussions** on patients with complex needs and **multi-source feedback**. There are other educational activities you can employ (see box diagram below).

Working with others								
Developing networks	Use the example of caring for a patient with complex needs. Identify the networks of other health professionals involved. Ask the trainee to find out the best way to communicate with each other.	**Building and maintaining relationships**	Ask the trainee to identify key people they interact with in the surgery – receptionist, manager and other GPs. How do they interact? How can they facilitate any communication? How will this impact on patient care, and how can this be demonstrated?	**Encouraging contribution**	Ask the trainee to draw a diagram of all those caring for a patient who is dying. Highlight the individuals they talk to regularly or have talked to once or have only had a letter from (and include the patient and their family in this). Find out if there is any contribution that could be encouraged – a discussion with a Macmillan nurse about chemo, etc. Look at the reasons why this was not done.	**Working with teams**	Look at an HDR planning event. Discuss how the GP training scheme works in terms of team dynamics. Use it as a discussion about team roles (for instance, Belbin). Review teams that have worked well, less well and discuss why.

Managing services

More junior, foundation year, ST1 and ST2 doctors find this difficult. They have usually been concentrating so hard on acquiring clinical competencies that the idea of being able to manage a service sounds very foreign indeed. The MLCF is designed to be learnt and adapted within the context of the individual; the junior doctors should be able to discuss this section from an educational or working activity angle, such as the on-call duty rota and so on.

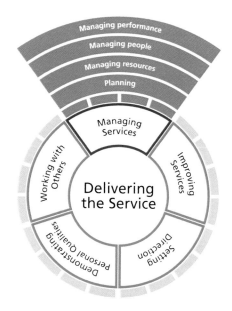

- This domain is useful for looking at chronic disease care in general practice.
- It can be used to move the discussion about care and the patient from outside the consulting room to the wider practice organisation.
- This domain can help a trainee (or anyone) develop a different service working with other practice staff members.

Managing services								
Planning	Dr S wishes to organise a study group for the MRCGP. What does she have to do to start?	Managing resources	What resources does she need? A room, a library, computers with Internet access, flip charts? What time is needed?	Managing people	How is she going to engage others? Are the local Training Programme Directors and Trainer supportive? How can they help?	Managing performance	One of her colleagues never turns up prepared, and it's starting to irritate the others. What should be done now? What could have been done to stop this happening in the first place?

Improving services

New members of a team can bring a fresh look to systems that have been operating in a practice for years. Encouraging debate, especially with a GP trainee who has spent time in other practices, can be valuable learning for everyone. The competency list for this domain provides:

- a structure for discussion and development (see example below)
- a review structure for the commissioning of new services
- a good opportunity for the GP to get some understanding of the intricacies and the complexity of Practice Based Commissioning and its interplay with patient safety and clinical governance.

This domain is particularly suitable for problem-based learning activities within a GP training scheme.

AN EXAMPLE OF 'IMPROVING SERVICES' – THE COMMISSIONING LEARNING SET

The Training Programme Director presented a scenario where a practice wishes to develop a GPwSI service in Dermatology. The group collectively came together with information they would need to know to carry this forward:

Facilitating transformation

- Are there any guidelines for GPwSI – in terms of training and delivery of services?
- What are the rules about who can, and can't be a provider?
- When would the PCT need to go out to tender?
- What is a commissioning cluster?

Encouraging improvement and innovation

- Are there any local GPs who would be able to deliver this service?
- What are the current commissioning plans?
- Which people in the PCT would be involved in commissioning this?

Critically evaluating

- Is there a need for this service?
- How could you use this to benefit patients?
- What financial issues or implications are there? What does 'tariff' mean?
- How could you evaluate such a service?

Ensuring patient safety

- Are there any issues of patient safety? Who would identify these?

Each of these questions was then taken up by a learning champion who agreed to research this for presentation at a future meeting. The group allowed individuals 15 minutes to give feedback on their findings and present a handout for their colleagues. Once the group had met again, they had obviously been able to learn a lot more about how GPs, PCTs and commissioning clusters work. They also identified that, as a group, they'd like to know more about what makes a good business case, and how you can manage a project like this.

Setting direction

This domain is possibly the most abstract of all.

- It's a good one to look at the understanding of what leadership means and its contextual approach in primary care.
- It certainly enables a discussion between what might be seen as management and what is leadership.
- This is a good one to discuss using a sudden untoward incident or a **significant event** as an example.

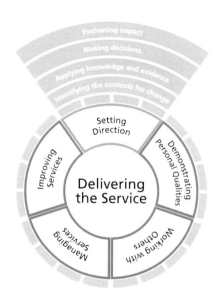

SETTING DIRECTION THROUGH A SIGNIFICANT EVENT

A practice team met to discuss a significant event. One of their elderly housebound patients had been recently discharged from the Medical Assessment Unit (MAU). However, the change in his medication hadn't been picked up, and as a result he'd gone back to his old doses of medicines; his condition deteriorated, and he needed to be readmitted. The following themes formed part of the discussion.

- Doctors reviewing letters and the problem of increasing paperwork.
- System issues – in this particular case the letter hadn't been reviewed by a doctor, who had taken three days' study leave. In fact, none of his letters had been forwarded for someone else to see. The new receptionist knew letters needed forwarding when someone was on leave but only equated that with annual leave and not study leave.
- The pros and cons of leaving the system as it is. However, it became clear that there had been several near misses.

The practice identified a GP, the attached pharmacist, the GP trainee (who wanted to be involved) and the reception manager to take this forward. The GP trainee then discussed potential outcomes using the four elements from the 'Setting Direction' domain. He was able to take a lead within the group for assessing workload implications and helping to decide a way forward for the team.

Other leadership group activities

Now that we've finished with the nuts and bolts of leadership (at least in terms of the requirements of the RCGP curriculum), we'd like to focus our attention on the multitude of educational activities and games that also help us *understand* leadership better. These have all been used in GP and other specialty groups. The obvious outward-bound type team building activities can also be used to look at leadership *issues*.

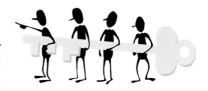

The Goleman Hat Game

Affiliative	• creates harmony and builds emotional bonds
Authoritative	• mobilises people towards a vision
Coaching	• develops people for the future
Democratic	• consensus through participation of all
Pace setting	• sets and expects high standards of performance
Coercive	• demands immediate compliance

This game looks at the six leadership styles that Goleman[17] (also famous for his writing on emotional intelligence[18]) identified. These are: Affiliative, Authoritative, Coaching, Democratic, Pace Setting and Coercive.

Method: The facilitator reads out a scenario, and the groups have to rush to identify a hat with the appropriate leadership style on it (use coloured paper crowns with each style written in with thick black ink).

Some of the scenarios are obvious (a patient requiring resuscitation – coercive), but some can be written to identify more than one style. And if more than one hat is grabbed and worn by an individual, he or she then needs to debate its merits with the person wearing one of the others.

It helps to put the definitions up on a flip chart or on a PowerPoint slide so that people can use it as a reference at the start. By the end, the group generally has a pretty good idea of how each style is defined and which scenario would require which style.

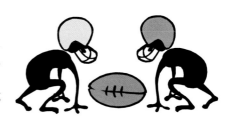

Variations: Goleman Chair game – with them rushing to sit on the appropriate chair rather than grabbing a hat. There are more Goleman scenarios on our website.

Chatterblocks

This learning activity was invented, and created and tested by Dr Peter Nightingale. Chatterblocks are **three** cubes, like large dice, designed to promote learning through narrative. Its objectives are to remind learners that networking is important, and not to discount informal discussions (which are just as important as formal presentations and meetings).

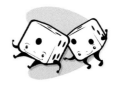

Method: Discuss an event or a planned change and tell a story around it.

● Divide a large group into three, each taking a cube.
● Each member of the group takes it in turn to roll the cube. The group then discusses the aspects of the case in terms of the word identified.

- Peter Nightingale has some beautifully crafted blocks with the words on them, but you could use three dice with each number on the dice being ascribed to one of the chatterblock words.

1 The Senses Cube
- Creating a compelling vision
- MLCF: setting direction
- Six sides representing (1) sight; (2) sound; (3) hearing; (4) touch; (5) smell; (6) intuition.

Leaders need a clear and communicable vision of a future state (better, safer, more efficient . . .). They need to be able to share that vision with all those involved – building a profile of the desired state using all relevant senses. For instance, some people like to see pictures and presentations. Some like to hear the spoken word and some like documents to read, take back and understand. Some individuals rely on a sixth sense or intuition.[19] Roll this cube and discuss how best to present an issue.

2 The Emotions Cube
- Emotional intelligence
- MLCF: aspects of developing personal qualities and working with others
- Six sides represent:
  1 Leaders need to build and maintain relationships.
  2 Leaders need to develop self-awareness.
  3 All change provokes emotional responses – in those who lead and in those who follow.
  4 Effective leaders take into account the emotional responses of themselves, and those who they work with.
  5 They plan how to deal with these emotions, often adapting their leadership style.
  6 They review how they have performed and whether they would change reactions in the future.

3 The What When, Where, How Why and Who Cube
- Creating a story of success
- MLCF: managing services and improving services
- The six words on this cube are based on 'well-formed outcomes'.[20]
  1 **What** do you want to happen?
  2 **Where** is each activity going to be located?
  3 **When** is each task going to be completed?
  4 **How** will I know when each goal is achieved?
  5 **Why** are we doing what we are doing; can we evaluate the process?
  6 **Who** do I need to influence to achieve this goal?

Get Out of Jail Game
This game was developed from an exercise we used for many years with GP and other specialty training groups.

Method: The facilitator sets a scenario (which needn't be medical) which the groups then have to find a way through. This game can be modified to look at current NHS systems, as well as discussing abstract ethical issues and working out how as a team the group works through problems. Things like the following.

- Which individuals from a list have to be saved from a flooding cave and in which order.
- Dividing up a pot of development money between new services (more dialyses, more district nurses, more GPS, more cancer drugs, increased availability of radiology and imaging services).
- Running a commissioning scenario; allocating a budget and the asking the trainees to work up a business case for a three or four scenarios. This enables them to think widely and about the whole team, as well as understanding what commissioning involves.
- Dragons' Den exercise: each trainee has to come up with a planned change in how the practice they work in offers services. They need to work out a business plan and a system of change and then present it to their colleagues to see if anyone will 'invest'.

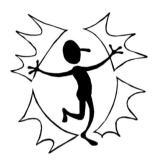

During the activity, you can stop the discussions halfway to see if any of the groups have worked out a strategy and then set the groups going again. The scenario can be as detailed as the facilitator wishes. It can be used to highlight the difficulty PCTs have in allocating new money and the way in which individual decision-makers need to look outside their own area in order to come to a rational and all-encompassing decision. Guidance by NICE (www.nice.nhs.uk) can help if economic considerations are going to be considered.

After the activity, discuss both the outcome *and* the process by which the team got there.

- How did they do the ranking?
- Was it done by voting (and can this be justified)?
- Was there any discussion of how decisions were made before the items were discussed?
- Were there clearly identified priorities set before consideration?

Practice Leaders Program[21]

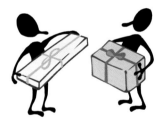

The Practice Leaders Program is a well-evaluated *practical* leadership training programme. Please look up reference 21 for more details. Something similar can be developed locally and it needn't be very complicated. For instance, in order to build leadership skills, a group of GP trainees, Trainers and TPDs could meet at an agreed time and work through a clinical commissioning issue.

Closing remarks

As soon as people adapt to change, another change is bestowed upon them. This adds to the uncertainty and complexity in our personal and professional lives. The effective leader can operate under rapidly mutating circumstances and sometimes this requires a rethink of one's own leadership concepts, frameworks and style.[22]

Whenever I think about leadership, I like to think also about followership. What behaviours make me a good or bad follower . . . particularly when the environment is challenging? I realise that I am fortunate to be surrounded by an excellent followership . . . people who are leaders too in their own right.'

Mark Purvis, GP Director (Yorkshire & the Humber Deanery)

A sample of resources on our website
- Leadership & Commissioning by Pete Smith.
- Entrusting and enabling GPs to lead change to improve patient experience.

Other chapters you may like to read
- Chapter 30: Quality – how good are we?

Please give us some feedback on this chapter to help shape it for the next edition.
Go to www.essentialgptrainingbook.com and simply click on the title of this chapter.

References

1 Darzi A. *High Quality Care For All.* London: Department of Health; 2008.
2 Cumming I. *The Little Black Book of Leadership Hints and Tips for Healthcare Staff.* Littleborough: Perfect Circle; 2008.
3 Cullinane N, Findlay G, Hargraves C, *et al. A Report of the National Confidential Enquiry into Patient Outcome and Death.* London: NCEPOD; 2005.
4 Reeves S, Lewin S. Interprofessional collaboration in hospital: strategies and meanings. *J Health Service Res Policy.* 2004; **9**: 218–25.
5 Firth-Cozens J. Leadership and the quality of care. *Qual Health Care.* 2001; **10**(Suppl. II): Sii3–ii7.
6 DoH. Available at: www.mmcinquiry.org.uk/MMC_FINAL_REPORT_REVD_4jan.pdf (accessed 2 May 2011).
7 Alimo-Metcalf B. Leadership in the NHS: what are the competencies and qualities needed and how can they be developed? In: Mark A, Dobson S, editors, *Organisational Behaviour in Health Care: the research agenda.* London: Macmillan; 1999.
8 Blanchard K, Hersey P, Johnson D. *Management of Organizational Behaviour.* 7th ed. New Jersey: Prentice-Hall; 1996.
9 Vroom VH, Deci E. *Management and Motivation.* London: Penguin; 1970.
10 Handy C. Trust and the virtual organisation. *Har Bus Rev.* 1993; **73**: 40–50.
11 Fletcher J. Shared leadership paradox and possibility. In: Pearce CJ, Conger JA, editors. *Shared Leadership: framing the hows and whys of leadership.* Thousand Oaks, California: Sage; 2003.
12 Bass B, Avolio B *Improving Organisational Effectiveness through Transformational Leadership.* New York: Sage; 1994.
13 Burns J. *Leadership.* New York: Harper and Row; 1978.
14 Martin A. The future of leadership: where do we go from here? *Industrial and Commercial Training.* 2007; **39**(1): 3–8.
15 NHS Institute. *Medical Leadership Competency Framework.* AORMC; 2008. Available at: www.institute.nhs.uk/assessment_tool/general/medical_leadership_competency_framework_-_homepage.html
16 NHS Institute. *Medical Leadership Curriculum.* 2009. Available at: www.institute.nhs.uk/images/documents/Leadership/Medical%20Leadership%20Curriculum.pdf
17 Goleman D. Leadership that gets results. *Harv Bus Rev.* 2000; **78**(2): 78–90.
18 Goleman D. *Emotional Intelligence.* New York: Bantam Books; 1995.
19 Myers P, Briggs I. *Gifts Differing: understanding personality type.* Mountain View, California: Davies-Black Publishing; 1980.
20 Henwood S, Lister J. *NLP and Coaching for Healthcare Professionals: developing expert practice.* Oxford: Wiley and Sons; 2007.
21 Lynch M, McFetridge N. Practice Leaders Programme: entrusting and enabling general practitioners to lead change to improve patient experience. *Perm J.* Winter 2011; **15**(1): 28–34.
22 Avery GC. *Understanding Leadership.* London: Sage; 2004.

Index

Note: page numbers in **bold** refer to tables and figures.